Planning & Designing Health Care Facilities in Developing Countries

Building a clinically integrated workplace with a high level of clinical competence requires careful considerations of Hospital Planning. For greenfield or brownfield hospital projects, clinicians and C-Suite executives need to acquire capabilities to address the planning needs of any organization.

This book aims to provide both theoretical and practical inputs for the *Planning & Designing of Health Care Facilities in Developing Countries*. It clearly indicates the steps to be followed, facts to be weighed, and components to be considered to arrive at a correct planning solution. With health reform looming and the revenue base shifting rapidly, we need to integrate patient safety concerns in the design process.

Key Features

- Liberal use of tables and figures to support conclusions, illustrate concepts, and display quantitative information, making it easier for readers to understand and refer to large quantities of data

- Integrates the international norms for planning and designing health care facilities into the developing country setting

- Handbook and ready reckoner for C-Suite executives, hospital engineers, project consultants, and hospital administration students

Planning & Designing Health Care Facilities in Developing Countries

Lt. Col. (Dr.) Shashikant Sharma, MD, MBA
Armed Forces Medical College
Ministry of Health & Family Welfare, Government of India

Dr. (Maj.) Saurabh Singh, MD
Armed Forces Medical College
PGIMS, Lucknow
NEIGRIHMS, Shillong

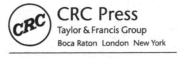

CRC Press
Taylor & Francis Group
Boca Raton London New York

CRC Press is an imprint of the
Taylor & Francis Group, an **informa** business

Designed cover image: Shutterstock

First edition published 2025
by CRC Press
2385 NW Executive Center Drive, Suite 320, Boca Raton, FL 33431

and by CRC Press
4 Park Square, Milton Park, Abingdon, Oxon, OX14 4RN

CRC Press is an imprint of Taylor & Francis Group, LLC

© 2025 Taylor & Francis Group, LLC

Library of Congress Cataloging-in-Publication Data
Names: Sharma, Shashikant, author. | Singh, Saurabh (Professor of hospital administration), author.
Title: Planning & designing health care facilities in developing countries / Shashikant Sharma,
    Saurabh Singh.
Other titles: Planning and designing health care facilities in developing countries
Description: First edition. | Boca Raton : CRC Press, 2024. | Includes bibliographical references
    and index.
Identifiers: LCCN 2023044581 (print) | LCCN 2023044582 (ebook) | ISBN 9781032561042 (hardback) |
    ISBN 9780367460877 (paperback) | ISBN 9780367460884 (ebook)
Subjects: MESH: Hospital Planning—organization & administration | Hospital Design and Construction |
    Developing Countries
Classification: LCC RA967 (print) | LCC RA967 (ebook) | NLM WX 140.1 | DDC 725/.51091724—
    dc23/eng/20231026
LC record available at https://lccn.loc.gov/2023044581
LC ebook record available at https://lccn.loc.gov/2023044582

ISBN: 9781032561042 (hbk)
ISBN: 9780367460877 (pbk)
ISBN: 9780367460884 (ebk)

DOI: 10.1201/9780367460884

Typeset in Warnock Pro
by Apex CoVantage, LLC

CONTENTS

FOREWORD

By Prof Anupam Sibal

"Form Follows Function" has been the cornerstone of good architecture for more than a century now. Buildings are no longer just inanimate structures but are increasingly seen as an integral part of overall well-being. Hospitals and health care facilities have also endorsed these concepts over the years. The concept of "Healing Architecture" is in vogue with increasing evidence of that hospital design can influence faster recovery.

Cognitive psychologists have identified the physical environment as having a significant impact on overall human performance. Humans do not always behave clumsily and do not always err, but they are more likely to do so when they work in a badly conceived and designed structure. This becomes more relevant to health care organizations wherein we are striving for patient safety. Anything that increases the chances of errors is a definite red flag and any aspect that helps in decreasing errors should be adopted. Therefore, thoughtful hospital designs become imperative to creating a "healing atmosphere," as well as a conducive work environment for health care workers to minimize errors.

The COVID-19 pandemic has taught us to be malleable and flexible. With changing demographics, explosion of noncommunicable diseases, resurgence of infectious diseases, and an aging population, we can certainly expect a rise in disease burden. Structural upgradation and remodeling are imminent to meet the evolving requirements with time. The sooner we adapt, the better equipped we will be to take on the new challenges.

Structural remodeling is often seen to be an added cost and financial burden. The authors avidly address these concerns and discuss how the cost of building or remodeling projects based on a design conducive to patient safety can result in organizational savings over time, without adversely impacting revenues. Thus, addressing one of the important concerns for key decision makers in both greenfield and brownfield projects.

This handbook can be useful for a wide range of stakeholders ranging from promoters, investors, hospital engineers, project consultants to students of hospital administration. The key insights on conducive designs can be implemented at all stages of hospital project planning, right from conception all the way up to commissioning. The modular design with liberal use of tables and figures to support conclusions makes it a quick and engaging read.

I wish the entire team behind this avid publication, all the very best.

Prof Anupam Sibal
Group Medical Director and
Senior Pediatric Gastroenterologist and Hepatologist
Apollo Group of Hospitals
President, GAPIO (2020–2022)

FOREWORD

By Atul Kotwal

"By failing to prepare, you are preparing to fail."
– Benjamin Franklin

The health care system in India is a mix of private and public with a wide range of types of health care facilities. At one end of the spectrum are the glittering steel and glass structures supplying high-tech facilities to the well-heeled, primarily metropolitan Indians; and on the other end, are small aspirational public health care facilities being upgraded to health and wellness centres in the public sector, and informal providers with single-room clinics in the private health sector.

Universal health coverage needs strengthening of all the building blocks of health systems. Health infrastructure is an important indicator for understanding the country's health care policy and implementation mechanisms. It signifies an investment priority regarding the creation of health care facilities.

To combat the health infrastructure issues in the public health care system, the Government of India launched the PM Ayushman Bharat Health Infrastructure Mission (ABHIM) in conjunction with health grants under the 15th Finance Commission. In the next 4 to 5 years, the goal is to improve the vital health care network from village to block to the district to regional and national levels. There are four sides to this mission. The first is the development of complex diagnostic and treatment facilities. The second is connected to the testing network for illness diagnosis. The third issue is the growth of current pandemic research centres, including the One Health approach; and the fourth aspect is infrastructure strengthening at the most peripheral health care facilities.

Good health care facility design integrates functional requirements with the human needs of its varied users. This need for diverse functions is reflected in the breadth and specificity of regulations, codes, and oversight that govern hospital construction and operations. However, most health care professionals are as unfamiliar with design and construction as architects and contractors are unfamiliar with the day-to-day realities of hospital operations.

Health care leaders at all levels must acquire the wherewithal to plan, design, build, and commission a health care facility at any level. This book will close the existing knowledge gap and equip administrators and clinicians to design a workplace that mimics the health care processes on the ground. I am sanguine that this book will add value to further the health care system in India and will serve as an expert resource for the mission of achieving Universal Health Care in India.

I wish the authors all the best in their excellent initiative to write this handbook and look forward to the success of the publication.

Maj Gen (Prof) Atul Kotwal, SM, VSM
Executive Director
National Health Systems Resource Centre
Ministry of Health & Family Welfare
Govt of India

PREFACE

For planners, design is what shapes the physical form of development. It is both a process and an outcome; it influences the success of both planning as an activity and the quality and usefulness of hospitals.

Influencing design is an immensely complex matter. It involves the skills and actions of a wide range of people; multiple economic factors; and many levels of policy, guidance, and processes in the public and private sectors. Design can be influenced by a wide range of strategies, delivery mechanisms, and systems of management and stewardship, operating from the short to the long term.

Most health care professionals are as unfamiliar with design and construction requirements as architects and contractors are unfamiliar with the day-to-day realities of hospital operations. This book aims to help people who are involved in planning—many of them early in their careers—to understand what design is and how it fits into health care planning. The health planner needs help in deciding what kind of facility is needed, where it should be situated, and what priority should be allocated to it. How to phase the erection of various facilities means realizing the availability of the material and human resources, understanding how to make use of scarce and often unreliable statistics, and recognizing which statistics are indispensable and which are merely helpful.

Although literature is available regarding the planning of health care services, a well-synthesized effort that incorporates all the requisites is found to be lacking. This book helps in presenting a clear and concise view on how to plan and design a health care facility up to the department level and is an elaborate first step. The contribution of the work in this publication reflects a way of thinking about various facts and elements of health care facilities. They are an addendum to the work of the government, architects, engineers, and construction agencies. Presenting a user perspective, the intention is to identify the key result areas in hospital planning.

Drawing on the authors' experience gained from hospital projects around the country, this book charts a readable path through everything from the planning of a new hospital to major refurbishment or the remodeling of an existing hospital. It clearly explains the hospital design language and processes needed by professionals overseeing any project and covers essential aspects including ensuring cost-effectiveness, eco-efficiencies, improved services, and patient safety in design. A chapter on "Enhancing Patient Safety by Design" is also incorporated.

Industry professionals, architects, engineers, and hospital planners involved in planning, designing, and construction of hospital and health care establishments will gain by reading the authors' perspective on the construction of the facility. Researchers and academicians involved in teaching this subject will also find it useful and helpful.

Comments and suggestions are always welcome.

Shashikant Sharma
Saurabh Singh

ACKNOWLEDGMENTS

Writing a comprehensive handbook on hospital planning and design for developing countries has been a journey filled with challenges, dedication, and unwavering support from countless individuals and organizations. As we present this handbook to the world, we wish to express our heartfelt gratitude to those who have played pivotal roles in its creation.

First and foremost, we extend our deepest thanks to the health care professionals and experts in the field who generously shared their knowledge, insights, and experiences. Your expertise has been the foundation upon which this handbook was built. I take this opportunity to thank our teacher and guide Lt Gen (Dr) Arindam Chatterjee, VSM, Director General Medical Services for inspiring and motivating us through this arduous journey.

The contributions of various institutions and organizations cannot be overstated. We are grateful to the Department of Hospital Administration at Armed Forces Medical College; All India Institute of Medical Sciences, Delhi; Kasturba Medical College; Manipal & NMIMS Mumbai among others, for providing us with access to vital research, data, and case studies. Your commitment to promoting health care excellence in developing nations is greatly appreciated.

Our sincere thanks also go to the National Health System Resource Centre, Ministry of Health & Family Welfare, Govt of India that have supported our research efforts and provided valuable data. Your dedication to improving health care accessibility and quality is making a significant impact on the lives of millions.

The process of creating this handbook involved countless hours of meticulous editing and design work. We thank the entire editorial team led by Ms Shivangi Pramanik, Senior Commissioning Editor, CRC Press/Taylor & Francis for their outstanding editorial contributions. Your keen eye for detail and commitment to clarity has elevated the quality of this publication.

Last but certainly not least, we want to acknowledge our families for their unwavering support and understanding throughout this journey. I would like to thank my wife Dr Jyoti Sharma, PhD for being the constant source of encouragement. Her unwavering belief in me, and this project has been the driving force behind the determination to see this book to completion. Your patience and encouragement have been our pillars of strength.

We hope that this handbook serves as a valuable resource in the ongoing efforts to improve health care infrastructure in developing countries.

AUTHORS

Dr. Shashikant Sharma is a clinician-turned-administrator, a TEDx Speaker, and Educator with over 19 years of experience in Armed Forces Medical Services. In addition to his vast experience in Hospital Planning & Designing, Hospital Operations, and Quality & Accreditation, he is External Consultant and National Assessor to the Ministry of Health & Family Welfare, Government of India. The author is associated with premier Health Care Institutes such as the Armed Forces Medical College, Pune, Kasturba Medical College, Manipal & School of Business Management, and NMIMS Mumbai.

Dr. Saurabh Singh is an alumnus of the prestigious Armed Forces Medical College, Pune, India, with rich experience of 13 years in Armed Forces Medical Services. Key areas of work experience include Hospital Administration, Operations & Quality Management. The author is concomitantly involved in scientific publications and various training and research activities. After a stint at PGIMS Lucknow, he is currently working as Assistant Professor, Department of Hospital Administration at NEIGRIHMS, Shillong, India.

Unit 1
Concepts of Planning & Designing

1A HOSPITAL PLANNING
Types and Steps of Planning

1.1 Background

Hospital design and build planning encompasses a multifaceted process involving various types and essential steps to ensure the creation of efficient and patient-centric health care facilities. Types of design and build planning may include architectural planning, engineering planning, and interior design planning, each crucial in creating a functional and healing environment. Architectural planning focuses on creating a structural layout that optimizes patient flow and enhances staff efficiency. Engineering planning entails the integration of advanced technological systems and infrastructure to support medical services. Interior design planning involves the development of patient-friendly spaces that promote comfort and well-being. These planning steps collectively contribute to the establishment of modern, state-of-the-art health care facilities that prioritize patient care and safety.

Planning is the first phase of most construction and renovation projects. This phase involves many activities, from incorporating goals for the future of the organization to steps such as analysing health care needs, assembling a team, gathering data, creating a project plan, determining a budget, and phasing in and documenting the facility plan. Project planning in health care facilities typically incorporates several types of planning: strategic planning, master facility planning, and project planning.

1.2 Strategic Planning

Given that most projects take more than two years from ideation to completion, today's new hospital projects are oppressed with uncertainties: How will such projects weave with the evolving needs of new models of care and the complexities of the continuous quality care? In this brittle, anxious, non-linear, incomprehensible (BANI) world, strategic planning is looking through a shorter than ten-year window.

The common element in each planning strategy is to identify an organization's SWOT factors: its strengths, weaknesses, opportunities, and threats. Planning a new facility or renovating existing facilities can be a strategic response to various factors identified through SWOT analysis. It can leverage societal strengths, address weaknesses such as obsolete structures or troublesome locations, support an expansion of services, or gain competitive advantages. Once the need for construction or renovation is identified, the planning phase can commence. This phase includes two types of planning: master facility planning, and project planning. Master facility planning involves developing an all-inclusive plan for the entire facility, while project planning focuses specifically on the details and requirements of the individual project.

1.3 Master Facility Planning

Master facility planning for constructing a hospital involves a comprehensive process aimed at strategically addressing the myriad complexities and requirements of creating a modern health care facility. This planning phase serves as the foundational framework for designing and developing a hospital that can effectively meet the health care needs of the community it serves.

The process begins with a detailed analysis of the health care demands and demographics of the target population. This initial assessment helps in understanding the specific medical services and resources required to cater to the community's health needs. Additionally, it involves identifying potential site locations that can accommodate the size and scope of the hospital project, considering factors such as accessibility, zoning regulations, and proximity to other medical facilities.

Furthermore, the master facility planning process involves the integration of various departments and services within the hospital, ensuring a cohesive and interconnected health care delivery system. This includes strategic allocation of space for patient care units, emergency departments, surgical suites, diagnostic imaging facilities, administrative offices, and other essential support services. The planning must also consider future expansion and scalability to accommodate potential growth and advancements in medical technology.

Moreover, a key aspect of master facility planning is the incorporation of state-of-the-art technology and infrastructure to support advanced medical treatments and procedures. This involves the integration of robust IT systems, specialized medical equipment, and cutting-edge communication networks to facilitate seamless information exchange and efficient patient care delivery.

In addition to the physical layout and infrastructure, the master facility planning process emphasizes the importance of incorporating sustainable and environmentally friendly design elements. Implementing energy-efficient systems, utilizing natural light, and incorporating green spaces contribute to creating a healing environment that promotes patient well-being and comfort.

Overall, an effective master facility planning process for hospital construction involves a holistic approach that considers the community's health care needs, the latest medical advancements, technological integration, and sustainability, all while creating a patient-centric environment that prioritizes quality care and safety.

For example, a campus plan incorporating various building projects and crucial infrastructure might extend over several years. Many organizations view the master facility plan as a dynamic document that undergoes periodic scrutiny, modification, and enhancements.

1.4 Individual Project Planning

Individual project planning, an integral component of master facility planning, meticulous attention is given to the specific details and requirements of the hospital construction project. This phase involves a detailed assessment of the project's unique needs, including the allocation of resources, budgeting considerations, and the development of a comprehensive timeline. It also includes a thorough analysis of

DOI: 10.1201/9780367460884-1A

the facility's layout, design requirements, and integration of advanced medical technology. Furthermore, this planning stage emphasizes the establishment of a cohesive team structure, comprising architects, engineers, contractors, and health care professionals, to ensure the seamless execution of the hospital project in alignment with the broader master facility plan.

Project pre-design planning, or pre-design, is a preliminary planning phase that takes place before the actual design drawings and construction, typically following the acquisition of some funding.

1.5 Separate or Combined Processes

Master facility planning and individual project planning can be distinct processes or merged depending on the scale and complexity of the health care project. In larger health care systems or multi-campus facilities, master facility planning serves as the overarching strategic framework that guides the development of multiple individual projects. It involves a comprehensive analysis of the organization's long-term goals, resource allocation, and the integration of various health care services and departments across different locations.

Conversely, in smaller health care settings or single-campus projects, the master facility planning and individual project planning stages may be combined into a singular, streamlined process. This approach involves integrating the specific requirements and objectives of the individual project into the broader framework of the master facility plan.

1.6 Steps of Planning a Hospital Project

Planning a hospital project involves several crucial steps to ensure its successful execution. Firstly, a comprehensive needs assessment is conducted, considering the health care demands and demographic factors of the community. The formulation of a project team, gathering related data and statistics, and the subsequent site selection and acquisition are carried out, accounting for accessibility, zoning regulations, and geographical considerations. The project scope is then defined, encompassing the layout, design, and integration of advanced medical technology. Budgeting and resource allocation are meticulously planned, followed by the establishment of a cohesive project team comprising architects, engineers, and health care professionals. Finally, a detailed timeline is developed, outlining the sequential phases of construction, infrastructure development, and commissioning to ensure the timely and efficient completion of the hospital project.

The following sections describe steps in the planning phase. The scope and nature of the project will determine whether organizations engage in all these activities or just some of them (Figure 1A).

1.6.1 Step 1: Comprehensive Needs Assessment

A comprehensive needs assessment for a new hospital involves a thorough analysis of the health care requirements and demographic trends of the target population. This assessment considers factors such as population growth, disease prevalence, and existing health care services to identify specific medical needs. It also takes into account the accessibility

STEP 1	• Comprehensive Need Assessment
STEP 2	• Formulation of a Project Team
STEP 3	• Related Data & Statistics
STEP 4	• Making a Project Plan
STEP 5	• Scheduling
STEP 6	• Financial analysis & Budgeting
STEP 7	• Mandatory Compliances
STEP 8	• Master Planning Document

FIGURE 1A   Steps of Planning.

and geographical distribution of health care facilities within the community. Furthermore, it delves into the identification of specialized medical services and treatment programs required to cater to the diverse health care demands of the population.

For example, when conducting a needs assessment for a geriatric unit, an organization should analyse population projections for population aged more than 65, including historical and projected morbidity rates based on geographical locations. Similarly, while evaluating the needs of a surgical service, an organization should examine the implications of payer-driven changes, such as the shift from inpatient to outpatient service provision, and predict the future population-based surgical rate for specific procedures, like heart or orthopaedic surgeries (Table 1A).

TABLE 1A: Information Obtained by Comprehensive Needs Assessment

Comprehensive Needs Assessment
Targeted area demographics and projections
Payer-payee mix
Expertise required
Competitor analysis
Probable location of a new facility

Results from this research should be considered to determine the technical feasibility of the project, as well as when determining the location, nature, timing, and financial impact of the project if it goes ahead.

1.6.2 Step 2: Formulation of a Project Team

Forming a project team involves assembling a diverse group of professionals with specialized expertise in health care infrastructure development. This entails recruiting skilled architects, engineers, and contractors, along with health care consultants and facility managers, to ensure a comprehensive understanding of the project's intricate requirements.

Effective team formation also necessitates the engagement of health care professionals, including physicians and administrators, to provide valuable insights into patient care and operational functionalities (Table 1B).

TABLE 1B: Formulation of a Project Team

User Representatives

Executive Project Team	• Representative of the administration, e.g. CEO, medical superintendent • Doctors and other practitioners • Nursing director • Infection control officer/nurse • Director of engineering • Information technology supervisor • Director of finance • Safety officer • Other user representatives
Project Lead	Primary contact on the team, preferably a hospital administrator with experience in hospital planning and designing
User Group Teams	• Clinical areas • One rep each from ancillary and auxiliary areas
External Groups	• Patients and community representatives • Vendors in key areas, such as information technology, imaging, and surgical specialties • Representatives from local regulatory or governmental organizations

Project Partners

Project Partners and Professional Consultants	• Architects • Engineers • Contractors • Hospital management consultants • Developers or development consultants • Financial consultants • Equipment and technology planners • Landscape architects • Interior designers • Wayfinding experts • Process flow experts • Green construction expert

1.6.3 Step 3: Related Data and Statistics

The data collection process familiarizes the project team with the organization, its services, and its facilities. Gathering data for a comprehensive needs assessment of a new hospital involves a meticulous approach to acquiring and analysing diverse sets of information. This process includes collecting demographic data, such as population growth, age distribution, and socioeconomic factors, to understand the community's health care needs. Additionally, it entails reviewing existing health care facilities, services, and infrastructure within the region, identifying gaps and opportunities for improvement. Conducting surveys, interviews, and focus groups with community members and health care professionals provides valuable insights into prevalent health issues and specific medical requirements (Table 1C).

TABLE 1C: Related Data and Statistics

Detailed Graphic and Written Documentation	Type and volume of existing services • Current and anticipated competitors • Current facility issues • Desired facility elements
Existing Facility and Site Conditions	Layout, size, and function of existing facilities Narrative and graphic histories of each facility Existing drawings On-site survey with measurements of each department, floor, building, and site may be necessary.
Workload Analysis	Five-year profile that details historical workload, staffing, and other measures for each service Analysis of operational policies, functional requirements, patient care objectives, and growth assumptions
Mandatory Requirements	Research the local, state, and national regulations that will affect the design, content, and layout of the facility

1.6.4 Step 4: Making a Project Plan

Preliminary project planning, also known as space programming, involves the initial delineation and allocation of functional spaces within the hospital facility. A preliminary facility plan is utilized to define the project's scope and projected facility requirements, as well as the sequencing and scheduling, and initial budget estimates for early phases. This process includes defining the spatial requirements for patient care units, administrative offices, diagnostic and treatment centres, and specialized medical services. It also encompasses the strategic arrangement of ancillary spaces, such as waiting areas, corridors, and support facilities, to ensure efficient patient flow and staff accessibility. Space programming serves as the foundation for the hospital's architectural design, guiding the development of a functional and patient-centric environment (Table 1D).

TABLE 1D: Making a Project Plan

1 Phasing and scheduling of the project
2 Spatial needs
3 Cost-benefit analysis
4 Future growth projections
5 Standards and regulations related to safety in health care facilities
6 Major equipment

1.6.5 Step 5: Scheduling

Scheduling involves the development of a comprehensive timeline outlining the sequential phases of the hospital project, from initial planning and design to construction and eventual commissioning. Effective scheduling requires the identification and organization of specific tasks and activities within each phase, including architectural design, infrastructure development, and installation of advanced medical equipment. It also incorporates the allocation of resources, budgeting considerations, and quality control measures to ensure the timely and efficient completion of the hospital project, facilitating the seamless transition to operational readiness and the delivery of high-quality patient care. It's prudent to incorporate some buffer time in the schedule as a contingency for unforeseen circumstances and delays (Table 1E).

TABLE 1E: Scheduling

Representing the Timeline	Program evaluation and review technique, critical path method, or GANTT charting
Detailed Space Plan	Develop estimates of space programming of various clinical and auxiliary areas
Room Data Sheet	At a minimum, this sheet should identify the name, number, and size of every room, space, area, and department that will be included in the project. For all key spaces, identifying how the size and character of each are determined.
Benchmarking	Teams should be wary of using simple rule-of-thumb guidelines to estimate schedules, space needs, budgets, and other aspects of the preliminary facility plan.

1.6.6 Step 6: Financial Analysis and Budgeting

Financial analysis and budgeting for a new hospital project involve a comprehensive assessment of the project's financial feasibility and resource allocation. This process includes evaluating the initial capital investment required for infrastructure development, medical equipment procurement, and technology integration. Additionally, it entails forecasting operational expenses, such as staffing costs, administrative overhead, and maintenance expenditures, over an extended timeline. Effective financial analysis and budgeting also consider potential revenue streams, including patient services, insurance reimbursements, and government funding, to ensure the project's long-term sustainability and profitability.

Underestimating or neglecting to anticipate the complete costs associated with a project poses a significant challenge to its successful completion. Hence, meticulous financial and data analysis plays a crucial role during the planning phase (Table 1F).

TABLE 1F: Financial Analysis and Budgeting

Anticipated Critical Costs	**Construction Costs:** 60% to 80% of total project costs
	Equipment Costs: 15% and 40%
	Finishing Costs: 32%
	Professional Fees: Planning/pre-design, design, construction, and commissioning services, including consultants not traditionally listed in the basic architectural or engineering categories
	Permit Fees: Local building department, the regional utilities, and the state's department of health each levy their own fees to review and approve the project plans and construction
	Cost of Delays
Budget Contingencies	For new construction, a rule of thumb is to initially budget construction contingencies at 2% to 4% of construction cost; for remodelling, 4% to 10% is typical.

1.6.7 Step 7: Mandatory Compliances

Adhering to regulatory and mandatory compliance for a new hospital is paramount to ensure ethical and legal operational practices. This process entails securing essential licenses and certifications from relevant health care authorities and regulatory bodies. Compliance with health care standards, patient safety protocols, and industry-specific guidelines is crucial in upholding quality care and service delivery. Additionally, adherence to labour laws, financial regulations, and environmental sustainability norms is essential for the hospital's ethical and sustainable functioning. By adhering to these stringent regulations and standards, the hospital can establish a trustworthy reputation, foster patient confidence, and contribute positively to the health care landscape.

1.6.8 Step 8: Master Planning Document

The master planning document serves as a critical reference point encapsulating the comprehensive strategic framework and operational blueprint of a health care facility. Documenting the master planning process facilitates transparent communication and knowledge dissemination among stakeholders, ensuring a unified understanding of the hospital's overarching goals and development strategies. This document outlines the key insights derived from the needs assessment, facility design, and infrastructure planning, providing a comprehensive roadmap for effective project management and resource allocation. Furthermore, it serves as a foundational reference for future expansions, renovations, and technology integrations, guiding the hospital's continued growth and evolution in alignment with the changing health care landscape.

All project plans must be documented in a manner that is not only easy to understand but also easy to use, share, and store. This documentation serves multiple purposes, such as providing the historical perspective of selection decisions and rationales and orienting new partners and organizational team members.

(a) **Form and Format:** This documentation typically takes the shape of a comprehensive report or digital document, incorporating detailed narratives, charts, graphs, and architectural drawings to illustrate the facility's layout and design. It includes an executive summary highlighting key objectives, findings, and recommendations, followed by a systematic breakdown of the planning phases, analyses, and proposed solutions. The inclusion of appendices containing supplementary data, research findings, and meeting minutes further enriches the master planning document, providing a holistic and transparent overview of the hospital's development trajectory.

(b) **For Communicating and Training:** Training and communication surrounding the master facility planning document are vital for ensuring effective implementation and stakeholder engagement. Comprehensive training programs are essential to familiarize key personnel with the document's strategic objectives, operational guidelines, and infrastructure development plans. Clear and concise communication strategies, including presentations, workshops, and interactive sessions, facilitate seamless knowledge transfer and foster a shared understanding of the hospital's overarching goals and development trajectory. Open dialogue and regular updates further promote transparency and collaboration, encouraging active participation and constructive feedback from all stakeholders. By prioritizing training and effective communication, the hospital can foster a unified and informed approach to realizing its strategic vision and delivering high-quality patient care.

1.7 Summary

Planning is the first phase of most construction and renovation projects. Most hospital projects take more than three years from inception to completion, and today's facility projects are fraught with uncertainties. Master facility planning that determines the building and/or campus needs to align with an organization's strategic plan. The project team analyses the project needs, gathers relevant data, and makes a budget, thereby finalizing and documenting the master facility plan. A well-made master facility plan goes a long way in ensuring a well-executed hospital project.

1B PRE-FEASIBILITY AND FEASIBILITY ANALYSIS

1.1 Pre-Feasibility Analysis

1.1.1 Background

A pre-feasibility analysis is a broad assessment of whether or not it is possible for your hospital to be built and operated the way that you and your partners envision. That is, a pre-feasibility analysis tests your project's viability and risk analysis at an early stage. In addition, it identifies key issues, it requires consideration and input related to downstream activities such as financing, marketing, and facility design, and it prioritizes important preparatory steps that will have a substantial impact on the project's progress.

1.1.2 Conducting the Pre-Feasibility Analysis

If you wish to retain an in-house/international consulting or advisory firm, then you need to ensure that it has a local/international team that is familiar with the economic, market, and regulatory environment in the country and area where your hospital will be located (Table 1G).

1.2 Feasibility Analysis

1.2.1 Background

Detailed feasibility analysis examines the details of the plan throughout the facility's construction and subsequent daily operation. It should develop the specifics of how to construct and operate the hospital to ensure the project's feasibility and viability, including identifying and minimizing risks.

To keep the concepts of process and output distinct, we refer to the process of analysing the project's feasibility as the *feasibility analysis* and to the resulting document as the *business plan*. The business plan presents all aspects of your project in detail. It has two main objectives: (a) to provide its readers with sufficient information about the project so that they can understand the project well, and (b) to convince its readers to make a positive decision to support and/or invest in the project.

In thinking through the details of your project's construction stage and subsequent daily operations, you and your partners will need to consider several different scenarios in terms of the services to be offered, prices to be charged, cost-efficient ways to design and construct your hospital, ways to finance the construction and raise working capital, and so on. You will

TABLE 1G: Key Questions Asked in the Course of a Pre-Feasibility Analysis

1 Does the prevailing regulatory and policy framework support the establishment of a new private facility?
2 What is the health status of the target population?
3 Is there sufficient market demand for your facility?
4 How is the patient referral system structured?
5 How will prices be structured, and will your target population be able to pay the prices?
6 How much investment will your hospital need, and how will it be financed?
7 How will your hospital be staffed?
8 What are the key risks?

need to reach an agreement on the best set of alternatives for construction, financing, and daily operation.

1.2.2 Conducting the Feasibility Analysis

The feasibility analysis should be conducted with an objective, realistic, and professional mindset. It is a dynamic process and requires numerous iterations as your analysis continues and your plans evolve. Often, entrepreneurs who set out to build health care facilities choose to retain an independent professional consulting firm to carry out the feasibility analysis and prepare the business plan. Should you decide to do this, you should make sure that the consultants will indeed prepare a thorough, objective, and professional analysis and will not simply seek to reinforce your desire to carry out the project. It can be conducted by in-house experienced partners or can be outsourced (Table 1H).

Following are some of the basic areas to be considered in the feasibility analysis. The list is not exhaustive, and you will need to add to it according to the particularities of your project.

1.2.3 Non-Financial Analysis

(a) Market and Competitive Landscape: (Table 1I)
   (i) Demand Analysis (Table 1J)
   (ii) Supply Analysis (Table 1K)
   (iii) Pricing (Table 1L)
   (iv) Payment System (Table 1M)
   (v) Hospital's Competitive Position

TABLE 1H: Parts of a Feasibility Analysis

Primary Data	Potential clients, existing hospitals, and consumer survey companies
Secondary Data (Major Source)	Reports and statistics published by government agencies, individual researchers, consulting firms, international organizations, or industry associations
Non-Financial Analysis	Market demand, competitive landscape, macroeconomic and political environment, legal and regulatory environment, technical and technological factors, environmental and safety factors, ownership structure, organizational and management structure, and corporate governance
Financial Analysis	Looks mainly at costs, revenues, working capital, and financing

TABLE 1I: Market and Competitive Landscape

1 Is there sufficient demand for the services that your hospital will provide?
2 Are there enough people who are willing and able to pay the prices that your hospital will need to charge in order to ensure its financial viability?
3 Who will pay for the services, and what will be the payment conditions?
4 Who will be your major competitors?
5 What will be your competitive advantage?

DOI: 10.1201/9780367460884-1B

TABLE 1J: Demand Analysis

Primary Catchment Area	Where 75% to 80% of your hospital's patients will come from (for example, within 100 km of the location of your facility)
Target Segment	For example, high-income, middle-income, or low-income; local population only or foreign residents and local population; ethnic groups, if applicable); any particular characteristics of this population; and the estimated number of people in the target groups
Health Care Expenses	The estimated average level of health care expenses incurred annually by each family or person in the target population
Quantity & Frequency of Interventions	Estimated quantity or frequency of health interventions needed by your hospital's primary target patients in the main catchment area

TABLE 1K: Supply Analysis: Key Information about Each Facility

1 Number of years in operation, reputation
2 Number of beds by department or by type
3 Number of operating rooms
4 Services offered and prices charged; quality of facilities
5 Key medical equipment
6 Main catchment area, how many patients are treated at the hospital each year, bed occupancy rates, and trends over recent years
7 Average waiting time for certain treatments or procedures, number of surgical operations by type of operation, and capacity and utilization rate of key equipment
8 Number of physicians and nurses; where the hospital's physicians come from
9 The hospital's business model, accessibility by public and private transportation, public or private ownership, for-profit or not-for-profit status, affiliation with a religious or other type of organization, ownership structure
10 Quality of management; expansion plans

TABLE 1L: Key Factors Determining the Pricing of Services

1 Prices charged by competitors
2 Prices mandated by government regulation
3 The target population's income levels and their willingness and ability to pay
4 Capital and operating costs of your hospital; hospital break even
5 The mix of payment types (out-of-pocket, publicly financed insurance, or privately financed insurance)
6 The image and reputation of your hospital, which will influence people's willingness to pay

TABLE 1M: Common Payment Mechanisms

Fee for service	Payment is made per individual item of service.
Case payment	The payment is for a package of services or an episode of care; for example, fees may be predetermined based on specific Diagnosis-Related Groups (DRGs).
Per diem arrangement	A flat charge is billed for each day of hospitalization and care.
Contracting arrangement	Agreed payment is determined for a selected group (or all) services in a given period.

Once you have determined that there is sufficient demand for the services that you plan to offer, you will need to assess each competitor's strengths and weaknesses and anticipated changes, if any, in the competitive position of each hospital that could diminish the chances of success for your hospital. You will need to document this analysis in as much detail as possible to serve as a reference for the future. You should also include it in the business plan for your hospital.

(b) Macroeconomic and Political Environment (Table 1N)

TABLE 1N: Feasibility Areas in the Macroeconomic and Political Environment

1 What is the outlook for overall economic growth in the country and your hospital's catchment area for the next three to five years?
2 What drives economic growth nationally and regionally in your hospital's target market area, and what is the outlook for the economic drivers, that is, key industries, in the country and in the region?
3 • What is the annual per capita income in the country and in your hospital's target market area and growth thereon?
4 • Is the health care sector a priority area for government spending?
   • What are the possible changes in government priorities in the next few years?
5 • What are the key features of the government's monetary policy?
   • Is the government planning to relax the money supply by decreasing the central bank reserve rates for commercial banks, or vice versa?
   • Is the government expected to lower or increase interest rates in the near future?
   • What will be the time frame for any action in this regard?
6 • What has been in the inflation rate nationally and regionally in the past three to five years, and what are the expected changes in inflation in the next three to four years?
   • How would the anticipated inflation rate changes affect the capital and operating costs of your project?
7 • What are the official exchange rates for major hard currencies? Are they close to market rates? If not, how large are the gaps between the two?
   • How stable have the official and market exchange rates been in the past three to five years? If the exchange rate has been stable in recent years, is any change expected in the near future?
   • What are the chances for a sudden devaluation of the local currency?
8 • How stable is the political climate?
   • How will a change in government affect the sustainability and profitability of your facility?
   • On average, how long do health ministers stay in power?

(Continued)

TABLE 1N: (Continued)

9   What political forces might influence the operations of your facility, including the choice of services to be provided by it?

10 How will the existence of, or potential for, corruption in the country affect your ability to conduct business?

TABLE 1O: Feasibility Areas in the Legal and Regulatory Environment

1   • How often do regulations relating to health care (including the pharmaceutical sector) change?
    • Are substantial reforms pending?

2   How feasible is it to work within the constraints of local government regulations?

3   Is there any regulation concerning capacity (number of institutions, beds, etc.)?

4   What are the regulations concerning treatment of emergency patients?

5   Are there regulations that affect patient referrals by physicians?

6   Is there any requirement that private health care facilities provide free services?

7   What kinds of licenses and permits will be needed to operate your facility?

8   What regulations govern the issuance (and revocation) of such licenses and permits?

9   • What are the costs related to obtaining such licenses and permits?
    • Do physicians have a choice in where they can practice?
    • Are hospitals allowed to take out loans?

10 • Does the government subsidize payments for private health care?
    • What regulations, if any, affect the choice and procurement of major medical equipment?

11 What are the laws and regulations governing the health care sector and financing concerning foreign investment, staffing and employment, agreements and contracts, trade and taxes, environmental and occupational safety matters?

(c) **Legal and Regulatory Environment (Table 1O)**

(d) **Technical and Physical Parameters**

The feasibility analysis should consider whether or not the construction of necessary buildings and auxiliary facilities can be completed according to the architectural plan and at an affordable cost. All elements relevant to construction of the facilities, including the location and condition of the site, the quality of construction companies available, the availability of construction materials, the timing of obtaining various permits, and so forth, must be examined. Attention should be given to the sequence of steps, the assignment of responsibilities, the time and costs involved in each aspect of construction, and any risks that may affect this process.

(e) **Information and Technology Factors**

A properly designed and installed management information system/hospital information system (MIS/HIS) is critical to the smooth and efficient operation of the hospital and collection of critical data. It will allow the hospital to integrate data inputs and information outputs that include, among other things, patient data, physician's notes, pharmacy operation, billing, accounts receivable, inventory management, and the production of financial statements.

A well-developed MIS/HIS package can cost $1 million or even more. Therefore, you will need to start the search for an information technology (IT) package supplier early in the feasibility analysis and obtain realistic price quotations that cover all activities needed for the smooth launching of the system.

(f) **Environmental and Safety Factors**

During the feasibility analysis, you will address issues such as how medical wastes will be disposed of and/or treated, the safe handling of various industrial gases, the safe handling of blood, the disposal of laboratory materials and supplies, and radiology safety. You will need to identify the major risks concerning these matters and prepare an action plan that meets international requirements. Documenting the discussions in the early stage will save time and effort later in developing the hospital's written policies and procedures for environmental and safety issues.

(g) **Ownership Structure**

During the feasibility analysis, you should also consider what ownership structure would provide the required flexibility if the facility should need to expand in the future, with a corresponding expansion of the capital structure. Various tax and accounting regulations must be taken into account, along with other legal and regulatory limitations on ownership of a health care facility in your country. Another consideration is the need to minimize the exposure of investors and founding partners to liabilities potentially arising from the project.

(h) **Organization and Management Structure and Staffing**

During the feasibility analysis, you need to start developing the details of how the hospital will be managed after it begins operation, including the overall organizational structure, the management team, corporate governance, and staffing.

1.2.4 Financial Analysis

A financial analysis should answer two critical questions.

• First, does it make financial sense to build and operate the hospital in the way that is being considered?
• Second, what conditions are required to ensure that the hospital can operate on a positive cash-generating basis (Table 1P)?

1.3 Summary

At the end of the feasibility analysis, you should be able to ascertain whether your hospital project is viable and sustainable or not. Can the hospital be built without major problems and within the overall budget and time frame? Can the

TABLE 1P: Financial Feasibility

Estimating Hard Costs	Most critical cost items include the acquisition and preparation of land, the construction of buildings and infrastructure, and the purchase and installation of equipment, furniture, and fixtures.
Estimating Soft Costs	These include project development, pre-opening and construction costs.
Estimating Permanent Working Capital	These are operating costs that are incurred before the payments for the hospital's services are collected in cash. Permanent working capital is so-called because once a business gets established and starts to grow, the amount of working capital will continue to grow accordingly.
Estimating Financing Cost	Financing costs (including interest and fees) that will be incurred during the period leading up to the hospital's full operation need to be estimated, and these estimates need to be included in the project cost and financial plan.
Contingencies	The two most important possibilities that require a good contingency plan are delays in completion of the physical facility (related to construction, equipment installation, setting up the IT system, connecting to communication channels, and so forth) and a slow build-up in operations that hampers revenue generation.
The Financial Plan	Consider various potential financial partners and the availability of financing and its conditions so that you can gain a reasonable sense of whether you will be able to obtain the financing necessary for your hospital.
Preparing Financial Projections	Prepare a financial projection model (using Excel worksheets or a similar software program) to help you analyse the financial implications of each scenario in your project plan.
Estimating Revenues, Operating Costs, and Expenses	Optimistic estimation of revenues, especially for the first two to three years of the project's operation, is one of the most common and serious mistakes in planning for any project. This should be strenuously avoided. The most important cash items in operating costs and expenses are staff salaries, supplies (pharmaceutical, medical, and other), and utilities.
Estimating Cash Flows	The cash flow generated from operations, after all operating costs and expenses have been paid off, is used for two main purposes: to reinvest in the business and to pay back the capital that was invested in the project.
Estimating Financial Viability	The most frequently used indicators of financial viability include gross operating margin, operating margin, debt-to-equity ratio, debt service ratio, financial rate of return of the project, and financial return on equity.
Sensitivity Analysis	Having completed the base case scenario projections, you will need to identify the major risk areas and modify the relevant assumptions negatively to see how the hospital's financial results will differ from the base case scenario.

hospital operate without serious worry of disruption (for example, power shortages, lack of necessary personnel, floods, social unrest, nearby construction, or serious pollution)? Will the hospital be able to generate enough cash to pay for all its operating expenses, increases in working capital, and capital expenditures required for the proper upkeep of its facilities? Will it be able to service its debts and pay dividends and other obligations associated with share capital? Can the hospital operate without serious concern about environmental or health hazards and/or worker safety issues? A feasibility report helps the organization to proactively identify the risks associated with the establishment of the hospital.

2 PLANNING MACHINERY AND ARCHITECT BRIEF

2.1 Background

Planning can be defined as the "specification of the means necessary for the accomplishment of goals and objectives before action towards these goals has begun. These are issues that must be addressed during the health care programming and design process. Planning machinery should provide a functional design that ensures efficient, safe, and appropriate workspaces. It should accommodate technical requirements for highly sophisticated equipment and create clear, segregated paths for the movement of people and materials within the building. Planning machinery should create a humane environment for patients and staff while developing building systems that can accommodate rapid change.

2.2 The Planning Team and the Process

The complex process of planning and designing a hospital requires that it be a multidisciplinary endeavour consisting of various stakeholders. This composition of teams depends on the scope and size of the project.

(a) **Needs assessment team**: Establishes an overall plan of the needs, range of services to be provided, the target population or catchment area, the financial feasibility of the project with a cost-benefit analysis and the scale of the hospital, etc.

(b) **Briefing team**: "The design brief", which translates the requirements into functions, activities, space distribution and/or any other information necessary for the design.

(c) **Design team**: Produces the instruments for implementing construction, starting from preliminary investigation to the final designs with technical specification, and tenders documents and detailed working drawings and estimates of cost. This team mainly consists of engineers, architects, quantity, surveyors, hospital staff, the community, and the approving authority.

(d) **Construction team**: This team consists of engineers, architects, and builders. The construction team implements the design from the approved drawings and technical specifications within the prescribed time and cost and produces facilities commissioned for waste disposal, which causes serious complications when left untreated.

(e) **Commissioning team**: The commissioning team in consultation with hospital staff are responsible of hospital commissioning and procures the equipment, furniture & supplies & prepares the hospital for operations.

2.3 Roles of Members of the Team

Table 2A gives a simplified version of the stages and their corresponding inputs and outputs and the role of working professionals at each stage.

2.4 Responsibilities of a Functional Planner

1. Physical evaluation of existing facilities along with architect
2. Functional evaluation of existing facilities
3. Preparation of workload projections
4. Functional programming
5. Space programming (along with architect)
6. Master site planning (along with architect)

Determination of the services to be provided in quantitative terms requires a consideration of the following:

(a) Functions
(b) Locations
(c) Relationships
(d) Utilization
(e) Staffing patterns
(f) Space requirements
(g) Workflow

TABLE 2A: Roles of Members of the Team

Stage	Task	Input	Output	Working Team Active	Working Team Consultative
One	Establish demand for new hospital or for expansion	Information, indicators, projections	Decision to construct, renovate, and expand	User, client Planners	–
Two	Preparing a design brief	Services to be delivered, functional requirements	Design brief	User, client	Architects, engineers
Three	Design	Design brief, additional data from consultants	Design of hospital, working documents	Architect, engineers	User, clients
Four	Construction	Design of hospital working drawings	Hospital in physical form	Architects, builders, engineers	User, clients
Five	Commissioning	List of staff/furniture/equip/supplies	Appointment and training of staff, procurement of furniture/equip/supplies	User, clients, procurement staff Personnel staff	–

DOI: 10.1201/9780367460884-2

Before an architect can develop a hospital design that will best serve its functions, they must be provided a written program explaining these requirements. This is the Architect Brief from which the architect prepares schematic drawings and sketch plans. The brief should contain the permission required from various regulatory bodies, spatial needs of various departments, manpower required, special requirements of various departments, and inter- and intra-departmental relationships.

The team also carries out market research for project conceptualization and a feasibility study.

2.5 Architect Briefs

An architect brief is defined as a written expression of a client's vision about the hospital project or a client's need with respect to the hospital project expressed as a written document. It represents the problem that a client may have, which an architect attempts to solve. It is a written brief formulated with the architect for design purposes, wherein problems are appraised and constraints are highlighted. It is also known as a client's brief, architectural brief, planning and design brief, design brief, functional brief, functional program, etc.

2.6 Responsibility for Preparing an Architect Brief

It may be developed by a trained hospital administrator in consultation with a board of trustees (client) and users, by a representative of trustees (client) in consultation with architects, engineers, and clinicians, or by an agency in consultation with the client.

2.7 Importance and Characteristics of an Architect Brief

An architect brief forms the basis of creation for the hospital. It may be possible to develop a state-of-the-art hospital out of a state-of-the-art design brief; however, this is not certain. Better briefing produces better hospital building. This point should be emphasized to the end users in the first design briefing meeting.

Table 2B shows the characteristics of an architect brief.

TABLE 2B: Characteristics of an Architect Brief

How much to brief	It must be detailed enough to enable a design team to interpret it correctly and translate it into a design that meets the objectives.
Quality of the brief	If the design brief is of poor quality, then a hospital can never be state of the art, irrespective of enormous resources.
Standardization	One cannot standardize a design because every hospital is unique. There should be a balance between briefing for general acceptable practices and the special requirements of end users. The brief should be clear with a broad strategic framework within which an architect designs the hospital.

2.8 Process of Making an Architect Brief

Making an architect brief should be an established procedure, and the following aspects should be decided beforehand.

(a) **In charge of briefing**: Should be one of the prime roles of a trained hospital administrator by virtue of their academic qualifications and training.

(b) **Project coordinator:** If a hospital administrator is available, then they can be given this additional role to function as an interface between the end users and design team.

(c) **Project management group:** Consists of end users, representatives of the administrator, the project coordinator, and the design team. In case a hospital administrator is not available in-house, they may be hired, or alternatively, a designated representative of the trustees can provide briefings and function as the project coordinator.

(d) **Date/time/place** for providing briefing/briefing documents should be decided.

In the early stages of the design process, the brief may be continuously reappraised as the requirements become clearer—this is known as "firming up the brief" (especially if the briefing is not conducted by a trained hospital administrator). Finally, a clear set of instructions setting out the key objectives and requirements emerge, which form the starting point of the architect's designs and will be continually tested against the brief as the design progresses. In the later stages of writing a brief, a schedule of accommodation is sometimes prepared that specifies the number and size of rooms/areas that are required.

2.9 Relationship between a Brief and Designing

(a) Ideally, a complete design brief should be created once after feasibility is ascertained.

(b) Briefing may extend throughout the design stages of a building project.

(c) The client compiles the brief gradually throughout the design process as a parallel activity to the architect.

2.10 Systems Approach to the Architect Brief

Compared to the traditional approach, the systems approach to an architect brief is designed to

(a) Handle rapid obsolescence;

(b) Reduce the briefing and design time;

(c) Facilitate design decision making; and

(d) Avoid fixed plans without losing the advantages of standardization.

We concentrate on the common features of the hospital. Complete requirements are divided into basic activity units, which provide information to the designer. The requirements are structured in terms of a predetermined hierarchy of functional levels as shown in Table 2D.

Approaches for Making an Architect Brief: Systematic Functional Programming

Developed countries	• No general agreement on the method to adopt for briefing
	• Client writes instructions to designer based on users' requirements
	• Drawbacks
	  • Designers work in isolation
	  • Subjected to conflicting demands
	  • Time consuming for user

Developing countries	• No detailed brief or briefing process
	• Medical planners prepare rudimentary brief, and both planners and designers are under different administrative control
	• Brief is mostly in the form of a schedule of accommodation
	• Drawbacks
	  • Medical planners take quasi-architectural decisions, and designers can make quasi-medical assumptions while interpreting a schedule of accommodation
	  • Current health facility guidelines are not taken into consideration
	  • In case of an existing structure, the schedule of accommodation may be derived from the existing building

2.11 Activity Units

A basic functional unit is independent of any specific program. Its requirements are defined in terms of space programming, services or functions, the environment, special requirements, and equipment. An example of an activity unit, an Intensive Care Unit (ICU) bed, is shown in Table 2C.

2.12 Traditional Approach to Architect Briefs

Details of the traditional approach to an architect brief are mentioned in Table 2E.

TABLE 2C: ICU Bed as an Activity Unit

Space	A 14-sq m, half-partitioned cubicle (by glazed tiles) is used to separate it from other beds.
Services	The Unit will accommodate a patient for critical care, requiring continuous monitoring and nursing with 360° access. Need space & facilities for 3–4 staff to provide care. Unit will be provided with bed head unit, handwashing basin, and ceiling-mounted IV fluid track.
Special requirements	Each bed is separated by other beds/environment by ceiling-fitted curtain track.
Environment	• Air conditioning with 15 air changes per hour • Light—indirect light with dimmers, one light in bed head unit, and one emergency light for procedures • Temperature—22°C • Floor—non-skid vitrified tiles of size 2' × 2'
Equipment	• 5 multi-sockets with 5 and 15 amperes, two in-bed units • Nurse call system • Cardiac monitor—wall mounted • Defibrillator—placed in a corner • BP equipment—standing • Stethoscope • Ophthalmoscope and laryngoscope • Ventilator—on a required basis

TABLE 2D: Hierarchy of Functional Levels

Functional Levels	Nomenclature	Example
Level 1	Activity unit	ICU bed, bed head unit, handwashing basin
Level 2	Activity set	• Patient care area in ICU (01 × ICU bed + 1 × bed head unit + 1 × handwashing basin) • Basic nursing activity area (nurse station + 1 WHB + nursing room + restroom)
Level 3	Activity section	(8 patient care areas in ICU + 2 isolation rooms + basic nursing activity area + support area in ICU + 3 × sanitary area)
Level 4	Activity organization	OT, ICU, and OPD
Level 5	Activity sub-system	Patient care services, diagnostic services, and ancillary and auxiliary services
Level 6	Activity system	Hospital

TABLE 2E: Architect Brief—Traditional Approach

Proposal / Objectives	To construct a multi-specialty hospital for the provision of patient care, medical education, and personnel training • Guidelines will be provided for the construction of a 1,000-bed multi-specialty hospital for high-quality patient care. • The hospital will be affiliated with a medical college with an intake of 120 students per year and will cater to the training needs of medical students. • The hospital will provide training to 400 paramedics in different specialties. • The hospital will support biomedical research.
Cost	The overall cost of the hospital has been estimated at 700 Crores.
Brief on what is existing	The present proposal pertains to a new hospital for which a plot is available. Or At present, approximately 500 beds and their associated debts are existing. From these, 300 beds are to be demolished along with associated departments.
Beneficiaries	The hospital will provide treatment to needy patients of all of society who belong to a large economic strata. It will also cater to the poor.
Facilities	The hospital will cater to an expected workload of 5,000 OPD patients and 1,000 inpatients. Or The hospital will provide accommodation to 120 trainees. The hospital will provide accommodation to 120—400 paramedics undergoing training. The hospital will provide accommodation to 120—200 attendants of patients. The hospital will have hospitality services and recreational facilities.
Additional facilities	• Guide Maps. • Signage/signposting. • Information kiosks. • Layout plans. • Touch screen. • Cafeteria for staff and visitors. • Flower shop. • Fruit shop. • Book store. • Souvenir shop. • Provision store. • Vending machine—tea, coffee, and juice; communication facilities—STD, ISD, and fax. • Cybercafé—internet. • Aquarium. • Water bodies. • Well-furnished waiting areas with basic amenities. • Security and safety system with CCTV. • Fire prevention, detection, and firefighting systems. • Post office. • Police post. • Banking/ATM and Xerox facilities. • Prayer room/facilities. • May I Help You counters. • Parking lots. • Public conveniences. • Biomedical waste disposal area. • Ramp. • Intelligent lighting system. • Intelligent lift and escalator system. • Fast food outlets. • Food junction. • Spa. • Shopping malls/complex. • Wellness/fitness centre. • Special facilities for geriatric and physically challenged. • Emphasis on blending architecture with local culture, traditions, and aesthetics. • Subway/foot bridge/connecting bridge between adjoining buildings.
Area availability	Availability of total plinth area— Area available for present construction The area earmarked for future expansion

Planning and engineering grid	• This will be decided in consultation with the board of trustees, architects, and engineers. • The hospital will be constructed by taking a hospital space module of 14 sq m. The minimum space unit will be 3.5 sq m. • The structural grid will be taken as 1.6 m. The planning grid is largely determined by the layout of the inpatient facilities. • It describes the accommodations desired for a single-bed patient room and a double-bed patient room and their toilets (viable space planning module = 14 sq m with space unit = 3.5 sq m).
Planning and engineering grid	• The structural grid is the network of lines defining the location of columns and is derived from the planning grid. It is the basic unit of architecture. • 1.6, six such grids, i.e., 3.2 m × 4.8 m leads to carpet area = 14 sq m, after deducting the wall thickness. • Structural grid need not be the same as the planning grid but is usually derived from it. • Structural grid continues downwards through the rest of the hospital. • The lower floors, which may house the X-ray dept, kitchen, laundry, and mechanical services in the basement, will need to be designed within these column positions. • The position of an additional column required would be derived from the structural grid. • In semi-urban or rural situations where the available land area is much larger concerning the built-up area desired, the planning grid has much greater flexibility and provides more elbow room to the architect. This freedom enables many different types of building layouts and forms. • Structural grid is a design tool subject to local variation in terms of the structure being single-story or high-rise. • Different parts of the hospital may have different planning grids derived from the functional planning requirements.
Departmental planning	• General Medicine • General Surgery • Obstetrics & Gynecology • Orthopedics & Traumatology • Paediatrics • Dermatology & STD • Oto-Rhinolaryngology (ENT) • Ophthalmology • Rheumatology • Pathology with Central Laboratory Services • Microbiology • Radiology Imaging • Anaesthesiology • Transfusion Medicine & Blood Bank • Cardiology • Cardio-Thoracic & Vascular Surgery	• Gastroenterology • GI Surgery • Nephrology (with Dialysis) • Urology (and Renal Transplantation) • Neurology • Neuro-Surgery • Medical Oncology • Surgical Oncology • Radiotherapy Services • Endocrinology & Metabolic Diseases • Clinical Haematology • Paediatric Surgery • Burns & Plastic Surgery • Pulmonary Medicine
Bed distribution	The policy of distribution of beds • Based on specialty. • Medicine. • Surgery. • Other disciplines. • Based on the payment system. • Suites. • Single room. • Double room, multiple patient cubicle.	• Resuscitation beds. • Beds with specialist centres. • Day care beds. • Chemotherapy centre. • ICUs/NICU/PICU. • Pre- and post-operative beds.
Support services	• Blood transfusion services. • Medical store and pharmacy services. • CSSD. • Laundry and linen services. • Dietary services.	

(Continued)

TABLE 2E: (Continued)

Proposal	To construct a multi-specialty hospital for the provision of patient care, medical education, and personnel training
Utility services	• Hospital communication and HIS • Housekeeping services • Electricity requirements for the facility • Stand by the power supply • Lighting • Water/steam requirements • Sewage disposal system • Bio-waste disposal system • Medical gases • Fire safety • Security system • Ventilation system • Medico-social services • Mortuary services • Biomedical engineering department
Miscellaneous	• Rainwater harvesting • Landscaping
Departmental requirements	• Description of functions. • Physical facilities. • Location. • Interdepartmental relationships. • Size—department/areas. • Intra-departmental relationships. • Construction requirements. • Engineering services. • Flow of various traffic. • Patient. • Staff. • Supplies. • Visitors. • Special requirement. • Zoning. • HVAC system. • Supervision. • Privacy. • Acoustic requirements. • Future expansion. Various areas—the details of various areas are enclosed as a schedule of accommodation in respective areas.
Barrier-free environment	The hospital should have an efficient layout for a barrier-free environment that helps patient mobility and wellness by providing ramps, lounges, worship places, gardens, kitchen activity rooms, parking places, restrooms, and drinking water facilities wherever required as per norms. Many of these details and facilities can be incorporated into the plan at little to no extra cost.
Equipment planning Specifications	

Ser No	Area	Floor	Walls	Ceiling	Door	Window
1	OT	Vinyl	Concrete epoxy paint	Gypsum bd	Ht -1.8m W - 1.2 m	Al frame

The detailed specifications for all the departments and other services are to be included.

2.13 Summary

Hospitals are complex health care facilities. Thus, it is important to plan and design their architecture down to the smallest detail. In addition, they need to provide healing support. Architects need to go beyond their conventional role and have a say in the planning process. With newer technologies comes complexity in the design process. Moreover, there is an increase in the number of specialized wards in hospitals. This makes the architect's job even more difficult. In order to create the functional environment, the architect brief provides the architect with inputs to accommodate the technical requirements for highly sophisticated equipment and creates clear, segregated paths for the movement of people and materials within the building. It should be able to blend technical and functional requirements into a design that brings delight to those who use the building and to those who pass by it.

3 ISSUES AND FACTORS TO CONSIDER WHILE PLANNING AND DESIGNING A HOSPITAL

3.1 Background

Hospitals are the most complex of building types as they provide a wide range of services and are made up of many functional units. Hospitals have diagnostic and treatment functions, such as clinical laboratories, imaging, emergency rooms, and surgery; hospitality functions, such as food service and housekeeping; and inpatient care or bed-related functions.

3.2 Issues and Factors to Consider While Planning and Designing a Hospital

The following issues and factors should be considered while planning and designing a hospital.

1. **Architecture and Campus Design:** Good campus planning and architecture allow the layout of streets, the building approach, and the building entries to serve as wayfinding devices. Vehicular access and approach roads should be designed to be intuitive and clear to alleviate stress on the commute. In addition, choices in scale, lighting, and materiality for the hospital's main entrance, parking structures, and medical office buildings put patients and their families on the quickest path to the front door.

2. **Welcoming Design Aesthetic:** Good hospital design should reflect both the region and the visual and cultural ethos of the institution. Today, many institutions reference elements of hospitality design when discussing their vision for new buildings. This includes covered drop-offs with valet parking, open and transparent lobbies and public spaces, and warm, natural materials that evoke a sense of comfort. Concierge and check-in services are becoming more common.

3. **Drop-Off and Parking:** There is no better way to feel that you are being taken care of—pampered even—than by eliminating worry of arrival, drop-off, and parking. Free valet services reduce the stress of finding a parking space, paying for, and returning to your car. An expanded vehicular drop-off and pick-up accommodate these services. It is also adaptable for ride-share and a potential autonomous car revolution.

4. **Internal Wayfinding:** Aligning the patient journey with key architecture and interior elements alleviates the need for excessive signage, which can become distracting. Less signage also means more room for a design that creates joy and delight. For example, bold colours or visually distinct changes at elevator banks pull people toward them. Using the concourse concept or promenade to connect departments is a way to intuitively organize wayfinding.

5. **Better Waiting Area:** The same holds for check-in desks and waiting areas—the spaces and their visual identities can be used to intuitively help patients navigate. The waiting room is one of the most stressful parts of a visit, so make it an amazing place to be: provide expansive views, windows for daylight, art, and beautiful, comfortable furniture.

6. **Pleasant Clinical Environment:** Patients and staff benefit from a well-designed space. Although it is tempting to focus only on lobbies and waiting areas, clinical areas need just as much attention. Imaging suites, procedure rooms where patients are conscious, and blood-draw stations benefit from natural daylight and positive distractions in art, a material palette, and views.

7. **Onstage/Offstage Environments (The Disney Effect):** Today, many health care institutions take cues from Disney's onstage/offstage concept, where impeccable service appears to happen seamlessly. When designing a new hospital, it is about not only separating experience areas from service areas but also designing a circulation and planning diagram that allows the separation of goods and services from patients and their families, both vertically and horizontally. There are varying degrees to this separation and many influential criteria. For example, adding service and patient transport elevators centred in the patient wing instead of at the end of units decreases the amount of crossover between patients and services.

8. **Healthy Building = Healthy Occupants:** Healing happens inside hospitals, and the building itself should participate in this healing process. Designing with Red List-free materials, providing clean and filtered air, and offering access to outside experiences with operable windows or terraces in places where immune systems are not compromised are all strategies for healthier buildings.

9. **Dignified Discharge:** Finally, consider how to give a dignified exit to patients who are leaving the hospital but who still require assistance. Provide a comfortable and private discharge route that does not go through the main hospital doors for those using crutches or a wheelchair for the first time or those recovering from a same-day procedure. Provide the departing patient a more dignified departure that can also calm the nerves of new patients entering the hospital.

10. **Enhanced Patient Expectations:** Patients have become more quality-conscious and price-sensitive. They expect clinical, administrative, and supportive services and the design of facilities to be conducive to their requirements.

11. **Epidemiological and Demographic Changes:** There has been a cascading pattern in the incidence of lifestyle diseases and geriatric-related health care problems. Hospitals of the future need to be more disabled-friendly, which is better suited for geriatric and vulnerable populations.

12. **Emphasis on Ambulatory/Day Care:** Hospital stays are gradually being programmed for only high-dependency cases admitted for inpatient care and for other cases; a greater emphasis is placed on a shorter hospital stay.

13. **Enhanced Standards:** There have been upgraded standards and norms in the delivery of health care in almost all aspects. More and more health care organizations are now opting for third-party certifications and accreditations.

DOI: 10.1201/9780367460884-3

14. **Changing Function of Hospitals:** Hospitals are an evolving system. Hospitals apart from curing the sick have the added functions of the maintenance of health, prevention of illness, biomedical research, and provision of community outreach services. The focus has shifted from treating illness to creating wellness.

15. **Health Insurance:** Health insurance is gradually permeating as an important facet of health care delivery systems. The providers of insurance and health care and the recipients view the hospital as an important hub for health care delivery.

16. **Advancement in Medical Science:** Advancements in medical sciences dictate/change the paradigm of health care delivery. Trends and dimensions in molecular biology, pharmaceuticals, and surgical interventions have changed medical management outcomes. New diagnostic and therapeutic modalities require a special controlled environment, energy requirements, and other engineering services.

17. **Design for Flexibility and Expandability:** Due to the complexity of hospital organization and diversity in various factors such as operations, functions, and development, alterations and expansions of buildings are varied and frequent. Buildings should be adaptable to changing requirements. Generally, 10–15% of the gross area is earmarked for future expansion.

18. **Anticipate Change in Demand Functions:** None of the varied elements are static, for as technology develops, medical understanding progresses, and their combined application expires, along with social demands and expectations. Demand will change due to increases in life expectancy, health becoming a norm, and health care that focuses on prevention and intervention rather than treatment.

19. **Emphasis on Patient-Focused Hospitals:** Patients until recently were more of an object on the scene than the focus of design. Hospitals are service organizations that are essentially facilitating systems that enable users to achieve their goals in direct interaction with providers. In a major paradigm shift, sensitivity to people's feelings and their need for sensory input has entered the lexicon of facility planning and design. The thought process has moved from improving "Patient Satisfaction" to enhancing the overall "Patient Experience".

20. **Focus on Energy Conservation and Creating a Healing Architecture:** Energy conservation must be planned and implemented. The hospital must have a humanizing architecture that can positively contribute to the healing process.

21. **Visualize the Hospital of the Future:** In the future, more common hospital functions will move close to patients, and only a few specific specialized functions will be concentrated at other places. The concentration of specialized facilities and dispersal of other hospital functions will influence the building design, planning, and facilities to support the continually changing hospital functions.

22. **Access:** If the public cannot reach a health care facility because of its location or lack of infrastructure, then it might as well not exist. Easy access by foot, bicycle, scooter, motorcycle, public transportation (buses, jitneys, taxis, vans, trains, and ambulances), automobiles, and/or helicopter is vital.

23. **Alignment of Care and Expertise:** Health facilities should not be designed and built without thoroughly thinking through the patient population and its health problems. Considering the type of allied professionals needed and the type and scope of health and hospital facilities needed is simply not solving the "whole" problem. Care providers must develop comprehensive disease-fighting strategies rather than just constructing new buildings. This requires an understanding of the causes of illness and death in the region of the world and how to prevent, diagnose, treat, and rehabilitate people from the effects of these diseases.

24. **Demographics:** Trends in demographic facts and the life expectancy of population sectors have to be determined. Some regional populations are accelerating at a higher rate, while others have a significant aged population and fewer births.

25. **New Channels for Continuous Care:** The widely acknowledged focus on disease prevention and wellness continues to be tremendously important. Non-communicable ailments such as heart disease, stroke, and chronic respiratory diseases are becoming more prevalent, and chronic diseases continue to account for many health care costs. In response to this, forward-thinking health care providers are expanding their services beyond the physical walls of hospitals and clinics. With strong informational and educational components, these services include virtual consultations, remote monitoring of vital signs, access to online medical records, and targeted community health screening events.

26. **Patient Safety:** One of the greatest issues in health care design and operation is patient safety, and a great amount of evidence demonstrates that planning and design decisions have a direct impact on this. Evidence-based design strategies to reduce safety concerns such as patient falls may include providing handrails, designing flush flooring transitions, and requiring direct, unobstructed pathways to frequently used areas such as bathrooms.

27. **Sustainability:** A hospital building is one of the highest energy consumers, and sustainable design is essential in reducing the consumption of natural resources and a facility's life-cycle costs. The principles of lean design, lean operations, and standardized design must be applied to minimize waste of all types.

28. **Innovations in Facility Planning and Management:** Hand in hand with design, construction, and operation, there must be qualified innovations in facility management and planning such as building information modeling and integrated project delivery.

29. **Medical Tourism:** Soaring costs in some countries are creating a new industry in other countries, specifically, medical tourism. Medical tourism means traveling to another country for medical procedures that can cost much less than in one's own country. There are parts of the world where medical care has become so expensive that people fly from one part of the world to another to receive medical care at a greatly reduced expense.

30. **Efficiency and Cost-Effectiveness:** An efficient hospital layout should promote staff efficiency by minimizing the distance of necessary travel between frequently used spaces that allows visual supervision of patients and provides an efficient logistics system for supplies and food

(and removal of waste) by making efficient use of multi-purpose spaces and consolidating spaces when possible.

31. **Security and Safety:** Hospitals have several particular security concerns, such as the protection of patients, staff, and hospital property and assets (including drugs) and vulnerability to terrorism because of high visibility. With these things in mind, security and safety must be built into the design.

32. **Distances:** Distances must be minimized for all movements of patients and medical, nursing, and other staff for supplies, aiming at a minimum of time and motion. Similarly, the routes that the patients will have to take on stretchers, wheelchairs or foot from their wards to the radiography department, laboratory, and physiotherapy require careful thought to minimize the length of these routes.

33. **Compactness:** Functional efficiency and economy also depend on the compactness of the hospital. Horizontal development demands more land involving extra costs in the development and installation of services, roads, water supply, sewage, electric lines, and so on. From this angle, multi-story construction has the advantage of being convenient because of compactness.

34. **Landscaping:** The psychological effect of the visual impact of attractive grounds, buildings, and surroundings on patients, visitors, and staff cannot be underestimated. If possible, the building is best located on relatively high ground, although the elevation should not be so great to be a handicap for those approaching on foot. The site should permit the orientation of the structure in such a way that most of the patient rooms will derive maximum benefit from natural light, and maximum advantage should be taken of the prevailing wind for natural ventilation.

35. **Linearity:** Linearity exhibits high stability with reasonable adaptability. The image of a hospital designed linearly will be low and not monumental. The problem of giving form to a hospital offers an opportunity for the architect to create a unique institution. The central problem for the architect is to understand the relationship between the hospital and its environment and how to mold this into the correct form.

36. **Efficient Material Transport Systems:** Hospitals have many materials—from food and medical supplies to computers and waste—that they must transport throughout the building. An efficient and accessible network of elevators and chutes should be created to streamline the transfer of materials. These networks should be separated from patient and visitor areas.

3.3 Summary

Good hospital design integrates functional requirements with the human needs of its varied users. This need for diverse functions is reflected in the breadth and specificity of regulations, codes, and oversight that govern hospital construction and operations. Each one of a hospital's wide-ranging and constantly evolving functions, including highly complicated mechanical, electrical, and telecommunications systems, requires specialized knowledge and expertise. Hospital design is also influenced by site constraints, opportunities, the climate, surrounding facilities, the budget, and available technology.

4 PREPARING A DETAILED PROJECT REPORT

4.1 Background

Detailed Project Reports (DPRs) are bankable sets of documents that show the results and outputs of working and projections while planning and designing a project. A DPR comprises detailed and elaborated projections and plans for the project that indicate the overall calculations, program, financials, roles and responsibilities, time planning for the project, details of required activities, and resources required for completion of the project.

During the planning stage, a blueprint is prepared on paper that gives a detailed study and analysis of what has to be performed to convert the investment into a feasible and profitable venture. In this set of documents, top management's policies and guidelines, their impact on the project span, and their appraisal of financial viability are estimated and addressed in-depth. The DPR mainly covers issues such as contract drawings, detailed technical feasibility studies, financial feasibility calculations, execution of the project from the practical point of view, the time period for completion of the project, and staff planning. The DPR also emphasizes the type and nature of inherited risks in the project and other foreseeable external risks that can influence the outcome of the hospital project.

The DPR should address and provide measures for risk management and risk mitigation. The DPR is a document that guides management about the progress of the project on a real-time basis. It also provides the tools to compare the actual vs. projected figures in terms of the costs, time period, milestone achievements, etc. Table 4A shows the questions that are answered by a DPR.

4.2 Template for Preparation of a DPR

Table 4B shows a sample of a template for the preparation of a DPR.

TABLE 4A: Questions Answered by a DPR

1. Estimated period of project completion
2. Actual cost of the project within reasonable limits of cost escalation
3. Quality and quantity of project deliverables

TABLE 4B: Template for Preparation of a DPR

Salient Features	• Title of the project.
	• Details of the project location.
	• Implementing agency.
	• DPR prepared by (Name of the person/agency).
	• Project outlay.
	• Budget provision.
	• Budget speech reference.
	• Administrative sanction.
	• Nature of project (new building/renovation).
	• Details of proposed building:
	• Number of blocks proposed.
	• Number of stories of building.
	• Total area of each block.
	• Other details of the building.
	• Details of investigation/surveys conducted.
	• Total estimated cost with item-wise cost breakup and details of the schedule of rates.
	• Whether a detailed estimate is attached.
	• Whether technical specifications of the medical equipment are attached.
	• Details of revenue stream.
	• Details of cost-benefit analysis (CBR value).
	• Details of project risks.
	• Details of project management organization strategy.
	• Details of contract management strategy.
	• Details of project implementation schedule (PIS) and work breakdown schedule (WBS):
	• Proposed time to complete the project.
	• Details of statutory clearances.
	• Quality control infrastructure and mechanism.
	• Operations and maintenance (O&M) arrangements of the project after completion.
	• Details of attached drawings.
	• Other attachments.
Executive Summary	This section should contain a brief of all relevant details discussed in the following chapters.

(Continued)

DOI: 10.1201/9780367460884-4

TABLE 4B: (Continued)

Introduction	• This section should provide a general introduction of the project being submitted. • The general introduction should include a written description of the type of the project, location of the project area, general description of topography, physiography, and geology of the project area, historical background of the project, need for the project, specification of the machines/equipment to be purchased, etc. • Aims and objectives of the project should also be briefed in this section.
Project Definition, Concept & Scope	The proposed project has to be clearly demarcated in terms of all of its subcomponents/elements including details of equipment to be purchased with Annual Maintenance Contract (AMC), the design, detailed engineering, and drawings of each physical infrastructure subcomponents, and environmental compliance/protection measures/improvement measures.
Project Background	A brief description of the existing facilities for serving the purpose, if any, in the project area, its present condition, and the need for the present project.
Project Details	Description of the equipment to be purchased, civil works to be performed to install the equipment, details of work relating to the modernization and upgradation of hospitals, rationale behind the project, etc. should be included.
Objective & Scope of the Work	A brief note about the necessity of the works proposed under the project and the main works to be carried out to fulfil the objective.
Status Feasibility Studies	Description of any feasibility study conducted earlier and its outcome should be discussed in this section.
Requirements/Demand Analysis	• This section should present the specific problem(s) or issue(s) faced by stakeholders, such as citizens, businesses, or governments, that would be addressed by the provision of improved services through the proposed project. • In this section, describe the proposed project in terms of the rationale behind the project by clearly focusing on the existing condition (how it will help in improving the situation and bring benefits to the stakeholders). • The rationale should be broad-based and supplemented with facts and figures. Information based on objective research, not subjective impressions, should be provided to justify the need or problem. The rationale should be written in a way that would lead to objectives.
Functional Design	• This section should present an analysis of different options available to achieve the objective, and the reasons for selecting the proposed option should be substantiated. • Both the form and structure of the existing hospital or institute and the proposed expansion should be detailed. • The functional design of the project is mainly achieved through field study and documentation using existing information and specifications from various standards. • In case of buildings, the area quantification of the requirements should be mentioned in the report. The methodology adopted in arriving at the total area of each building should also be clearly specified. • The location should generally be governed by several factors such as easy accessibility and minimum requirements of land acquisition/demolitions, if any. • History of the functioning of existing/nearby building/equipment in the project location, if any, under adverse conditions, damage to structure, maintenance problems, etc. should be considered. • The structure should be planned not only to obtain the most economical design but also to satisfy specific requirements, if any. • The design of the building/installation space for medical equipment should result in minimum construction costs and simultaneously achieve and maintain an acceptable standard of quality of care. • The building proposed should satisfy all the rules and regulations in the codes and manuals published by concerned authorities such as the Bureau of Indian Standards (BIS), National Medical Commission, Ministry of Health & Family Welfare (Indian Public Health Standards), etc.
Engineering Design	• This section should elaborate the technology choices, structural aspects, foundation options, evaluation of the technology option, and the basis for the technology for the proposed project. • A detailed description of the site including topographical and geotechnical investigations adequate to choose the suitable foundation should be furnished. • The structural layout should be planned so that the viability of adopting state-of-the-art large span arrangements, for example, flat slab, grid floor slab, ribbed slab, pre-stressed panels, etc., is explored with a view to bring in maximum utility, aesthetics, economy, etc. • The preliminary design for a typical building project should consist of architectural drawings of the proposed buildings, including floor plans, elevations, sections, site plans, etc., that conform to the guidelines established in relevant building bylaws and manuals. • A detailed technical specification of goods, hospital equipment, furniture, etc. should be furnished in the report. Equipment planning should be conducted as required for a standard health facility. • Environmental pollution control, biomedical waste treatment and disposal, etc. should be included in the design. • New innovations such as green building concepts may be incorporated in the design of the buildings.

(Continued)

TABLE 4B: (Continued)

Financial Estimates & Cost Projections	• This section should focus on the cost estimates, budget for the project, means of financing, and phasing of expenditure. • Cost estimates have to be worked out on the basis of a detailed bill of quantities (with detailed measurements of the length, breadth, and depth/height for each item), using the current Schedule of Rates (SOR) of the State Government (PRICE) or relevant SOR as applicable. • Applicable taxes, contingencies, investigation charges, including any O&M cost for a specific period, should be clearly specified. • AMC of medical equipment should be duly projected and budgeted. • Lump sum provisions for land acquisition, medical equipment, etc. should be explained in detail.
Revenue Streams	Options for cost recovery, if any, should be explored. Innovative ideas for additional revenue generation may be indicated.
Cost-Benefit Analysis & Investment Criteria	• Cost-benefit analysis (CBA) is a technique whereby the costs of and benefits from a scheme are quantified over a selected time horizon and evaluated by a common yardstick. • A financial and economic CBA of the project should be undertaken when such returns are quantifiable and are possible for infrastructure buildings such as hospitals. • The cost-benefit ratio (CBR—benefit-to-cost ratio), Economic Internal Rate of Return (EIRR), etc. should be worked out in detail with all supporting primary and secondary data. • The project cash flow projections for the life cycle along with underlying assumptions must be presented.
Environmental & Sustainability Aspects	• An Environmental Management Plan (EMP) is developed that explains the possible environmental issues that may arise during the construction and operation of the infrastructure and associated facilities depending upon the size of the project. • Environmental impact assessment study, if mandatory, and measures identified to mitigate the adverse impact, if any, should be conducted and documented in detail. • Issues relating to land acquisition, rehabilitation, and resettlement should be addressed in this section. • Inclusion of international best practices in sustainable infrastructure management including green building concepts, potential low-carbon, low-energy, zero-pollution features, etc. are desirable.
Risk Assessment & Mitigation Measures	• For projects that involve a large capital outlay and various issues relating to land acquisition, environmental aspects and a detailed and systematic risk analysis may be needed. • Identification and assessment of implementation risks that can lead to time overrun, cost escalation, scope reduction, etc. constitute the primary stage of risk assessment. • Risk analysis should include legal/contractual risks, environmental risks, revenue risks, project management risks, regulatory risks, etc. • Mitigation plans including risk avoidance, risk transfer, and risk elimination are to be well-analyzed and documented. • For complex projects with multiple risk profiles, numerical modelling and simulation may be adopted.
Project Management Organization	• Responsibilities of different agencies for project management should be elaborated. The organization structure at various levels, human resource requirements, and monitoring arrangements should be clearly identified. • Management arrangements refer to the institutional structures and mechanisms that should be established to ensure effective project management. • The involvement of an external consultant, if any, should be documented.
Contract Management Strategy	• The contracting methodology for the execution of the project should be specified in detail (e.g., the item rate, lump sum, EPC, etc.). • The system followed in the bidding document, reference manuals, etc. should be explained (PWD/CPWD/FIDIC, etc.). • Any contract clause that may likely lead to additional financial liability should be identified and reported with suggestions to overcome such an issue.
Implementation Schedule & WBS	• The time-bound work schedule is an important part of every project because it helps in the better handling of projects in planning, implementation, etc. • This section should indicate the proposed zero date of commencement and provide a bar chart/project schedule when relevant. • The phasing of project activities, proposed contract packages, and schedule of implementation should be described for each phase. • Critical dependencies in the project, expected timelines for completion of key milestones, and associated process indicators for the same should be identified. • The DPR should provide a time-bound action plan that includes tendering, appointment of contractors, construction schedule, quality assurance, quality control and, post-construction activities, including project delivery.
Statutory Clearances	• This section should elaborate the statutory clearances to be obtained from the various authorities. • Statutory approvals as per bylaws, the master plan, fire safety norms, environmental clearance, etc. as applicable to the project are to be documented.

(Continued)

TABLE 4B: (Continued)

Quality Management Plan	• The DPR should include information relating to the institution to be engaged in the quality assurance and quality control of the project execution. • The methodology to be adopted to ensure the quality of construction should be clearly mentioned in the report. • A quality management plan including the internal inspection and testing procedure should be documented. • If a third-party quality control mechanism is adopted, then its structure and the plan should be specified in detail.
Operations & Maintenance Plan	• The DPR should incorporate/include information relating to the institution to be engaged in the O&M of the created infrastructure asset/enhanced infrastructure assets. • A brief description/analysis of the key issues and obstacles regarding O&M (including billing/collection issues) and proposed countermeasures to overcome them for the project should be explained. • Requirements of funds for operation and maintenance of assets should also be included in the report.
Annexures	• Detailed architectural drawings of the buildings (including floor plans, sections, elevations, site plans, etc.). • Detailed estimate. • Geo-technical investigation report. • Copies of statutory approvals.

4.3 Summary

A DPR includes the project definition, concept, scope, background, and objective, as well as the scope of the work, status feasibility studies for requirements/demand analysis, functional and engineering design, financials, cost projections, projecting revenue streams, CBA and investment criteria, and environmental and sustainability aspects. It also includes a risk assessment and mitigation measures, project and contract management strategy, implementation schedule, and work breakdown structure. The DPR is the go-to document for the all of the details pertaining to a hospital project. A diligently made DPR will become the primary basis of the contract agreement and will ensure that the project is completed as per the requirements of the entire scope of the hospital.

5 SITE SELECTION AND SITE PLANNING

5.1 Background

Site selection is one of the most important steps that health care organizations take when embarking on the development of a new facility. More than just choosing a plot of ground, many factors that are considered in the selection of a facility site—from the size and cost of a parcel of land to its visibility, its proximity to other health care facilities, and how quickly it can be developed.

5.2 Site Selection Process

The site selection, or facility location, decision is triggered when organizations seek to locate, relocate, or expand their operations. The process involves the identification of alternative potentially viable locations and an analysis thereof, followed by an evaluation and ranking of the sites. Part of the business activities of the project team is to search for and select the optimal location.

A four-phase approach is usually followed for site selection, including screening, site work, negotiations, and finalization, as shown in Figure 5A. The screening phase includes a fatal flaw analysis to reduce the list of candidate sites to only those that are viable. Site work and negotiations are necessary to obtain the information that will be used in the selection and acquisition stage.

5.3 Site Selection Criteria and Considerations

The criteria and considerations for site selection are given in Table 5A.

5.4 Decision Matrix for Site Selection

To be able to make an unbiased site selection, a decision matrix is used where site criteria are weighted and scored for each of the candidate sites.

A decision matrix for site selection is shown in Table 5B. Any consistent scoring and weighting system can be used. To keep it simple, it is suggested to use ranking scores of 1 to 5 and weights of 1 to 5. Once the scoring is completed, the scores are multiplied by the weights, and the answers are recorded in the column S × W (Score × Weight). The S × W results are totaled for each of the sites, and the preferred site should be the one with the highest total score.

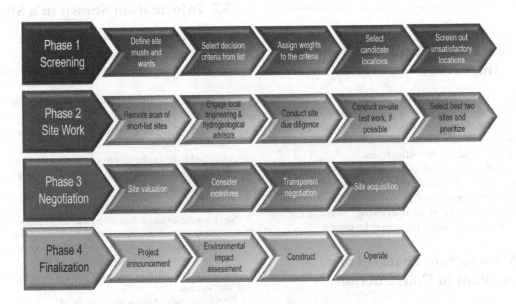

FIGURE 5A Site Selection Process (Adapted from Greyhill Advisors, undated).

TABLE 5A: Criteria and Considerations for Site Selection

Setting Priorities	• Set a clear vision. • Anticipate current or target patient base and volume. • Identify specific requirements for the facility site.
General Considerations	• Ensure area is large enough to enable future expansion and growth. • Collaborate closely with local town planning authorities and National Building Code. • Hospital should be situated in the heart of society. • In crowed localities, there will seldom be a building site of the usually accepted acreage (2.5 to 5 acres per 100 beds) available in a central place.

(Continued)

DOI: 10.1201/9780367460884-5

TABLE 5A: (Continued)

Land Requirements Floor Area Ratio	• In urban areas, the only available avenue is vertical growth. • Floor Area Ratio (FAR) is the ratio of the total covered area on all floors of a building to the total area of the site, that is, if a hospital building standing on a plot of land measuring 12,000 sq m has four floors and each floor has a 1,500 sq m floor area (total floor area on all floors is 6,000 sq m), then the FAR at this site will be two. • A FAR of one represents a building whose total floor area of all floors equals the area of the plot of land. This means that if a hospital is a two-story structure, then half of the area is covered with a building, and the remaining half is available as open space for parking, approach, internal roads, lawns, gardens, etc. • A plot ratio of 2:1 is the highest that should be considered for hospital development, and this ratio is acceptable only in the centres of cities, where a high density of buildings is the rule. When a limited site is an inevitable choice for a new hospital, the hospital size must be limited. • Generally, hospitals that have a plot ratio of 2:1 will have a crowded site, high buildings close to one another, very little open space, and a certain amount of overshadowing and over-looking between the buildings.
Soil Structure	A preliminary soil survey to determine the subsoil water level and "bearing" quality of the soil will help determine the type of foundation, the possibility of constructing a basement, and the effectiveness of the sewage plant (if it is to be built on the site).
Public Utilities	The availability of water supply, sewage disposal system transportation, and electric power should be identified.

TABLE 5B: Decision Matrix for Site Selection

		Site 1		Site 2		Site 3	
Site Criteria	Weight	Score	S × W	Score	S × W	Score	S × W
		Total		Total		Total	

5.5 Site Plan: Introduction and Important Features

A site plan is a large-scale drawing that shows the full extent of the site for an existing or proposed development. Site plans, along with location plans, may be necessary for planning applications. In most cases, site plans will be drawn following a series of desk studies and site investigations.

Typically, depending on the size of the project, site plans are likely to be at a scale of 1:500 or 1:200. However, for very small projects, larger scales may be used, and for large projects, smaller scales, or even several drawings perhaps pulled together on one very small-scale plan, may be used.

5.6 Important Features of a Site Plan in Construction

• A site plan is prepared by personnel who are either licensed engineers, design consultants, land surveyors, or architects.
• A site plan shows a visual representation of the arrangement of the buildings, parking, driveways, and landscaping details. All of the important details that surround and are related to the development project are shown on a site plan.
• A site plan is a combination of construction drawings that are the basis on which the builder or the contractor makes improvements to the property.

• A site plan is the standard document that is checked by the legal authorities for the legal building structure rules and regulations of the region and is hence developed based on the standard rules and regulations provided by the national building code.

5.7 Information Shown in a Site Plan

The information shown in a site plan will vary depending on the size and nature of the project; however, certain information is likely to appear on most site plans (Table 5C).

TABLE 5C: Information Shown in a Site Plan

1 Title block, giving the project name, drawing type, author, revision number, status, the scale used, etc.
2 Notes highlighting changes from previous revisions.
3 Directional orientation. This can be a compass or a north-pointing arrow.
4 Key dimensions. Key materials.
5 Site boundaries and delineation of adjacent properties, including where necessary, adjoining, or adjacent structures, and surrounding streets, trees, tree protection orders, and the main elements of the landscape.
6 Parking areas with dimensions or capacities, traffic flows, and signage.
   Roads, footpaths, ramps, paved areas, etc.
   Easements such as rights-of-way, right of support, etc.

Site plans might also include the following information:

7 Buildings to be demolished or removed.
8 The general extent of earthworks, included, cutting and filling, the provision of retaining walls, etc.
9 The general layout of external services, including drainage, water, gas, electricity, telephone, manhole covers, etc.
10 The layout of external lighting. Fencing, walls, and gates.
11 The location of miscellaneous external components such as bollards, fire hydrants, signage, litter bins, etc.

Where the site is complex, some of this information might be shown on additional specialist site plans, such as structural site plans, site history, site lines, services site plans, landscape drawings, access and traffic flows, ground conditions and geology, etc. Site plans may be accompanied by site sections showing the topography of the site.

5.8 Site Plans versus Floor Plans

The difference between a site plan and a floor plan is that a site plan demonstrates all the structures on a property area or piece of land whilst a floor plan illustrates the interior layout of a building. Both site plans and floor plans are useful in presenting a property, with site plans having the added benefit of including the surrounding grounds and plot.

A site plan drawing begins with clear property lines and precise measurements between key buildings and landscaping. It includes everything that will exist within the property lines. The focus is on the exterior of the building or home. A floor plan is a scaled drawing of the interior of a home that depicts details such as room sizes, doors, windows, fixtures, and relationships between spaces. The focus is on the inside of the building.

5.9 Types of Site Plans

- **2D Site Plan:** A 2D site plan is a sketch that shows the layout of the building/land/facility from above. It includes the location of buildings and structures, driveways, landscaping, walkways, and more. These are especially useful for new development projects, as sales representatives can show clients how their property fits into the neighborhood. This design provides a clear, flat diagram of the layout of the property, and it may be colour-coded to distinguish various areas. It is a simple design and the first step in drawing a site plan.
- **3D Site Plan:** A 3D site plan makes it easier to show clients the texture and contrast of various materials. It is the pop-up book version of the 2D plan. Images are rendered in a more immersive way that allow the viewer to imagine walking through the site once completed. Designers can show clients how their home and landscaping will look at different times of the day, with details that cannot be viewed in 2D. For clients who are unfamiliar with reading site plans, the 3D site plan is easier to understand. It creates a lasting impact and a wow factor for clients, making them more eager to invest in the construction.

5.10 Purpose of a Site Plan

The main purposes of a site plan include:

- To represent how the land is utilized and the details of the surrounding area.
- To submit the document of reference to the zoning or government administrator to check and approve for construction of the project. The administrator checks whether the proposed building or structure meets the standards of the respective zone or region.
- The administrator checks whether the proposed structure meets the requirements of and serves the public through facilities such as roads, water, emergency services, sewage disposal, schools, etc.
- To protect the landowners by complying with government procedures. If not, then the project can attract lawsuits and complaints.

5.11 Summary

Site selection is one of the many important steps in the construction of a health care facility. Site selection is a scientific process based on numerous factors to determine the long-term suitability of the land for the purposes of longevity and future scope of expansion. Well-made site plans can pre-emptively identify and mitigate many structural and procedural risks in hospital building management.

6 FUNCTIONAL AND SPACE PROGRAMMING

6.1 Background

A functional program is a multi-purpose document that describes, in detail, the proposed services to be addressed in a capital project, specifying human, technical, and building resources necessary for it to function as intended. Overall, the functional program documents the scope of services, objectives, and basic operational description of each component to be addressed in a capital project, workload, and staffing of the components, together with an estimate and description of the facility resources (space) required to support them. It provides a comprehensive understanding of the activities and the functional needs of each component, the relationships between the components that must be accommodated within the capital project, and the relation of the capital project components to the broader systems external to it.

The functional program is a coherent, meaningful compilation of the information needed to develop facilities. It is required to effectively support the health care facility's (HCF) operations and organizational goals by directing (without limiting or dictating) design. It should permit design latitude and provide necessary criteria against which the design consultant can assess the validity and vitality of the design solution. It is

- the critical link between strategic/operational development and building facility design;
- the use of experience and coordination for future planning to facilitate good control over the proposed project design and development; and
- a vital stage in Health Care Facility (HCF) planning, which results in information to inform design (Table 6A).

TABLE 6A: Characteristics of a Functional Program

1. Concise and detailed
2. Sound methodology for analysis and projection of activity (e.g., functions determine workload, which ultimately determines space)
3. A detailed listing of the functions to be undertaken in the completed facility and of the physical requirements for the performance of these functions
4. Comprehensive to allow the development of operational management plans (e.g., staff and facility), budgets for each component, and a determination of overall operational cost impact
5. Incorporates fixed and loose equipment elements to list the items of furnishings/equipment that were considered during the programming of each component and that will be required to make each space operational

Steps to Create a Functional Program: There are five broad steps to create a functional program, which are given as follows (Table 6B).

TABLE 6B: Steps to Create a Functional Program

Step 1 **Create Project and Determine Required Information**
- Create a project to address shortcoming(s) or to attain the desired goal(s); assign project identifiers.
- Identify the scope and general description of project understanding to define an order of magnitude.
- Determine the need for a functional program.
- Assemble a multi-disciplinary team.
- Identify functional and clinical information and input required for the project and input required to inform the project that has been identified.

Step 2 **Define Purpose, Project Initiatives, and Intentions**
- Define the purpose of the project, and discuss the environment of care components.
- Discuss the layout and operations.
- Establish a care delivery model, and identify infrastructure and system requirements.
- Articulate project requirements, project vision, and goals and how these will influence patients, staff, providers, and occupants.
- A functional program will clearly define the intended purpose of the project, how it will influence facility users, and the balance of the organization and local region/community.

Step 3 **Perform Needs Assessment and Establish Project Documents and Context**
- Provide a project overview.
- Determine demand and utilization data necessary to justify and support the proposed project.
- Identify the project type, scope, and scale.
- Identify the applicability of FGI and other standards that govern functional, operational, and space requirements.

Step 4 **Define Operational and Functional Requirements**
- Identify operational requirements and functional support.
- Determine how materials management supports the care model.
- Perform a systems evaluation.
- Explore planning efficiencies and workflow improvements.
- Consider quality improvement metrics, such as LEAN.
- Coordinate logistics.
- Conduct a life-cycle cost analysis.
- How will the project function, and what performance improvement benefits are desired?

Step 5 **Collect Data and Produce Functional Program**
- Synthesize information from steps 1–4.
- Integrate the needs assessment (step 2) with project requirements (step 3) to create the most reasonable project.
- The published functional program and executive summary should clearly identify the who, what, and why of a project and how it will be created.

DOI: 10.1201/9780367460884-6

6.2 Elements of a Functional Program

Functional program documentation will be developed for each identified component within a project. The following may be brief or quite detailed depending on the complexity of the project—generally, the elements to be included in the functional program are shown in Table 6C.

6.3 Health Care Space Programming: Calculation Methodology

The approved projections of censuses, outpatient visits, and workloads are the basic starting point for developing master/function programming. Following this, detailed space programming takes place to develop appropriate net and gross space programs for the HCF. All of these planning processes precede the beginning of the design stage.

6.4 Calculation Methodology for Space Programming

- From a space programming point of view, spaces in a health care project can be classified into two major groups:
  - Workload-driven spaces
  - Support spaces

- The workload-driven space is the activity space in the department that can be translated and calculated from the projected workloads. To be able to perform the transformation, the applicable workload units (patient days, visits, procedures, etc.) and the space function planning unit (such as patient beds in nursing units and operating theatres in surgical departments) should be identified and utilized to calculate the required workload-driven spaces.
- By summing all workload-driven spaces and support spaces, the department net area can be calculated.
- The department grossing factor represents an allowance for the spaces additional to the primary department net spaces, such as vertical and horizontal circulation areas (corridors, stairways, and elevators), wall and partition thicknesses, and public restroom facilities.
- The building gross area can be calculated by following the same methodology by totaling up all departments' gross area and applying the building conversion/grossing factor. This factor introduces an allowance for the building's main circulation/corridors, wall and partition thickness between departments, public restroom facilities, stairways, and elevators.
- An overview of the space programming process is shown in Figure 6A.

TABLE 6C: Elements of a Functional Program

Assumptions	Premise(s) for the future, upon which the project is based (e.g., occupancy at 90%, population growth, and change in treatment protocols), key costs, schedule, and implementation assumptions.
Planning Parameters	• Strategic intent, project vision; guiding principles for the project (e.g., integrated and coordinated service). • Strategy of how change will be implemented and the operational principles/business process; how the facility will operate and how the individual services interface or integrate with existing services/facilities.
Activities/Functions for Each Component within the Project	• Operational/service planning model organization and management. • Service delivery principles and methods. • Hours of operation; client/patient flow; scope of service (current and future); client/patient profile; clinical roles and activities; education roles and activities; and research roles and activities.
Workload/Volumes	• Detailed description of current components and projected workload (clinical and para-clinical). • Current and projected FTEs, staff workload patterns, and projections at maximum occupancy—based on equivalent full-time positions including relief needs.
Functional Relationships	• External to the component—e.g., diagram/descriptions describing critical relationships to other programs/services/components within the facility (e.g., patient transport from emergency department to component, material management flow to and from the component, etc.). • External to the facility—relationships with other facilities to provide the program context within the greater health care system (e.g., patient transport for a specialized diagnostic procedure and sending/receiving lab specimens). • Internal: Relationships of sub-units within the component space (e.g., location of nurse station to patient rooms, waiting area to reception) to facilitate flow, functionality, etc. within the component.
Design Criteria/Physical Requirements	Space requirements and description of each space type, activities, what is contained within (furniture, fixtures, and equipment), special features, number of people, etc.
Schedule of Accommodation	Room-by-room space list or schedule of accommodation of space types that identify the number or units required and the area in net sq m, with reference to the number of occupants and major equipment; and component gross-up factors.

(Continued)

TABLE 6C: (Continued)

Assumptions	Premise(s) for the future, upon which the project is based (e.g., occupancy at 90%, population growth, and change in treatment protocols), key costs, schedule, and implementation assumptions.
Equipment	Preliminary list of equipment to determine space sizes, which assists in preliminary costing, completed in detailed design (depending on the project, it could be a detailed list); and overview of the fixed or large loose equipment (e.g., diagnostic imaging, sterile processing, and medical gas/electrical service columns in patient cubicles).
Impact Analysis	Impacted services assess the additional workload added by the service and what resources staff, space, equipment, etc. are required to support the component.
Appendices Can Include	• Applicable guidelines and standards. • Planning teams and committees.

TABLE 6D: Health Care Function Zones

James and Tatton-Brown (1986) Group	Zilm and Spreckelmeyer (1995)	Dickerman (1992)
• The nursing zone for patient services • The clinical zone for diagnosis and treatment • The support zone for other spaces serving the previous two zones	• Patient care area • Diagnostic treatment areas • Support areas	• Inpatient nursing services • Ancillary medical services • Administrative services • Support services • Other services areas

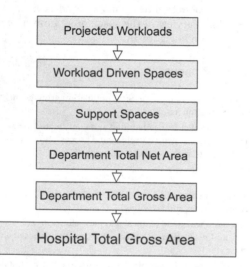

Health Care Function Zones: Hospital spaces and departments can be zoned and classified using different approaches (Table 6D).

6.5 Summary

A detailed project report documents the various structural layouts and requirements of a hospital project. As a subsequent activity, functional and space programming provides a comprehensive understanding of the activities and the functional needs of each component, the relationships between the components that must be accommodated within the capital project, and the relation of the capital project components to the broader systems external to it. This is conducted to ensure seamless structural and process integration so that the form follows function.

FIGURE 6A An Overview of the Space Programming Methodology for Health Care Projects (Al Zarooni S, Abdou A, Lewis J. Improving the client briefing for UAE public health care projects: space programming guidelines. Architectural Engineering and Design Management. 2011 Nov 1;7(4):251–65).

7 ANTHROPOMETRY IN HOSPITAL ARCHITECTURE

7.1 Background

Anthropometry is the comparative study of the measurements and capabilities of the human body. It derives from the Greek words "Anthropos" (meaning human) and "metron" (meaning measure). Anthropometry influences a wide range of industries, processes, services, and products and has a considerable importance in optimizing the design of buildings.

Human dimensions and capabilities are paramount in determining a building's dimensions and overall design. The underlying principle of anthropometrics is that building designs should adapt to suit the human body rather than people having to adapt to suit buildings.

There are two basic areas of anthropometry:

• **Static Anthropometry:** It is the measurement of body sizes at rest and when using devices such as chairs, tables, beds, mobility devices, etc.
• **Functional Anthropometry:** It is the measurement of abilities related to the completion of tasks, such as reaching, manoeuvring, and motion, and other aspects of space and equipment use.

The use of anthropometrics in building design aims to ensure that every person is as comfortable as possible. In practical terms, this means that the dimensions must be appropriate, ceilings must be sufficiently high, doorways and hallways must be wide enough, etc. In recent times, it has come to have particular significance for workplace design and the relationship among desk, chair, keyboard, and computer display.

Building regulations provide a range of standard requirements and approved solutions for designers to help develop suitable designs. However, it is important to consider the specific purpose and requirements of end users. Attempts to apply standardized dimensions may not reflect the true need of the space requirements.

Older people, children, people with mobility issues, wheelchair users, and so on may have specific requirements. In particular, good accessibility and easy maneuverability around the building must be considered when designing stairs, lifts, ramps, and other features.

Anthropometry may also impact the space requirements for furniture and fittings. For example, a bathroom must have enough space to comfortably fit a bath and sink; a bedroom must have enough space to comfortably fit an average-sized bed; and an office building must have enough space to fit desks, air conditioning units, communal areas, meeting rooms, etc. Anthropometric data are regularly updated to reflect changes in the population.

7.2 Anthropometric Measurements

Anthropometric data vary considerably between regional populations. Anthropometric dimensions for each population are ranked by size and described as percentiles. It is common practice to design for the 5th percentile (5th%) female to the 95th percentile (95th%) male. The 5th% female value for a particular dimension (e.g., sitting height) usually represents the smallest measurement for design in a population. Conversely,

a 95th% male value may represent the largest dimension for which one is designing. The 5th% to 95th% range accommodates approximately 90% of the population. To design for a larger portion of the population, one might use the range from the 1st% female to the 99th% male (Figure 7A).

7.3 Universal Design Considerations

Most people experience some degree of physical limitation at some point in life, such as broken bones, sprained wrists, pregnancy, or aging. Others may live with a limitation or impairment every day. When considering designing buildings/hospitals, designers can recognize the special needs of different users, including individuals with disabilities. Adequate space should be allocated for persons using mobility devices, for example, wheelchairs, crutches, walkers, white canes, etc. and those walking with the assistance of other persons.

(a) **Mobility Devices and Space Allowances:** Figure 7B shows the standard parts of a wheelchair.
   (i) **Dimensions of a Manual Wheelchair** (Table 7A and Figures 7C–7E).
   (ii) **Wheelchair User:** The minimum clear floor or ground area required to accommodate a single, stationary wheelchair and occupant is 900 mm (W) × 1,200 mm (L) (Figure 7F).

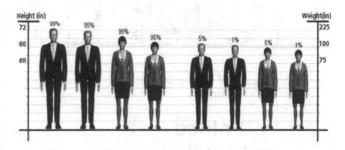

FIGURE 7A The Relative Sizes of Different Percentiles in Humans (Courtesy of Scott Openshaw, Allsteel et al. Ergonomics and Design: A Reference Guide).

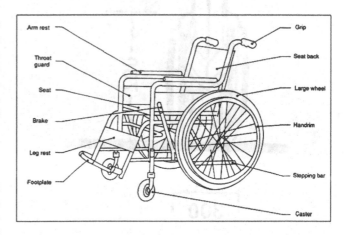

FIGURE 7B Parts of a Wheelchair (Harmonized Guidelines and Space Standards for Barrier-Free Build Environment for Persons with Disability and Elderly Persons; February 2016).

DOI: 10.1201/9780367460884-7

TABLE 7A: Dimensions of a Manual Wheelchair

When the Wheelchair Is Open

Length	1,000–1,200 mm
Width	650–720 mm
Height	910–950 mm
Wheelchair Footrest	350 mm deep
Wheelchair Castor Width	12 mm
Seat Height	480 mm
Arm Rest Height	760 mm
Lap Height	675 mm

When the Wheelchair Is Folded

Width	300 mm
Arm Rest Height	760 mm

A wheelchair has a footplate and leg rest attached to the front of the seat. (The footplate extends approximately 350 mm in front of the knee.) The footplate may prevent a wheelchair user from getting close enough to an object. Hence, at least 350 mm deep and 700 mm high space under a counter, stand, etc. should be given.

(iii) **Circulation Dimension:** The minimum clear floor ground area for a wheelchair to turn is 1,500 mm, but it may be ideal to provide 2,000 mm (Figure 7G).

(b) **Space Allowances for a Crutch User:** Although people who use walking aids can manoeuvre through door openings with a 900-mm clear width, they need wider passageways, such as 920 mm, for a comfortable gait (Figure 7H). Crutch tips often extend out and down at a wide angle and are a hazard in narrow passageways where they might not be seen by other pedestrians.
- Width: 920 mm
- With no obstruction, up to 300 mm in height

(c) **Space Allowance for Cane Users:**
- Protruding objects, such as directional signs, tree branches, wires, guy ropes, public telephone booths, benches and ornamental fixtures should be installed with consideration of the range of a person with vision impairment as indicated by a white cane.

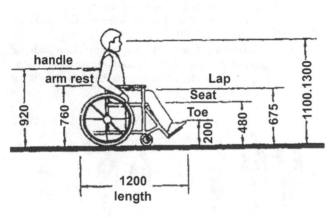

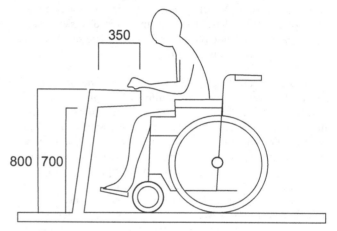

FIGURE 7E Knee Clearance (Harmonized Guidelines and Space Standards for Barrier-Free Build Environment for Persons with Disability and Elderly Persons; February 2016).

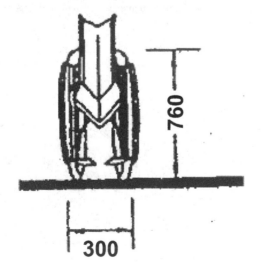

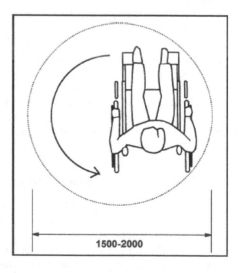

FIGURES 7C AND D Dimensions of a Manual Wheelchair in Usable and Folded Condition (Harmonized Guidelines and Space Standards for Barrier-Free Build Environment for Persons with Disability and Elderly Persons; February, 2016).

FIGURE 7F Turning Radius (Harmonized Guidelines and Space Standards for Barrier-Free Build Environment for Persons with Disability and Elderly Persons; February 2016).

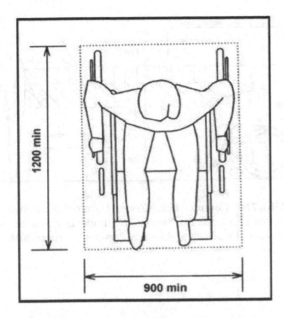

FIGURE 7G Clear Floor Space (Harmonized Guidelines and Space Standards for Barrier-Free Build Environment for Persons with Disability and Elderly Persons; February 2016).

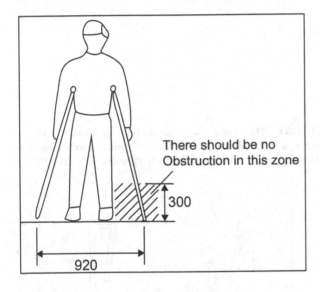

FIGURE 7H Space Required for Crutch User (Harmonized Guidelines and Space Standards for Barrier-Free Build Environment for Persons with Disability and Elderly Persons; February 2016).

- A barrier to warn blind or visually impaired persons should be provided under stairways or escalators.
- Walkways, halls, corridors, passageways, aisles, or other circulation spaces should have clear headroom to minimize the risk of accidents.
- The radial range of the white cane is a band that is 900 mm wide (Figure 7I).
- Any obstacle above 600 mm cannot be detected by a white cane. If there are projections above this height, then the projections have to be reflected at the floor level in terms of level or textural differences (Figure 7I).

(d) Reach Range: A wheelchair user's movement pivots around his or her shoulders (Figure 7J). The range of reach (forward and side, with or without obstruction) of a wheelchair user should be taken into consideration.

    (i)   **Reach without Obstruction (Table 7B and Figures 7K–7L)**

   (ii)   **Reach over Obstruction (Table 7C and Figure 7M)**

  (iii)   **Common Reach Zone**

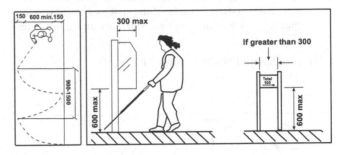

FIGURE 7I Radial Range and Object Detection by the Visually Impaired (Harmonized Guidelines and Space Standards for Barrier-Free Build Environment for Persons with Disability and Elderly Persons; February 2016).

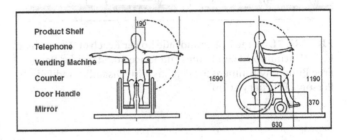

FIGURE 7J Range of Reach of Wheelchair User (Harmonized Guidelines and Space Standards for Barrier-Free Build Environment for Persons with Disability and Elderly Persons; February 2016).

TABLE 7B: Reach without Obstruction

Max. Forward Upper Reach	1,200 mm
Max. Forward Lower Reach	380 mm
Max. Side Upper-Level Reach	1,300 mm
Max. Side Lower-Level Reach	250 mm

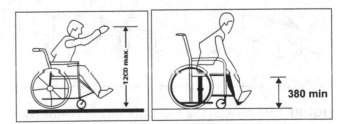

FIGURE 7K Forward and Lower Reach of Wheelchair User (Harmonized Guidelines and Space Standards for Barrier-Free Build Environment for Persons with Disability and Elderly Persons; February 2016).

- The comfortable reach zone when seated in a wheelchair is between 900 mm and 1,200 mm.
- The maximum reach zone is between 1,200 mm and 1,400 mm (Figure 7N).

(e) **Vision Zone:** Different fields of vision are given in Figure 7O. All signage should be designed based upon these dimensions (vision zone: 900–1,800 mm). The smallest letter should not be less than 15 mm. Map and information panels along pathways should be placed at a height between 900 mm and 1,800 mm (Figure 7P).

(f) **Heights and Widths (Table 7D)**

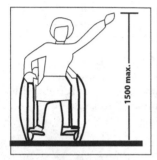
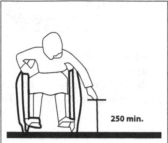

FIGURE 7L Side Upper and Side Lower Reach of Wheelchair User (Harmonized Guidelines and Space Standards for Barrier-Free Build Environment for Persons with Disability and Elderly Persons; February 2016).

TABLE 7C: Reach over Obstruction

Max. Forward Reach over Obstruction	1,000 mm from the floor
Max. Side Reach over Obstruction (Upper)	1,200 mm from the floor
Max. Side Reach over Obstruction (Lower)	500 mm

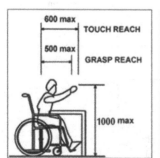
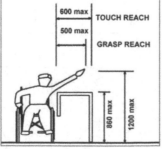

FIGURE 7M Forward and Side Reach over an Obstruction (Harmonized Guidelines and Space Standards for Barrier-Free Build Environment for Persons with Disability and Elderly Persons; February 2016).

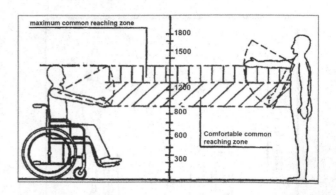

FIGURE 7N Common Reach Zones (Harmonized Guidelines and Space Standards for Barrier-Free Build Environment for Persons with Disability and Elderly Persons; February 2016).

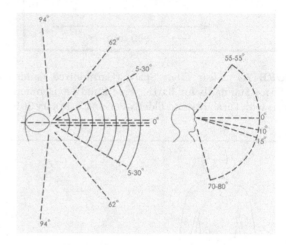

FIGURE 7O Field of Vision (Harmonized Guidelines and Space Standards for Barrier-Free Build Environment for Persons with Disability and Elderly Persons; February 2016).

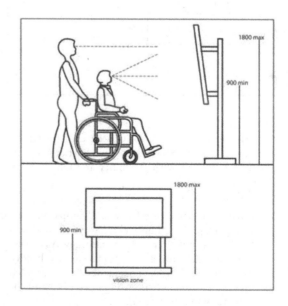

FIGURE 7P Vision Zone (Harmonized Guidelines and Space Standards for Barrier-Free Build Environment for Persons with Disability and Elderly Persons; February 2016).

TABLE 7D: Heights and Widths

Wheelchair Users	The average height of a person seated in a wheelchair is generally less than 1,200 mm.
Standing Person	The average height of a standing person is generally less than 2,000 mm.
Height of Controls	• Height of controls from floor level: 400–1,200 mm • Height for switches (power): 400–500 mm • Height for switches (light): 900–1,200 mm • Height of door handles: 900–1,000 mm • Opening controls for windows: 900–1,000 mm • Space required under the counter for wheelchair footrest: 350-mm deep
Entrance/Exit Doors	• Min. width of entrance/exit door: 900 mm • Min. front approach doorway space: 600 mm • Min. latch approach doorway space: 1,250 mm

7.4 Summary

The use of anthropometrics in building design aims to ensure that every person is as comfortable as possible. In practical terms, this means that the dimensions must be appropriate, ceilings sufficiently high, doorways and hallways wide enough, etc.

The National Building Code provides a range of standard requirements and approved solutions for designers to help develop suitable designs. Older people, children, people with mobility issues, wheelchair users, and so on may have specific requirements. In particular, good accessibility and easy maneuverability around the building must be considered when designing stairs, lifts, ramps, and other features.

Anthropometry may also impact space requirements for furniture and fittings. For example, a bathroom must have enough space to comfortably fit a bath and sink; a bedroom must have enough space to comfortably fit an average-sized bed; an office building must have enough space to fit desks, air conditioning units, communal areas, meeting rooms, and so on.

8 SCHEMATIC DESIGN

8.1 Introduction

Schematic design is the phase of the project during which the client's requirements and desires determined in the pre-design phase are resolved into physical, architectural form. The purpose of this phase is to transform the results of the pre-design investigation into a concept of "what will be built". At this stage, the architect and the client begin by agreeing on an architectural expression representing a synthesis of the following elements:

- The character of the site (including physical features, local surroundings, neighborhood and landscape features, and regulatory restrictions)
- The space planning requirements described in the client's functional program
- The image or philosophical objectives that the client wants to project
- The design approach of the architect

Throughout the schematic design phase, the architect tests the client's program by studying various planning and massing relationships, always within the constraints of the project budget. Ideally, the schematic design will conclude with a design that is the best possible synthesis of all the factors being considered.

There are several methods to document design decisions. Traditional sketch overlays may still assist in the depiction of program concepts. Current technical software allows architects to undertake preliminary modeling, develop rapid prototypes, and document the building as a three-dimensional model. For example, building information modeling (BIM) allows the architect to model the anticipated energy performance of a design, but it can also be time-consuming to generate all the information that the model requires to be accurate, so the design fees should be calculated with this additional effort in mind.

As the design character emerges, the need to change program details may become evident. Although the program typically drives the schematic design, there are instances where design drives the program. Throughout the schematic design phase, the assumptions made during pre-design should be tested to uncover any inconsistencies or conflicts and new opportunities for the more effective use of space. Assumptions made earlier need to be validated so that the design time and effort can be focused on solid, viable initiatives.

8.2 Client–Architect Relationship

During schematic design, the architect–client dialogue continues as proposals for specific responses to the project's requirements are put forward by the architect. It is important for the parties to remain in agreement over the fundamental issues outlined in the functional program. To facilitate effective client participation and to maintain trust among all project stakeholders, the architect must manage communication and ensure that all design issues and construction budgets are presented as open to discussion. These communications need to be fully recorded and documented. Minutes of design meetings should be taken by the architect and circulated for review and approval by all.

8.3 Pre-Design Information Required before Beginning a Schematic Design

The client is responsible for providing a functional program/architect brief that defines the following:

- Functional requirements and spatial relationships (adjacencies)
- Flexibility and provision for expansion
- Special equipment and systems
- Site requirements and/or restraints
- A feasible construction budget
- Sustainability goals
- Time frame or schedule

In addition to the functional program, the client is responsible for providing full documentation of site conditions, including:

- Legal and physical surveys
- Zoning bylaw considerations
- On subsurface conditions, including the presence of hazardous materials or other pollutants
- Any assessment/condition reports and hazardous material assessment if the project is a renovation to an existing building
- Any other professional reports or opinions from specialist consultants that will have an impact on the work

If the client does not have all of this typical pre-design documentation, then the architect may help procure it by acting as the client's advisor. As this approach requires additional work on the part of the architect and implicates additional professional liability for the architect, the overall compensation for the schematic design should reflect this additional effort.

As the schematic design process continues, the architect confirms technical and regulatory considerations by:

- Incorporating appropriate construction materials and methods (with research into durability and life cycle considerations);
- Consulting with the engineering members of the design team to consider the technical requirements of their disciplines;
- Compliance with applicable building codes;
- Dealing with occupational health and safety codes; and that local zoning and urban design requirements are met.

To complete the schematic design, architects must fully investigate the planning and technical requirements and the regulations of authorities that have jurisdiction (such as environmental impact, site plan control, zoning, parking requirements, and limiting distances). Generally, an overview rather than a detailed analysis of building code compliance is necessary at this stage.

DOI: 10.1201/9780367460884-8

8.4 Space, Circulation, and Massing Studies

As part of the preliminary analysis, the architect will often prepare a series of space plans to identify the comparative size, relationships, and optimal adjacencies of the functional areas and spaces anticipated. Relative proportions and volumes can be established, and with the data rationalized to this extent, the preliminary architectural planning and designing can be commenced with greater confidence.

In addition, the pedestrian and vehicular circulation layouts linking the relevant spaces and applicable site constraints can be examined, usually concurrently. Subconsultant input, especially related to mechanical and electrical space requirements, vehicular traffic, and vertical transportation systems may be added to the research agenda at this time. The engineering disciplines' input helps determine the area and volume needed for service rooms at this very preliminary stage.

On large and complex projects, the architect should ask the client periodically to approve the conceptual drawings as they are developed. These "sign-offs" enable the architect to monitor the schedule milestones and legitimately request additional fees if the client subsequently makes changes to previously approved work.

Having undertaken and established some basic planning relationships through these flow and space plans, the architect, with input from the integrated design team, then begins creating the overall form that the project will take.

Using sketches, block models, and other design approaches, the architect explores various forms and relative volumes for the building project. From such studies, the architect

- Establishes the form and massing qualities of the building
- Visualizes the space between buildings (proposed and existing)
- Determines the effect of sun, shade, snow, rain, and wind on the project and its surrounding environment

8.5 Integrated Design Process

No part of a site, building, or system is unaffected by the other parts. A change of a window results in changes to the heating, ventilation, and air conditioning (HVAC) systems, changes to the controls, and changes to the electrical system. Sustainable and regenerative design objectives are driving the demand for higher performing buildings and sites, which requires greater levels of design effort, including testing, collaboration, thoughtfulness, and detailing. High performance building certification systems now require that design processes demonstrate integrative methods where all disciplines work together to solve complex and interrelated problems that cannot satisfactorily be solved by each discipline working in isolation.

The integrated design process (IDP) requires deep understanding of the natural systems present in the environment and evidence-based design. It also requires a shift in thinking about design methodology, processes, and firm operations. Numerous concepts, models, and methodologies have been proposed to implement the IDP, and each architectural practice, with its engineering and special consultant partners team, must develop and refine their own methodology to achieve best-in-class performance and competitive advantage in an ever more demanding marketplace.

As the general form of the facility emerges from programmatic data, engineers from the various disciplines work with the architect to develop a design and building system concept that is appropriate to the project goals. Early involvement by design engineers is a significant factor in obtaining the synthesis of building elements that can lead to reduced capital costs and improved building performance.

The IDP requires the seamless movement of data and information across firms' corporate boundaries. It is important to analyse technological approaches to communication and information management and knowledge generation and distribution. BIM processes, and the software that makes them possible, provide the design and construction teams with the means of generating and communicating complex design, construction, and operational information.

8.6 Design Alternatives: Evaluation and Selection

The project program may include more than one possible path to follow for planning or for developing architectural concepts. In these circumstances, the architect may prepare design alternatives for the client to consider. Design alternatives should be evaluated and selected through an unbiased discussion and analysis of the pros and cons of each choice based on the

- Completeness of response to the program and budget
- Success in resolving functional relationships and adjacency requirements
- Compliance with previously established sustainable goals
- The merits of any proposed alternative structural assemblies and mechanical or electrical systems
- Comparisons of building efficiencies including the
  - ratio of net to gross floor areas
  - ratio between circulation and usable floor areas
  - wall surface to floor area ratios
  - capital, operating, and maintenance costs (although at this phase, cost calculations will be speculative and remain so until the design is detailed)

The architect should receive a formal "sign-off" of the selected alternative from the client before proceeding with further work.

8.7 Building Cost Analysis

During schematic design, the architect prepares preliminary cost evaluations (or works closely with a specialist costing subconsultant) usually based only on the area or volume of the proposed building multiplied by the appropriate regional unit costs. In the instances where the IDP is utilized, the IDP team should all have acknowledged the budget figure at the outset of design and appreciate the contractual obligations to not over-design or choose materials, assemblies, or systems that are beyond the client's reach. In cases where the budget and program are unachievable, the IDP team may need to consider a "go/no-go" decision regarding continuation with the project.

8.8 Documentation and Presentation

Schematic design documents illustrate the functional relationships of the project elements and the project's scale and character based on the final version of the functional program, the schedule, and the construction budget. For this presentation and report, each team member's discipline may be at different stages of concept design. It is important that the report captures the client's and design team's objectives, so an understanding of the client's expectations beforehand is important. Sharing previous schematic design presentations and reports with the client beforehand can be useful. The design presentation documents are recommended to include the following:

- A site plan showing the proposed location and site circulation
- Functional block plans showing relative spatial areas and relationships (adjacencies) and circulation routes
- Vertical sections to depict building height and initial space conjecture for structural support
- Outline building elevations to display massing and image
- Illustrative sketches, perspectives, or computer-generated presentations (these should be at the concept level and avoid conveying a finished product, which would be misleading at this phase)
- Three-dimensional massing models

In addition to design presentation documents, it is often appropriate to prepare a report (not always required but always recommended and generally referred to as a schematic design report) that contains the following:

- Design approach or philosophy
- Description of how the design fits with the pre-design goals or the client's expectations
- An executive summary that supports the decisions made and looks forward to the next phase's activities
- Description of identified sustainable targets and environmental features (special materials or assemblies planned and highlighting any operational or energy savings that these elements might produce)
- Probable construction cost that identifies any potential cost risks
- Summary of the status of design with respect to applicable environmental, planning, and zoning regulations and building codes
- Preliminary schedule for design and construction start and completion and a recommendation of the form of construction delivery (lump-sum, design-build, construction management, etc.)
- Description of the structural, mechanical, and electrical systems and a depiction of the space needed to accommodate these elements (including vertical shafts)
- Confirmation of basic area calculations and analyses
- Site data
- Product and material descriptions and samples of key construction materials or finishes

The architect reviews the documents with the client and should obtain formal, written approval from the client before beginning design development.

8.9 Suggested Contents for a Schematic Design Report

(a) Introduction and background to the project (executive summary)
(b) List of drawings (appended to the schematic design report)
(c) Design objectives
(d) Assumptions, constraints, limitations, and uncertainties
(e) Description of the design
  (i) **Site design:**
  - Local context and site characteristics
  - Site servicing capacity requirements
  - Environmental and storm water management requirements
  - Landscaping design requirements and site design conceptual design
  - Site circulation requirements including vehicular and pedestrian traffic
  (ii) **Architectural design:**
  - Schematic layout, spatial and massing relationships
  - Conceptual elevations
  - Conceptual building sections
  - Summary of programmed areas (usually in spreadsheet format)
  (iii) **Structural design:**
  - Structural requirements and challenges
  - Conceptual structural foundation and framing systems
  - Special structural systems
  (iv) **Mechanical design:**
  - Interior space environmental requirements
  - Energy usage and generation requirements and operating costs estimates
  - HVAC systems requirements
  - Building automation systems
  - Conceptual HVAC systems design
  - Conceptual plumbing systems design
  (v) **Electrical design:**
  - Functional power and lighting requirements
  - Communications, security, and fire alarms and fire suppression requirements
  - Conceptual electrical system design
  (vi) **Special considerations:**
  - Requirements related to specific functions concerning acoustics, laboratory, medical, performance, exhibitions, etc.
  - Conceptual plans, sections, elevations, and descriptions addressing specific functions
(f) **Sustainability and regenerative design requirements and objectives**
(g) **System descriptions (standard formats are available for these)**
(h) **Preliminary regulatory analysis (recommended)**
(i) **Design and construction program cost estimate**
(j) **Construction project procurement approach (if appropriate)**
(k) **Design project management approach:**
  - BIM approach (if appropriate)

8.10 Summary

Design is a learning process for all involved. Throughout developing the schematic design, new ideas emerge, and assumptions are challenged. The client may find that their original intent and vision are now questionable, which leads to a lack of clarity of project objectives. Schematic design should be delayed until the appropriate level of shared understanding of project objectives is established. Active client involvement will help resolve difficulties with program elements and facilitate decision making if the design needs adjustment as it evolves. However, the general principles of effective stakeholder engagement and open and transparent communication will support obtaining the needed approvals to advance design decision making.

9 DESIGN AND CONSTRUCTION DRAWINGS

9.1 Background

Drawings are essential documents at any construction project site. Without a detailed drawing of different building components, no work can be done on-site. Different types of construction drawings serve as the guide to the site engineer in charge and give detailed information such as the size, dimensions, material, and location of a component of the structure. Construction drawings provide guidelines for the development of a building.

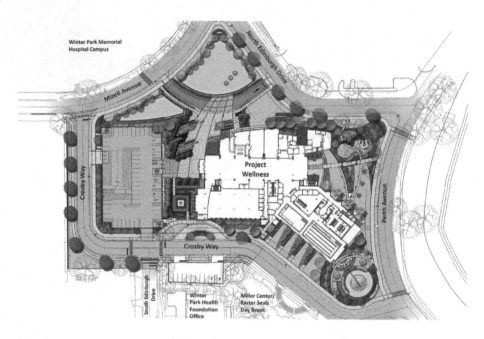

FIGURE 9A Site Plan (Centre for Health and Well Being Site Plan [Internet]; www.wphf.org/portfolio-item/site-plan/).

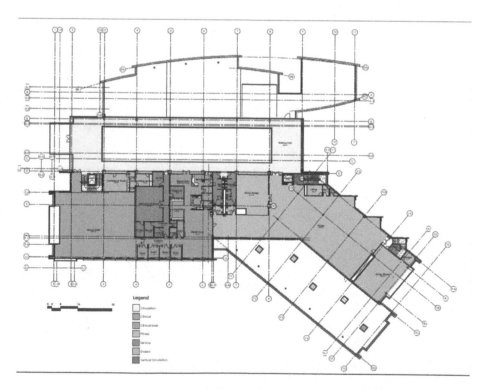

FIGURE 9B Floor Plan (Centre for Health and Well Being Site Plan [Internet]; www.wphf.org/portfolio-item/second-floor/).

DOI: 10.1201/9780367460884-9

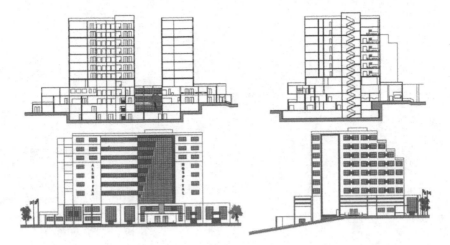

FIGURE 9C Elevation and Section Drawing (Cadbull. Hospital Elevation and Section Plan [Internet]; https://cadbull.com/detail/31952/Hospital-Elevation-and-Section-plan).

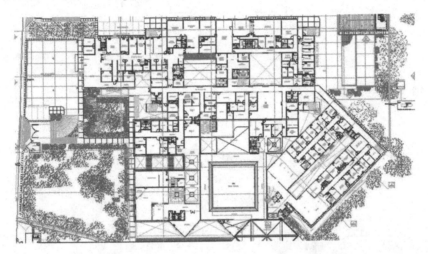

FIGURE 9D Landscape Drawing (Cadbull. Landscaping of General Hospital Project [Internet]; https://cadbull.com/detail/30128/Landscaping-of-General-Hospital-Project-dwg-file).

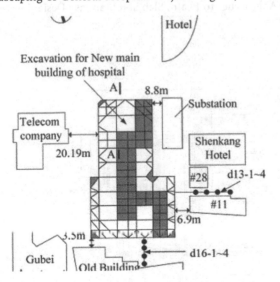

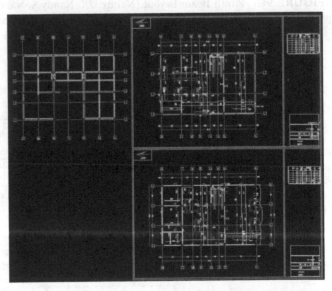

FIGURE 9E Excavation Drawing (Zhang HB, Chen JJ, Zhao XS, Wang JH, Hu H. Displacement performance and simple prediction for deep excavations supported by contiguous bored pile walls in soft clay. Journal of Aerospace Engineering. 2015 Nov 1;28(6):A4014008).

FIGURE 9F Column Layout (Cadbull. Hospital Building Column Layout Design [Internet]; https://cadbull.com/detail/382/Hospital-building-column-layout-design-DWG-2D-CAD-Drawing.Download-the-CAD-file-now).

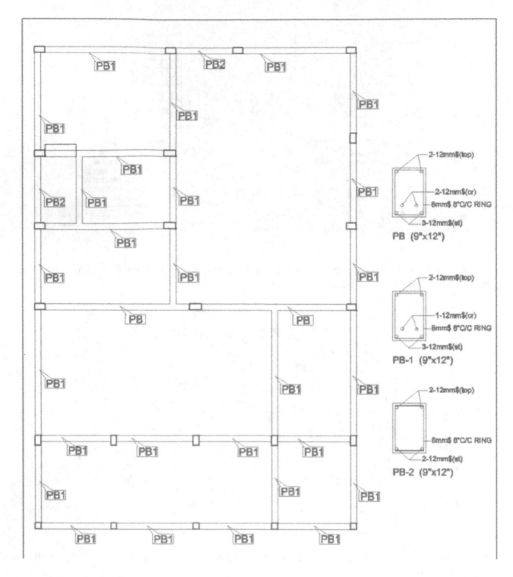

FIGURE 9G Plinth Beam Layout (Nandy UK, Nandy S, Nandy A. Approaches to Beam, Slab and Staircase Designing Using Limit State Design Method for Achieving Optimal Stability Conditions).

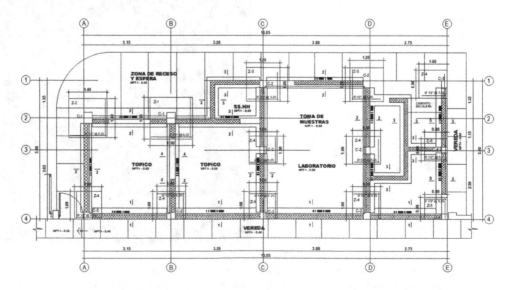

FIGURE 9H Foundation Plan (Cadbull. Clinic Foundation Plan [Internet]; https://cadbull.com/detail/182204/Clinic-Foundation-Plan-AutoCAD-Drawing-Download-DWG-File).

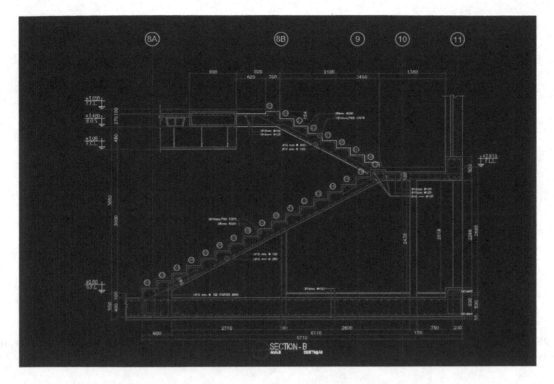

FIGURE 9I Staircase Layout and Reinforcement Details (Civil Engineering. Stair Reinforcement Details [Internet]; https://sonatuts.blogspot.com/2020/12/stair-reinforcement-details.html).

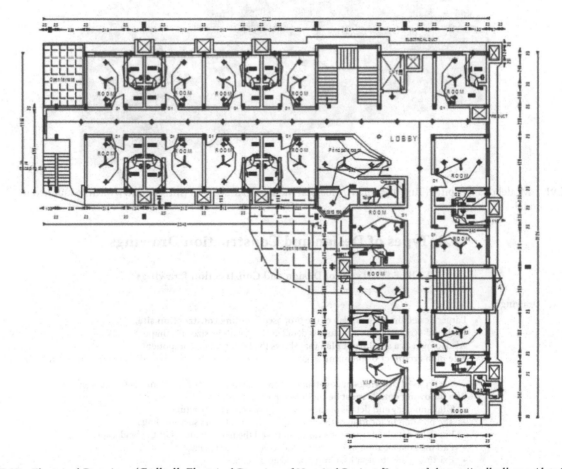

FIGURE 9J Electrical Drawings (Cadbull. Electrical Drawing of Hospital Project [Internet]; https://cadbull.com/detail/83312/Electrical-drawing-of-hospital-project-dwg-file).

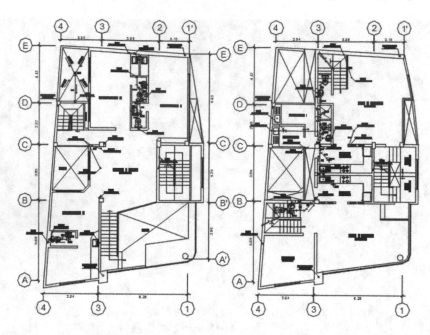

FIGURE 9K Plumbing Drawings (Cadbull. Plumbing Layout of the Clinic [Internet]; https://cadbull.com/detail/68568/Plumbing-layout-of-the-clinic-in-AutoCAD-drawing).

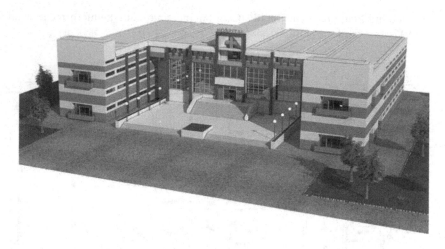

FIGURE 9L Model of a Hospital (TurboSquid. 3D Hospital Model by Anurozgen [Internet]; www.turbosquid.com/3d-models/3d-hospital-model-1370361).

9.2 Types of Design and Construction Drawings

TABLE 9A: Types of Design and Construction Drawings

Architectural Drawings

Site Plan
(Figure 9A)

- Larger-scaled drawing or plan of the proposed **building construction site.**
- Each and every existing structure is detailed along with its size and shape.
- Also known as a **site layout plan** that shows the layout of site components.
- **Site plan architect or planning** to get an idea about existing features of the site, to plan accordingly, and to make the decision for demolition, if it is required.
- These **types of drawings in construction** are prepared first before planning the building.
- **The following details must be included in the site plan:**
  - Site boundary and details of surrounding properties or structures.
  - The position or location of the building with respect to its surroundings.
  - Location details of tree protection orders and the main elements of the landscape.
  - Parking area location or capacities, traffic flows, and signage.
  - Existing roads, footpaths, ramps, paved areas, etc.

(Continued)

TABLE 9A: (Continued)

Architectural Drawings

Floor Plan (Figure 9B)
- One of the most important types of construction drawings.
- Two-dimensional drawing that shows the position of different components of the room with their dimensions.
- Sometimes, the floor plan also shows furniture, appliances, or anything kept in the room.

Sectional Drawing (Figure 9C)
- **Section drawing** is the same line elevation of the building, but it is cut in a vertical plan inside the building plan. Moreover, it represents the building details when it is cut vertically inside the building.
- Similarly, **sectional drawing** is important to get details of the inside components, so they are visible in the sectional drawing of the building.

Elevation Drawing (Figure 9C) Finishing Drawing
Elevation drawings help an architect understand the facing of the building. It is useful to know about the direction of the sun and the wind corresponding to the building. They also **indicate the height of the building** and the external and internal markings that include the doors and sizes of the windows.
The finishing drawing has a close relationship with the elevation drawings as it also shows the **smaller details of a building.**
The patterns of the floor, type, shape of the false ceiling, paint colours, plaster, textures, etc. can be included.

Landscape Drawing (Figure 9D)
The landscape drawing is the aerial of the whole area in which the building is built. It includes the areas designated for trees, street lights, parks, pools, etc.
More often, it is used to depict the external aesthetics of the building.

Working Plan
For contractors to **help them understand the scope of the project.**
Convenient to fabricate the construction material according to the overall design.
A legend provides information about the different components.

Section Drawings
Section drawings **show the structure in a sliced form.**
They help identify the primary structures in relation to other surrounding structures of the building along with information on the types of materials to be used in the construction.

General Note
Includes the bylaws, codes, length, mapping forms, construction type, legends, abbreviations, etc. that are essential.

Excavation Drawings (Figure 9E)
Excavation drawings are needed to know the length, depth, and width of the building excavation. They show the extent of excavation, removal of soil, and process of excavation. The different processes used for excavation comprise trenching, wall shafts, tunnelling, and others.

Structural Drawings

Column Layout (Figure 9F)
The column layout plan is the plan that includes the details of the column size, shape, and location with dimensions.

Plinth Beam Layout (Figure 9G)
This is a **type of drawing in construction** that shows the details of the plinth beam position, layout, size, and reinforcement details.

Roof Beam and Shuttering Layout
A roof beam is made to strengthen the building's overall structure. A roof beam is a triangular structure that is usually made on the top of a building that supports the roof. Roof beams are usually comprised of wood but can also be made from steel or concrete.

Block Plan
A block plan is the **representation of a wider area that is in proximity to the main building under construction.** A block plan may include the adjoining buildings, roads, boundaries, and other such components. More importantly, a block plan is represented in scales, which also means that it covers a wide area.

Component Drawings
The component drawings are primarily referred to as the drawings supplied by the manufacturer of a product. These kinds of plans are replete with the drawings of the components and thus provide detailed insight into their markings and different sub-parts.

Concept Drawings
Concept drawings are more like the first draft of a construction project that is made in the first instance. They are not very detailed or distinguished. Concept drawings are like **rough sketches of the building and the nearby areas.** They are more prominently used to describe an overview of the building to potential clients or stakeholders.

Engineering Drawings
Any building may require the installation of some engineered objects or components. So, an engineering drawing is **targeted toward the convenient construction or placement of these types of structures.** They are more of a guide to help the contractor and the engineer work in sync with one another and obtain the desired results.

Foundation Plan (Figure 9H)
The **foundation layout plan** is the most important **type of construction drawing.** It is a plan that has details of the foundation of the building. The foundation plan includes the following:
- **Type of foundation** to be constructed;
- Size and shape of the foundation.
- Dimension and distance between the length and width.
- Centreline of building and component.
- Details of PCC and excavation work.

Flooring Detail Drawings
The **flooring plan in building construction** shows the details of the flooring size, thickness, types of material, and types of flooring to be used. It also shows the flooring base material details.

Staircase Layout and Reinforcement Details (Figure 9I)
This shows the details of the stair layout with standard dimensions. It includes the **details of the stair length, width, size of landing, number of risers, number of treads, etc.** It is an important drawing while constructing stairs. A staircase plan and section show the details of the reinforcement, angle-to-stair flight, and cover to be used.

(Continued)

TABLE 9A: (Continued)

Electrical and Plumbing Drawings

Electrical Drawings (Figure 9J)	• This is a graphical representation of the exact location of various electrical fixtures such as switch boards, light points, fan points, and ceiling points with a wiring diagram. An electrical engineer can read this layout plan and calculate the material required for the electrification of the building.

Plumbing Drawing (Figure 9K)	• This is an important type of construction drawing. **Plumbing work** is related to the water supply system in the house. It includes the layout plan of different types of pipes that run in the house to supply water to various rooms.
	• A plumbing plan includes the following:
	  • Size of pile.
	  • Material of pile.
	  • Position of sanitary fittings.
	  • Outlet point location.

HVAC and Fire Drawings

HVAC Drawing	Also called mechanical drawings, HVAC drawings provide information about the heating and ventilation systems. They also include the air conditioning patterns and layout that are to be constructed inside the building. The HVAC drawings provide an insight into these complex systems and help the builders plan their construction process accordingly.
Firefighting Drawing	Firefighting drawings are drawn before the construction of a building. They depict the pattern of the placement of the fire hoses, points, water outlets, etc. They also describe the fire protection plan and safety systems that are to be put in place.

Other Types of Construction Drawings

Finishing Drawings	Finishing drawings show the final finish details of each component such as the flooring pattern, painting colour, false ceiling shape, plastering texture, and elevation design.
Detail Drawings	These are drawings of any type of geometric structure that has to be constructed. Detail drawings can include anything from a small building to a large bridge or even a tunnel. These drawings are more detailed and **give attention to the intricate designs and details of any construction project.**
Perspective Drawings	A perspective drawing **highlights the spatial aspects of a building and shows its three-dimensional volumes.** These are the realistic images of the building that is under construction. In addition, there are different types of perspectives based on vanishing points.
Production Drawings	Production drawings are guides that convey information to the workers and supervisors about the construction process. Along with the materials, they include the dimensions, tools, assembly, etc. The production documents provide instructions and indicate how to meet these requirements.
Scale Drawings	Scale drawings demonstrate the larger objects, as it is not possible to draw them in the original size. Therefore, this means that every drawing of a building is a type of scale drawing. For instance, a location plan has a scale of 1:1,000, a site plan's scale is 1:200, a floor plan's scale is 1:100, etc. **When the size of the object under construction is larger, the propensity of the scale will be higher.**
Technical Drawings	Technical drawings also convey the broad meaning regarding a construction project. The **basic purpose of technical drawings is to indicate how an object functions.** Unlike artistic drawings, these drawings are made with one specific purpose. In this sense, almost every drawing that is prepared before, during, and post-construction can be referred to as a technical drawing.
Submission Drawings	Submission drawings are **prepared with reference to the bylaws drafted and implemented by an authority.** They are sent to the authorities for their approval and include index plans, detailed drawings, elevation drawings, and other sectional plans.
Model (Figure 9L)	Models come after the drawings. They are prepared for the larger building and demonstrate how the building will look when it is completed. The benefit of making models is that it helps architects identify difficulties. Everything is clear in a model, including the design, elevation, and internal and external detailing.
Environment Plans	Some projects are built around rivers or streams. In this case, environmental plans offer insights into how erosion and sedimentation will be managed. Moreover, these drawings also discuss plant removal procedures and chemical disposal mechanisms. Environment plans also contain the procedures and plans to attenuate the harmful effects.
Presentation Drawings	Presentation drawings are prepared as a part of proposals, for exhibitions, or even for publications. These types of drawings may include any kind of drawing that has been discussed previously.

9.3 Summary

Drawings are essential documents for any construction project. A hospital construction will have structural, architectural, electrical, plumbing, HVAC, fire, and medical gas pipeline system (MGPS) drawings, to mention a few. These drawings are prepared by an architect in consultation with the construction engineer. The client and the various consultants for specialized services should be actively involved in finalizing these drawings. Early involvement of all of these stakeholders will avoid major renovations and refurbishments during the hospital commissioning phase.

10 CONSTRUCTION DOCUMENTS

10.1 Introduction

The construction documents phase bridges the gap between conceptual ideas and built reality. Here, the client's initial aspirations, meticulously etched during pre-design, transform into a meticulously detailed roadmap for construction. This roadmap not only encapsulates the architect's design intent meticulously honed through earlier stages but also meticulously aligns with all technical specifications and building regulations. This meticulousness serves a dual purpose: ensuring clarity and consistency from vision to construction and equipping the architect with the tools to safeguard the project's integrity throughout construction administration.

By the culmination of this phase, a comprehensive design symphony emerges, seamlessly orchestrating all building elements and components across disciplines. Each note, meticulously rendered in these documents, adheres to the chosen procurement, construction, and delivery methods. Meticulous diligence and attention to detail are of paramount importance here, as they not only minimize professional liability risks but also pave the way for a thriving project.

The quality of this meticulous score directly impacts the architect's role during contractor selection and construction phases. It further serves as the key to unlocking essential permits from relevant authorities. Hence, clear and concise communication of regulatory compliance within these documents is fundamental.

10.2 Understanding Construction Documents

Construction documents are the meticulous blueprints that translate conceptual ideas into tangible reality. They encompass detailed drawings, precise specifications, and supporting documentation, meticulously crafted by design professionals or the client themselves. The exact definition of these documents is typically enshrined in both the tender documents and the construction contract, ensuring a clear roadmap for project execution.

In the event of any discrepancies within these vital documents, a hierarchical order of priority reigns supreme. Information and instructions for bidders take the highest precedence, followed by the general and special conditions of the contract. Each subsequent element, from the detailed assignment and scope of work to material schedules and drawings, plays its crucial role in ensuring project consistency.

Drawings, the visual architects of the project, hold a special place in this hierarchy. Larger-scale drawings trump their smaller counterparts of the same date, while dimensions directly specified on them supersede those scaled from the drawings. Time also plays its part, with newer documents superseding their earlier counterparts.

The intricate dance between drawings and specifications is central to the success of any project. Meticulous coordination is paramount to avoid inconsistencies, overlaps, or gaps, both within individual disciplines and across different ones. As a rule of thumb, drawings define the scope of the design, while specifications meticulously prescribe its quality.

Construction documents are the culmination of a well-defined design journey. They are built upon the design documentation meticulously produced and approved by the client in earlier phases. This ensures the following:

- Adopted solutions are grounded in feasibility, minimizing surprises during construction.
- Critical design decisions have been addressed upfront, preventing costly delays and rework.

Critical design issues, those heavily impacting other elements or systems, are tackled head-on before reaching this stage. User requirements, regulatory compliance, and building code adherence are all meticulously addressed and resolved to ensure a smooth transition into the construction phase.

10.3 Process of Preparing Construction Documents

The construction documents phase is where the building and site design, conceptualized in the schematic design stage and elaborated upon in the design development stage, undergoes further refinement and development to a level of comprehensive detail, accuracy, and interdisciplinary coordination. This process ensures that technical design choices for building materials, systems, and technologies align with the project's governing requirements and are validated for feasibility.

Before being finalized and issued as bid or contract documents, construction documents in progress are often referred to as "progress documents" (drawings or specifications). These interim versions of design information serve as communication tools within the design team and are distributed to relevant stakeholders as needed throughout the development process.

10.4 Construction Documents: Essential Outputs

Outputs of the construction documents essentially, but not exclusively, comprise the following:

- **Drawings**: Visual representations of the building's layout, dimensions, and details. They provide a clear picture of the spatial arrangement of building elements and their interconnections.
- **Specifications**: Written documentation that outlines the quality, materials, and workmanship required for each element of the project. They serve as a detailed guide for construction contractors, ensuring adherence to the project's design intent.
- **Schedules**: Tabular presentations of essential project information, such as building code compliance, door and frame details, floor, wall, and ceiling finishes, electrical panel configuration, and air–handling unit specifications. They provide a concise overview of project requirements and their coordination.
- **Complementary Documents**: Additional documentation tailored to the project's specific needs, highlighting

DOI: 10.1201/9780367460884-10

interdisciplinary or multiple trade–based design information. They integrate information from drawings and specifications, ensuring a comprehensive understanding of the project.

All these deliverables work together to direct the construction process and ensure that the completed building conforms to the design's intent, technical performance requirements, and owner's expectations outlined in the contract documents.

10.5 Guiding Principles for Effective Construction Documents

Effective construction documents are the cornerstone of successful project execution. They serve as the primary means of communicating design intent to all project stakeholders, ensuring that the constructed building aligns with the client's vision and meets all performance requirements. Key criteria for effective construction documents include the following:

Editorial defects can lead to misinterpretations, disagreements, and disputes among project stakeholders. Utmost care must be taken in drafting and reviewing construction documents to ensure accuracy and clarity.

10.6 Ensuring the Quality of Construction Documents

Effective construction documents are crucial for project success, influencing both client satisfaction and the efficiency of subsequent stages. Improper construction documents can lead to costly rework, delays, and disputes, highlighting the importance of thorough quality assurance and quality control (QA/QC) measures.

The initial planning and organization of construction document development play a pivotal role in ensuring the desired level of quality. Key QA/QC considerations include the following:

- **Consistency and Compatibility**: Ensure seamless alignment with approved design development documents and procurement requirements. Maintain consistent document format, form, and presentation standards established at the outset.

Sl. No.	Key Criteria	Details
1	Clarity	• **Comprehensiveness**: The documents should provide all relevant information necessary for contractors to accurately interpret and execute the design. • **Redundancy Avoidance**: Avoid excessive duplication of information across different documents. • **Consistency**: Maintain consistent graphic standards (scales, line styles, symbols, etc.) throughout the documents. • **Terminology and Language**: Use appropriate terminology, phrasing, and grammar that is consistent throughout the documents. • **Legibility**: Ensure drawings are legible and easily readable, with clear annotations and consistent line weights.
2	Readability	• **Logical Organization**: Arrange information in a logical and sequential manner, making it easy for users to navigate and find the information they need. • **Visual Clarity**: Use clear and uncluttered layout, avoiding unnecessary graphics or distractions. • **Key Information Emphasis**: Highlight key information and design elements visually to enhance readability.
3	Intelligibility of Design Solutions	• **Transparency**: Clearly represent design intent, especially for architectural features and complex assemblies. • **Lack of Ambiguity**: Avoid ambiguity or misinterpretations in drawings and specifications. • **Coordination**: Ensure proper coordination between different disciplines and trades to avoid conflicts or inconsistencies. • **Self-Explanatory Nature**: Construction details should be self-explanatory to qualified and experienced users.
4	Constructability	• **Feasibility**: Ensure the design is constructible within the project's context, considering available materials, resources, and labour availability. • **Work Sequencing**: Consider the sequencing of construction activities to avoid conflicts or delays. • **Innovation**: Evaluate the feasibility of innovative or unique construction methods or techniques. • **Site-Specific Conditions**: Adapt the design to site-specific conditions and constraints.
5	Usability	• **Adequacy**: Provide sufficient information to meet the needs of different stakeholders throughout the project life cycle. • **Bidding Phase**: Clearly define materials, specifications, and quantities for accurate cost estimation and bidding. • **Construction Phase**: Guide contractors in the execution of construction activities and ensure adherence to design intent. • **Project Completion**: Facilitate building commissioning, handover, and final occupancy.

6	Quality of Graphic and Written Language	• **Accuracy**: Ensure drawings and specifications are free from errors, including grammatical, syntactic, or semantic mistakes.
		• **Cross-Referencing**: Provide accurate and consistent cross-referencing between drawings, specifications, and other relevant documents.
		• **Written Material**:
		  • **Correct Grammar and Spelling**: Maintain correct grammar, spelling, and punctuation throughout the written documentation.
		  • **Appropriate Terminology**: Use appropriate terminology and phrasing consistently across all documents.

7	Graphic Material	• **Standardized Representation**: Use standardized graphic symbols, line types, and hatch patterns consistently throughout the drawings. • **Clear Navigation**: Implement clear navigation indicators (cross-referencing symbols, tile placement, fonts, etc.) on all drawings.

- **Accuracy and Completeness**: Eliminate errors, omissions, and ambiguities in both drawings and specifications. Provide sufficient, complete, relevant, and internally consistent construction information.
- **Disciplinary Coordination**: Harmonize detailed design solutions between different disciplines and trades, ensuring alignment for specific building elements or systems.
- **Field Feasibility and Constructability**: Address actual, physical field feasibility and constructability concerns. Even for standardized or generic solutions, ensure compatibility with building envelope integrity, building code compliance, and desired finish quality.
- **Error Prevention**: Implement preventive measures, such as peer review, checklists, and regular internal audits, to minimize errors and inconsistencies.
- **Documentation Control**: Establish a robust document control system to track revisions, maintain version history, and ensure accessibility to the most up-to-date information.

- **Training and Expertise**: Invest in the training and expertise of the construction document team to ensure they possess the necessary skills and knowledge to produce high-quality documents.

By adhering to these QA/QC principles, architects can significantly enhance the quality of construction documents, leading to satisfied clients, streamlined project execution, and minimized risks and liabilities.

10.7 Summary

The construction documents stage of the design services is generally where the client's project objectives as defined at the pre-design stage are captured for construction, especially with respect to costs, time, and overarching considerations, such as sustainability, durability, life cycle, etc. These are legally valid documents that keep the project on track and viable for the entire duration of project management.

11 CONSTRUCTION OF THE HOSPITAL

11.1 Introduction

Safety during construction of the health care facility becomes a primary concern because the construction work itself poses safety risks, in particular infection control and life safety. Proactive risk assessments and implementation of various measures address these risks, as do other construction activities.

11.2 Construction Documentation

In addition to written records, the planning phase can be documented using multimedia presentations, slides, and detailed models, including three-dimensional representations that vividly portray the physical implications of the plan. Thorough documentation becomes especially vital in cases of staff turnover, as new team members need to swiftly familiarize themselves with the project's history, objectives, components, phases, and current status. A lack of comprehensive documentation could lead to the loss of valuable time and knowledge, potentially resulting in uninformed decisions and increased costs due to delays and the need for error rectification.

11.3 Proactive Risk Management

Before physical construction begins, however, a number of activities must be completed to ensure adequate construction risk management.

(a) **Preconstruction Phase:** Meticulous attention to the risks posed to patients, visitors, staff, and construction workers needs to be taken into consideration and addressed. A preconstruction risk assessment is an important exercise and documentation becomes imperative. As a result, mitigating risks to patients, visitors, hospital, and construction staff.

(b) **Infection Control Risk Assessment (ICRA):** The American Institute of Architects (AIA) Academy of Architecture for Health. The new AIA Guidelines strongly support infection control input at the initial stages of planning and design by requiring a new element termed an infection control risk assessment (ICRA) for broad and long-range involvement of infection control/epidemiology leadership. An ICRA provides for strategic, proactive design to mitigate environmental sources of microbes and for prevention of infection through architectural design (e.g. handwashing facilities, separation of patients with communicable diseases), as well as specific needs of the population served by the facility. An ICRA should be an ongoing process, commencing during the planning stage and continuing throughout the design and construction phases.

(c) **Implementing Preconstruction Risk Assessment Measures:** The measures derived from the assessment must be actively implemented and monitored. It is crucial for the organization to continuously reassess the risks during the construction phase to ensure comprehensive risk management. Additionally, documenting the entire risk assessment process is imperative. While the organization bears the ultimate responsibility for conducting the assessment and implementing measures, the contractor involved in the project also shares responsibilities for specification and execution, which should be clearly delineated in the contract.

11.4 Safety Measures

Conducting an assessment to ensure compliance with the applicable safety codes is a crucial preconstruction measure for addressing project risks. According to the National Building Code of India, hospitals are classified as institutional buildings. Construction and renovation projects are particularly susceptible to non-compliance issues. Notably, common deficiencies observed during construction pertain to the safety and accessibility of patient rooms, fire exits, and emergency departments, as well as the proper operation of alarm and sprinkler systems (Table 11A).

TABLE 11A: Safety Measures

	Safety Measure Options
Exits	Are all exits free from obstructions or impediments?
	Are all exits unlocked and can be readily open in direction of travel?
	Can all egress doors open fully?
	Are exits signs in place, visible, and illuminated?
	Are the shafts and electrical cable openings in the floors/walls sealed with fire stop material?
Electrical Safety	Are all electrical system maintained, and are there no loose or open wirings?
	Is the installed electrical load in the building per the sanctioned load?
	Are air conditioner and ventilators present in the hospital building maintained?
Firefighting Systems	Are all emergency power systems tested and inspected on regular basis?
	Is the fixed fire protection system (fire pumps, downcomers, wet risers, hydrant valves, first aid hose reels, automatic sprinkler systems) maintained and in working condition?
Fire Detection System	Is the fire detection system installed in building and in working condition?
Emergency Preparedness	Are regular fire evacuation drills conducted in building?
	Are all hospital staff trained in usage of fire extinguishers / fixed fire protection systems?
	Are all hospital staff provided training on emergency preparedness?
	Are all hospital staff aware of the roles and responsibilities during emergency and whether the same has been documented?
	Are emergency evacuation plans pasted in building?
	Is there a public address system installed in building, and is it working?
General Points	Are all curtains, bedsheets, ceiling and wall claddings made of fire-retardant materials?
	Are all ventilators and filters installed at ground level and fresh air intake ducts inducted at terrace level?
	Is fire safety executive appointed in building?

DOI: 10.1201/9780367460884-11

11.5 Construction Activities

The construction process is multifaceted and requires participation from all members of the project team, including organization leadership, staff, architects, engineers, contractors, and construction personnel. The specific responsibilities of each member or group of members will vary according to the size and scope of the project; however, certain activities must be performed during the construction phase of any project. These may begin before physical construction begins and will continue throughout the construction phase—and some may continue beyond into the commissioning phase (Table 11B).

11.6 Risks during Construction and Measures to Minimize the Risks

(a) **Risks during Construction (Table 11C)**
(b) **Measures to Minimize the Risks during Construction**

TABLE 11B: Construction Activities

Project Team Kick-Off Meeting	• Review project procedures, schedules, and budget. • Determine actions for establishing project site security. • Confirm that site conditions are acceptable for completing the project as proposed. • Storage of building materials • Contractors' access to occupied areas • Relocation of furniture and equipment • Above-ceiling access in occupied areas • Barrier construction and placement • Reaction or disaster plans for undesirable events • Travel paths for contractors and deliveries • Contractor and construction worker education • Contractor parking
Educating Staff on Safety Measures	• Educating staff could involve training staff members on any identified safety risks, measures to address those risks and infection control measures, and how to report activities that occur without the proper risk prevention measures. Organization leaders, facility directors, infection control professionals, and safety officers may learn of a hazardous condition that needs prompt attention. These individuals should have the authority to stop all work until the issue is addressed, if that is what is warranted.
Cleaning Up	• Insufficient clean-up has led to instances where soda cans and cigarette butts have been inadvertently sealed within walls, resulting in potential mould, fungus, and bacterial issues. Establishing clear cleaning agreements before the commencement of construction is therefore essential to prevent such issues.
Cleaning during Construction	• Have staging areas properly allocated for materials being delivered to and stored on the site. • Keep absorbent materials protected from moisture. • Suppress dust with wetting agents or sweeping compounds. • Clean up immediately after activities that produce high dust levels (or at the end of each day the activity continues). • Replace any absorbent materials that become exposed to moisture during construction. • Vacuum stud tracks prior to application of a second surface of gypsum board, to remove dirt and potential mould food sources. • Maintain temperature and humidity levels whenever possible. • Keep duct ends sealed with plastic to reduce dust infiltration into the mechanical system when the system is not in use. • Cover return air registers with filter material if the mechanical system must be used during construction. • Restrict food and beverage consumption (except water) to a designated area that can be maintained daily.
Cleaning after Construction	• Remove barriers carefully to minimize the spread of dust and debris (do before other cleaning tasks). • Dispose of barriers properly. • Clear, clean, and decontaminate the area. • Vacuum the work area with high-efficiency particulate air (HEPA)-filtered vacuums. • Mop the area with disinfectant. • Bag construction waste or transport it in covered carts. • Unblock air vents.

TABLE 11C: Risks during Construction

Dust and Fumes	Volatile organic compounds (VOCs), which are chemicals typically contained in cleaners, paint, adhesives, and the off-gas of new carpeting and upholstered furniture, can cause a variety of adverse health effects.
Mould	Organizations must dry materials completely before use or remove them within 72 hours.
Fungi	The phases of construction that usually create the greatest fungi risk include demolition, window or wall removal, ventilation and utility outages, application of volatile chemicals, and placement of combustion engines.
Hazardous Materials	A renovation process can sometimes disturb existing materials, and some of these materials could be hazardous to patients' health. For example, asbestos and lead paint are still present in some facilities, and they have well-documented health risks across all populations. A common mistake is that facilities may look only at lead paint. During construction, these instruments sometimes break, releasing the highly toxic substance into the surrounding environment.
Water Contaminants	During projects, bacteria can enter and contaminate the water system. Many existing water systems already contain contaminants such as *Legionella* in the biofilm. This does not pose a threat if left undisturbed. However, during construction, vibration can release *Legionella* into the water supply.
Noise and Vibration	Organizations should be aware of and work to minimize the negative effects of construction noise on patients and staff.
Utilities Disruption	During the course of construction, an organization may be required to shut off the main power, heat, water, or air conditioning. Organizations must consider the effect of these shutdowns on system and patient levels. For example, if the water must be shut off for two hours, how will patients, staff, and equipment be affected? When can the shutdown be scheduled so as to have the least effect?

TABLE 11D: Measures to Minimize Risks during Construction

Isolate the Project Site	Large-scale projects, such as constructing a new wing or renovating an old one, might be easier to isolate than small-scale projects, such as painting a few rooms or repairing ceiling tiles
Effective HVAC System	This includes contamination from dust, fumes, or other airborne particles. To prevent contamination from the construction site, air must flow from clean to dirty. The facility's HVAC engineer must determine how to isolate the system. This may include sealing vents, adding additional filters, or using other means. Elevator shafts require special consideration because of their tendency to function like a chimney, drawing odours, dust, and fumes up through the shaft onto other floors.
Use Negative Pressure Areas	
Set Up Clean and Dirty Anterooms	Just outside the construction site, organizations may wish to set up clean and dirty rooms. This can minimize the transfer of such particles outside the construction zone.
Use Low-Emitting Materials	By using low-emitting materials during construction, organizations can prevent off-gassing of VOCs and carcinogens into the air. This can preserve the environment as well as the safety of construction staff, health care staff, patients, and visitors.
Carefully Plan Traffic Control	Preconstruction planning defines how workers will enter and exit a building and the route they will take to the construction area. If possible, separation of patient, visitor, and staff traffic from construction traffic is highly desirable.

11.7 Summary

The construction of hospitals demands meticulous attention to safety measures, ensuring the protection of patients, staff, and construction personnel. A comprehensive approach to hospital construction safety is critical, encompassing thorough risk assessments, compliance with safety codes, and the implementation of effective cleaning practices. Furthermore, the active involvement of all project stakeholders, including organizational leadership, architects, engineers, and contractors, is imperative for the successful execution of safety protocols. With the implementation of these stringent safety measures, hospitals can foster an environment conducive to quality health care delivery, promoting the well-being and security of all individuals involved in the construction process.

12 COMMISSIONING OF THE HOSPITAL

12.1 Introduction

Building commissioning is a professional practice that ensures that a building's systems and assemblies perform interactively according to the Owner's Project Requirements (OPR). It is a quality-focused process that begins during the design phase and continues through construction, occupancy, and operations. Commissioning is an ongoing process that continues throughout the life cycle of the facility.

Building commissioning activities include, but are not limited to, the following:

- Developing and documenting the OPR
- Verifying that the design documents meet the OPR
- Overseeing the installation and testing of building systems
- Training building staff on how to operate and maintain the building systems
- Documenting the commissioning process and findings

Building commissioning can be performed on new construction projects, as well as existing buildings. It is a valuable tool for ensuring that buildings operate efficiently and effectively, meet the needs of their occupants, and achieve the owner's goals.

According to the Building Commissioning Association, commissioning is a systematic process for investigating, analysing, and optimizing the performance of building systems through the identification and implementation of low-/no-cost and capital-intensive facility improvement measures and ensuring their continued performance.

12.2 Objectives of Commissioning

The objectives of commissioning are as follows:

- Include the commissioning process in the OPR document.
- Verify that the OPR, including commissioning, is in the project design and construction documents for new projects.
- Facilitate the delivery of buildings and construction projects that meet the OPR.
- Prevent or eliminate problems in a cost-effective manner through proactive quality techniques.
- Verify that systems are installed and working as intended and benchmark their operation.
- Provide and collect documentation and records on the design, construction, and testing to facilitate the operation and maintenance of the facility.
- Facilitate training functions, system operation documentation, and commissioning tools for operations and maintenance (O&M) staff performance and implementation of ongoing commissioning.
- Lower overall first costs and life-cycle costs for the owner.
- Maintain facility performance throughout the building's entire life cycle.

12.3 Types of Commissioning

New Building Commissioning	It is a quality-assurance process that ensures that all building systems and assemblies are planned, designed, installed, tested, operated, and maintained to meet the OPR. It includes thorough design reviews, functional testing, system documentation, and operator training to ensure that the building operates properly and efficiently.

Extended Commissioning

Retro— Commissioning	It is the systematic process of investigating, verifying, improving, and optimizing the performance of building systems and assemblies in existing buildings that have not previously undergone commissioning.
Re-Commissioning	It is a process of using the original functional performance tests to verify that building systems and equipment continue to operate as designed. It is an important part of building commissioning and maintenance, and it can help to identify and address problems before they lead to costly failures.
Ongoing Commissioning Process	It is a continuation of the commissioning process in an operating building to verify that it continues to meet the current and evolving needs of its occupants. Ongoing commissioning activities occur throughout the life of the building, some of which are continuous in implementation, while others are scheduled or unscheduled.

12.4 Process of Commissioning

The commissioning process varies by project, but it typically begins in the planning phase and continues for a year or more after construction is completed. Different aspects of the process are emphasized at different phases of the project:

- **Pre-Design Phase:** The process of commissioning should start in this phase. Early involvement of the commissioning professional in this phase is essential for the successful commissioning of a building. The commissioning professional can help to develop the OPR, the Basis of Design, the Commissioning Plan, and the Operations and Maintenance Systems Manual. These documents are critical for ensuring that the building meets the owner's needs and operates efficiently and effectively throughout its life cycle. If these tasks are delayed until later in the process, the commissioning professional will have to "reverse engineer" them to fit the design. This can reduce the effectiveness of the OPR, the Basis of Design, and the Commissioning Plan as tools for communication, cost and risk management, and quality assurance.
- **Design Phase:** During this phase, the project design is finalized and documented for construction, ensuring compliance with the OPR. The commissioning professional develops commissioning requirements, including system selection, scope, and contractor and

DOI: 10.1201/9780367460884-12

manufacturer responsibilities. The commissioning professional also refines the commissioning plan, verifying design and performance requirements and developing field observation, functional testing, and performance requirements, as well as documentation formats.

- **Construction Phase:** During construction, the commissioning process shifts from planning to implementation. Schedules are integrated, submittals reviewed, and testing and functional requirements finalized. The commissioning team, including the general contractor, subcontractors, manufacturers, and suppliers, coordinates through scoping and systems integration meetings. An issues log is created to communicate problems to the team and owner. Contractors complete field observations and checklists, which are reviewed by the commissioning professional. Functional performance tests are conducted with the commissioning professional as a witness, and a preliminary commissioning report is drafted.
- **During the Commissioning Phase:** Commissioning activities continue from earlier phases, with new ones added to address the following key elements:
  - Documenting system and workflow design intent, operating sequences, and testing and monitoring procedures
  - Verifying system and staff performance through extensive operational testing and measurement
  - Training building operations staff on system operation and maintenance procedures, and orienting staff to the new spaces and processes
  - Monitoring system and staff performance on an ongoing basis

Once the facility is operational, the organization can measure the outcomes of the goals set in the DOP (Design-Operation Plan) and evaluate the performance of the systems and processes identified during commissioning, as well as any other quality measures established. Some processes may have fluctuating measurements during the first few months of operation as they stabilize.

12.5 The Commissioning Team

The commissioning team is a group of professionals who work together to ensure that a building or facility is designed, constructed, and operated to meet the OPR. The team typically includes (but is not limited to) representatives from the following disciplines:

- Owner
- Architect/engineer
- Commissioning professional
- Contractors and subcontractors
- Representatives of project team dealing with particular services/systems
- Representatives of equipment agencies
- Infection prevention and control specialist
- Facilities engineers and representatives from the maintenance team
- Staff representative(s) from the area(s) under construction

Who should commission a building depends on the type and scope of the project, the organization's preferences, and the budget and timeline for commissioning. A common approach is to appoint a commissioning authority to manage, coordinate, execute, and document the commissioning process. The commissioning professional can be an independent third party, a member of the organization's staff, or someone working under contract with the construction manager. The commissioning professional should represent the owner's interests and ensure that the building meets the OPR.

12.6 Commissioning a Building

Commissioning a building or a facility, as previously explained, pertains to the assessment and validation of the physical structures, components, and systems within a project. The commissioning plan designed for building commissioning is typically initiated at the commencement of the construction phase, and it undergoes periodic updates as equipment is progressively installed and tested. This comprehensive process involves a meticulous examination of project schedules, thorough scrutiny of contractor documents, and the evaluation of operation and maintenance manuals.

- **Performance Tests during Commissioning:** Commissioning plan must include comprehensive performance tests for each system and equipment, considering construction complexities. Commissioning personnel must work with contractors to conduct pre-functional performance tests throughout construction, prioritizing key systems, such as (but not limited to) the following:
  - Building envelope
  - Life safety
  - Heating, ventilation, and air conditioning (HVAC) systems
  - Controls
  - Plumbing systems
  - Medical gas and other specialty gas systems
  - Electrical system
  - Fire alarm system
  - Information technology
  - Fire protection system
  - Interior and exterior lighting
  - Refrigeration
  - Vertical transport
  - Materials and pharmaceutical handling
- **Maintaining and Using a Commissioning Issues Log:** The Commissioning Issues Log is a critical document in the process of commissioning a building. It is a collaborative effort between the design team and the organization to ensure that the building looks and functions as intended. The Commissioning Issues Log lists all deficiencies and malfunctions that must be addressed before the building can be fully occupied, such as malfunctioning equipment, incorrect finishes, and improper hardware. The contract requires the contractor to address all Commissioning Issues Log items before the organization accepts the facility and releases final payment.

- **Using Checklists in Commissioning Process Management:** The checklists for commissioning a building help organization in managing the building commissioning process as the using checklists verify all aspects of building design, construction, and systems. Organizations can customize checklists for each project, using construction documents and changes made during construction. Creating checklists is a time-consuming process, but checklists can be an invaluable tool for streamlining the commissioning process.
- **Documenting the Commissioning Process:** In order to streamline the process of commissioning the building and ensuring comprehensive oversight, it is imperative for organizations to meticulously document the entire process of commissioning, encompassing acceptance parameters and Commissioning Issues Log items. Project personnel or the commissioning team should conduct regular reviews of this documented process during the commissioning phase, facilitating ongoing awareness of Commissioning Issues Log concerns and the corresponding steps taken to address them.

12.7 Familiarization with the Building

Organizations must plan extensive orientation for all staff using the new facility.

Orientation should be documented individually for each staff member and cover all aspects of the new space, including equipment, access to supplies, and cleaning procedures. Support staff are often overlooked in orientation, but they should be included as their duties may be significantly affected by the new space. Checklists of all new equipment, systems, and processes should be complete and documented before orientation begins. These lists can be formulated throughout the design process and updated as needed. Staff orientation and training records must be available for the post-occupancy evaluation. These records must show complete documentation of the training process, including content and dates of completion. In addition to intradepartmental training, all staff users of the new facility should learn the location, transport pathways, and access methods to all departments. This will enable them to confidently assist patients and visitors with wayfinding.

12.8 Simulations

Building simulation is a computer-based process that uses mathematical models to test how building design elements will perform under real-world conditions. It enables architects and engineers to evaluate the performance of their designs before construction begins. Users provide information such as climate data, lighting requirements, and occupancy profiles to the simulation software. The software then uses this information to calculate factors such as indoor temperature, fresh air rates, CO_2 levels, and energy consumption. Building simulation is a valuable tool for simplifying the complexity of modern buildings, especially as they become more intelligent and interconnected. It can help designers to ensure that buildings are comfortable and safe for occupants while also meeting energy efficiency and cost requirements. Simulations are important during commissioning because they can do the following:

- Reveal interactions between the building, occupants, HVAC systems, and the outdoor climate.

- Facilitate the use of environmentally and energy-efficient design solutions.
- Predict the performance of a building, including its impact on occupants and its site.
- Characterize and assess proposed new equipment and system integration ideas.
- Evaluate wind loads externally and ensure indoor air quality.
- Test operational and safety factors on-site.

12.9 Commissioning of Clinical Operations

Commissioning of clinical operations is the process of preparing a new or renovated health care facility for clinical operations. It is a complex and multidisciplinary process that involves a variety of stakeholders, including health care providers, clinical engineers, architects, and construction managers. Commissioning of clinical operations typically includes the following steps:

- **Planning:** The commissioning of clinical operations team develops a plan that outlines the scope of work, timeline, and budget for the commissioning process.
- **System Testing:** The commissioning of clinical operations team tests all of the clinical systems in the facility to ensure that they are functioning properly. This includes testing medical equipment, building management systems, and communication systems.
- **Integration:** The commissioning of clinical operations team integrates the clinical systems with each other and with the facility's overall infrastructure.
- **Training:** The commissioning of clinical operations team provides training to health care staff on how to use the new clinical systems.
- **Validation:** The commissioning of clinical operations team validates the clinical systems to ensure that they are meeting the needs of health care providers and patients.
- **Seven Medical Flows:** The seven types of medical flows compose the majority of routine and clinical work flow processes in a health care facility
  - Patients
  - Providers
  - Visitors and families
  - Supplies
  - Equipment
  - Medication
  - Information

Commissioning of clinical operations is an essential part of ensuring that new or renovated health care facilities are safe and efficient for clinical operations. It helps to identify and resolve any potential problems before they can impact patient care. Here are some specific examples of tasks that may be performed during commissioning of clinical operations:

- Testing and calibration of medical equipment
- Verifying building management systems, such as temperature control and ventilation
- Integrating clinical systems with electronic health records (EHRs) and other IT systems
- Training health care staff on how to use new clinical systems
- Conducting mock drills and simulations to test the facility's readiness for emergency situations

Commissioning of clinical operations is a critical step in ensuring that new or renovated health care facilities are able to provide high-quality care to patients.

12.10 Shifting to the New Building

Opening a new or renovated health care facility is a complex process. Organizations must decide which services to open first and how to move existing services. This planning should begin months in advance and involve an interdisciplinary team which can help manage the transition and resolve issues quickly. This team should be staffed by personnel from all relevant departments, including clinical operations, facilities management, and IT.

Once shifted to the new building, commissioning tasks from the initial commissioning contract continue throughout the typical one-year warranty period, known as the shakedown period or the defect liability period. During this time, the building will usually be managed and maintained by the contractor. The focus is on closing out the commissioning for the project, clearing defects, and finalizing any outstanding documentation/reports.

12.11 Post-Occupancy Evaluation

Evaluating a facility's operation against the original brief, planning policies, and design can identify both successes and deficiencies in the building and its operational systems, providing valuable feedback for future projects. A post-occupancy evaluation (POE) is not an exercise in fault-finding; it recognizes that many decisions made throughout the project life cycle have varying levels of success. A POE should reveal the following:

- Deficiencies in the design that can be remedied easily
- Where previously accepted design principles are giving trouble in practice
- Design features that have proved to be expensive in terms of running costs
- Where accepted design principles are working well

The results of a POE should be used to do the following:

- Assess the design principles and space allocation.
- Identify issues that require further research or expert input.

- Promote successful solutions in future projects.
- Avoid costly errors or mistakes that compromise functionality or efficiency in capital works projects.

12.12 Commissioning Budget

Commissioning has both monetary and time costs. Organizations must hire a third-party commissioning professional or pay the contractor for commissioning efforts, and organization representatives who perform commissioning tasks must be given time in their schedules to do so effectively. This may require temporarily reassigning their regular job duties to others. Organizations should therefore factor the timing and monetary aspects of commissioning into their project budget.

12.13 Benefits of Commissioning

Commissioning a building can have several benefits:

- Lower energy and operational costs
- Fewer change orders and other claims
- Fewer deficiencies at substantial completion
- Managed and documented start-up procedures
- Smoother building turnover
- Value-added construction quality and fewer project delays
- Preventing expensive breakdowns
- Creating better indoor conditions for occupants
- Improving occupant comfort
- Leading to more stable occupancy rates and higher rents
  Commissioning can also help to do the following:
  - Optimize energy and water use.
  - Facilitate O&M staff orientation and training.
  - Improve installed building systems documentation and operations.

12.14 Summary

Building commissioning is a critical process that ensures that a building's systems and equipment perform as intended. Building commissioning is an investment that pays off in the long run, resulting in reduced energy costs, improved occupant comfort, extended life of building assets, and a more sustainable building.

References

Chapter	Reference
1A.	International Facility Management Association (IFMA). *Strategic Facility Plan: A White Paper*. IFMA, 2009. https://community.ifma.org/cfs-file/__key/telligent-evolution-components-attachments/13-463-00-00-01-05-69-96/2009_5F00_Strategic-Facility-Planning_5F00_White-Paper.pdf.
	Reno K, Okland K, Finis N, LaMantia G, Call R, Cardon K, Gerber D, Zeigler J. Lessons learned: Clinicians' post-occupancy perspective of facility design involvement. HERD: Health Environments Research & Design Journal. 2014;7(2):127–139.
	Lavy S, Dixit MK. Wall finish selection in hospital design: A survey of facility managers. HERD: Health Environments Research & Design Journal. 2012;5(2):80–98.
1B.	The World Bank. *Establishing Private Healthcare Facilities in Developing Countries: A Guide for Medical Entrepreneurs*. The World Bank, 2007. The Prefeasibility Analysis and the Feasibility Analysis; pp. 19–66.
2.	WHO. District hospital facilities: guidelines for development and operations; Western Pacific Series No. 22; 1998. https://apps.who.int/iris/bitstream/handle/10665/207020/9290611219_eng.pdf?sequence=1&isAllowed=y.
	Varnawalla H, Desai V. Hospital design guide: How to get started. www.academia.edu/4237726/Hospital_Design_Guide_How_to_get_started_Contents.
3.	10 Elements of the Perfect Hospital Design—Architizer Journal 2019 [Internet]. https://architizer.com/blog/practice/details/perfect-hospital-design/.
	Hospital design challenges: Now and into the future [Internet]. http://hospitalhealth.com.au/content/design-in-health/article/hospital-design-challenges-now-and-into-the-future-1050121645.
	Indmedica—Journal of the Academy of Hospital Administration [Internet]. www.indmedica.com/journals.php?journalid=6&issueid=25&articleid=238&action=article.
	Major issues and trends impacting health and hospital planning, design, construction, operation and maintenance [Internet]. www.asianhhm.com/facilities-operations/issues-trends-hospital-planning-design.
	Factors to consider in hospital design and construction [Internet]. https://philippiqualityconstruction.com/factors-to-consider-in-hospital-design-and-construction/.
	6 Things to consider before planning and designing of a new hospital [Internet]. www.shareyouressays.com/knowledge/6-things-to-consider-before-planning-and-designing-of-a-new-hospital/115954.
	Hospital design and planning guide [Internet]. www.jrmcm.com/jrm-news/hospital-design-planning-guide/.
4.	HSCC (India) Ltd. Detailed project report for proposed Advanced Neuroscience Centre at PGIMER, Chandigarh. www.environmentclearance.nic.in/writereaddata/EC/050720199ML2ZKG7DPRPGIMER.pdf.
	Detailed project report for operation and management services at Narayana Hrudayalaya Bharuch Hospital. http://gcsra.org/writereaddata/images/pdf/Bharuch-Hospital-Project.pdf.
	Ram Sharada Healthcare Pvt. Ltd. Multi-Specialty Hospital Project report. www.codexgpo.com/upload/consultancy/codex_report.pdf.
	KIIFB. Template for preparation of detailed project report. www.google.co.in/url?sa=i&rct=j&q=&esrc=s&source=web&cd=&cad=rja&uact=8&ved=0CAQQw7AJahcKEwiAx7-s2-P4AhUAAAAAHQAAAAAQAg&url=https%3A%2F%2Fkiifb.org%2Fincludes%2FfileViewer.jsp%3Ffmde%3Dres%26did%3D29%26fname%3DHealthDPRTemplate.pdf%26dPrfx%3DDWD&psig=AOvVaw1daPtsnhonYBorS0x3Tlp9&ust=1657177865984650.
	Hospital with teaching facility—detailed project report. www.entrepreneurindia.co/Document/Download/pdfanddoc-579263-.pdf.
5.	Steyn JW, Buys CP. Project optimisation techniques: Site Selection for Process Plants. Owner Team Consultation; 2017 Mar. [Accessed 2022 June 17].
	Greyhill Advisors. The site selection process, Undated. http://greyhill.com/site-selection-process.
	Deloitte Touche Tohmatsu Limited. 12 mistakes to avoid in the site selection process: Implementing an effective corporate location strategy. https://www2.deloitte.com/us/en/pages/operations/articles/twelve-mistakes-to-avoid-site-selection-process.html.
	Four criteria for selecting health care sites: Setting priorities will help to streamline the facility site selection process. www.hfmmagazine.com/articles/3116-four-criteria-for-selecting-health-care-sites.
	Site Plan. www.designingbuildings.co.uk/wiki/Site_plan.
	What is an Architectural Site Plan. www.firstinarchitecture.co.uk/what-is-an-architectural-site-plan/.
	Site plans—what they are and how to create one. www.roomsketcher.com/site-plans/.
	Site Plan. https://cedreo.com/site-plans/.
	Site plans: Purpose, types and requirements. www.prodyogi.com/2020/04/what-is-site-plan-what-is-purpose-of.html.
6.	Al Zarooni S, Abdou A, Lewis J. Improving the client briefing for UAE public healthcare projects: Space programming guidelines. Architectural Engineering and Design Management. 2011;7(4):251–265.
	Alberta Health Services. Functional program framework for health capital projects. https://open.alberta.ca/dataset/31eb4a0d-b5ae-4979-8889-56ed732dfbda/resource/5883d89c-277d-4cec-97f9-5208cecf9891/download/appendix-7.pdf.

The Centre for Health Design. Functional program process guide. www.healthdesign.org/tools/functional-program-guide.

Colliers Project Leaders. Why is functional programming important in healthcare? www.colliersprojectleaders.com/insights/why-is-functional-programming-important-in-healthcare#gref.

7. Ministry of Urban Development, GoI. Harmonized guidelines and space standards for barrier free build environment for persons with disability and elderly persons, February 2016. https://cpwd.gov.in/publication/harmonisedguidelinesdreleasedon23rd-march2016.pdf.

Scott Openshaw, Allsteel et al. Ergonomics and design: A reference guide [Internet]. https://ehs.oregonstate.edu/sites/ehs.oregon-state.edu/files/pdf/ergo/ergonomicsanddesignreferenceguidewhitepaper.pdf.

Anthropometry in architecture design [Internet] https://urbandesignlab.in/anthropometry-in-architecture-design-urban-design-lab/.

8. Allen E, Iano J. *The Architect's Studio Companion: Rules of Thumb for Preliminary Design*, 6th Edition. John Wiley & Sons, 2017.

Boecker J, Horst S, Keiter T, Lau A, Sheffer M, Toevs B. *The Integrative Design Guide to Green Buildings: Redefining the Practice of Sustainability.* Hoboken, NJ: John Wiley & Sons; 2009.

Hamilton DK, Watkins D. *Evidence-Based Design for Multiple Building Types.* John Wiley & Sons, 2009.

Ostime N. *RIBA Job Book*, 9th Edition. RIBA Publishing, 2013.

Royal Architectural Institute of Canada. *Canadian Standard Form of Contract for Architectural Services Document Six.* RAIC, 2018.

Sinclair D. *Guide to Using the RIBA Plan of Work 2013.* RIBA Publishing, 2013.

Sinclair D. *Assembling a Collaborative Project Team: Practical Tools Including Multidisciplinary Schedule of Services.* RIBA Publishing, 2014.

WBDG Aesthetics Subcommittee. *Engage the Integrated Design Process.* Whole Building Design Guide, October 17, 2016. www.wbdg.org/design-objectives/aesthetics/engage-integrated-design-process

9. A master class in construction plans: Blueprints, construction safety plans, and quality plans [Internet]. www.smartsheet.com/how-to-read-construction-plans.

Types of drawings used in building construction [Internet]. https://theconstructor.org/building/drawing-types-construction/24524/.

Building drawing and its types: A comprehensive guide [Internet]. https://civilseek.com/building-drawing/.

List of civil drawings required for building construction [Internet]. www.aboutcivil.org/list-drawings-buildings.html.

Types of drawing for building design [Internet]. www.designingbuildings.co.uk/wiki/Types_of_drawings_for_building_design.

Different types of drawings used in building construction [Internet]. https://civiconcepts.com/blog/construction-drawings.

Zhang HB, Chen JJ, Zhao XS, Wang JH, Hu H. Displacement performance and simple prediction for deep excavations supported by contiguous bored pile walls in soft clay. Journal of Aerospace Engineering. 2015;28(6):A4014008.

Nandy UK, Nandy S, Nandy A. Approaches to beam, slab & staircase designing using limit state design method for achieving optimal stability conditions. International Journal of Engineering Research. 2016; Feb 1:545–548.

Dhoopati S, Chenna R. Seismic performance assessment of a G+ 4 school building in Gujarat, Ahmadabad. Asian Journal of Civil Engineering. 2021;22(2):205–215.

10. Afsari K, Eastman CM. *A Comparison of Construction Classification Systems Used for Classifying Building Product Models.* 52nd ASC Annual International Conference Proceedings, April 2016.

Demkin JA (ed.). American Institute of Architects. *The Architect's Handbook of Professional Practice.* John Wiley & Sons Inc., 2013.

Guthrie P. *Cross-Check: Integrating Building Systems and Working Drawings.* McGraw-Hill, 1998.

Nigro WT. *RediCheck Interdisciplinary Coordination*, 6th Edition. The RediCheck Firm, 2015. www.redicheck-review.com/TheSystem/RedicheckBook.aspx.

"United States National CAD Standard—V6." National Institute of Building Science, 2017. www.nationalcadstandard.org/ncs6.

Canadian Construction Documents Committee (CCDC). *CCDC 23–2018: A Guide to Calling Bids and Awarding Construction Contracts.* CCDC.

Klien RM (ed.). The American Institute of Architects. *The Architect's Handbook of Professional Practice*, 15th Edition. John Wiley & Sons, 2014.

Environmental Protection Agency. Federal green construction guide for specifiers. *Whole Building Design Guide.* www.wbdg.org/ffc/epa/federal-green-construction-guide-specifiers.

National Research Council Canada. *Canadian National Master Construction Specification (NMS).* https://nrc.canada.ca/en/certifications-evaluations-standards/canadian-national-master-construction-specification.

National Research Council Canada. *NMS User's Guide*, 2017. https://nrc.canada.ca/en/certifications-evaluations-standards/canadian-national-master-construction-specification/nms-users-guide.

Stitt FA. *Construction Specifications Portable Handbook.* McGraw-Hill, 1999.

11. Bartley JM. APIC state-of-the-art report: The role of infection control during construction in health care facilities. American Journal of Infection Control. 2000;28(2):156–169.

Premier Inc. Definition of ICRA. www.premiersafetyinstitute.org/safety-topics-az/building-design/infection-control-risk-assessment-icra.

Premier Inc. Tools & resources for ICRA. www.premiersafetyinstitute.org/wp-content/uploads/ICRA-MatrixColorRevised-091109.pdf.

12. ASHRAE. The strategic guide to commissioning. www.ashrae.org/file%20library/technical%20resources/bookstore/english-ashrae_bpa-brochure_fnl_6-24-14.pdf.

Whole Building Design Guide. Building commissioning: The process. www.wbdg.org/building-commissioning.

GSA. The building commissioning guide. www.gsa.gov/cdnstatic/BCG_3_30_Final_R2-x221_0Z5RDZ-i34K-pR.pdf.

BCA. Essential attributes of building commissioning. www.bcxa.org/about-us/essential-attributes.html.

American Society of Healthcare Engineers (ASHE). *Health Facility Commissioning Handbook: Optimizing Building System Performance in New and Existing Health Care Facilities*. ASHE, 2012.

Operations Commissioning: Putting New Healthcare Buildings to the Test. https://healthcaredesignmagazine.com/architecture/operations-commissioning-putting-new-healthcare-buildings-test/.

Status in Whales. Capital investment manual: Commissioning a healthcare facility. www.wales.nhs.uk/sites3/documents/254/CIM%20Commissioning.pdf.

13 EMERGENCY DEPARTMENT (ED)

The public needs a service for dealing with accidents and emergencies 24 hours a day throughout the year. The Emergency Department (ED) in a hospital is the main institutional provider of emergency treatment for major accidents and illness. EDs are designated clinical areas in which patients receive immediate and urgent care, ideally provided by specialists in Emergency Medicine, with support from other specialties as required. It is the health care entry point responsible for receiving, sorting, assessing, stabilizing, and managing patients arriving at its door with different degrees of urgency and complexity. Conditions of patients requiring emergency care vary from major trauma and stroke to intoxication and mental disorders. Therefore, an ED is considered to be an extremely complex system.

The Accident & Emergency (A&E) Reference Group of the London Implementation Group defined the primary tasks of an A&E department as providing the following:

- Resuscitation and immediate treatment for the critically ill and injured.
- A diagnostic and treatment service for the less seriously ill and injured patients who merit urgent hospital attention.
- A diagnostic and treatment service for those with conditions that allow them to be subsequently discharged.

ED design is influenced by the needs of patients, ED staff requirements and the characteristics of Emergency Medicine (Table 13A and Figure 13A).

13.1 ED and Wider Hospital Context

EDs need to be placed in an area of the hospital that is easily accessible to emergency vehicles entering the site. The situation must allow ease of access and egress from the department. ED clinical areas should be on the ground floor. An ED department operates in the context of an entire hospital, whose parts are interdependent in function. ED is a mini hospital within a hospital.

13.2 Models of Care

Operational Models: The Emergency Unit may be configured in a number of models that are aimed at improving efficiency

TABLE 13A: Characteristics of Emergency Medicine That Influence ED Design

- High levels of activity
- High patient turnover
- Varied case mix
- Large multi-disciplinary workforce
- Need for efficiency of process
- Infection control requirements
- Access issues
- Interface with pre-hospital services
- Multiple interactions with in-hospital specialties/patient transfers
- Communications issues
- Potential for growth
- Teaching activities
- Major incident capacity
- Responsiveness to local service demands/social issues
- Administrative functions—Emergency Medicine specific
- Possibility of aggression/assault—security issues

of treatment and may influence facility design. The majority of Emergency Units will have a number of these models in operation.

(a) **Triage & Registration:** Patient assessment in Triage occurs first followed by initial registration by clerical staff. In this model, Reception and Triage are collocated. The patient is rapidly assessed and assigned to the appropriate care zone. A variation of this model includes a senior nurse to manage patients in the waiting room to continually review patients who have been triaged and are awaiting treatment. This initiative may be implemented to improve patient safety and quality of care as the nurse can escalate access to care as needed.

(b) **Patient Streaming:** In this model, the patient is first triaged and registered in a rapid triage model and transferred to a streaming zone for assessment by a senior Emergency Physician. A streaming zone nurse coordinates patients through the streaming area into an Early Treatment Zone.

(c) **Early Treatment Zone:** The Early Treatment Zone is a separate clinical area where patients are managed for a short time and then moved to another area of the Emergency Unit such as acute care or the waiting area for patients waiting on results before discharge. This model works in conjunction with other models such as Acute Care, Non-Acute Observation, Fast Track, and Short Stay Units, as well as mental health assessment.

(d) **Fast Track:** Specific patient groups may be assessed and treated via a separate "fast" track to other Emergency Unit presentations. This may occur at the triage point or immediately after triage but in a separate zone. Patient types suitable for this area are ambulant with non-complex conditions such as contagious diseases, minor injuries, and paediatric illnesses. Assessment and treatment may be carried out in consult/examination rooms and the majority of patients discharged to home.

(e) **Grouping by Patient Acuity:** Patients of similar acuity (urgency) or staff intensity may be treated in the same zone. Facilities for this model include separate areas for resuscitation, acute monitored beds, acute non-monitored beds and ambulatory treatment spaces. There may be separate entry points (or triage points) for the different areas. Staff may be separately allocated to different areas for each shift and may require separate staff stations and private workspace. Examples of Grouping by Patient Acuity include the following:

(i) **Resuscitation & Trauma:** This model sets out how resuscitation and trauma patients are assessed and managed in order to streamline the process and ensure that the correct team and diagnostic services are available. This model ensures that when emergency or trauma patients arrive, trained staff are available to attend.

(ii) **Acute Care:** The Acute Care model is aimed at assessment and treatment of patients who are acute or unstable with complex illnesses. Acute care may be provided in a separate zone or allocated beds that require a higher level of care and endeavours to improve the patient's access to specialist care and minimize delays. The acute care environment typically uses a standardized clinical environment for each treatment space by using the principles of lean thinking.

DOI: 10.1201/9780367460884-14

(iii) **Non-Acute Care:** Non-acute care involves assessment of the patient to determine their need for monitoring or interventional care. Patients in this category do not require acute care or monitoring but have complex conditions that require observation, investigation, discharge planning, or follow-up and are not suitable for Fast Track care. Non-Acute Care patients are allocated to a separate treatment area or a Short Stay Unit.

(f) **Grouping by Specialty:** Patients may be managed in different areas according to the specialty of service that they require, for example, paediatric assessment and observation or mental health assessment and emergency care. Patients may be triaged from a central arrival point or from separate ambulance and ambulant entry points. Within each functional area, patients would be prioritized according to acuity. In this model, separate specialist staffing for each area is required, which would also include workspaces for staff.

(g) **Short Stay Unit:** The Short Stay Unit is also known as an Emergency Medical Unit or Clinical Decision Unit and is a separate unit located adjacent to or incorporated into the Emergency Unit. This may allow sharing of administrative, staff, and support facilities. Patients suitable for the Short Stay Unit require observation, diagnostic services, therapy, or follow-up that may take up to 24 hours. These patients are typically discharged home or admitted to an Inpatient Unit if their condition remains unresolved. Short Stay Units provide efficiency by improving both the patient flow through the Emergency Unit and bed management in the hospital by avoiding short-term inpatient admissions.

(h) **Urgent Primary Care/Urgent Care Centre:** Hospitals with a Role Delineation Level of 1 to 3 may provide an Urgent Primary Care Unit also known as an Urgent Care Centre instead of an Emergency Unit that can undertake basic resuscitation, stabilization, and minor procedures with medical services provided by local General Practitioners (GPs) supported by Registered Nurses. The Urgent Care Centre generally operates on a long-day basis, and some operate 24 hours per day, providing an extended late-hour GP service. The Urgent Care Centre should have links to a network of local health services so that patients requiring more specialized care can be transferred to a higher-level Emergency Unit.

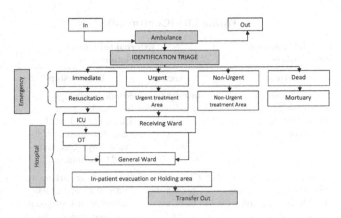

FIGURE 13A Flowchart for the Emergency Department.

TABLE 13C: Key Result Areas and Quality Indicators for the Emergency Department

Key Result Areas

- Policies and procedures on "dead on arrival", transfer/discharge process, non-availability of beds
- Identified area for emergency care, defined beds
- Triage
- Medicolegal Case
- Access to ED
- Disaster management
- Quality assurance
- BMW
- Ambulance communication
- Infection control
- Medication management
- Case records—documentation
- Cardiopulmonary resuscitation
- Fire safety
- Equipment/furniture maintenance
- Medical gas

Quality Indicators

- Time for initial assessment of patients
- Percentage of medication charts with error-prone abbreviations
- Return to ED within 72 hours with similar presenting complaints
- Hand hygiene compliance rate
- Time taken for discharge
- Patient fall rate
- Compliance with medication prescription in capitals
- Number of variations in mock drills (disaster management)

TABLE 13B: Factors in Planning of ED Services

1	Location: Rural/Semi-Urban/Urban
2	Industries in drainage areas
3	Population Characteristics
4	Communication Facilities
5	Patient Load/Morbidity Patterns
6	Regional Emergency Services
7	Architectural Design of Hospitals

Other Planning Parameters

8	ED visits increase by 5% to 6% every year.
9	Admissions through ED are 16% to 30% and include 10% of the OPD workload.
10	Peak load of ED is 1700 h to 0100 h.

TABLE 13D: Functional Relationships of the Emergency Department

Internal Functional Relationships	External Functional Relationships	
Area	Area	Relationship
Entrance/waiting room/reception area	Hospital access/egress	Close relationship desirable for patient and relative wayfinding after-hours access and egress parking/public transport

(Continued)

TABLE 13D: (Continued)

Internal Functional Relationships	External Functional Relationships	
Area	Area	Relationship
Triage area resuscitation area; acute treatment area; consultation area	Investigative modalities	Satellite radiology Satellite laboratory Larger ED: dedicated radiology units with plain radiology, ultrasound, and CT scanning
Adjunctive areas (x-ray, Short Stay Unit, allied health, investigation room (point-of-care testing)) Staff/amenities areas Administrative areas Storage areas	Close proximity to other acute services	Reserved car parking for on-call anaesthetists, obstetricians, surgeons; helipad; angiography suite; high-dependency unit; coronary care; intensive care; operating theatre; and clear unencumbered route to wards
Clean preparation and drug preparation room(s); Dirty utility and disposal areas Patient amenities areas, e.g., a food storage fridge that meets OH&S standards for patient sandwiches (for after hours) Toilet (for staff and patients including disabled patients) and bathroom/shower facilities Teaching and research areas	In the event of mass casualty incidents	Communications/ command/media centre; outpatient areas (for ambulatory patients); and open areas, e.g., car parks for mass decontamination requiring state/regional emergency services

TABLE 13E(i): Major Space Determinants and ED Size

Clinical Est Act of India

Level 2 Hosp	Emergency bed and surrounding space	10.5 sq m/bed
	Other areas such as a nurse station, doctor duty room, clean and dirty utility areas, dressing area, toilets	Nurse station out of circulation Doctor duty room of 7 sq m and a toilet of 3.5 sq m Store of 7 sq m
Level 3 Hosp	Emergency bed and surrounding space	10.5 sq m/bed: in addition circulation space of 30% as indicated in total area should provide for a nurse station, doctor duty room, clean and dirty utility areas, dressing area, toilet, etc.

TABLE 13E(ii): Provision for Various Floor Areas in the Accident and Emergency Department

S No.	FACILITY	CATEGORY A		CATEGORY B		CATEGORY C		CATEGORY D		CATEGORY E	
		ROOM (NO.)	Area (m²)	ROOM (NO.)	Area (m²)	ROOM (NO.)	Area (m²)	ROOM (NO.)	Area (m²)	ROOM (NO.)	Area (m²)
(1)	(2)	(3)	(4)	(5)	(6)	(7)	(8)	(9)	(10)	(11)	(12)
EMERGENCY DEPARTMENT											
(a)	Drive in ambulance		—		—	1	17.5	1	17.5	1	17.5
(b)	Doctor duty room with toilet	1	10.5	2	10.5	3	10.5	4	10.5	4–6	10.5
(c)	Examination cubicle		—		—	1	10.5	1	10.5	1	10.5
(d)	Medicolegal specimen and records room	—			—	1	10.5	1	10.5	1	10.5
(e)	Brought in dead room	—		1	10.5	1	10.5	1	14	1	17.5
(f)	Retiring room for ambulance driver and nursing assistant	—		1	10.5	1	14	1	14	1	14
(g)	ECG room		—	1	10.5	1	14	1	14	1	14
(h)	Fracture treatment room with plaster preparation		—	1	17.5	1	17.5	1	17.5	1	17.5
(i)	Treatment room		—		—	1	14	1	14	1	14
	Operating theatre		(OT)								
(j)	OT	1	17.5	1	21	2	21	1	33	1	33
(k)	Instrument sterilization	1	7.0	1	7.0	1	10.5	1	10.5	1	10.5

(Continued)

TABLE 13E(ii): (Continued)

S No. (1)	FACILITY (2)	CATEGORY A		CATEGORY B		CATEGORY C		CATEGORY D		CATEGORY E	
		ROOM (NO.) (3)	Area (m²) (4)	ROOM (NO.) (5)	Area (m²) (6)	ROOM (NO.) (7)	Area (m²) (8)	ROOM (NO.) (9)	Area (m²) (10)	ROOM (NO.) (11)	Area (m²) (12)
(l)	Scrub-up		—	1	7.0	1	7.0	1	10.5	1	10.5
(m)	Dirty wash		—	1	7.0	1	7.0	1	10.5	1	10.5
(n)	Anaesthesia room		—		—	1	10.5	1	10.5	1	10.5
(o)	Resuscitation room		—	1	21	1	35	1	42	1	63
(p)	X-ray with dark room facilities		—	1	21	1	28	1	35	1	35
(q)	Clinical laboratory	1	17.5	1	17.5	1	17.5	1	21	1	21
(r)	Blood storage area	—			—	1	10.5	1	10.5	1	10.5
(s)	Drug-dispensing facility		—		—	1	10.5	1	10.5	1	10.5
(t)	Stores		—		—	1	14	2	14	3	14
(u)	Sluice room and janitor closet		—	1	10.5	1	10.5	1	10.5	1	10.5
(v)	Nurse station with toilet		—		—	1	17.5	1	17.5	1	17.5
(w)	Observation room	1	14	1	21	1	28	1	35	1	52.5
(x)	Emergency ward	—		1	8 BEDS	1	12 BEDS	1	20 BEDS	1	14 BEDS
(y)	Pantry	—		1	10.5	1	10.5	1	10.5	1	10.5

Layout & Zoning (Figure 13B)

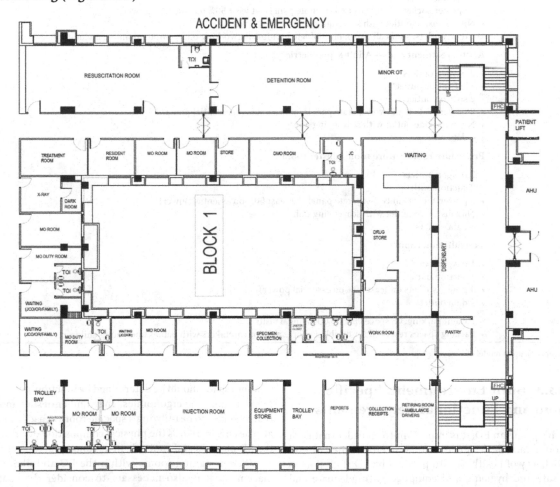

FIGURE 13B   Sample Layout of an Emergency Department.

Built Environment: General Considerations (Table 13G)

TABLE 13G: General Considerations for Built Environment in an Emergency Department

Wayfinding	**Purpose** • Integrated with the hospital-wide system • Utilizes the same styles and conventions • Major intersection and destination • Electronic wayfinding and/or information kiosks are becoming common **Other considerations** • Wayfinding lines on the floor: infection control issues, so wayfinding directions may need to be on the wall • Braille signage for visually impaired • Hearing loop system or an infrared system to assist people using hearing aids
Finishes & Robustness	• Robust and easily cleaned with hospital disinfectants, without deterioration • Bed bumpers and reinforcing in walls are desirable
Lighting	**Purpose** • Mimic the diurnal rhythm through the dimming of lights at night-time • Glare should be eliminated • Electric lighting should be designed to supplement and balance incoming daylight • Clinical area equipped with task lighting (30,000 lux) • General lighting to minimize glare • Dimmable lighting in patient treatment spaces is ideal
Infection control standards & hand hygiene	**Purpose** • Basins with hands-free taps/sensors based in all clinical areas and patient cubicles • **Alcohol-based hand rubs (ABHRs)** • Readily available and mounted on walls, trollies, etc. in all clinical areas
Service panels	**Resuscitation room (for each patient space)** • 3 oxygen outlets • Medical air outlet* • 3 suction outlets • 16 power sockets in at least two separate panels (at least 50% on essential power) • Nitrous oxide outlet with scavenging unit* • 6 data outlets: staff call panel; physiologic monitor networking plus remote monitor; includes phone and computer **Acute treatment beds—Adult & paediatric** • 2 oxygen outlets • Medical air outlet* • 2 suction outlets • 8 power sockets in two separate panels (at least 50% on essential power) • Nitrous oxide outlet with scavenging unit* • 4 data outlets **Procedure room/suture room/plaster room** • 2 oxygen outlets • 2 suction outlets • 8 power sockets in two separate panels (at least 50% on essential power) • Nitrous oxide outlet with scavenging unit* • 6 data outlets **Consultation room** • 1 oxygen outlet • 1 suction outlet • 4 power sockets (at least 50% on essential power) • 4 data outlets
Parking	• Patient parking: 06 spaces per 10,000 annual visits • Parking spaces reserved for disabled people and for caretakers with babies and young children

* Desirable/depends upon model of care

13.3 Built Environment: Specific Room and Functional Requirements

When designing an ED, it is important to consider that each specific room must be designed in order to ensure the safe and efficient delivery of health care to patients by ED staff. Rooms must be safe and hygienic and equipped with adequate and secure storage and the required medical equipment.

Room space should be determined by function, activity, equipment, station, and ergonomics. The number of staff and patients that are likely to be utilizing a specific room at a given time must also be considered, as the physical composition of a room within the ED plays a significant role in its functional capacity.

When designing rooms within the ED and planning their placement, it is also necessary to consider the spatial relationships between these rooms. Direct access from one specific room within the ED to another is often required, and it is therefore important to consider that swift access must be facilitated to and from rooms by both staff and patients (Table 13H).

TABLE 13H: Specific Room and Functional Requirements for Built Environment in the Emergency Department

Ambulance Bay/Ambulance Reception

Purpose	• At least 02 × Ambulance space with covered porch • Separate entrance for delivery of both ambulant and non-ambulant patients to the ED by the ambulance service • For size and specifications, refer to the National Ambulance Code of India • Secondary function as a decontamination zone and as a triage and/or treatment area for mass casualty incidents (MCIs)
Size	• Minimum of two spaces for each 4 × 6 m per vehicle is required • Allowance for an unloading space at the rear of the vehicle's side-door opening; manoeuvre stretchers and pedestrian access along both sides of a parked vehicle • Refer to the National Ambulance Code for India for patient ambulance specifications
Functional requirements	• Dedicated and separate ambulance vehicle access and egress • Signage including ground marking for vehicle bays • Adequate lighting • Ability to off-load and load patients safely • CCTV—usually with feedback to security, triage, and staff station where the nurse in charge is situated • Overhead and weather protection
Spatial relationships	• Direct access to triage or a dedicated ambulance triage area • Ideally, direct access to trauma/resuscitation rooms • Access to an ambulance-dedicated storeroom with cleaning facilities

Decontamination Room/Area

Purpose	To decontaminate patients who have CBRN agents; a decontamination area consists of • A de-robing area • A decontamination area including a water hose • A drying-off area • Entry to the ED proper
Size	Depends on a hospital's role in the regional or state emergency CBRN response to MCIs
Functional requirements	Flexible water hose, floor drain, and contaminated water trap with ventilation and drainage systems (independent and isolated); area to perform immediate life-saving measures by staff in PPE
Spatial relationships	Directly accessible from the ambulance bay with ingress to ED

Ambulance store

Purpose	• Re-stocking of ambulances that require rapid turnaround • Secure area for the return of ambulance equipment • A cleaning facility for ambulance and ambulance equipment • Rest area for ambulance personnel
Functional requirements	Space and equipment used to re-stock ambulances and cleaning equipment, including outside tap
Spatial relationships	• Ambulance bay • Internal access from triage area may be an advantage

Triage & Reception Area

Purpose	• Initial clinical assessment of patients and allocation of an urgency score • Single point of entry for acute patients • Provides controlled access to treatment areas and to the wider hospital • Should be designed so that the first point of contact for patients is the triage doctor/nurse
Size	The size is governed by the maximum number of triage staff expected to be present at any given time, in proportion to patient census
Functional requirements	• Triage assessment • Administration of simple treatment measures, e.g., dressing, analgesia, ice, and splinting • Security for staff and patients, e.g., duress alarm system and CCTV
Spatial relationships	• Ambulance and walk-in entrances • Internal hospital entrances if ED bypass from triage systems is in operation • Reception, incorporating the concept of "triage first" • Waiting room • Relationship of triage to areas used by nurses to rapidly perform electrocardiography (ECG) or take blood • Relationship of triage Fast Track/discharge areas • Location with respect to advanced Nurse Practitioners providing care • Relationship to x-ray department and wheelchair route for nurse-initiated x-rays • All acute treatment and assessment areas • Resuscitation, adult and paediatric assessment, and consultation areas

(Continued)

TABLE 13H: (Continued)

Other considerations	• The need for design to allow for staff to have a clear line of sight into the waiting room • The adoption of models of care incorporating medical triaging and RAT systems necessitate an appropriate increase in size in order to accommodate these additional functions • The ability to accommodate an additional Triage Nurse during busy periods • The ability to accommodate a waiting room nurse and their equipment requirements • Pneumatic tube system in the triage/reception area • Two-sided triage with the secondary triage assessment areas to reassess waiting room patients

Current trends	• A pneumatic tube system in the triage area for pathology specimens to be sent to a lab
	• Some EDs have placed less emphasis on traditional triage practices, adopting instead
	  • Arrival time-based initiation of treatment
	  • Streaming of patients to an appropriate area within the department
	  • Mobile triage and bedside triage

Patient Registration & Reception Area

Purpose	Electronic recording of the demographic details and generation of an Electronic Medical Card; at Reception, hard copy medical records are also retrieved
Size	Size is governed by the number of Reception workstations required for patient census
Functional requirements	• Dedicated registration area co-located with triage • Access to an electronic patient information entry portal • Mechanisms to ensure privacy for disclosed patient details and/or displayed patient information • Security of staff from any aggressive patients • Duress alarm • Online registration at the bedside
Spatial relationships	• Relationship with retrieval of hospital medical records • Relationship to a Triage Nurse, either as a triage and a registration pairing or as a separate area for registration only (following triage) • Relationship to the ambulant entrance of the ED (often a Registration Clerk is responsible for regulating entry and exit to the ED) • Relationship to the entrance of the hospital after hours • Design must allow for clinical staff to have a clear line of sight into the reception area

Waiting Room

Purpose	For patients to wait in both before and after triage, for entry to treatment areas, for waiting for transportation post-discharge, or for accompanying persons waiting
Size	Governed by the annual census and models of care

Functional requirements	• Observation of waiting patients for clinical and security reasons
	• Minimize patient agitation, e.g., décor including appropriate artwork, and lighting and seating arrangements
	• Maximize patient comfort by providing
	  • Ambient temperature control
	  • Access to food and drink
	  • Toilets
	  • Special requirements for the disabled, children, and mothers
	  • Patient information including signage and indication of wait times; access to written material and public health information
	  • Distractions from waiting, e.g., public television, magazines, and video entertainment for children
	  • Emergency call system, e.g., patient-activated in toilets
	  • External vehicle drop-off area and provision for short-term parking
	  • Facilities for communication, e.g., public phone and free taxi phone
	  • Facilities for the disabled
	  • Adequate signage and wayfinding
	  • Seating to accommodate mobility-aiding wheelchairs

Spatial relationships	• Triage • Reception • Ambulance and walk-in entrances • Clinical areas of the ED
Other considerations	• Colour-coded seating for zoning • An electronic display with current waiting times • Sub-waiting areas within the ED • Facilities for charging mobile phones and electronic devices • Electronic systems that allow patients to be in other areas of the hospital whilst waiting and then be recalled when they can be seen by a clinician

(Continued)

TABLE 13H: (Continued)

Trauma & Resuscitation Rooms

Purpose	• A trauma room provides reception, assessment, and initiation of treatment of patients who have been subjected to major trauma
	• A resuscitation room provides reception, assessment, and initiation of treatment for patients who have life-threatening or time-critical illness
Size	• Trauma room should be at least 30 m²
	• Resuscitation room should be at least 252 m²
Functional requirements	• Assembly area for the trauma team with ability to assign roles and gown up
	• Rapid reception of patients from waiting room, ambulance bay, or helipad
	• Rapid off-loading from ambulance stretcher to ED trolley with minimal manoeuvres
	• A central mobile trauma trolley with 360-degree access to patients
	• All medication and equipment at hand and stored in or immediately adjacent to the room
	• Adequate floor space to accommodate mobile equipment, e.g., ultrasound machine
	• Adequate shelving to accommodate medication and equipment required for trauma care
	• Adequate space to accommodate the maximal personnel concurrently involved in treating a patient
Spatial relationships	• Access from the waiting room, ambulance bay, or helipad
	• CT scanner should be close to resuscitation room
	• Ready access to the radiology department and operating theatre/Intensive Care Unit
	• Desirable for resuscitation rooms to be equipped for radiology
	• Relationship to the distressed relatives' room that provides for privacy of relatives in the room and in transit to the trauma/resuscitation rooms
Other considerations	• Fully digital radiology may improve the function of a trauma/resuscitation area
	• An example of excellent resuscitation design is several identical rooms that are all interconnected
	• The ability to maintain patient privacy whilst allowing ready access and monitoring by clinical staff
	• Use of pendants rather than wall-mounted service panels
	• Adjacent equipment stores for portable equipment and other commonly used items
	• Ceiling rail for IV fluids (though trolleys with IV poles incorporated make transport much easier)
	• Plumbing to accommodate for haemodialysis
	• Adequate floor space to accommodate for Extracorporeal Membrane Oxygenation Equipment (ECMO) in certain institutions

General/Acute Treatment Cubicles

Purpose	Assess, manage, and initiate treatment on patients with a high likelihood of admission
Size	Minimum treatment area should be 12 m²
Functional requirements	• Space to fit a standard mobile trolley and essential equipment, e.g., oxygen masks
	• Accompanying persons to sit comfortably (minimum of two people)
	• Allow procedure trolleys to be at the bedside and functional
	• Cubicle should have solid partitions to provide privacy for the patient
	• Storage for limited amounts of linen and easy access to bedside equipment
	• Direct observation is possible from the staff position
Spatial relationships	Ready access to clean and dirty utility rooms, medication room, and patient toilets/shower
Other considerations	• Ceiling rail for IV fluids (though trolleys with incorporated IV poles make transport much easier)
	• A defined number of cubicles fitted with lifting equipment for the disabled or bariatric patient
	• Cubicles catering to the elderly or children
	• Internal decoration of the room, e.g., colour, health promotion posters, and art/television on the roof for people with spinal precautions
	• Natural light, wherever possible

General Consultation Area & Fast Track/Ambulatory Area

Purpose	Area dedicated to the management of patients without major illness who do not require resuscitation or monitoring; often these patients are non-complex, presenting with single-system conditions and traumatic injuries
Functional requirements	Assessment and treatment of patients who are mostly ambulatory and anticipated to go home; design should be based on a rapid turnover of patients
Spatial relationships	Direct access from Reception/Triage and waiting room areas without having to pass through other areas; ready access to x-rays
Other considerations	Area should be fully reticulated with gas, suction, power, and data points
Current trends	Some EDs have non-private rooms but have common areas with chairs allowing several patients to be treated and larger consultation areas, with their own sub-waiting areas; this demonstrates the nature of EDs changing business and the way that ED staff work

(Continued)

TABLE 13H: (Continued)

Plaster Room

Purpose	• Application of splints, plasters, and mobility aids associated with musculoskeletal injuring, dislocations, and fractures • Procedural sedation and reduction of dislocations and fractures also commonly occur
Size	The room should be at least 20 m² in size (unless combined with other rooms, e.g., procedure room)
Functional requirements	• Adequate size to allow a trolley • Appropriate physiological monitoring systems and resuscitation equipment to allow safe analgesia and sedation • Adequate room/storage capacity to allow for procedure trolleys and equipment, e.g., tourniquet matching • Room to accommodate portable x-rays of image intensifier • Access to the patient from both sides
Spatial relationships	• Close to both minor and major areas of the ED if sedation is likely to occur in the room • Close proximity of the plaster room to the medication area allows for ready access to local anaesthetics and take-home analgesics
Other considerations	Enough floor space to accommodate an image intensifier or portable x-ray machine; dimmable lights

Procedure Room

Purpose	Performance of procedures such as suturing, phlebotomy, lumbar puncture, tube thoracotomy, thoracocentesis, abdominal paracentesis, bladder catheterization, etc.
Size	The procedure room should be at least 20 m² in size (unless combined with other rooms, e.g., plaster room)
Functional requirements	• Adequate size to allow a bed • Appropriate physiological monitoring systems to allow safe analgesia and sedation • Adequate room/storage capacity to allow suture trolleys/procedure, trolleys/dressing, and trolleys/resuscitation equipment
Spatial relationships	Close to both minor and major areas of the ED
Other considerations	Furnished to accommodate for paediatric patients, e.g., has glow-in-the-dark stars in the room

Interview Room

Purpose	Conduct patient (including psychiatric patient), relative, and carer interviews safely, comfortably, and privately
Size	At least 12 m² (comfortably fits at least three people without feeling crowded)
Functional requirements	• Sound-proof (from external auditory stimuli) • Can be directly seen by observers (one-way mirrors and CCTV) • Does not contain objects that can be thrown at staff, e.g., light-weight chairs • Furniture should have soft corners and no hard edges • There should be no parts of the furniture that can be removed and used as a potential weapon • A functional duress/panic alarm is needed within easy reach of the interviewer and at each exit • Two doors, opening outwards and able to be locked from the outside but not from the inside • The room should be square and not have any narrow corners in which people could become cornered • Has low stimuli décor and muted colours • The room does not require medical gases or suction • There should be no vents or lights or other apparatus that could be used as a hanging point • Smoke detector(s)
Spatial relationships	• The interview room should be in a highly visible part of the ED • Near a treatment/examination room for physical assessment

Distressed Relatives' Room

Purpose	• Private, quiet room for distressed relatives, caretakers, or friends of all ages and cultural backgrounds to gather • A space to obtain a collateral patient history and potentially to deliver bad news about a patient
Size	Comfortably seats at least four relatives, friends, or caretakers and has seating room for a nurse or doctor to enter and deliver news regarding a patient
Functional requirements	• A private and sound-proof space • A space where distressed relatives, friends, or caretakers can gather and support one another • A space that is culturally neutral and inoffensive • A space that is aesthetically calming and peaceful
Spatial relationships	• Close to the resuscitation area • Should not be so close that people can see or overhear clinical care being delivered to the patient (or to other patients) • Ready access to refreshments and toilets
Other considerations	• Calming, peaceful music may or may not be appropriate • Cultural- or religion-specific needs • Unrestricted access to waiting room but controlled access to the ED

(Continued)

TABLE 13H: (Continued)

Staff Workstations

Purpose	• Staff can undertake work that is not performed at a patient's bedside • Used for discussion, advice, and referrals and for the entry or writing of notes • Separate consulting rooms are provided specifically for patient consultation
Terminology	• Work desk—an individual area for a single staff member to work at • Workstation—group of conjoined work desks with associated storage and other facilities
Size	• A desk area minimum of 1.2 m wide by 600 mm deep, per individual work desk • A minimum number of work desks equals 1.5 × (average number of Emergency Physicians + average number of Emergency Nurses on daytime weekday shifts) • Additional dedicated work desks for the nurse and doctor in charge of the shift and the clerk dedicated communications personnel (optional)
Functional requirements	• Aspects to be factored in include ergonomics, such as computer monitors being 800 mm from eyes and at a correct height • Bench space around computers must be adequate to allow for papers to be on the desk; desk height is ideally adjustable • Sufficient space to allow for an adequate number of chairs and circulation within the staff area (opposing work desks should have minimum of 2 m between desk edges) • Workstation(s) ideally should have clear vision of the ED clinical areas that they are serving • Consider separate workstations for different areas of ED • Consider local work desks for cubicle groups (e.g., on the end of a dividing wall) as this allows data entry without leaving the patient • Design needs to consider security for staff and privacy for conversations
Spatial relationships	• Design needs to facilitate staff flow between workstation and cubicles • Clear views of nurse call displays
Other considerations	• Enclosing part of the workstation to increase privacy • Under desk brackets/shelves for computers with cable tidying systems • One or two x-ray viewing boxes if the department is not equipped for PACS/radiological films originating from outside the hospital; note that rapid progress is eliminating film-based radiology systems and rapidly making x-ray viewing boxes redundant • Need to allow staff to perform appropriate hand hygiene between patients and between patients and workstation

Department Corridors

Purpose	Corridors provide patients, relatives, and staff not only access to all parts of the ED and to service areas of the ED but also access to and storage of equipment that is needed frequently or urgently	
Size	• Clinical areas—the minimum must be to allow 2 trolleys/wheelchairs to easily pass with associated equipment, e.g., IV stands • A minimum width of 3 m is recommended • Access to service areas will need a width suitable for the purpose, e.g., disposal areas may need access for large refuse bins, and equipment stores need access for trolleys (supermarket style or dressing); consider the need for storage of mobile patient hoists and other large equipment	
Functional requirements	Parking/storage of ECG and ultrasound machines, IVs, dressing, and procedure trolleys	• Parking/storage of clean linen trolleys and used linen bags • Equipment bays need GPOs to plug power cables into for battery charging
	Beverage bay(s) with	Hot and cool drinking water, beverage preparation equipment, and waste disposal
	Patient meal delivery area	Consideration regarding the process for managing patient meals and parking of patient meals trolley
	Consideration of infection control/hygiene is necessary	• The need for wash basins depends on cubicle design and staff flows • The need to allow staff to wash hands between patient and workstation • If suitable basins are in all cubicles, then hand sanitiser dispensers may suffice
Other considerations	• Ensure sufficient room for trolleys to enter/leave cubicles • Notice boards and/or decorations (photographs or paintings), if appropriate • Kitchenette facilities if reheating of food is required	

Dirty Utility/Disposal Room

Purpose	The dirty utility/disposal room is used for the disposal of clinical and other waste and soiled linen; for testing and disposal of patient specimens; for decontamination and storage of patient utensils such as pans, urinals, and bowls; for cleaning and holding of used equipment for collection and sterilization elsewhere
Size	Minimum of 12 m²
Functional requirements	There must be a sink for handwashing and a rim sink that can be flushed

TABLE 13H: (Continued)

Spatial relationships	Access to this room should be available from all clinical areas
Other considerations	• A macerator for disposable bedpans/urinals rather than washer/sanitizers • Two or more dirty utility rooms may be required to minimize travel distance in a large ED • Consider single patient pan cleaners and macerators in isolation room en suites

Equipment/Storeroom

Purpose	Used to store equipment and disposable supplies for the ED; portable equipment may also be stored and recharged in this room
Size	The total area of dedicated storerooms must take into account central and decentralized storage of equipment and disposables with the presence of equipment at the bedside
Functional requirements	• The room should be secure with access limited to authorized personnel only • Sufficient space and power sockets to store and charge battery-powered equipment, e.g., infusion pumps
Other considerations	• Decentralized storage solution in large EDs, including separate storage for disposables, trauma resuscitation equipment, mobile equipment, and stationery • Separate room for equipment servicing should be considered • Bar code systems allowing toping up of supplies on a daily basis thus reducing the need for larger amounts of stock to be kept in the equipment room

Pharmacy/Medication Room/Clean Utility

Purpose	Storage and dispensing of medications and the preparation of drugs (including IV-administered)
Size	Minimum 12 m²
Functional requirements	Secure electronic medication storage solution and open access to pharmacy/medication room (preferable) • Centralized—single medication area serving the entire ED; or • Decentralized—multiple medication areas, which is more common in larger EDs or those with electronic medication storage solutions
Spatial relationships	The pharmacy/medication room needs to be situated to allow easy access to all clinical areas
Other considerations	• Space for the storage and charging of IV infusion pumps • Cold water dispenser, e.g., hydro tap • Refrigerator monitor and alarm (linked to security) to prevent warming of temperature-sensitive medications • Consider space for a medication trolley • Wall-mounted push button alert indicating to staff outside the pharmacy/medication room that the controlled drug cupboard keys are required • If an automated dispensing machine is installed, then consider omitting swipe card door access in favour of open access to room with secure storage of medication

Disaster Equipment Room

Purpose	Storage room for equipment that would be used in an MCI/mass disaster incident or chemical, biological, or radiation (CBR) incident or for retrieval of patients from the ED
Size	Consistent with the role of the individual ED in a major incident or disaster
Functional requirements	This room should be easily accessible and have sufficient supplies to fully equip the disaster team for on- or off-site incidents
Spatial relationships	Close to ambulance bay (ideally, door access via the ambulance entrance); accessible to the helipad if appropriate

Short Stay Units (SSUs)

Purpose	• SSUs serve an important function in the diagnosis and management of ED patients; a number of criteria apply to SSUs, including that they
	  • Are designated and designed for the short-term treatment, observation, assessment, and reassessment of patients initially triaged and assessed in the ED
	  • Have specific admission and discharge criteria and policies
	
	  • Are designed for short-term stays no longer than 24 hours
	  • Are physically separated from the ED's acute assessment area
	  • Have a static number of beds with oxygen, suction, and patient ablution facilities
	  • Are not a temporary ED overflow area and are not used to keep patients solely awaiting an inpatient bed or awaiting treatment in the ED
	• There should be the ability to monitor each bed to the same level as an acute cubicle and dedicated staff bases; hospital beds, not ED trolleys, should be used

Administration Areas

Purpose	Offices provide space for the administrative, managerial, safety, quality, teaching, and research roles of the ED
Functional requirements	• Offices should be located close to one another and close to secretarial services • Wi-Fi should be available throughout • There should be ready access to printing and scanning/photocopying
Spatial relationships	• Staff members who are mostly office workers should, if possible, have offices with natural light • The area should be accessible to authorized staff only • The administration area should have room(s) in which private meetings can be held

(Continued)

TABLE 13H: (Continued)

Other considerations	• The total office space should be sufficient for future expansion of staff numbers and new roles • There is an emerging trend for common and shared office areas • Some hospitals have common meeting areas for all departments to share
Teaching Facilities	
Purpose	• The ED requires dedicated facilities for formal education, tutorials/mannequin simulation, and meetings • This area may be used by medical, nursing, or other staff and undergraduates; it should be a private, non-clinical area with noise attenuation, often near the staff room and offices, with access to toilets and amenities
Other considerations	• Natural light • Teaching rooms that can be adequately darkened for viewing projected material • An ability to expand the area of the room to cater to large groups; large EDs may benefit from having more than one room or a room that can be divided, and the divider should be of high quality to ensure adequate sound attenuation • Projectors offer better viewing than large television displays • The size of the room should be calculated based on the maximum number of people likely to use it at any one time, e.g., a combined medical and nursing meeting or a network teaching session
Staff Room	
Purpose	• Well-designed staff facilities provide time out and relaxation and add to morale and proper staff functioning • The staff room is used by staff to consume meals, for social events, and for the celebration of achievements • The kitchen area may be incorporated within the staff room or immediately adjacent to it; staff should be able to prepare hot and cold drinks and prepare or heat food • Depending on the size of the ED, the kitchen area may also be used for the preparation of beverages for patients
Size	The size of the staff room should be large enough to seat all staff on a rostered meal break
Functional requirements	• Preparation and consumption of meals • Located away from patient care areas • Natural lighting is desirable • Secure • Access to an outside area if possible • Other aspects of relaxation, e.g., music, television
Spatial relationships	• Toilets in close proximity • Offices usually located in the same area of the ED
Other considerations	• ABHR or hand basin at the entrance to the staff room • Multiple microwaves allow faster preparation of food • Industrial-grade, fast-cycle dishwashers and industrial refrigerators • A managed beverage service negates the need for replenishment and maintenance of tea and coffee
Staff Amenities	

Purpose	• To provide staff with an area to store personal items securely, change clothes, and attend to personal grooming and hygiene; there should be
	  • An adequate number of staff toilet facilities in the staff and clinical areas
	  • Separate male and female shower and change facilities
	  • Secure bicycle lock up (if not provided by hospital in general)
	  • A sufficient number of lockers for staff members' personal belongings
	  • Overnight room with a desk, computer, or Wi-Fi access
	  • Staff mail boxes and notice boards

13.4 Summary

The ED is said to be the hospital's hospital. Designing an effective ED in a hospital requires meticulous planning and attention to detail. Key considerations include optimizing patient flow; creating distinct zones for triage, treatment, and observation; and ensuring adequate space for medical staff and equipment. Safety and infection control measures are essential to safeguard patients and health care providers. An efficient ED can be the shop window for a hospital, thus bringing in trust and patient satisfaction.

14 OUTPATIENT DEPARTMENT (OPD)

Outpatient Department: Facility of the hospital with allotted physical facilities, regularly scheduled hours, and personnel in sufficient numbers designed to provide care for patients who are not registered as inpatients. An OPD is also known as a hospital's shop window.

Polyclinic: A group of outpatient clinics housed under one roof that functions at the same time for quick interaction (Indian Standard 13808 [Part 1]: 1993).

14.1 Reasons for Shifting Focus from Inpatient to Outpatient Treatment

- Rising costs of hospital care
- Shortage of hospital beds
- Economic importance
- Technology
- Developments in medical sciences
- Emphasis on home care post-COVID-19

TABLE 14A: Characteristics of OPD That Influence Its Design

- Convenient ground floor access to outpatient entry
- Demarcated parking areas for ambulances, patient support vehicles, and private cars
- Effective wayfinding signage throughout the facility and enquiry points at entrances
- Facilities for patient refreshment, pharmacy, and toilets
- Waiting areas to accommodate patients, caretakers, children, and differently abled persons
- Patient flow patterns to enable clinical pre-assessment, medical consultation, pathology, and radiology services
- Storage facilities for patient belongings
- Clustering procedure rooms with service consultation rooms
- Furniture, fittings, equipment, services, and hydraulics to meet specific clinical requirements
- Patient attendance numbers
- Number of specialties
- Medical, allied health, and support staff numbers
- Anticipated usage of medical suites and potential to share rooms between specialties
- Population profiles that drive specialty service delivery
- Consultation with medical specialists, examination, and investigations
- Treatment on a same-day basis
- Facility for minor procedures
- Follow-up review consultation and ongoing case management
- Patient screening prior to surgery—peri-operative services
- Health education or counselling sessions for patients and families
- Referral of patients to other units or disciplines for ongoing care and treatment
- Referral for admission to a hospital for inpatient services

TABLE 14B: Scope of Services That Influence OPD Design

- General Practitioner (GP) clinics
- Primary Care centres
- Women and child health services
- A comprehensive range of surgical specialties
- Medical specialties including diabetes and multidisciplinary team reviews, e.g., chronic disease clinics, infectious diseases services, etc.
- Pain management
- Genetics clinics
- Health promotion initiatives

14.2 OPD and Wider Hospital Context: Location & Access

The facility should be planned to keep in mind the maximum peak hours for patient load and should have a scope for future expansion. The OPD should approach from the main road with signage visible from a distance.

(a) **Reception and Enquiry**: An Enquiry/Help Desk should be available with competent staff fluent in the local language. The service may be outsourced. Services available at the hospital are displayed at the enquiry.

(b) **Waiting Spaces**: A waiting area with adequate seating arrangements should be provided. The main entrance, general waiting area, and subsidiary waiting spaces are required to be adjacent to each consultation and treatment room in all clinics. A waiting area at the scale of 1 sq ft/per average daily patient with a minimum 400 sq ft of area should be provided.

(c) **Patient Amenities** (norms given in the following pages):
  - Potable drinking water
  - Functional and clean flushable toilets with running water
  - Fans/Coolers
  - Seating arrangement as per patient load

(d) **Clinics**: Clinics should include General, Medical, Surgical, Ophthalmic, ENT, Dental, Obstetrics and Gynaecology, a Post-Partum Unit, Paediatrics, Dermatology and Venereology, Psychiatry, Neonatology, Orthopaedic, and the Social Service Department. Doctor chambers should have ample space to seat four to five people. A chamber size of 12.0 sq m is adequate. Clinics for infectious and communicable diseases should be located in isolation, preferably in a remote corner with independent access. For the National Health Programme, adequate space should be made available. An immunization clinic with a waiting room that has an area of 3 m × 4 m in the PP centre/Maternity centre/Paediatric Clinic should be provided. One room for HIV/STI counselling should be provided. The pharmacy should be in close proximity of the OPD. All clinics should be provided with an examination table, X-ray view box, screens, and handwashing facility. An adequate number of wheelchairs and stretchers should be provided.

DOI: 10.1201/9780367460884-15

(e) **Nursing Services**: Various clinics under Ambulatory Care require nursing facilities in common, which include a dressing room, side laboratory, injection room, social service room, treatment rooms, etc.

(f) **Nurse Station**: Need-based space required for the nurse station in the OPD for dispensing nursing services (based on the OPD patient load).

14.3 Models of Care

Planning models applicable to the Outpatient Unit include a discreet unit within a hospital facility or located on a hospital campus that shares the support services of the hospital facility; an integrated unit such as a private medical practice within a commercial development, such as a shopping centre or an office building; and a stand-alone unit not connected with a hospital or commercial facility.

(a) **Two types of OPD services**
  • Centralized OPD
  • Decentralized OPD
(b) **Based on type of patients**
  • General OPD
  • Emergency OPD
  • Referred OPD
(c) **Types of OPD services**
  • Ambulatory care centre
  • Polyclinic
  • Health centre
  • Walk-in clinic
  • Day care
  • Dispensary, etc.
(d) **Depending upon outpatient visit**
  • New outpatient visit
  • Repeat outpatient visit

Separate and combined consult/examination rooms: Consult and examination take place within a single room. The room should have a desk and chairs in the consultation zone and a screened examination area with a couch. The layout of the rooms should ensure patient privacy particularly in the examination area. Another option is to have a separate consult and examination room.

14.4 Patient Flows

The patient flow in an OPD is shown in Figure 14A.

14.4.1 Needs Assessment

(a) **The size of the facility**—depends upon
  • The size of the population served by the unit and demographic trends
  • The number of clinical practitioners available
  • The average length of consultation or treatment
  • The number of referrals and transfers from other local regions or hospitals
  • The number of other Outpatient Units in the vicinity
(b) **Expected workload**—depends upon
  • Transport facilities
  • Geographic and topographical factors
  • Rough criterion—every hospital bed attracts five to six patients/day in the OPD of which 50% are

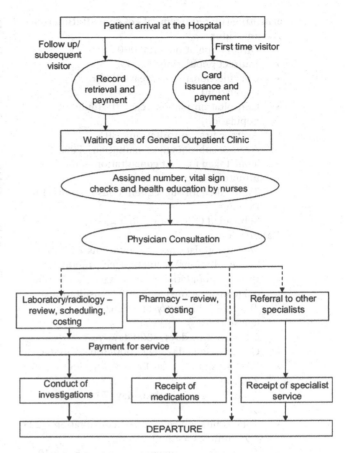

FIGURE 14A Patient Flow in an OPD (Ogaji DS, Mezie-Okoye MM. Waiting time and patient satisfaction: Survey of patients seeking care at the general outpatient clinic of the University of Port Harcourt Teaching Hospital. Port Harcourt Medical Journal. 2017 Sep 1;11(3):148).

follow-up patients and 50% are new patients, e.g., for 200 civil beds, the expected OPD/day = 1,000 to 1,200 patients/day (*Indian Standard* IS 13808 (Part 1): 1993; Quality Management Procedures for Outpatient Department & Emergency Services-Guidelines)

(c) **Factors to be considered when assessing needs include:**
  • Number of clinic staff to be accommodated (including doctors, nurses, and other professional and technical staff)
  • Number of rooms required for each clinic based upon the working methods of the staff concerned
  • Time to be used for consulting/examination rooms
  • Availability of staff to conduct and support clinics

14.5 Indexes Relevant to OPD Planning

(a) **In deciding the number of consultation rooms required**
  • Room hours (service time) = Number of doctor examination rooms available × Number of hours that the OPD is scheduled
(b) **For planning the waiting area**
  • Holding capacity = Maximum expected number of patients in the main or subsidiary waiting area and clinics (should cater to at least one attendant/patient)

(c) **Determining the requirements of consultation rooms**
  - **Assumptions**
    - Direct population—100,000
    - Indirect population—50,000
    - Consultation/person/year—2 (direct population)
    - Consultation/person/year—0.5 (indirect population)
    - Average first consultation—30%
    - Average subsequent consultation—70%
    - Time taken for first consultation—20 minutes
    - Time taken for subsequent consultation—10 minutes
    - Scheduled OPD hours—6 hours
  - **Calculations**
    - Direct population × consultations = 100,000 × 2 (consultations) = 200,000 (consultations)
    - Indirect population × consultations = 50,000 × 0.5 (consultations) = 25,000 (consultations)
    - Total consultations/year = 225,000 (consultations)
    - OPD working days = 300 days/year
    - Consultations/day = 225,000/300 = 750/day
    - First consultation/day (30% of all) = 750 × 30% = 225/day
    - Follow-up consultations/day (70% of total) = 525/day
    - Total time required for first consultation = 225 × 20 minutes = 4,500 minutes
    - Time for follow-up consultations = 525 × 10 minutes = 5,250 minutes
    - Total consultation time required = 9,750 minutes
    - Consultation room hours/day (required) = 9,750/60 = 162 hours
    - **Number of consultation rooms required = 162 hours/6 hours = 27 rooms**

TABLE 14C: Key Result Areas and Quality Indicators for an OPD

Key Result Areas

- Patient admission from OPD
- Managing non-availability of beds
- Patient transfer
- Access prioritized patients according to clinical needs
- Referral of patients
- Predefined and time for initial assessment
- Outpatients are informed of their next follow-up where appropriate
- Care of vulnerable patients
- Antenatal care; frequency of visits; maternal nutrition assessment
- Care of paediatric patients
- Mechanism for physician's sample
- Medication errors
- High-risk medications defined
- Drug reconciliation
- Patient rights displayed, staff awareness
- General consent for treatment

- Patient and/or their family members are interviewed for the scope of general consent
- Uniform pricing policy; availability of tariff list to patients
- Instructions for handwashing displayed near every handwashing area
- Adherence to safe injection and infusion practices
- Availability of PPEs, soap, and disinfectants and their correct usage
- Segregation of biomedical waste
- Documented plan for handling fire and non-fire emergencies
- Identification of hazardous materials; sorting, labelling, handling, storage, transporting, and disposal of hazardous materials
- Spills management plan for hazardous materials, staff awareness
- Communication with patients and relatives
- Staff awareness on these policies and procedures
- Patient interview

Quality Indicators

- Patient fall rate
- Hand hygiene compliance rate
- Patient satisfaction index
- Waiting time for an OPD consultation
- Needle stick injury rate
- Compliance rate to medication prescription in capitals

Internal & External Functional Relationships (Table 14D & Figure 14B)

TABLE 14D: Functional Relationships of an OPD

Internal Functional Relationships	External Functional Relationships
• Reception area should allow patients to move conveniently to and from the consult and treatment areas and accommodate a high volume of patients, support staff, care takers, and mobility aids.	• Drop-off zone/car park and main entry.
• Sub-waiting areas may be located close to treatment areas for patient and staff accessibility.	• Admission Unit (satellite, stand alone, or central) for patient referrals.
• Staff must be able to move easily to and from treatment areas, Reception/registration, and waiting areas.	• Clinical Information Unit for delivery/return of clinical records unless digital records are used.
• Discreet and private work areas away from patients are recommended.	• Day Surgery/Procedure Unit.
• Staff areas may have restricted access to patients.	• Emergency Unit for patient referrals.
	• Medical imaging for diagnostic procedures.
	• Pharmacy for patient medications.
	• Pathology and specimen collection for diagnostic studies.
	• Rehabilitation Unit/Allied Health for patient follow-up.
	• Transit lounge for patients awaiting transport.

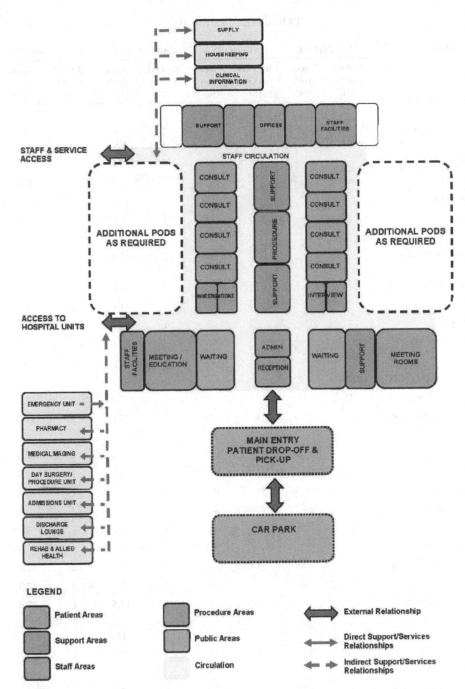

FIGURE 14B Functional Relationship Diagram of an OPD (Courtesy: iHFG).

Major Space Determinants of an OPD (Table 14E)

TABLE 14E: Provisions for Various Floor Areas in an OPD

S No.	FACILITY	CATEGORY A		CATEGORY B		CATEGORY C		CATEGORY D		CATEGORY E	
		ROOM (NO.)	Area (m²)	ROOM (NO.)	Area (m²)	ROOM (NO.)	Area (m²)	ROOM (NO.)	Area (m²)	ROOM (NO.)	Area (m²)
(1)	(2)	(3)	(4)	(5)	(6)	(7)	(8)	(9)	(10)	(11)	(12)
(a)	Dark room			1	10.5	1	14	1	17.5	1	17.5
(b)	Waiting room	1	14	1	14	1	21	1	28	1	42

(Continued)

TABLE 14E: (Continued)

S No.	FACILITY	CATEGORY A		CATEGORY B		CATEGORY C		CATEGORY D		CATEGORY E	
		ROOM (NO.)	Area (m²)	ROOM (NO.)	Area (m²)	ROOM (NO.)	Area (m²)	ROOM (NO.)	Area (m²)	ROOM (NO.)	Area (m²)
(1)	(2)	(3)	(4)	(5)	(6)	(7)	(8)	(9)	(10)	(11)	(12)
ENT CLINIC											
(a)	Consultation and examination room	To be shared with surgical clinic		1	28	1 1	28 17.5	1 1	28 17.5	1 2	28 17.5
(b)	Treatment room			1	14	1	14	1	17.5	1	17.5
(c)	Audiometric room			—		1	14	1	17.5	1	17.5
(d)	Electronystagmography			—		—		—		1	17.5
(e)	Waiting room			1	14	1	21	1	28	1	42
DENTAL CLINIC											
(a)	Consultation and examination room			1	17.5	1	17.5	2	17.5	3	17.5
(b)	Dental hygienist room			1	10.5	1	14	2	17.5	3	17.5
(c)	Recovery room			—		1	14	1	21	1	28
(d)	Dental workshop			—		1	17.5	2	17.5	3	17.5
(e)	Processing room for x-rays			—				—		1	10.5
(f)	Waiting room			1	14	1	21	1	28	1	35
OBSTETRIC AND GYNAECOLOGICAL CLINIC											
(a)	Reception and registration	1	14	1	14	1	17.5	1	17.5	1	21
(b)	Consultation and examination	1	17.5	1	17.5	2	17.5	2	17.5	3	17.5
(c)	Treatment room	1	17.5	1	17.5	1	17.5	1	17.5	1	21
(d)	Clinical laboratories			1	10.5	1	14	1	17.5	1	21
(e)	Toilet-cum-changing	1	10.5	1	10.5	1	10.5	1	10.5	1	10.5
(f)	Mother craft demonstration	—		—		—				—	
(g)	Waiting room	1	21	1	21	1	28	1	35	1	42
FAMILY PLANNING CLINIC											
(a)	Consultation and examination	1	17.5	1	17.5	1	17.5	2	17.5	2	17.5
(b)	Treatment room	1	10.5	1	14	1	17.5	2	17.5	2	17.5
(c)	Health educator and social worker room			—		1	17.5	1	17.5	1	17.5
(d)	Recovery room			—		1	14	1	21	1	28
(e)	Waiting room	1	10.5	1	14	1	21	1	28	1	35
PAEDIATRIC CLINIC											
(a)	Consultation and examination	1	17.5	1	17.5	2	17.5	2	17.5	3	17.5
(b)	Dressing treatment and dispensing room	1	14	1	14	1	17.5	2	17.5	2	21
(c)	Therapy room	—		—				1	10.5	1	17.5
(d)	Immunization room	1	14	1	14	1	17.5	1	17.5	1	21
(e)	Recreation and play room							1	14	1	17.5
(f)	Waiting room	1	14	1	21	1	28	1	35	1	42
SKIN & STD CLINIC											
(a)	Consultation and examination	—		—		1	17.5	2	17.5	2	17.5
(b)	Treatment rooms	—		—		2	17.5	3	17.5	3	17.5
(c)	Biopsy room	—		—		—		1	10.5	1	10.5
(d)	Superficial therapy	—		—		1	14	1	17.5	1	17.5

(Continued)

TABLE 14E: (Continued)

S No. (1)	FACILITY (2)	CATEGORY A		CATEGORY B		CATEGORY C		CATEGORY D		CATEGORY E	
		ROOM (NO.) (3)	Area (m²) (4)	ROOM (NO.) (5)	Area (m²) (6)	ROOM (NO.) (7)	Area (m²) (8)	ROOM (NO.) (9)	Area (m²) (10)	ROOM (NO.) (11)	Area (m²) (12)
(e)	Skin laboratory		—	—		1	21	1	28	1	28
(f)	Barber's room		—		—	—		1	7	1	7
(g)	Waiting room		—	—		1	21	1	28	1	35
PSYCHIATRIC CLINIC											
(a)	Consultation and examination	—	—	1	17.5	2	17.5	2	17.5		
(b)	ECT room	—	—	1	21	1	17.5	1	17.5		
(c)	Recovery room	—	—	1	17.5	1	17.5	1	17.5		
(d)	Psychologist room	—	—	1	17.5	1	17.5	1	17.5		
(e)	Social worker room	—	—	1	17.5	1	17.5	1	17.5		
(f)	Electroencephalography room	—	—	—	—	1	17.5				
(g)	Occupational therapy room	—	—			—	1	28			
(h)	Waiting room	—	—	1	21	1	28	1	35		
SUPPORTING FACILITIES											
(a)	Central injection room	1	14	1	14	1	14	1	17.5	1	21
(b)	Specimen collection room	1	14	1	14	1	17.5	1	17.5	1	21
(c)	Clinical laboratory							1	17.5	1	21
(d)	Social worker room	—	—	1	14	1	17.5	1	17.5		
(e)	Waiting room	1	10.5	1	14	1	21	1	28	1	35

14.6 Layout & Zoning

(a) **Single Corridor Access Model:** This examination/ treatment model permits multidisciplinary rooms with similar configurations accessed by a single entry point. Common reception and waiting areas enhance efficient staffing and resourcing (Figure 14C).

(b) **Double Corridor Access Model:** Where space permits, the double corridor model enables staff support and service areas to remain discreetly separate from public access. In this model, waiting areas can be located centrally, but this may reduce patient privacy and confidentiality (Figures 14D and 14E).

(c) **Multidisciplinary Consult Rooms:** The adoption of modular consult rooms enables efficient use by multidisciplinary practitioners on a sessional basis (Figure 14 F).

(d) **Single Specialty Consult Rooms:** Where a range of highly specialized equipment is required during each consultation, rooms can be configured to accommodate these special requirements. Examples of specialties that this model suits include ENT/Ophthalmology, Endoscopy specialties, Cancer Centre (Chemotherapy, Radiotherapy, and Consulting), and Specialist Medical Suites.

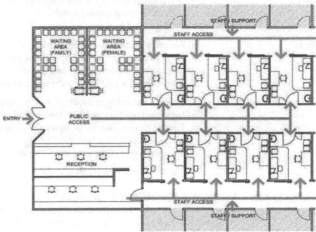

FIGURE 14D Double Corridor Access Model with Waiting Area at the Entry (Courtesy: iHFG).

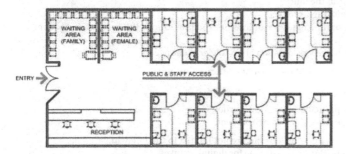

FIGURE 14C Single Corridor Access Model (Courtesy: iHFG).

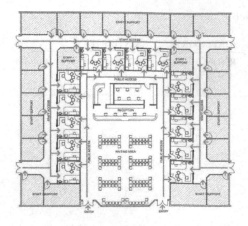

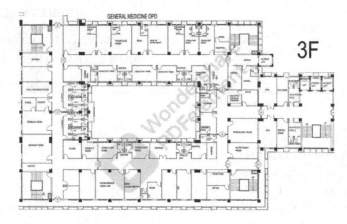

FIGURE 14E   Double Corridor Access Model with Centralized Waiting Area (Courtesy: iHFG).

FIGURE 14F   Schematic Diagram of Layout of OPD.

Built Environment: General Considerations

TABLE 14F: General Considerations for the Built Environment in an OPD

Location	• Separate entrance and situated close to, and accessed via, the main entrance • Should be located on the ground floor • Parking areas for disabled people and wheelchairs close to the main entrance • There should be separate dropping-off points close to the OPD entrance for patients arriving by ambulance and by car
Wayfinding	• Clear signposts from the entrance(s) to the hospital site, from the car park, and from the main entrance to the hospital
Acoustics	• Acoustic privacy is required in consult, interview, and treatment rooms and any rooms where confidential information will be discussed • Noisy areas such as waiting rooms and play areas should be located away from consult, treatment, and staff areas
Natural Light/Lighting	• The use of natural light should be maximized within the unit (windows/skylights) • Windows are particularly desirable in waiting areas and staff lounges
Privacy	• Discreet and non-public access to medical records • Privacy screening for all patient bays • Location of doors to avoid patient exposure in consult and treatment rooms
Interior Décor	• Interior décor refers to colour, textures, surface finishes, fixtures, fittings, furnishings, artwork, and atmosphere that are combined to create a calming, non-threatening environment • Colours should be used in combination with lighting to ensure that they do not mask skin colours as this can be a problem in areas where clinical observation takes place
Accessibility	• Wheelchair access is required in all patient areas • The unit should require suitable seating and provisions for patients with special requirements, e.g., elderly, disabled, and pregnant patients
Doors	• All entry points, doors, or openings should be a minimum of 1,200 mm wide and unobstructed • Larger openings may be required for special equipment • Doors used for emergency bed transfer to Operating Units must be appropriately positioned and sized; a minimum of a 1,400-mm clear opening is recommended for doors requiring bed/trolley access
Safety and Security	• Control the entry and exits points to and from the unit • Improve the observation of patient and clinical areas for staff • Reduce duplication by grouping functions, optimizing space utilization, and promoting efficient staff and patient management • The perimeter of the unit should be secured and consideration given to electronic access

Finishes	• The following aspects should always be considered when specifying internal finishes:
	  • Cleaning and infection control
	  • Fire safety of the materials
	  • Patient care and comfort and staff safety, particularly for floor finishes
	  • Cultural/social perceptions of a professional health care environment

Communications	• Patient information and image management systems include but are not limited to the following:
	  • Picture archiving communications systems (PACS) and storage for digital archives
	  • Voice/data cabling and outlets for phones, fax, and computers
	  • Network data requirements and wireless network requirements to support remote reporting
	  • Video- and tele-conferencing capability

(Continued)

TABLE 14F: (Continued)

	• CCTV surveillance if indicated
	  • Patient, staff, emergency call, and duress alarms and paging systems
	  • Communications rooms and server rooms
	• Patient, staff assist, and emergency call facilities should be provided in all consult, examination, procedure, and treatment rooms and patient areas (including toilets) so that patients and staff can request urgent assistance
	• Close collaboration with the IT Unit and obtaining advice from consultants early in the design phase are recommended

Windows	• Clear glazing, providing an outlook for patients and staff, should be supplied in as many spaces as possible • Privacy in consult, examination, and treatment rooms should be maintained • Windows should be easy to clean, both inside and out • Consideration of thermal loss or solar gain, energy conservation, and the prevention of glare
Heating, Ventilation, and Air Conditioning	The unit should have appropriate air conditioning that allows the control of temperature and humidity for patient and staff comfort
Medical Gases	Medical gases may be provided within consult, procedure, and treatment rooms as required by the facility's operational policy
Flooring	• Use non-slippery tiles in order to avoid causing further injuries to patients or medical staff • Must be water-resistant so that the flooring does not bloat • OPD-Kota Stone/Vitrified/Ceramic are preferred
Walls	• Selected with infection control in mind and to resist bacterial growth • Hard, seamless, non-absorbent, scrubbable surfaces are recommended • Finishes should be unaffected by colour changes, staining, and mildew • Wall protection at drinking fountains and lavatories: provide solid surface panels on mold-resistant gypsum board on rear walls of drinking fountain alcoves where wallboard or plaster finishes occur and behind lavatories and end walls

Water	• Number of water outlets required and quantity of water required calculated on assumptions such as
	  • Number of patient load
	  • Number of relatives accompanying the patients
	• In Indian conditions, the average Indian adult consumes approximately 4 L of water per day; during a hospital visit, he will use about ½ L of water for drinking

Electricity	• Electrical supply from two sources • Care should be taken to avoid interference in intensity and frequency affecting diagnostic and monitoring equipment, computers, and other sensitive electrical equipment • Fix electrical points for permanent equipment as per requirements of various specialties • Minimum 2 electrical outlets in an OPD—one 5 amp and one 15 amp for temporary equipment • Corridors should have electrical outlets at fixed distances—for attachment of cleaning equipment

Lighting	• Adequate illumination must be ensured by using artificial and natural/daylight
	• Illumination in lux
	  • Reception—300 Lux
	  • Waiting area—200 Lux
	  • Corridors—200 Lux
	  • Consultation rooms—300 Lux
	  • Examination/procedure room—1,000 Lux
	• Limiting glare index: 19–22
	• Colour rendering index > 85
	• Colour temperature: 4,000–5,000 K
	• Luminaire: LED

TABLE 14G: Specific Room and Functional Requirements for an OPD

Entrance	• Located prominently • Free from any obstruction to access • Covered porch • Wheelchair/trolley bay • Well-illustrated guide map • Steps/ramp with handrails
Registration counter	• Registration-cum-info counter with a minimum area of 6 sq m per receptionist • Colour-coded OPD ticket • Availability of PRO/education handouts • Notification of patient rights

(Continued)

TABLE 14G: (Continued)

Entrance	• Located prominently • Free from any obstruction to access • Covered porch • Wheelchair/trolley bay • Well-illustrated guide map • Steps/ramp with handrails

Waiting area	• An adult male human body occupies an area of approximately 1.5 sq ft (0.14 m²); an average adult male human body occupies a 0.22-sq m area
	  • However, when considering queues, the body buffer zone is to be expanded to an inter-person spacing of 3.5 ft (1.07 m)
	• Waiting area recommended
	  • 0.7 sq m per person (HBN)
	  • 8–10 sq ft per patient in an OPD session (McGibony)
	  • 18 sq ft per person—Jain Malkin
	  • 15 sq ft per each of half of the total not attending an OPD session (HBN 12)
	• Spacious comfortable chairs
	• Well-lit/ventilated/non-institutional character
	• Soothing interior décor
	• Display board for staff availability/waiting status/miscellaneous information
	• Magazines/newspapers/snack counter/telephone booths
	• Prayer hall
	• TV and background music
	• Adequate sanitary facilities

14.7 Summary

For many years, the health care system has experienced a continuing decline in the number of beds required for inpatients. As inpatient care is reduced, there is a corresponding trend toward increased outpatient health care. An outpatient clinic is less expensive to build and operate than a hospital. OPDs can be in a polyclinic away from hospital inpatient areas or in a separate building connected horizontally with respective inpatient areas. Whatever the model of construction is, the OPD should be planned and designed according to the expected future OPD load with every specialty finding a representation in the OPD.

15 INTENSIVE CARE UNIT (ICU)

15.1 Introduction

An ICU is a highly specialized, specified, and sophisticated area of a hospital that is specifically designed, staffed, located, furnished, equipped, and dedicated to the management of critically sick patients or those with injuries or complications. It is a department with dedicated medical, nursing, and allied staff. It is emerging as a separate specialty and can no longer be regarded purely as part of anaesthesia, medicine, surgery, or any other specialty. An ICU has to have its own separate team in terms of doctors, nursing personnel, and other staff who are tuned to the requirements of the specialty. The characteristics of an ICU that influence its design are listed in Table 15A.

TABLE 15A: Characteristics of an ICU That Influence Its Design

Level I ICU

(Recommended for hospitals including nursing homes up to 50 beds and district hospitals/community health centres up to 100 beds)

- Number of beds—6 to 8.
- Should be able to perform cardiopulmonary resuscitation including intubation and short-term cardiorespiratory support with non-invasive ventilation and defibrillation.
- Provision for short-term mechanical ventilation (desirable).
- Has syringe pumps/infusion pumps.
- Has multipara monitors with SPO2, HR, ECG, NIBP, and temperature facility.
- Access to ABG facility.
- Access to ultrasound, x-ray, and basic clinical lab (CBC, blood sugar, electrolytes, LFT, and RFT).
- Desirable to have access to CT scans and microbiology.
- Access to ambulance (ACLS desirable) and trained manpower for safe transport of patients to higher level centres.
- Doctors should be encouraged to participate in short-term training courses/workshops such as FCCS/4C/ACLS/mechanical ventilation, etc.
- Access to 24 × 7 blood bank/pharmacy/nutrition (desirable).
- Provision for telemedicine consultations (desirable).
- At least one book and one journal of critical care medicine should be available as ready readers.
- General infection control and safety measures for patients and staff should be observed.

Level II ICU

(Recommended for larger general hospitals from 100 to 150 beds)

It includes all recommendations of Level I in addition to the following requirements:
- Number of beds 8 to 12.
- Head of Department (HOD)/Director in-charge of the ICU should be an intensivist and qualified/trained/certified in critical care.
- Facility for multisystem organ support.
- Central nurse station (CNS)/central monitoring facility.
- Provision of both invasive and non-invasive ventilation (preferably up to one-half to two-thirds of bed strength).
- Access to renal replacement therapy (RRT).
- Transcutaneous pacing facility.
- Microbiology support with facility for fungal identification (desirable).
- Nurses and duty doctors are trained/certified in critical care.
- Should have ABG, bedside x-ray, and ultrasound 24 × 7.
- Access to CT and MRI.
- ICU protocols and policies must be present and observed.
- Research should be encouraged.
- Should have access to super-specialties of medicine and surgery.
- High-Dependency Unit (HDU) facility and telemedicine are desirable.
- Should have access to e-journals, databases, and books.

Level III ICU

(For tertiary care hospitals >150 Beds including medical colleges and corporate hospitals)

It includes all Level II recommendations; in addition, it must have following facilities/provisions (Level III is further sub-classified into A and B on the basis of provision of extreme care services. Level III B provides extracorporeal therapies in addition to facilities available in Level III A):

Level III A

- Critical Care Unit should preferably be a closed ICU.
- Protocols and policies are defined.
- Must have provision of advanced cardiorespiratory monitoring—both invasive and non-invasive.
- Intra- and inter-hospital transport facilities available.
- Multisystem care and referral available 24 × 7.
- Should become lead centre for teaching and training in critical care.
- Ultrasound and echocardiography in the ICU 24 × 7.
- In-house blood bank, pharmacy, and canteen services 24 × 7.
- In-house CT scan and MRI facilities strongly recommended.
- Bedside flexible bronchoscopy facility is desirable.
- Bedside RRT.
- Continuous renal replacement therapy (CRRT) and plasma exchange facility are recommended.
- Optimum patient/nurse ratio (1:1 when patients are on organ support, e.g., mechanical ventilation, RRT, and multiple inotropes; and 1:2 at least when patient is on non-invasive ventilation and/or requires less-intense monitoring).
- Should follow guidelines of a professional body of critical care (ISCCM) or equivalent in terms of ICU structure.
- Should act as a centre for research, training, and teaching, including teleconsultations and a telemedicine centre.
- Should be equipped for both long-term acute care and palliative care.
- Team should be well-versed in transplant critical care.

Level III B

Includes all recommendations of Level III A plus ECMO-, ECCO2R-, and LV-assist devices.

DOI: 10.1201/9780367460884-16

15.2 ICU and Wider Hospital Context: Location & Access

The ICU should be a separate unit within the hospital with access to the ED, operating theatre, recovery room, surgical and medical wards, and diagnostic radiology department. There should be easy access to the High-Dependency Unit(s). This has advantages to units as a step-up or (more usually) step-down facility and for patient evacuation in the event of fire or for decanting in the event of closure.

Careful placement of departments can help to minimize the distances that patients are moved. Where there is a lot of patient flow, large lifts and extra-wide corridors are mandatory. Those hospitals that transfer or receive patients to and from specialist units in other hospitals or those that receive frequent transfers from outside the hospital must consider the position of the ICU in relation to ambulance or helicopter access, which may require dedicated external access.

15.3 Models of Care

There are two widely recognized arrangement systems of patient beds and services in ICUs, namely, open and closed models.

(a) **Open system**: Most old ICUs were designed on the recovery room model, with the head of the bed against the wall. Utilities such as oxygen, compressed air, vacuum, and electricity are also delivered from the wall at the head of the bed. Unfavorably, they are commonly blocked by the position of the patient.

(b) **Closed system**: Modern ICUs are built like operating rooms with a patient's bed away from the wall or in the case of a private cubicle, in the middle of the room. Utilities can be delivered from a power column that stands at one corner of the head of the bed or from an overhead boom (pendants) while in an operating room.

Other critical care centres define their ICUs as open or closed or a combination of both types based on the type of health care team and services provided.

(a) **In the open system**, nursing, pharmacy, and respiratory therapy staff are ICU-based. In contrast, the caring physicians of the ICU patient may have obligations at a site distant from the ICU such as the operating room.

(b) **In the closed system**, care is provided by an ICU-based team of critical care physicians, nurses, pharmacists, respiratory therapists, and other health professionals.

The number of operational models applicable to ICUs include the following.

(a) **Combined Critical Care**: Combined Critical Care may include a High-Dependency Unit, Intensive Care, and/or Coronary Care and is often located in a rural or regional hospital where flexibility of bed utilization is important. This allows short- and medium-term intensive care patients to be managed appropriately when required, and at other times, the unit can be used for more common cardiology or high-dependency patients. These units have lower medical and nursing demands and are usually staffed on a nurse/patient ratio of significantly less than 1:1.

(b) **Combined General Intensive Care**: In this model, intensive care consists of all patient specialties such as cardiothoracic surgery, orthopaedics, neurosurgery, and general medical patients. These units usually have a combination of intensive care and high-dependency beds. This model may be adopted where there are limited numbers of sub-specialty critical patients. The disadvantage of this model is that if the general intensive care is fully occupied, critical sub-specialty cases may need to remain in standard Inpatient Units for treatment.

(c) **Hot Floor**: The Hot Floor model of intensive care can be collocated with specialty ICUs, such as cardiothoracic, neurosurgical, and general intensive care, and may include a High-Dependency Unit. A comprehensive Hot Floor model may include the collocation of ICU with the Operating Unit, emergency, CCU, and parts or all of medical imaging. The Hot Floor model has the principal advantage of collocating services and avoiding duplication and with a single management structure, allowing a more efficient medical and nursing overview.

(d) **Separate ICUs**: This model covers a range of specialty ICUs provided as disconnected units in separate locations, with an independent management structure for each unit. Advantages of this model include helping to avoid bed blockages by allowing different groups to control the intensive care resources and encouraging the development of sub-specialty medical and nursing skills. Disadvantages include the duplication of management, policies, and procedures and physical isolation of units that may make staffing more difficult.

15.4 Patient Flows

Key Result Areas & Quality Indicators: Key result areas and quality indicators for an ICU are given in Table 15B.

TABLE 15B: Key Result Areas and Quality Indicators for an ICU

Key Result Areas

- Process KRA
  - Initial assessment and reassessment of patients
  - Admission and discharge criteria
  - Care plan for each patient
  - Discharge and discharge summary
  - Nursing care
  - Identification of early warning signs
  - CPR
  - Case records—documentation
- Structural KRA
  - Narcotics
  - Blood transfusions
  - Restraint policy
  - Vulnerable patients
  - Hazardous materials
  - Patient feedback
  - Fire safety
  - Medical gas

(Continued)

TABLE 15B: (Continued)

- Hand hygiene
- Documentation of handover
- Infection control
- Safe transfer of patients
- Medication orders
- Pain management
- Medication management
- Nutritional assessment

- BMW
- End-of-life care
- Engineering controls
- Credentialing and privileging
- Compressed air purity
- Equipment/furniture maintenance
- Referrals
- Quality assurance
- Patient rights

Quality Indicators

- HCAI Rates: VAE, SSI, CAUTI, and CLABSI
- Hand hygiene compliance rate
- Time taken for initial assessment of admitted patients
- Percentage of medication charts with error-prone abbreviations
- Percentage of patients developing ADRs
- Standardized mortality ratio of ICU
- Incidence of hospital-associated pressure ulcers after admission
- Nurse-to-patient ratio for ICU
- Time taken for discharge
- Patient fall rate
- Percentage of near misses
- Appropriate handovers during shift change (to be performed separately for doctors and nurses)—(per patient per shift)

Internal & External Functional Relationships (Table 15C and Figure 15A)

TABLE 15C: Functional Relationships of an ICU

Internal Functional Relationships *Optimal internal relationships to be achieved include those among*	External Functional Relationships *It is desirable that the ICU has ready access to*
Patient-occupied areas, which form the core of the unit, require direct access and observation by staff	Emergency Unit, for urgent admissions
Staff station(s) and associated areas that need direct access and observation of patient areas and ready access to administration areas	Operating Unit, for urgent patient transfers
Clinical support areas such as utility and storage areas that need to be readily accessible to both patients and staff work areas	Medical Imaging, particularly for chest x-rays and CT scanning
Public areas located on the perimeter of the unit with access to lifts and circulation corridors	Pathology Services (also via pneumatic tube)
Shared support areas that should be easily accessible from the units served	Pharmacy
—	Biomedical Engineering to ensure availability and functioning of monitoring and life support equipment

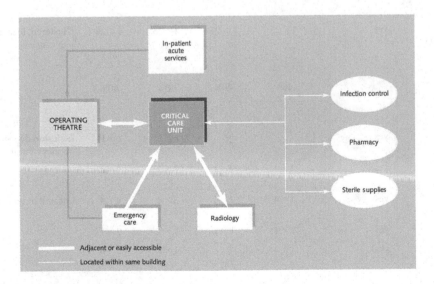

FIGURE 15A   Functional Relationships of an ICU (Courtesy: HBN 04-02).

Major Space Determinants and ICU Size

TABLE 15D: Major Space Determinants and ICU Size

ROOM/SPACE	Standard Component	Levels 2&3 Qty × m²	Level 4 Qty × m²	Level 5 Qty × m²	Level 6 Qty × m²	Remarks
ENTRANCE/ RECEPTION AREA:						
MEETING ROOM — 12 m²	yes		1 × 12			
MEETING ROOM—MEDIUM	yes			1 × 15	1 × 15	
TOILET—PUBLIC	yes	Shared	2 × 3	2 × 3	2 × 3	
WAITING	yes	2 × 10	1 × 15	1 × 20	1 × 30	1.2 m² per able-bodied person; 1.5 m² per wheelchair occupant
WAITING FAMILY	yes	1 × 20	1 × 25	1 × 30	1 × 5D	
DISCOUNTED CIRCULATION		25%	25%	25%	25%	
PATIENT AREAS:						
ANTEROOM	yes	1 × 6	1 × 6	2 × 6	4 × 6	Use for 1 bedroom—Isolation Class N (Negative Pressure Ventilation)
BATHROOM	yes	1 × 16'	1 × 16'	1 × 16*	1 × 16*	* Inclusion depends on operational policy of unit
BAY—LINEN	yes	1 × 2	1 × 2	2 × 2	4 × 2	
BAY— RESUSCITATION TROLLEY	yes	1 × 2	1 × 2	1 × 2	1 × 2	
BAY/ ROOM—BEVERAGE	yes	1 × 4	1 × 4	1 × 5	1 × 5	5 m² allows for enclosed room
EN SUITE	yes	1 × 6	1 × 6	2 × 6	4 × 6	Size for "full assistance", i.e., 2 staff plus medical equipment
PATIENT BAY—CRITICAL	yes	2 × 16	4 × 16	6 × 16	8 × 16	Group of not more than 12, within easy observation of staff station
PATIENT BAY—CRITICAL	yes	2 × 24	4 × 24	6 × 25	8 × 25	Group of not more than 12, within easy observation of staff station
PATIENT BAY—CRITICAL ENCLOSED (CLASS S ISOLATION)	yes	1 × 25	2 × 25	4 × 25	12 × 25	Group of not more than 12, within easy observation of staff station
PATIENT BAY— CRITICAL ENCLOSED (CLASS N ISOLATION)	yes	1 × 25	1 × 25	2 × 25	4 × 25	Clustered, located away from unit entrance
DISCOUNTED CIRCULATION		40%	40%	40%	40%	
STAFF AREAS:						
BAY—BLANKET WARMING	yes			1 × 1*	2 × 1*	Inclusion depends on operational policy of unit
BAY— HANDWASHING	yes	1 × 1	2 × 1	3 × 1	6 × 1	
BAY—MOBILE EQUIPMENT	yes	1 × 4	2 × 4	3 × 4	4 × 4	Located in quiet low traffic areas
BAY—PPE	yes	1 × 1	1 × 1	1 × 1	2 × 1	
BAY/ ROOM—BEVERAGE	yes			1 × 6	1 × 6	

(Continued)

TABLE 15D: (Continued)

CLEANER'S ROOM	yes	1 × 5	1 × 5	2 × 5	2 × 5	
CLEAN UTILITY	yes	1 × 12	1 × 12	2 × 12	2 × 12	
DIRTY UTILITY	yes	1 × 10	1 × 10	1 × 10	2 × 10	
DISPOSAL	yes	1 × 8	1 × 8	1 × 8	2 × 8	Inclusion depends on bed numbers and waste management policies
EQUIPMENT CLEAN UP/SUB-PATHOLOGY	yes similar	1 × 8	1 × 8	1 × 18	1 × 18	Similar to Clean-Up Room, 12 m²
MEETING—LARGE	yes	Shared	Shared	1 × 20	1 × 20	Education/Resources—may include library; 24-hour access perimeter of unit
MEETING—MEDIUM/ LARGE	yes	Shared	1 × 15	1 × 30	1 × 35	Seminar/Training/Library; 24-hour access perimeter of unit
OFFICE—CLINICAL/ HANDOVER	yes			1 × 15	1 × 15	Inclusion depends on operational policy of unit; close to staff station
OFFICE—SINGLE PERSON 9M²	yes	1 × 9	1 × 9	1 × 9	1 × 9	NUM
OFFICE—SINGLE PERSON 9M²	yes	1 × 9	1 × 9			Staff Specialist
OFFICE — 2 PERSON SHARED	yes			1 × 12	1 × 12	Staff Specialists—2 x workstations, may be open plan or in enclosed office
OFFICE—SINGLE PERSON 12M²	yes			1 × 12	1 × 12	Medical Director
OFFICE- WORKSTATION	yes	2 × 6	4 × 6	6x 6	8 × 6	Registrars—workstation/s, open plan or in enclosed office; number is determined by staffing
OFFICE—SINGLE PERSON 12M²	yes			1 × 12	1 × 12	Medical Director
OFFICE— WORKSTATION	yes	2 × 6	4 × 6	6 × 6	8 × 6	Registrars—workstation/s, open plan or in enclosed office; number is determined by staffing
OFFICE— WORKSTATION	yes	2 × 6	2 × 6	2 × 6	2 × 6	CNC/Educator—workstation/s, open plan or in shared office; number is determined by staffing
OFFICE— WORKSTATION	yes	1 × 6	1 × 6	2 × 6	2 × 6	Research—workstation/s, open plan or in shared office; number is determined by staffing
OFFICE— WORKSTATION	yes	1 × 6	1 × 6	2 × 6	2 × 6	Secretarial—workstation/s, open plan or in shared office; number is determined by staffing
OFFICE— WORKSTATION	yes	1 × 6	1 × 6	2 × 6	2 × 6	General—workstation/s, open plan or in shared office; Number is determined by staffing
OVERNIGHT STAY—BEDROOM	yes				1 × 12	
OVERNIGHT STAY—EN SUITE	yes				1 × 4	
RESPIRATORY/ BIOMEDICAL WORKROOM	yes similar			1 × 20*	1 × 20*	Inclusion depends on operational policy of unit
SHOWER—STAFF	yes	Shared	Shared	1 × 3	1 × 3	
STAFF ROOM	yes	1 × 15	1 × 18	1 × 30	1 × 35	
STAFF STATION	yes	1 × 12	1 × 18	1 × 25	2 × 20	
CHANGE—STAFF— FEMALE	yes	Shared	1 × 10	1 × 20	1 × 35	Includes toilets, showers, lockers; size depends on staffing per shift

TABLE 15D: (Continued)

ROOM/SPACE	Standard Component	Levels 2 & 3 Qty × m²	Level 4 Qty × m²	Level 5 Qty × m²	Level 6 Qty × m²	Remarks
CHANGE—STAFF—MALE	yes	Shared	1 × 10	1 × 20	1 × 25	Includes toilets, showers, lockers; depends on staffing
STORE—DRUG	yes	1 × 5*	1 × 10*	1 × 10*	1 × 10*	Inclusion depends on operational policy of unit
STORE—EQUIPMENT	yes	1 × 15	1 × 20	1 × 25	1 × 30	
STORE—FILE	yes				1 × 10	
STORE—GENERAL	yes	1 × 16	1 × 20	1 × 20	1 × 30	
STORE—PHOTOCOPY/ STATIONERY	yes	1 × 8	1 × 8	1 × 10	1 × 10	
STORE—RESPIRATORY	yes				1 × 20*	Inclusion depends on operational policy of unit
STORE—STERILE STOCK	yes		1 × 15	1 × 30	2 × 30	
X-RAY VIEWING & REPORTING	yes			1 × 12*	1 × 12*	Inclusion depends on operational policy of unit
DISCOUNTED CIRCULATION		25%	25%	25%	25%	
ENTRANCE/ RECEPTION AREA:						
MEETING ROOM — 12 m²	yes		1 × 12			
MEETING ROOM—MEDIUM	yes			1 × 15	1 × 15	
TOILET—PUBLIC	yes	Shared	2 × 3	2 × 3	2 × 3	
WAITING	yes	2 × 10	1 × 15	1 × 20	1 × 30	1.2 m² per able-bodied person: 1.5 m² per wheelchair occupant
WAITING FAMILY	yes	1 × 20	1 × 25	1 × 30	1 × 50	
DISCOUNTED CIRCULATION		25%	25%		25%	
PATIENT AREAS:						
ANTEROOM	yes	1 × 6	1 × 6	2 × 6	4 × 6	Use tor 1 Bedroom—Isolation Class N (Negative Pressure Ventilation)
BATHROOM	yes	1 × 16*	1 × 16*	1 × 16*	1 × 16*	* Inclusion depends on operational policy of unit
BAY—LINEN	yes	1 × 2	1 × 2	2 × 2	4 × 2	
BAY—RESUSCITATION TROLLEY	yes	1 × 2	1 × 2	1 × 2	1 × 2	
BAY/ROOM—BEVERAGE	yes	1 × 4	1 × 4	1 × 5	1 × 5	5 m² allows for enclosed room
EN SUITE	yes	1 × 6	1 × 6	2 × 6	4 × 6	Size for full assistance, i.e., 2 staff plus medical equipment
PATIENT BAY—CRITICAL	yes	2 × 16	4 × 16	6 × 16	8 × 16	Group of not more than 12, within easy observation of staff station
PATIENT BAY—CRITICAL	yes	2 × 24	4 × 24	6 × 25	8 × 25	Group of not more than 12, within easy observation of staff station
PATIENT BAY—CRITICAL ENCLOSED (CLASS S ISOLATION)	yes	1 × 25	2 × 25	4 × 25	12 × 25	Group of not more than 12, within easy observation of staff station
PATIENT BAY—CRITICAL ENCLOSED (CLASS N ISOLATION)	yes	1 × 25	1 × 25	2 × 25	4 × 25	Clustered, located away from unit entrance

(Continued)

TABLE 15D: (Continued)

		40%	40%	**40%**	**40%**	
DISCOUNTED CIRCULATION						
STAFF AREAS:						
BAY—BLANKET WARMING	yes			$1 \times 1^*$	$2 \times 1^*$	Inclusion depends on operational policy of unit
BAY—HANDWASHING	yes	1×1	2×1	3×1	6×1	
BAY—MOBILE EQUIPMENT	yes	1×4	2×4	3×4	4×4	Locale in quiet, low-traffic areas

Layout & Zoning (Figure 15B)

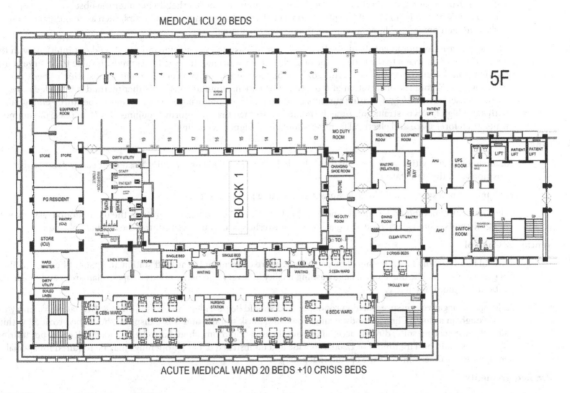

FIGURE 15B Sample Layout of ICU.

Built Environment: General Considerations

TABLE 15E: General Considerations for Built Environment in an ICU

Acoustics	• Signals from patient call systems, alarms from monitoring equipment, and telephones add to the sensory overload in Critical Care Units. Without reducing their importance or sense of urgency, such signals should be modulated to a level that will alert staff members yet be rendered less intrusive. • Floor coverings that absorb sound should be used while keeping infection control, maintenance, and equipment movement needs under consideration. • Walls and ceilings should be constructed of materials with high sound absorption capabilities. • Doorways should be offset rather than being placed in symmetrically opposed positions to reduce sound transmission. • Counters, partitions, and glass doors are also effective in reducing noise levels. • The International Noise Council recommends that the noise level in an ICU be under 45 dBA in the daytime, 40 dBA in the evening, and 20 dBA at night. For example, 16 A watch ticks at about 20 dBA, normal conversation is at approximately 55 dBA, and a vacuum cleaner produces about 70 dBA.
Natural Light	Natural light and views should be available from the unit for the benefit of staff and patients. Windows are an important aspect of sensory orientation, and as many rooms as possible should have windows to reinforce day/night orientation. If windows cannot be provided in each room, then an alternate option is to allow a remote view of an outside window or skylight.

(Continued)

TABLE 15E: (Continued)

Space Standards and Components	Where an open plan arrangement is provided, bed spaces should be arranged so that there is a clearance of at least 1,200 mm from the side of the bed to the nearest fixed obstruction (including bed screens) or wall. At the head of the bed, at least a 900-mm clearance should be allowed between the bed and any fixed obstruction or wall. When an open plan arrangement is provided, a circulation space with a 2,200-mm minimum clear width should be provided beyond dedicated cubicle space. Separate cubicles and single-patient bedrooms including isolation rooms should have minimum dimensions of 3,900 mm × 3,900 mm.
Finishes	The aesthetics of the unit should be warm, relaxing, and non-clinical as far as possible. The following additional factors should be considered in the selection of finishes: (a) acoustic properties (b) durability (c) ease of cleaning (d) infection control (e) fire safety (f) movement of equipment, as floor finishes should be resistant to marring and shearing by wheeled equipment. In all areas where patient observation is critical, colours should be chosen that do not alter the observer's perception of skin colour. Wall protection should be provided where bed or trolley movement occurs, such as corridors, patient bedrooms, equipment and linen storage areas, and treatment areas.
Equipment	Bedside monitoring equipment should be located to permit easy access and viewing and should not interfere with the visualization of or access to the patient. The bedside nurse and/or monitor technician must be able to observe at a glance the monitored status of each patient. This goal can be achieved by either a central monitoring station or bedside monitors that permit the observation of more than one patient simultaneously. Neither method is intended to replace bedside observation. Weight-bearing surfaces that support the monitoring equipment should be sturdy enough to withstand high levels of strain over time. It should be assumed that monitoring equipment will increase in volume over time. Therefore, space and electrical facilities should be designed accordingly.

Fixtures & Fittings

Clocks	An analogue clock with a second sweep hand should be provided and conveniently located for easy reference from all bed positions and the staff station.
Bedside Storage	Each patient bed space should include storage and writing provisions for staff use.
Window Treatments	Window treatments should be durable and easy to clean. Consideration can be given to the use of double glazing with integral blinds, tinted glass, reflective glass, exterior overhangs, or louvers to control the level of lighting

Infection Prevention & Control

Hand Basins	Clinical handwashing facilities should be provided that are convenient to the staff station and patient bed areas. The ratio of provision should be one clinical handwashing facility for every two patient beds in open-plan areas and one in each patient bedroom or cubicle.
Isolation Rooms	At least one negative pressure isolation room per ICU should be provided in Levels II, IIIA, & IIIB facilities. Entry should be through an airlock. Clinical handwashing, gown and mask storage, and waste disposal should be provided within the airlock. A special en suite, directly accessible from the isolation room, should also be provided. All entry points, doors, or openings should be a minimum of 1,200 mm wide and unobstructed. Larger openings may be required for special equipment, as determined by the operational policy.

Building Service Requirements

Mechanical Services	The unit should have appropriate air conditioning that allows control of temperature, humidity, and air changes.
Communications	It is vital to provide reliable and effective IT/communications services for efficient operation of the unit. The following items relating to IT/communications should be addressed in the design of the unit: (a) Electronic patient records—patient information systems. (b) Electronic forms and requests (e.g., scripts and investigative requests). (c) Picture archiving communications systems (PACS). (d) Telephones including cordless and mobile phones. (e) Computers and hand-held computers. (f) Paging for staff and emergencies. (g) Duress system. (h) Bar coding for supplies, x-rays, and records. (i) Wireless network requirements. (j) Video-conferencing requirements. (k) Communications rooms and server requirements. (l) Nurse and emergency call facilities should be provided in all patient and treatment areas in order for patients and staff to request urgent assistance. (m) The individual call buttons should alert to an annunciator system. Annunciator panels should be located at strategic points within the circulation area, particularly staff stations, staff rooms, and meeting rooms, and should be of the "non-scrolling" type, allowing all calls to be displayed at the same time. The audible signal of these call systems should be controllable to ensure minimal disturbance to patients at night. The alert to staff members shall be conducted in a discreet manner at all times.
Security	Entrance doors need to be secured to prevent unauthorized access. A video intercom with speech should be provided from the entrance and exit doors to the main staff reception complete with a door release button for staff access control. Security surveillance of the unit may include CCTV cameras and monitors.

TABLE 15F: Specific Room and Functional Requirements for Built Environment in an ICU

Entry/Reception/Waiting Areas	• As determined by the size of the ICU and hospital operating policy, Reception and visitor/relative waiting area. • Waiting areas should be provided immediately outside the entry to the ICU but away from patient and staff traffic areas. • It is desirable that this room has provision for a drink dispenser, radio, television, and comfortable seating. • An interview room and a separate area for distressed relatives should be available.
Patient Treatment Areas	• Patient bed bays, enclosed bays, isolation rooms, en suites and bathrooms provided according to the service plan. • All patient areas are to comply with standard components. • It is recommended that en suites be provided at a ratio of 1:6 beds and 1 for each isolation room. Patients must be situated so that health care providers have direct or indirect visualization at all times, such as by video monitoring. • The preferred design is to allow a direct line of vision between the patient and the central staff station. In ICUs with a modular design, patients should be visible from their respective nursing substations. • Sliding glass doors and partitions facilitate this arrangement and increase access to the room in emergency situations.
Procedures Room	• A procedures room should be provided if required by the operational policy. • If a special procedures room is provided, then it should be located within, or immediately adjacent to, the ICU. One special procedures room may serve several ICUs in close proximity. • Consideration should be given to ease of access for patients transported from areas outside the ICU. • Room size should be sufficient to accommodate the necessary equipment and personnel. • Monitoring capabilities, equipment, support services, and safety considerations must be consistent with the services provided in the ICU proper. • Work surfaces and storage areas must be adequate enough to maintain all necessary supplies and permit the performance of all desired procedures without the need for staff to leave the room. • Procedure rooms are to comply with Standard Components—Procedure Room.
Support Areas	
Biomedical Workshop	• Depending upon the size and intended use of the ICU, either a dedicated electronic and pneumatic equipment maintenance service may have to be accommodated within the hospital or a 24 hour on-call emergency service made available. • This same service would cover the Operating, Emergency and Medical Imaging Units. • If a dedicated workshop is provided, its location should be in an area that is equally accessible to all of the previously mentioned departments. The facility should have a degree of sound-proofing and be accessible from a non-sterile area.
Laboratory Facilities	• The ICU must have available 24-hour clinical laboratory services. • When this service cannot be provided by the central hospital laboratory, a satellite laboratory within or immediately adjacent to the ICU must serve this function. • Satellite facilities must be able to provide minimum chemistry and haematology testing, including arterial blood gas analysis.
Overnight Accommodation	• Depending upon the availability of nearby commercial accommodations, consideration should be given to the provision of overnight accommodation for relatives and staff, preferably near the unit.
Storage Areas	• Mobile equipment such as cardiopulmonary resuscitation trolleys and mobile x-ray that are used and located within the ICU should have storage areas that are outside traffic paths but conveniently located for easy access by staff. • Consideration should be given to the ever-increasing amount of equipment used in the unit.

Staff Facilities	• Offices/workstations should be required for senior staff in full-time administrative roles according to the approved positions in the unit.
	• Offices/workstations for medical staff and some nursing staff (manager/specialists/registrars/educators) may be located as part of the ICU where required for clinical functions or adjacent to an administrative area to facilitate unit coordination and educational and research activities.
	• A staff lounge should be provided within the unit for staff to relax and prepare beverages.
	• Inclusion of a window to the outside is desirable.
	• A library/reference area with an appropriate range of bench manuals, textbooks, and journals for rapid 24-hour access should be available within the ICU.
	• Staff will need close access to
	  • Toilets and showers
	  • Lockers
	  • Meeting room/s

15.5 Summary

The ICU of the hospital is equipment- and staff-intensive for the continuous monitoring and titrated life support of potentially salvageable and critically ill patients. The success of an ICU hinges on interdisciplinary collaboration involving health care professionals, architects, engineers, and other stakeholders. The design should prioritize patient safety, infection control, and efficient workflow while providing a supportive environment for health care staff. Optimizing space allocation, implementing advanced medical technologies, and ensuring adequate ventilation and lighting are essential. Flexibility and scalability should be integrated into the design to accommodate future advancements in medical practices and changing patient needs. Ultimately, a well-planned and designed ICU contributes to improve patient outcomes and enhances the overall quality of care provided.

16 OPERATING THEATRE (OT)

The OT provides a safe and controlled environment. The hospital operating theatre, also known as the operating room, is a vital and controlled environment where operative care of patients undergoing diagnostic/surgical procedures under anaesthesia and peri-operative care, including post-procedure recovery surgical procedures, are performed. It serves as a specialized workspace for surgical teams to carry out complex medical interventions, ensuring the utmost safety and sterility. Equipped with advanced medical technology, anaesthesia equipment, surgical tools, and monitoring devices, the operating theatre plays a pivotal role in ensuring successful surgeries and patient outcomes. Strict protocols are in place to maintain aseptic conditions, reducing the risk of infections. The seamless coordination among surgeons, nurses, anaesthesiologists, and support staff is crucial for effective and efficient surgical procedures within this critical medical setting (Table 16A).

16.1 OT and Wider Hospital Context: Location & Access

The location of the OT complex plays a vital role in deciding its features. It should be located close to critical areas but away from general traffic. It should not be located on the ground floor except for special operating rooms in the Accident and Emergency department and minor operating rooms in small hospitals. An OT should not be located on the top floor as it will increase the load on HVAC.

16.2 Models of Care

There are three basic models of surgery:

(a) Inpatient Surgery
(b) Day Surgery (outpatient or ambulatory care surgery), which may include
  • Catheter lab procedures
  • Endoscopy procedures
(c) Same-Day Surgery

All of these models should ideally be operated from the same integrated facility in the interests of efficiency, safety, and economy. These models require the following basic facilities and services:

  • Reception
  • Pre-operative facilities

TABLE 16A: Characteristics of OT That Influence OT Design

• High levels of activity
• High patient turnover
• Varied case mix
• Large multi-disciplinary workforce
• Infection control requirements
• Access issues
• Interface with pre-hospital services
• Multiple interactions with in-hospital specialties/patient transfers
• Communications issues
• Potential for growth
• Teaching activities
• Major incident capacity

• Operating room (or procedure room)
• Recovery Stage 1
• Recovery Stage 2
• Inpatient Unit (IPU)
• Intensive Care Unit (ICU)

The difference among the models is the flow of patients from one unit to the next. The models may utilize some facilities and bypass other facilities.

Inpatient Surgery: Patients undergoing elective or emergency surgery are first admitted to an Inpatient Unit or ICU or transferred from the Emergency Unit. After surgery, patients return to the ICU but not to the Emergency Unit. Inpatient surgery may start early (e.g., 7 am) and continue into the late hours of the evening. Longer hours of operation are highly efficient as they increase the throughput for the same physical facility investment. A 30% increase in the hours of operation is almost exactly the same as having 30% more operating rooms than every other support facility. In some Asian countries, operating 24 hours is the norm (Figure 16A).

Day Surgery (Outpatient Surgery): Up to 70% of all surgery may be performed as Day Surgery. Every surgical case performed as Day Surgery will save between 1 and 3 bed days as no IPU bed will be occupied by the patient. This will save costs whilst preserving valuable IPU beds for major inpatient surgery (Figure 16B).

Same-Day Surgery: This is also known as a peri-operative model and is similar to Day Surgery. However, there is no expectation for the patient to recover and go home the same day. This model allows the patient to be admitted to the hospital on the day of surgery, not earlier (Figure 16C).

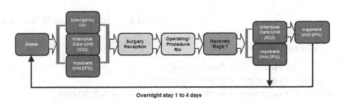

FIGURE 16A Inpatient Surgery Model Patient Flowchart (Courtesy: iHFG).

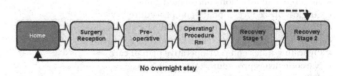

FIGURE 16B Day Surgery Patient Flowchart (Courtesy: iHFG).

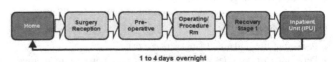

FIGURE 16C Same-Day Surgery/Patient Flowchart (Courtesy: iHFG).

DOI: 10.1201/9780367460884-17

16.3 Planning Models

The Operating Unit must be located and arranged to prevent non-related traffic through the suite. The number of operating rooms and recovery beds and the sizes of the service areas should be based on the service plan and expected surgical workload. A number of planning models can be adopted.

(a) **Single Corridor**: The single corridor model involves the travel of all supplies (clean and used) and patients (pre- and post-operative) in one main corridor. There is ongoing debate as to the suitability of this approach. However, this option is considered suitable provided that:
   - The main corridor is sufficiently wide in order to permit separation of the passage of goods and patients and
   - Handling of clean supplies and waste is carefully managed to avoid cross-contamination.

A major disadvantage of this planning model is that a patient awaiting surgery may be exposed to post-operative patients.

(b) **Dual Corridor or Racetrack**: The dual corridor or "Racetrack" model allows for all operating rooms to be accessed from an external corridor for patients and directly from a central set-up/sterile stock room for sterile goods. This model aims to separate "dirty" from "clean" traffic by controlling the uses of each corridor. In this design, there must not be cross traffic of staff and supplies from the decontaminated/soiled areas to the sterile/clean areas. In this model, stock and staff can be concentrated in one location, preventing duplication of equipment stock and staff.

(c) **Clusters of Operating Rooms**: In this model, operating rooms can be clustered according to specialty, with a shared sterile stock and set-up room for each group or cluster. Disadvantages of this model include
   - Additional corridor and circulation space is required for corridors around clusters of rooms, which reduces the available space for stock; potential duplication of stock and additional staff requirements may result in increased operating costs.

(d) **Dedicated Theatres with Fixed or Mobile Equipment**: In this model, operating rooms are dedicated to specific types of surgery such as hybrid operating/imaging rooms, urology, vascular, neurology, or other specialties requiring specific equipment. This may be beneficial in larger suites where the case volume justifies specialization; however, smaller suites may favour flexibility of operating room use. Fixed equipment can preclude the multifunctional use of the room.

(e) **Theatre Sterile Supply Unit (TSSU)/Sterile Supply Unit (SSU)**: The Operating Unit is a major user of sterile stock, and the location of the instrument processing area and sterile stock is of high importance. Two main options are available for supply of sterile stock to the Operating Unit:
   - A dedicated TSSU serving only the Operating Unit; and
   - An SSU that also serves other areas of the hospital.

Size of the Unit: The size of the Operating Unit will be determined by the Clinical Services Plan establishing the intended services scope and complexity. Schedules of Accommodation have been provided in the following for typical units at role delineation levels 2 (less complex services) to 6 (teaching/research facilities).

TABLE 16B: Key Result Areas and Quality Indicators for OT

Key Result Areas

- Nursing Plan of Care documented
- Rational use of blood and blood products
- Monitoring, managing, and reporting transfusion reactions
- Pre-anaesthesia assessment, anaesthesia plan
- Immediate pre-op assessment
- Informed consent for anaesthesia obtained by the anaesthesiologist
- Criteria for transfer/discharge from the recovery area
- Adherence to infection control guidelines
- Surgical procedures—policy and procedure
- Pre-op assessment and provisional diagnosis documented
- Informed consent for surgery obtained by a surgeon
- Operating notes and post-operative plan of care
- Narcotic drugs procedure
- Adherence to safe injection and infusion practices
- Pre- and post-exposure prophylaxis
- Segregation of biomedical waste and use of PPE
- Colour-coding of gas pipelines
- Medical gases safe handling, storage, and usage

Quality Indicators

- Percentage of unplanned returns to the OT
- Percentage of surgeries where the organization's procedure to prevent adverse drug events such as the wrong site, wrong patient, and wrong surgery have been adhered to
- Hand hygiene compliance rate
- Percentage of cases that received appropriate prophylactic antibiotics within the specified timeframe
- Percentage of rescheduling of surgeries

Internal & External Functional Relationships (Table 16C and Figure 16D)

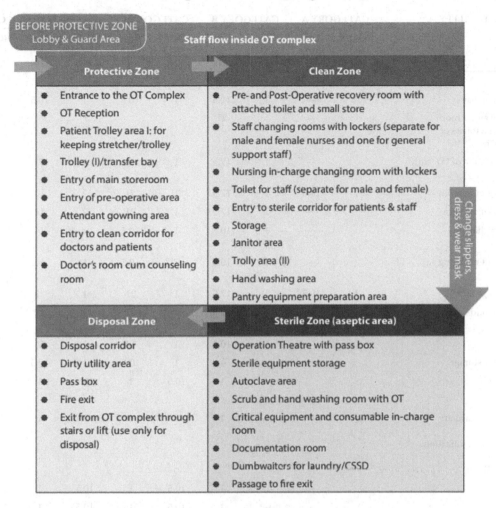

Protective Zone	Clean Zone
• Entrance to the OT Complex • OT Reception • Patient Trolley area I: for keeping stretcher/trolley • Trolley (I)/transfer bay • Entry of main storeroom • Entry of pre-operative area • Attendant gowning area • Entry to clean corridor for doctors and patients • Doctor's room cum counseling room	• Pre- and Post-Operative recovery room with attached toilet and small store • Staff changing rooms with lockers (separate for male and female nurses and one for general support staff) • Nursing in-charge changing room with lockers • Toilet for staff (separate for male and female) • Entry to sterile corridor for patients & staff • Storage • Janitor area • Trolly area (II) • Hand washing area • Pantry equipment preparation area
Disposal Zone	**Sterile Zone (aseptic area)**
• Disposal corridor • Dirty utility area • Pass box • Fire exit • Exit from OT complex through stairs or lift (use only for disposal)	• Operation Theatre with pass box • Sterile equipment storage • Autoclave area • Scrub and hand washing room with OT • Critical equipment and consumable in-charge room • Documentation room • Dumbwaiters for laundry/CSSD • Passage to fire exit

BEFORE PROTECTIVE ZONE — Lobby & Guard Area

Staff flow inside OT complex

Change slippers, dress & wear mask

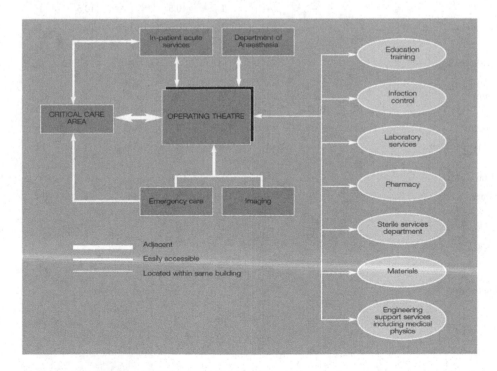

FIGURE 16D   Functional Relationship of OT (Courtesy: HBN 26).

TABLE 16D: Provision for the Various Floor Areas for the Operating Theatre

S No. (1)	FACILITY (2)	CATEGORY A ROOM (NO.) (3)	Area (m²) (4)	CATEGORY B ROOM (NO.) (5)	Area (m²) (6)	CATEGORY C ROOM (NO.) (7)	Area (m²) (8)	CATEGORY D ROOM (NO.) (9)	Area (m²) (10)	CATEGORY E ROOM (NO.) (11)	Area (m²) (12)
ZONE A											
(a)	OT reception bay		—	1	10.5	1	10.5	1	10.5	1	10.5
(b)	Relatives' waiting room (including 2 toilets of 3'5 m² each)		—	1	21						
(c)	Officer-in-charge of OT with toilet		—	1	17.5	1	17.5	1	17.5	1	17.5
(d)	Doctor changing room	1	10.5	1	17.5	1	21	2	14	2	14
(e)	Nurse changing room		—	1	17.5	1	21	2	14	2	14
(f)	Technician changing room		—	1	10.5	1	10.5	1	14	1	17.5
(g)	Class IV staff changing room		—	1	10.5	1	10.5	1	14	1	17.5
(h)	Sterile storage area	1	10.5	1	17.5	1	21	1	28	1	35
(i)	Instrument and linen room		—	1	17.5	1	21	1	28	1	35
(j)	Trolley bay		—	1	10.5	1	14	1	14	1	14
(k)	Gas cylinder storage		—		—	1	10.5	1	10.5	1	10.5
(l)	Switch room	.			—	1	10.5	1	10.5	1	14
ZONE B											
(a)	Fracture-cum-casualty theatre a) Instrument sterilization b) Scrub up c) Dirty wash up		—		—	1	28	1	28	1	28
			—		—	1	10.5	1	10.5	1	105
			—		—	1	10.5	1	10.5	1	10.5
			—		—	1	10.5	1	10.5	1	105
(b)	Plaster preparation		—		—	1	10.5	1	10.5	1	10.5
(c)	Splint store		—		—	1	10.5	1	10.5	1	10.5
(d)	Pre-operative room with toilet		—	1	14	1	21	1	28	1	28
(e)	Recovery room	1 (2 BEDS)	21	1 (4 BEDS)	35	1 (6 BEDS)	52.5	1 (10 BEDS)	87.5	1 (12 BEDS)	10.5
(f)	Nurse duty room			1	10.5	1	10.5	1	14	1	14
(g)	Theatre pack preparation room		—	1	10.5	1	14	1	14	1	17.5
(h)	Frozen section		—		—	1	10.5	1	10.5	1	10 5
(i)	X-ray with dark room		—	1	10.5	1	14	1	14	1	14
(j)	Pantry		—		—	1	10.5	1	10.5	1	10.5
ZONE C											
(k)	a) Operating theatres (major) b) Operating theatres (minor)	1	35	2	35	3–4	35	4–6	35	6–8	35
		1	20	1	28	2	28	2–3	28	3–5	28

(Continued)

TABLE 16D: (Continued)

S No.	FACILITY	CATEGORY A		CATEGORY B		CATEGORY C		CATEGORY D		CATEGORY E	
		ROOM (NO.)	Area (m²)	ROOM (NO.)	Area (m²)	ROOM (NO.)	Area (m²)	ROOM (NO.)	Area (m²)	ROOM (NO.)	Area (m²)
(1)	(2)	(3)	(4)	(5)	(6)	(7)	(8)	(9)	(10)	(11)	(12)
(l)	Instrument sterilization	1	10 5	2	10.5	3	10.5	3–5	10.5	5–7	10.5
(m)	Scrub up	1	10.5	2	10.5	3	10.5	3–5	10.5	5–7	10.5
(n)	Anaesthetist room		—	1	14	1	14	1	14	2	14
(o)	Anaesthetic storage		—	—		1	10.5	1	10 5	1	10.5
(P)	Anaesthesia room		—	1	21	2	21	2	21	3	21
q)	Doctor work room	1	10.5	1	17 5	1	21	2	14	2	17.5
(r)	Nurse work room		—			1	10.5	1	14	1	17.5
ZONE D											
(a)	Janitor room	1	10.5	2	10.5	3	10.5	3–5	10 5	5–7	10.5
(b)	Soiled utility room		—	1	70	1	7.0	1	10 5	1	10.5

Layout & Zoning (Table 16E and Figures 16E–F)

TABLE 16E: Functional Zoning and Pressure Gradient in OT

Sl. No.	Zone in OT	Pressure
1.	Sterile Zone	+25 Pa
2.	Clean Zone	+14 Pa
3.	Protective Zone	+5 Pa
4.	Disposal Zone	+ 3 or 0 Pa

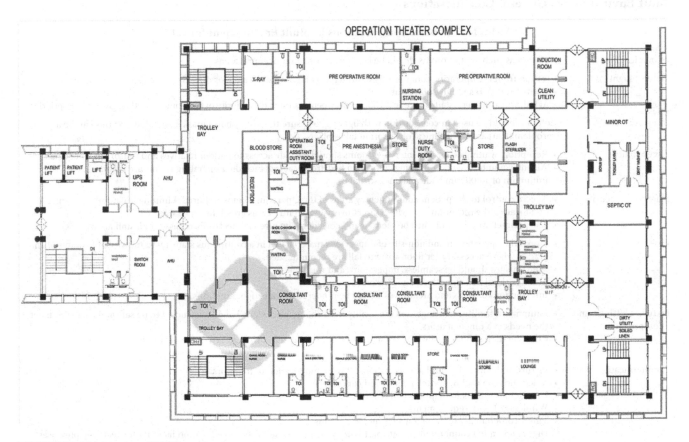

FIGURE 16E   Layout of OT Complex.

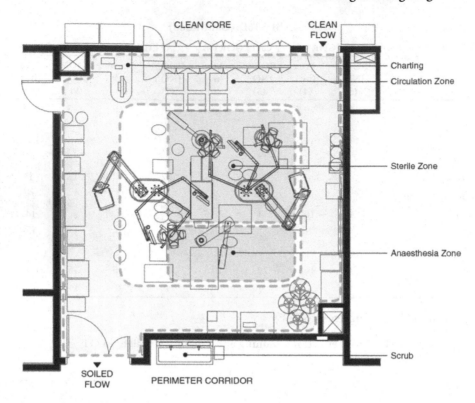

FIGURE 16F Zoning in OT (Barach PR, Rostenberg B. Design of cardiac surgery operating rooms and the impact of the built environment. In Pediatric and Congenital Cardiac Care 2015 [pp. 411–424]. Springer, London).

Built Environment: General Considerations

TABLE 16F: General Considerations for Built Environment for OT

Acoustics	Noisy areas such as staff rooms should be located away from procedural areas.
Natural Light	• Vision from the operating room could be through a corridor, set-up area, or directly to the external environment. • Many procedures require black-out. • Windows to recovery, staff lounge and TSSU areas where staff spend a majority of their time should be given a high priority.
Interior Décor	Colours should be used in combination with lighting to ensure that they do not mask skin colours as this can be a problem in areas where clinical observation takes place.
Accessibility	• Reception, waiting areas, and interview rooms should provide access to patient relatives and visitors in wheelchairs. • All entry points, doors, or openings requiring bed/trolley access including operating rooms are recommended to be a minimum of 1,400 mm wide and unobstructed.
Safety and Security	• Access control to the patient and staff entry areas of the Operating Unit is required. Limiting the number of entries and locating the reception area with a direct overview of entry areas are highly desirable. • The perimeter of the unit must be secured and consideration given to electronic access for all staff areas.
Finishes	• Floors that are smooth and non-slip of impervious material laid in a continuous stain-resistant washable material and graded where necessary for floor waste to fall are recommended. • Wall finishes should be seamless, impervious, and washable. • Ceilings should be smooth and impervious. • Intersections of walls and architraves should be rendered as watertight junctions.
Fixtures, Fittings, and Equipment	• Equipment, furniture, fittings, and the facility itself should be designed and constructed to be safe and robust to meet the needs of a range of users. • Consideration should be given to compact units for sterile items, storage and movement of loan equipment, and shelving for storing heavy items.
Communications	• Picture archiving communications systems (PACS) and location of monitors. • Voice and data cabling for telephones and computers. • Bar coding systems for supplies and records. • Wireless network requirements. • Video-conferencing requirements for meeting rooms. • Digital operating room requirements particularly linkages to seminar and education facilities for teaching purposes. • Communications rooms and server requirements.

(Continued)

TABLE 16F: (Continued)

HVAC	HVAC standards for an OT are given in Table 16 G.
Medical Gases	• Gas and suction outlets should be self-sealed when not in use. • Outlets from different gases should have non-interchangeable connections, for fear of giving the wrong gas during anaesthesia. • Filters on air and gas supplies should be capable of removing all particles larger than 5 microns. • Standardizing the position of gas outlets throughout the hospital ensures that accidents cannot occur, so outlets should supply oxygen, air, suction, and nitrous oxide in this order from left to right. • Portable anaesthesia machine should provide one oxygen, one air, one suction, and one nitrous oxide gas outlet in the anaesthetic room. • There must be three suction outlets per room for operative rooms and three outlets per bed in the recovery room.
Radiation Shielding and Radiation Safety	• Operating rooms that are used for undertaking imaging procedures require radiation shielding. • Relevant AERB guidelines should be followed. • Consideration should be given to the provision of floor and ceiling shielding when rooms immediately above and below are occupied.
Infection Control	• Infection control issues are paramount in the Operating Unit and require careful attention to planning models and separation of clean and dirty workflows. • The need for isolation rooms (positive and negative pressure) in holding and recovery areas is to be evaluated by an infection control risk assessment and should reflect the requirements of the service plan. • Clinical handwashing facilities should be provided within all patient holding and recovery areas and convenient to the staff stations.

TABLE 16G: HVAC Standards for OT

Sl. No.	Parameters	Requirements for Super Specialty OT	Requirements for General OT
1.	Temperature	18°C +/− 2°C	23°C +/− 2°C
2.	Relative Humidity	55%	55%
3.	Air Change Per Hour	20	20
4.	Fresh Air Allowance	100% Fresh Air	20% Fresh Air and 80% Recirculated Air
5.	Air Velocity	25–35 FPM	25–35 FPM
6.	Air Handling in the OT Including Air Quality	Through HEPA	Through HEPA

TABLE 16H: Specific Room and Functional Requirements for OT

Reception/Waiting	• Receiving hub of the unit for patients and visitors from the IPU, ICU, or Emergency Unit on beds/trolleys. • Access control. • The waiting area should be located to avoid conflict with patient traffic entering the Operating Unit.
Pre-operative Holding	• Patients received are placed in a curtained holding bay or private cubicle with solid side walls and curtain front. • The recommended number of bays/cubicles is a ratio of 1:1 for each operating room (or procedure room). • The bed bay/cubicle has facilities such as a bedside locker, medical gases, and patient toilets. • Patient pre-operative holding bays should be supervised from a staff base.
Anaesthetic Induction Rooms	• The anaesthetic room may be used for administration of local and spinal anaesthetics, patient monitoring, or patient preparation prior to the procedure. • General anaesthetics and sedations are typically administered in the operating room.
Operating/Procedure Room/s	• The procedures may be highly invasive, minimally invasive, sterile, or non-sterile. The design may vary slightly according to the intended procedure. • A very high level of specialization can lead to inefficiency in surgical throughput due to the number of useable operating rooms. Under this definition, a procedure room includes a catheter lab, endoscopy procedure room, etc.
Dental Surgery	In addition to the standard operating room equipment and services, items considered essential for dental procedures are the following: • One compressed dental air outlet situated close to the service panels for medical gases, suction, and electrical outlets, with the provision of a regulated bottle of appropriate compressed air for emergency backup or secondary use. • Facilities for dental x-rays.
Stage 1 Recovery	• Following general surgery, patients recover in Stage 1 Recovery. • Patients with complicated surgery may bypass Stage 1 Recovery and recover directly in an ICU. • The recommended ratio of beds in Stage 1 Recovery is 2:1 per general operating/procedure room and 1.5:1 per day surgery operating/procedure room.

(Continued)

TABLE 16H: (Continued)

Stage 2/3 Recovery	• Day patients and short-stay patients may progress to Stage 2 Recovery or be taken directly to Stage 2 Recovery following some procedures requiring minimal sedation or local anaesthetics.
	• In Stage 2 Recovery, patients will have regained consciousness following a procedure but still require observation and management.
	• Stage 2 Recovery may be provided as bed bays, chair bays, or a combination of both.
	• The recommended ratio of beds/chairs in Stage 2 Recovery is 3:1 per operating/procedure room. A higher number of beds/chairs per operating/procedure room allows for a rapid turnover for day surgery patients, particularly for procedures that take 15 minutes or less.
	• Stage 3 Recovery is a lounge area, where patients recover and are dressed in street clothes, awaiting collection by relatives.
	• The recommended ratio of chairs in Stage 3 Recovery is 3:1 per operating/procedure room. This number of chairs allows for patients to await relatives to arrive and transport them home without compromising the number of recovery bed bays required for patients undergoing procedures.
Support Areas	
Pathology Area	Depending on the service plan and unit policy, an area for preparation and examination of frozen sections may be provided.
Flash Sterilizing Facilities	A flash sterilizer should be located in the unit; however, the use of this method of sterilizing should be restricted to situations where a single instrument has been dropped, and no sterile duplicate is available.
Storeroom	• Adequate equipment storerooms for equipment and supplies used in the Operating Unit should be provided including sterile stock, consumables, anaesthetic supplies, drugs, and equipment such as operating table accessories, mobile microscopes and other mobile equipment.
	• Equipment bays are best designed as elongated rectangular shapes and may be combined for space efficiency.
Administration/Staff Amenities	• Offices and workstations may be located within a discreet zone remote from the operational areas.
	• Adequate access to meeting rooms should be provided to facilitate education and research activities within the unit.
	• Staff amenities:
	• Appropriate changing rooms, toilets, and showers should be provided for male and female personnel (nurses, doctors, and technicians) working within the Operating Unit.
	• The changing rooms should contain adequate lockers, showers, toilets, hand basins, and space for donning surgical attire and booting.
	• The changing room entrance door should be provided with locks or electronic access devices to prevent the entry of unauthorized persons into the Operating Unit.

16.4 Summary

In the present era of evidence-based medicine, it becomes imperative to give maximum importance to planning an operating theatre complex. Within the limitations of finances and space, the best results can be obtained, and anaesthesiologists with multiple roles inside the operating theatre complex should be consulted in the process. Efforts should be made to conform to the standards established by local bodies and international agencies, as health care facilities in India are now catering to an increasingly more international clientele.

17 MATERNITY UNIT

17.1 Background

Maternity care is provided in several different health care settings such as a hospital site, in the community, or at home. Maternity care is decided on a local basis by commissioning bodies, and there is an increasing call for woman-centred, user-friendly services offering choice and continuity of care.

Each setting should be designed so that it is appropriate for use by the family and the staff who are providing care. Whatever the setting and model of care, the main objective is to provide for the safe care of both mother and baby in a comfortable, relaxing environment that facilitates this normal physiological process, enables self-management in privacy whenever possible, and enhances the family's enjoyment of an important life event.

In all units, rooms should be designed to give women choice and control over their labour and birth, to normalise the process, and to welcome family participation. The "normality" of the experience is a key driver, but appropriate facilities are needed for intervention when complications occur. Table 17A shows the characteristics of the Maternity Unit that influence its design.

The Maternity Unit incorporates

- Birthing Unit
- Inpatient accommodation—Antenatal
- Inpatient accommodation—Postnatal
- Nurseries:
  - General care
  - Special care

17.2 Maternity Unit and Wider Hospital Context: Location & Access

The Maternity Unit should be located to ensure 24-hour easy access for ambulances and other vehicles, and it should have its own separate entrance. It should be located adjacent or close to the birthing unit and neonatal unit. Critical Care Units and the High-Dependency Unit (HDU) should be close enough for direct transfer in case of need. Access to external spaces is important for all units. The location should protect other patients and visitors from the noise of women in labour. Maternity Units should not be located near A&E and Mental Health Unit for safety and security reasons.

TABLE 17A: Characteristics of a Maternity Unit That Influence Its Design

- High-risk obstetric cases
- Medical termination of pregnancy (MTP)
- Pre-, peri-, and postnatal monitoring and care

17.3 Models of Care

The Birthing Unit may be either a

- Unit within a hospital facility or a
- Stand-alone facility in a community setting.

Size of the Unit: The number of beds will be determined by the facility's service plan. The preferred maximum number of beds in the Maternity Unit is 20–25 beds in order to accommodate additional rooms such as the general care nursery, feeding room, formula room, and communal activities areas. The number of cots in the nursery areas will be determined by the service plan depending on the number of beds in the unit.

The number of cots in a newborn nursery should not exceed 16 cots. Where the operational policy of the Maternity Unit includes rooming babies with mothers, then the number of cots in a general care nursery should accommodate the expected number of babies that are not rooming with the mother.

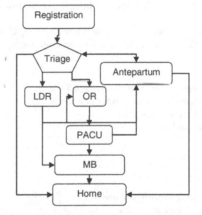

FIGURE 17A Patient Flow Patterns in a Maternity Unit (Griffin J, Xia S, Peng S, Keskinocak P. Improving patient flow in an obstetric unit. Health Care Management Science. 2012 Mar;15(1):1–4).

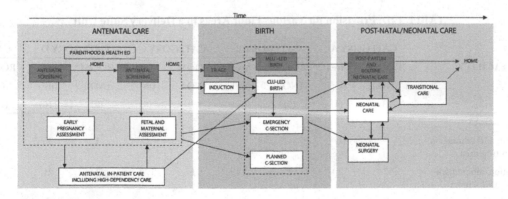

FIGURE 17B Care Pathway for Pregnant Females (Courtesy: HBN 09-02).

DOI: 10.1201/9780367460884-18

Key Result Areas

TABLE 17B: Key Result Areas for a Maternity Unit

Key Result Areas

- MTP: register, consents, confidentiality
- Obstetric services—policy and procedure
- Care of high-risk obstetrical patients: display of scope—whether high risk obstetric cases are cared for or not
- Obstetrical patient assessment including maternal nutrition
- Competence of staff handling high-risk obstetrical cases
- Pre-, peri-, and postnatal monitoring and documentation
- Documented procedures on provision of antenatal services
- Facilities to take care of neonates of high risk pregnancies

Internal & External Functional Relationships

TABLE 17C: Functional Relationships of a Maternity Unit

External Functional Relationships	Internal Functional Relationships
Principal relationships with other units include ready access to	*Optimum internal relationships in all models include*
• Short-term parking/drop-off bay for dropping off expectant mothers. • Drop-off and parking bays for florist deliveries. • Emergency Unit. • Birthing Unit. • Operating Unit. • Neonatal ICU and special care nurseries. • ICU and HDU for mothers requiring advanced care. • Diagnostic facilities such as medical imaging, laboratories, and pharmacy. • Supply, Housekeeping, Catering and Waste Handling Units. • Outpatient/Women's Health Units and community support services.	• Reception to supervise security to the entire unit with restricted access to maternity inpatient accommodation, Birthing Unit, and NICU/SCN nursery areas. • The staff station and associated areas need direct access and observation of patient areas. • Utility and storage areas need ready access to both patient and staff work areas. • Nursery areas to be accessible from postnatal inpatient areas particularly the general care nursery. • Feeding and formula rooms should be accessible to both the nursery and postnatal inpatient areas. • Public areas should be located in the entry area, prior to entry into restricted access zones. • Shared support areas should be easily accessible from the units served.
Principal relationships with public areas include	*Clear goods/service/staff entrance*
• Easy access from the main entrance of a facility. • Easy access to public amenities. • Easy access to parking.	• Access to/from key clinical units associated with patient arrivals/transfers via service corridor and lifts. • Access to/from key diagnostic facilities via service corridor and lifts. • Entry for staff via public or service corridor. • Close access to staff support areas that may be shared with adjacent areas. • Access to/from Supply, Housekeeping, Catering and Waste Units via service corridor and lifts.
Principal relationships with staff areas	*Clear public entrance*
• Ready access to staff amenities	• Entry for ambulant patients and visitors directly from dedicated lifts and public corridor. • Access to/from key public areas, such as the main entrance, parking, and outpatients. • Units from the public corridor and lifts.

TABLE 17D: Provision for Various Floor Areas in a Delivery Suite Unit

S No.	FACILITY	CATEGORY A ROOM (NO.)	CATEGORY A Area (m²)	CATEGORY B ROOM (NO.)	CATEGORY B Area (m²)	CATEGORY C ROOM (NO.)	CATEGORY C Area (m²)	CATEGORY D ROOM (NO.)	CATEGORY D Area (m²)	CATEGORY E ROOM (NO.)	CATEGORY E Area (m²)
(1)	(2)	(3)	(4)	(5)	(6)	(7)	(8)	(9)	(10)	(11)	(12)
FUNCTIONAL AREAS											
(a)	Reception and admission with waiting area	—		—		1	21	1	35	1	42
(c)	Examination and preparation room with toilet	1	14	1	14	1	17.5	1	21	1	21
(d)	Doctor changing room	1	10.5	1	10.5	1	10.5	1	10.5	1	10.5

(Continued)

TABLE 17D: (Continued)

S No.	FACILITY	CATEGORY A ROOM (NO.)	CATEGORY A Area (m²)	CATEGORY B ROOM (NO.)	CATEGORY B Area (m²)	CATEGORY C ROOM (NO.)	CATEGORY C Area (m²)	CATEGORY D ROOM (NO.)	CATEGORY D Area (m²)	CATEGORY E ROOM (NO.)	CATEGORY E Area (m²)
(1)	(2)	(3)	(4)	(5)	(6)	(7)	(8)	(9)	(10)	(11)	(12)
(e)	Nurse changing room	1	10.5	1	10.5	1	10.5	1	10.5	1	10.5
(f)	Class IV changing room	—		—		1	10.5	1	10.5	1	10.5
(g)	Technician changing room	—		—		—		1	10.5	1	10.5
(h)	Sterile storage	—		1	14	1	21	1	28	1	28
(i)	Instrument linen store	—		—		1	10.5	1	10.5	1	10.5
(j)	Trolley bay	—		—		1	10.5	1	10.5	1	10.5
(k)	Switch room	—		1	7.0	1	10.5	1	10.5	1	10.5
(l)	Recovery room	—		1	14	1	21	1	28	1	35
(m)	Pack preparation room	—		1	10.5	1	10.5	1	14	1	17.5
(n)	Anaesthesia room	—		—		1	14	1	21	1	21
(o)	Labour room	1	10.5	1	21					4	21
(p)	Delivery room	1	21	1	21	2	21	3	21	1	35
(q)	Operating delivery room	—		1	28	1	28	1	35	1	17.5
(r)	Instrument sterilizing	—		1	10.5	1	14	1	17.5	3	10.5
(s)	Scrub up	—		1	7.0	2	7.0	2	10.5	1	10.5
(t)	Children birth	—		1	7.0	1	10.5	1	10.5	1	10.5
(u)	Eclampsia room	—		—				1	14	1	21
(v)	Dirty utility	1	7.0	1	10.5	1	10.5	1	14	1	17.5
(w)	Janitor's closet	—		1	3.5	1	3.5	1	7.0	1	7.0
(x)	Bank	—		—		1	21	1	28	1	42
(y)	Post office	—		—				1	21	1	28
(z)	Library for patients	—		—		1	21	1	28	1	35

Layout & Zoning (Figure 17C)

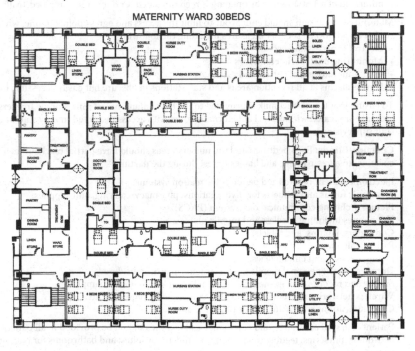

FIGURE 17C Layout of a Maternity Unit.

Built Environment: General Considerations

TABLE 17E: General Considerations for Built Environment

Acoustics	**Inpatient Areas:** Inpatient accommodation should be designed to minimize the ambient noise level within the unit and the transmission of sound among, patient areas, staff areas, and public areas. Acoustic treatment will be required for the following: • Patient bedrooms. • Interview and meeting rooms. • Treatment rooms. • Staff rooms. • Toilets and showers. **Nursery Areas:** Sound levels for all services installed within the nursery areas, particularly special care nurseries, should be controllable to provide minimal noise intrusion, ideally less than 40 dB.
Natural Light/Lighting	• External windows will require shading, and babies must be positioned away from windows to prevent excessive light and radiant heat gain. • Artificial lighting must be colour-corrected to allow staff to observe natural skin tones and dimmable for night lighting.

Observation and Privacy	• Factors for consideration include:
	  • Use of windows in internal walls and/or doors.
	  • Location of beds that may affect direct staff visibility.
	  • Provision of bed screens to ensure the privacy of patients undergoing treatment.
	  • Location of sanitary facilities to provide privacy for patients while not preventing observation of the bed area by staff.

Interior Décor	Interior décor includes furnishings, style, colour, textures, and ambience influenced by perception and culture. The delécor of the unit should be of a standard that meets the expectations of the clients using the services and make every effort to reduce the look of an institutional atmosphere. Patient treatment and reception areas should be open and inviting with delécor that is domestic and casual rather than institutional. Access to outdoor areas is desirable.
Room Capacity and Dimensions	• Maximum room capacity for a Maternity Unit should be two patients. • Minimum room dimensions are based on overall bed dimensions (buffer to buffer) of 2,250 mm long × 1,050 mm wide. • **Bed Spacing/Clearances:** In all bedrooms, there should be a clearance of 1,200 mm available at both sides and at the foot of each bed to allow for easy movement of equipment and beds. • In multiple-bed bedrooms, the minimum distance between bed centre lines should be 2,400 mm.
Accessibility	• Design should provide ease of access to wheelchair-bound patients in all patient areas including lounge rooms and nurseries.
Doors	• Doors used for emergency bed transfers within the unit or to the Birthing or Operating Units must be appropriately positioned and sized. • A minimum of a 1,400-mm clear opening is recommended for doors requiring bed/trolley access.

Safety and Security	• Maternity Unit design should endeavour to limit the access and egress points to one, which are supervised by staff, with additional security measures including the following:
	  • Electronic access and egress.
	  • Monitoring of all perimeter doors.
	  • CCTV monitoring of entries and exits.
	  • Duress alarms at all reception areas and staff stations in obscure but easily accessible locations.

Milk Storage	• To ensure that the correct milk is provided to the right infant, breast milk storage freezers and fridges should be lockable or located within a lockable formula room with access restricted to only staff or also to mothers under staff supervision.
Privacy Screens	• **Curtains/Blinds:** Each bedroom and the nursery areas should have partial blackout facilities (blinds or lined curtains) to allow patients and babies to rest during the daytime.
Communications	• Electronic patient records and patient information systems. • Electronic forms and requests for investigations, pharmacy, catering, and supplies. • Picture archiving communications system (PACS). • Telephones including cordless and mobile phones. • Computers, laptops, and tablets. • Patient call, nurse assist call, and emergency call systems. • Paging for staff and emergencies. • Duress systems; personal mobile duress systems may be considered. • Supply and records management systems including bar coding for supplies. • Wireless network requirements and video-conferencing requirements. • Communications rooms and server requirements.
Staff/Emergency Call	• Patient call, staff assistance, and emergency call facilities should be provided in all patient areas including bedrooms, nurseries, feeding rooms, lounges, toilets, en suites, and bathrooms for patients and staff to request urgent assistance.

(Continued)

TABLE 17E: (Continued)

Patient Entertainment Systems	Patient bedrooms and lounge areas can be provided with the following entertainment/communications systems according to the operational policy of the facility: • Television. • Telephone. • Radio. • Internet, wireless internet access.
Heating Ventilation, and Air Conditioning (HVAC)	• Nurseries should be serviced by HVAC systems that allow the temperature to be controllable between 21 and 30°C. • Inpatient accommodation areas should be air conditioned and maintain a temperature range comfortable for mothers and babies.
Medical Gases	• Table 17F shows the number of medical gas terminal units, AVSUs, and alarms for a Maternity Unit. • Table 17F shows the design flow for medical gas terminal unit (L/minute).
Pneumatic Tube Systems	If provided, the station should be located in close proximity to the staff station or under direct staff supervision.
Infection Control	• Each nursery should have a hand basin at the point of entry for staff and parents. Within the nursery, a minimum of one hand basin should be provided per four cots in general care nurseries and one per two cots in special care nurseries.
Isolation Rooms	• At least one "Class S—Standard" isolation room should be provided for each Inpatient Unit. • The need for negative pressure isolation rooms is to be evaluated by an infection control risk assessment and will reflect the requirements of the service plan.

TABLE 17F: Number of Medical Gas Terminal Units, AVSUs, and Alarms

Area/Room	Oxygen	Nitrous Oxide	Nitrous Oxide/ Oxygen Mixture	Medical Air	Surgical Air	Vacuum	Gas Scavenging	Heliox	AVSU	Alarms
Birthing Room										
Mother	1	0	1	0	0	2	0	0	1 set per 6–7 rooms	-
Baby (per cot space)	1	0	0	1	0	1	0	0		
Operating Suite										
Anaesthetist	1	1	0	1	0	1	1	0	1 Set	1 Set
Obstetrician	0	0	0	0	0	2	0	0		
Paediatrician	1	0	0	1	0	1	0	0		
Post-Anaesthesia Recovery	1	0	0	1	0	1	0	0		
Inpatient Accommodation										
Single bed	1	0	0	0	0	1	0	0	1 Set for ward unit	1 Set
Multiple-bed bedroom	1	0	0	0	0	1	0	0		

TABLE 17G: Design Flow for a Medical Gas Terminal Unit (L/minute)

Room/Area	Oxygen	Nitrous Oxide	Nitrous Oxide/ Oxygen Mixture	Medical Air	Surgical Air	Vacuum
Birthing Room						
Mother	10	0	275	0	40	—
Baby (per cot space)	10	0	0	40	40	—
Operating Suite						
Anaesthetist	100	15	0	40	40	Max—130 Min—80
Obstetrician	0	0	0	0	40	—
Paediatrician	10	0	0	0	40	—
Post-Anaesthesia recovery	10	0	0	40	40	—
Inpatient Accommodation						
Single bed	10	0	0	0	40	—
Multiple-bed bedroom	10	0	0	0	40	—

TABLE 17H: Specific Room and Functional Requirements for a Maternity Unit

Reception Area	• Reception is the receiving hub of the unit and may be used to control the security of the unit. • A waiting area for visitors may be provided with access to separate male/female toilet facilities and prayer rooms.

Bathing/Examination	• The bathing/examination area should include a bench with a baby examination area and baby weighing scales and a sink for baby bathing.
	• Special considerations include
	  • Provision of heating over the examination/bathing area.
	  • Provision of temperature-controlled warm water.
	  • Provision of good lighting levels; lighting should permit the accurate assessment of skin colour.
	  • The baby bathing sink should be manufactured from a material that will not retain heat or cold (stainless steel is not recommended).
	  • Staff will require access to an emergency call button for use in emergencies.

Patient Accommodation	• Patient rooms may be grouped together in zones corresponding to different levels of dependency. • Antenatal accommodation will preferably be separated from postnatal beds and be provided in single bedrooms. • Single bedrooms assist with infection control and patient privacy.
Patient Treatment Areas	• Antenatal accommodation may be provided in a quiet zone within the postnatal unit, preferably separated from postnatal patients. • Single bedrooms are preferred for patients with high-risk pregnancies that will require rest and quiet. • Support areas may be shared with postnatal accommodation. • Postnatal accommodation will generally include a combination of single and two-bed bedrooms and may include communal areas where mothers can gather to socialize or attend educational sessions. • Nursery areas, feeding rooms, and formula rooms should be readily accessible to mothers in postnatal accommodation.
Support Areas	Support areas include utility, disposal, and storerooms, which should be located conveniently for staff access. Meeting rooms and interview rooms for education sessions and interviews with staff, patients, and families may be shared with adjacent areas where possible.

Staff Areas	• Staff areas should consist of
	  • Offices and workstations.
	  • Staff room.
	  • Staff station and handover room.
	  • Toilets, shower, and lockers.
	• Staff areas, particularly staff rooms, toilets, showers, and lockers may be shared with adjacent units as far as possible.

Nursery Areas	The general area nursery will accommodate healthy newborn babies as required for short-term care. The nursery should include
	• A bathing/examination area where newborn babies can be examined, weighed, and bathed.
	• A staff station with direct observation of all cots in the nursery and a resuscitation trolley in close proximity; sterile stock and medications may be co-located with the staff station.
	• Support rooms including cleaner's room, utilities, and linen holding and storage areas.
	• A special care nursery will provide facilities for.
	  • Short-term care, including the provision of assisted ventilation, for babies who suffer from complications and while they are waiting to be transferred to a neonatal intensive care unit/facility.
	  • Isolation room as required.
	  • Resuscitation and transfer to a neonatal intensive care unit.
	  • Feeding, bathing, changing, and weighing the baby.
	  • Darkening the area and dimmable lighting to allow babies to sleep during the day.
	  • Education of staff and parents.
	  • Phototherapy.
	  • Care for premature newborns who are ill or who are simply recovering; due to their prematurity and/or low weight, they will be cared for in humidicribs and bassinettes.
	  • Nurseries will require access to public amenities for parents.

Feeding and Formula Room/s	The feeding room provides an area close to nurseries for mothers to feed under the supervision of staff. The feeding room will include • Comfortable chairs suitable for breast feeding. • Provision for use of breast pumps. • Privacy screening for patients. • Space for assistance from nursing personnel. • Access to a formula room for milk storage. The formula room should be located close to the nurseries and include facilities for holding milk supplies, specifically, both breast milk and prepared formula milk. The formula room will include • Bench with sink for rinsing equipment. • Cupboards for storage. • Refrigerator with freezer. • Baby milk warmer or microwave oven.

17.4 Summary

The Government of India adopted the Reproductive, Maternal, New-born, Child and Adolescent Health (RMNCH+A) framework in 2013, which essentially aims to address the major causes of mortality and morbidity among women and children. In order to further accelerate a decline in MMR in the coming years, MoFHW has recently launched "LaQshya—Labour Room Quality Improvement Initiative". LaQshya is a focused and targeted approach to strengthen key processes related to labour rooms and maternity operating theatres that aims to improve the quality of care around birth and ensure respectful maternity care. Construction of good quality facilities for childbirth will help reduce maternal mortality and thus improve the provision of maternity services.

18 INPATIENT UNIT AND ITS CONTEXT

The prime function of the Inpatient Unit is to provide appropriate accommodation for the delivery of health care services including diagnosis, care, and treatment to inpatients. The unit must also provide facilities and conditions to meet the needs of patients and visitors and the workplace requirements of staff.

The Inpatient Unit is for general medical and surgical patients. In larger health facilities, this unit includes specialist medical and surgical patients, for example, cardiac, neurology/neurosurgery, integrated palliative care, and obstetric patients. Patients awaiting placement elsewhere may also be accommodated in this type of unit.

18.1 Inpatient Unit and Wider Hospital Context: Location & Access

A bedroom and en suite should be provided with full accessibility compliance, and the number of accessible rooms should be determined by the service plan. Accessible bedrooms and en suites should enable normal activity for wheelchair-dependent patients, as opposed to patients who are in a wheelchair as a result of their hospitalization.

18.2 Models of Care

Models of care for an Inpatient Unit may vary depending upon the patients' acuity and numbers and skill level of the nursing staff available.

Examples of the models of care that could be implemented include:

- Patient allocation
- Task assignment
- Team nursing
- Case management
- Primary care
- Combination of these models

The physical environment should permit of a range of models of care to be implemented, allowing flexibility for future change.

Levels of Care: The levels of care range from highly acute nursing and specialist care (high dependency), with a progression to intermediate care prior to discharge or transfer (self-care). Patients requiring 24-hour medical intervention or cover are generally not nursed or managed within a general Inpatient Unit.

18.3 Planning Models

(a) **Bed Numbers and Complement**
   (i) Each Inpatient Unit may contain up to 32 patient beds and should have bedroom accommodation complying with the standard components.
   (ii) Additional beds up to 16 as an extension of a standard 32-bed unit may be permitted with additional support facilities in proportion to the number of beds, for example, 1 extra sub-clean utility, sub-dirty utility, and storage.

(iii) For additional beds of more than 16, additional support facilities for a full unit (32 beds) is required and located to serve the additional beds.
(iv) The preferred maximum number of beds in an acute Inpatient Unit in Maternity or Paediatric Units is 20–25 beds.
(v) A minimum of 20% of the total bed complement should be provided as single bedrooms in an Inpatient Unit used for overnight stay; the current trend is to provide a greater proportion of single bedrooms largely for infection control reasons.

(b) **Swing Beds**
   (i) For flexibility and added options for utilization, it may be desirable to include provisions for swing beds. This may be a single bed or a group of beds that may be quickly converted from one category of use to another. An example might be long-stay beds that may be converted to acute beds.
   (ii) At any given time, swing beds are part of an Inpatient Unit in terms of the total number of beds and the components of the unit. For example,
   - Unit A + Swing Beds = One Inpatient Unit
   - Unit B + Same swing beds = One Inpatient Unit

(c) **Unit Planning Options:** There are a number of acceptable planning options for Inpatient Units including the following:
   (i) **Single Corridor:** Patient and support clustered along a single corridor.
   (ii) **Double Corridor** (Racetrack): Patient rooms are located on the external aspects of the space, and support rooms are clustered in the central areas in a Racetrack configuration (Figure 18A).
   (iii) **Combinations:** L-, T-, and Y-shaped corridors and patient rooms are located along external aspects, and support areas may be located in a central core area (Figures 18B and 18C).

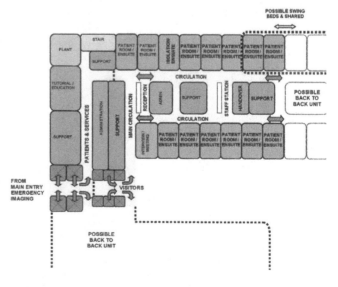

FIGURE 18A Double Corridor—Racetrack Model (Courtesy: iHFG).

DOI: 10.1201/9780367460884-19

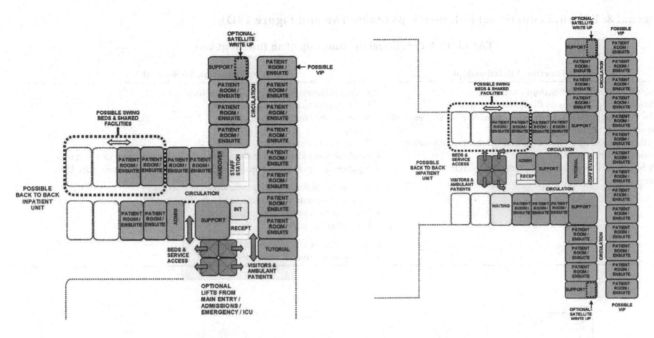

FIGURE 18B   L-Shaped Corridor Model (Courtesy: iHFG).   **FIGURE 18C**   T-Shaped Corridor Model (Courtesy: iHFG).

18.4 Patient Flows

Key result areas and quality indicators for an Inpatient Unit are given in Table 18A.

TABLE 18A: Key Result Areas and Quality Indicators for an Inpatient Unit

Key Result Areas

- *Process KRA*
  - Initial assessment and reassessment of patients
  - Admission and discharge criteria
  - Care plan for each patient
  - Discharge and discharge summary
  - Nursing care
  - Identification of early warning signs
  - CPR
  - Case records—documentation
  - Hand hygiene
  - Documentation of handover
  - Infection control
  - Safe transfer of patients
  - Medication orders
  - Pain management
  - Medication management
  - Nutritional assessment

- *Structural KRA*
  - Narcotics
  - Blood transfusion
  - Restraint policy
  - Vulnerable patient
  - Hazmat
  - Patient feedback
  - Fire safety
  - Medical gas
  - BMW
  - End-of-life care
  - Engineering controls
  - Credentialing and privileging
  - Compressed air purity
  - Equipment/furniture maintenance
  - Referrals
  - Quality assurance
  - Patient rights

Quality Indicators

- HCAI Rates: VAE, SSI, CAUTI, and CLABSI
- Hand hygiene compliance rate
- Time taken for initial assessment of admitted patients
- Percentage of medication charts with error-prone abbreviations
- Percentage of patients developing ADRs
- Incidence of hospital-associated pressure ulcers after admission
- Nurse-patient ratio for Inpatient Unit
- Time taken for discharge
- Patient fall rate
- Percentage of near misses
- Appropriate handovers during shift change (to be done separately for doctors and nurses)—per patient per shift

Internal & External Functional Relationships (Table 18B and Figure 18D)

TABLE 18B: Functional Relationship of an Inpatient Unit

Internal Functional Relationships	External Functional Relationships
Optimum internal relationships include	*Principal relationships with other units include*
• Patient occupied areas as the core of the unit	• Ready access to diagnostic facilities
• The staff station and associated areas need direct access and observation of patient areas	• Ready access from Emergency Unit
	• Ready access to critical care units
• Utility and storage areas need ready access to both patient and staff work areas	• Ready access to pharmacy
	• Ready access to material management, housekeeping, and catering units
• Public areas should be easily accessible from the units served	• Inpatient surgical units require ready access to OT/Day Procedure Unit
	Principal relationships with public areas include
	• Easy access from main entrance of a facility
	• Easy access to public amenities
	• Easy access to parking
	Principal relationships with staff areas
	• Ready access to staff amenities

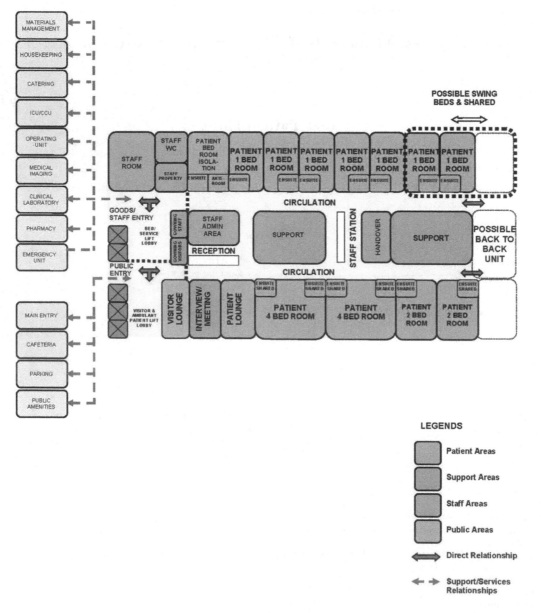

FIGURE 18D Functional Relationship Diagram of an Inpatient Unit (Courtesy: iHFG).

TABLE 18C: Major Space Determinants and Inpatient Unit Size

S No.	FACILITY ·	CATEGORY A 8–15 Beds		CATEGORY B 16–23 Beds		CATEGORY C 24–30 Beds	
		ROOM (NO.)	Area (m²)	ROOM (NO.)	Area (m²)	ROOM (NO.)	Area (m²)
(1)	(2)	(3)	(4)	(5)	(6)	(7)	(8)
GENERAL WARD							
(a)	Nurse station with work area and toilet	1	14	1	17.5	1	17.5
(b)	Doctor duty room with toilet	—		1	17.5	1	17.5
(c)	Treatment room	1	10.5	1	10.5	1	14
(d)	Laboratory	1	10.5	1	7	1	7
(e)	Ward pantry	1	10.5	1	10.5	1	10.5
(f)	Ward store	1	10.5	1	10.5	1	14
(g)	Trolley bay	—		—		1	10.5
(h)	Sluice room	1	10.5	1	10.5	1	14
(i)	Janitor's closet		—	1	3.5	1	3.5
(j)	Day space		—	1	14	1	14
(k)	Patient's relatives' waiting area with toilets	1	14	1	17.5	1	17.5
ADDITIONAL FOR PAEDIATRIC WARD							
(l)	Formula room	1	10.5	1	10.5	1	10.5
(m)	Clothes room	—		1	14	1	14
(n)	Play room	1	10.5	1	14	1	21
(o)	Dining room	—		—		1	10.5
(p)	Classroom	—		1	10.5	1	10.5
ADDITIONAL FOR ANTENATAL WARD							
(q)	Additional to play room	1	7.0	1	7.0	1	7.0
(r)	Additional to dining room	1	7.0	1	7.0	1	7.0

S No.	FACILITY	UP TO 32 MATERNITY BED		OVER 32 MATERNITY BED	
		ROOM (NO.)	Area (m²)	ROOM (NO.)	Area (m²)
(1)	(2)				
NEONATAL UNIT					
(a)	Nursery				
	• Premature	1	10.5	1	21
	• Septic	1	10.5	1	14
	• Normal	1	10.5	1	14
(b)	Nurse station with toilet	1	14	1	17.5
(c)	Doctor duty room with toilet	—	—	1	17.5
(d)	Formula-cum-breast feeding room	1	10.5	1	10.5
(e)	Store	1	7.0	1	10.5
(f)	Phototherapy room	1	7.0	1	10.5
(g)	Sluice room	1	7.0	1	10.5

Layout & Zoning (Figure 18E)

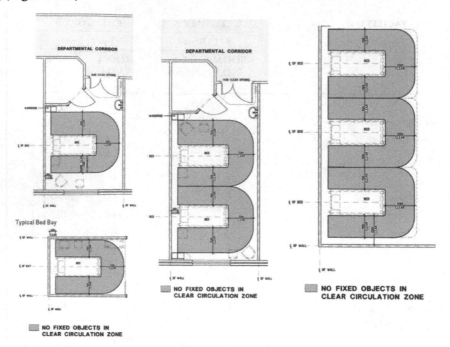

FIGURE 18E   Bed Spacing/Clearances in an Inpatient Unit (Courtesy: iHFG).

Built Environment: General Considerations

TABLE 18D: General Considerations for Built Environment in an Inpatient Unit

Acoustics	• Acoustic treatment is required for the following:
	  • Patient bedrooms
	  • Interview and meeting rooms
	  • Treatment rooms
	  • Staff rooms
	  • Toilets and showers

Natural Light	The use of natural light should be maximized throughout the unit.

Observation and Privacy	• Factors for consideration include
	  • Use of windows in internal walls and/or doors
	  • Location of beds that may affect direct staff visibility
	  • Provision of bed screens to ensure privacy of patients undergoing treatment
	  • Location of sanitary facilities to provide privacy for patients while not preventing observation by staff

Space Standards and
Components

Room Capacity & Dimensions

Room Type	Width (mm)	Length (mm)
Single-Bed Bedroom	3,450	3,600
Two-Bed Bedroom	3,450	5,600
Four-Bed Bedroom	6,100	5,600

Minimum room dimensions are based on overall bed dimensions (buffer to buffer) of 2,250 mm long × 1,050 mm wide. Minor encroachments including columns and hand basins that do not interfere with functions can be ignored when determining space requirements.

Bed Spacing/Clearances (Figure 18F)

• **Single-Bed Bedroom:** There should be a clearance of 1,200 mm available at the foot of each bed and ideally to one side to allow for easy movement of equipment and beds.

• **Double-Bed Bedroom:** The minimum distance between beds should be 900 mm to each side of each bed and 1,200 mm at the foot of each bed; the distance between bed centrelines should not be less than 2,400 mm. Paediatric bedrooms that contain cots may have reduced bed centres, but consideration must be given to the spatial needs of visiting relatives. Consider allowing additional floor area within the room for children to play.

• **Multiple-Bed Bays:** The minimum distance between beds should be 900 mm to each side of each bed and 1,200 mm at the foot of the bed; the distance between bed centrelines should not be less than 2,400 mm.

• **Bariatric Patient Facilities:** The provisions include a large single bedroom and large single en suite. All fixtures and fittings for bariatric patients need to accommodate up to 350 kg of weight. Ceiling suspended lifting system can be considered between the bedroom bed area and the adjacent en suite.

(Continued)

TABLE 18D: (Continued)

Finishes	The aesthetics of the unit should be warm, relaxing, and non-clinical as far as possible. The following additional factors should be considered in the selection of finishes: (a) acoustic properties (b) durability (c) ease of cleaning (d) infection control (e) fire safety (f) movement of equipment, and floor finishes should be resistant to marring and shearing by wheeled equipment In areas where clinical observation is critical such as bedrooms and treatment areas, the colour selected must not impede the accurate assessment of skin tones.
Safety and Security	• The arrangement of spaces and zones should offer a high standard of security through the grouping of like functions, control over access and egress from the unit, and the provision of optimum observation for staff. The level of observation and visibility has security implications.
Drug Storage	Each Inpatient Accommodation Unit should have a lockable storage area or cupboard containing • Benches and shelving • Lockable cupboards for the storage of restricted substances • A lockable steel cabinet for the storage of drugs of addiction • A refrigerator, as required, to store restricted substances that must be lockable or housed within a lockable storage area • Space for medication trolley

Fixtures & Fittings

Clocks	An analogue clock with a second sweep hand should be provided and conveniently located for easy reference from all bed positions and the staff station.
Bedside Storage	Each patient bed space shall include storage and writing provision for staff use.
Curtains/Blinds	Each room shall have partial blackout facilities (blinds or lined curtains) to allow patients to rest during the daytime.
Bed Screens	In multiple-bed bedrooms, visual privacy from casual observation by other patients and visitors should be provided for each patient. The design for privacy must not restrict patient access to the entrance, toilet, or shower.

Infection Control

Hand Basins	Handwashing facilities should not impact minimum clear corridor widths. At least one is to be conveniently accessible to the staff station.
Isolation Rooms	At least one "Class S—Standard" isolation room should be provided for each 32-bed Inpatient Unit.

Building Service Requirements

IT/Communications	Unit design should address the following information technology/communications issues: • Electronic records • Hand-held computers • Picture Archiving Communication System (PACS) • Paging and personal telephones replacing some aspects of call systems • Data entry including scripts and investigation requests • Bar coding for supplies and x-rays/records • Data and communication outlets, servers, and communication room requirements
Nurse Call	Hospitals must provide an electronic call system that allows patients and staff to alert nurses and other health care staff in a discreet manner at all times.
Patient Entertainment System	Patients can be provided with entertainment/communications systems according to the operational policy of the facility including television, bedside telephone, radio, and internet access.
Dialysis Station	The Inpatient Unit should provide one bedroom with a dialysis drain for use with mobile dialysis equipment, as needed by the unit operational policy.
Pneumatic Tube Systems	The Inpatient Unit may include a pneumatic tube station, as determined by the facility operational policy. If provided, the device should be located in close proximity to the staff station or under direct staff supervision.
Hydraulics	Warm water supplied to all areas accessed by patients within the Inpatient Unit must not exceed 43°C. This requirement includes all staff handwash basins and sinks located within patient-accessible areas.

TABLE 18E: Specific Room and Functional Requirements for an Inpatient OPD

Entry/Reception/ Waiting Areas	• Reception is the receiving hub of the unit and may be used to control the security of the unit • A waiting lounge for visitors can be provided with access to separate male/female toilet facilities and prayer rooms • If visitor and staff gowning and protective equipment are immediately adjacent to the unit, then they can also be located here for infection control during ward isolation
Patient Areas	Patient areas include • Bedrooms • En suites • Lounge areas • Patient laundry in some units
Support Areas	Support areas include • Handwashing, linen and equipment bays • Clean utility, dirty utility, and disposal rooms • Beverage bays and pantries • Meeting room/s and interview rooms for education sessions, interviews with staff, patients, and families, and other meetings
Staff Area	Staff areas consist of • Offices and workstations • Staff room • Staff station and handover room • Toilets and lockers Offices and workstations are required for administrative and clinical functions to facilitate educational/research activities. Staff areas, particularly staff rooms, toilets, showers, and lockers, may be shared with adjacent units as far as possible.
Shared Areas	In addition to the shared staff areas mentioned previously, shared areas include • Patient bathroom • Treatment room • Public toilets • Visitor lounge

18.5 Summary

Technological advances in health care are rapidly occurring, requiring the law and regulations to change and adapt for particular spaces. These changes are eminently present in modern diagnostics and surgery wards. Hospital bed wards, as spaces primarily utilized for recovery, rehabilitation, therapy, and observation of patients, are among the largest of a hospital's areas of functionality and are a place of work for a diverse staff of hospital employees. Work ergonomics in a bed ward are critical not only for nurses and physicians but also for technical, cleaning, and administration employees.

19 MEDICAL IMAGING UNIT

19.1 Introduction

The Medical Imaging Unit is a discreet unit that provides radiology and diagnostic investigations. Depending on the level of service and the clinical service plan, the unit may also provide diagnostic screening (fluoroscopy), ultrasound, mammography, computed tomography (CT), magnetic resonance imaging (MRI), or interventional radiographic procedures such as angiography.

The primary role of a Medical Imaging Unit is to support and serve other departments in a hospital or health care practice in providing diagnostics and treatment. It is estimated that up to 40% of new outpatient visits may result in radiological investigations. Therefore, due consideration should be given for ready accessibility from all wards, outpatient departments (OPDs), and casualty department.

The general Medical Imaging Unit may be co-located with or incorporate other specialties including Nuclear Medicine, Positron Emission Tomography (PET), and Oncology—Radiotherapy Units in a fully integrated imaging suite.

The (not limited to the) following acts, rules, and regulations must be adhered to during planning and designing the Medical Imaging Unit:

(a) Atomic Energy Act, 1962 and Amendments
(b) Environmental Protection Act, 1986
(c) Radiation Protection Rules, 1962
(d) Mines Minerals Prescribed Substance (MMPS) Rules, 1984
(e) Atomic Energy Safe Disposal of Radioactive Waste Rules, 1987
(f) PC&PNDT Act, 1994
(g) Clinical Establishment Act Standards for Medical Imaging Services (Diagnostic Centre)
(h) BMWM Rules, 2016 and Amendments Thereof

19.2 Medical Imaging Unit and Wider Hospital Context: Location & Access

(a) **Models of Care**
   (i) **Size of the Unit:** The size of the Imaging Unit will depend on the level of service and will be determined by the facility's service plan and operational policies.
   (ii) **Imaging Room/s:** Size of the imaging rooms will be influenced by the following:
      a. Ease of movement, in and around the room, for patients, staff, and equipment
      b. Number of staff required in and around the room to operate the equipment and support the patient
      c. Equipment to be installed—design will need to consider the manufacturer's recommended room sizes, equipment placement, and services requirements
      d. Potential future upgrading of equipment

TABLE 19A: Key Result Areas and Quality Indicators for Medical Imaging Units

Key Result Areas

- Service in scope should have appropriate diagnostic backup
- Compliance with BARC/AERB legal requirements
- Adequate and appropriate infrastructure and human resources
- Technician qualified as per AERB
- Identification and safe transportation of patients to the imaging services
- Turnaround time
- Reporting of critical results (including outsourced investigations also)
- Standardized reporting of results
- Mechanism to address recall/amendment of reports
- Monitoring of waiting time, time for tests, and time for reports
- Documented policies and procedures
- Quality assurance and quality control
- Regular training of staff
- Feedback to stakeholders
- Calibration and maintenance of all equipment
- Corrective and preventive actions
- Safety program documented including usage of safety equipment
- TLD badges provided and periodically sent to the appropriate authority for monitoring radiation exposure
- Usage and disposal of radioactive and hazmat as per statutory requirements
- Maintenance and storage of records
- Imaging signage: radiation hazard, PC-PNDT Act, etc.
- Informed consent
- Biomedical waste management
- Fire safety
- Uptime of equipment

Quality Indicators

- Number of reporting errors per 1,000 investigations
- Percentage of adherence to safety precautions by staff working in lab
- Rate of re-do's
- Percentage of reports correlating with a clinical diagnosis
- Waiting time for diagnostics
- Equipment downtime

19.3 Patient Flows

Important Key Result Areas and Quality Indicators for Medical Imaging Unit are given in Table 19A.

19.4 Internal and External Functional Relationships

Distances must be minimized for all movements of patients, medical, nursing, other staff and supplies. The department should be located at a place that is accessible to OPD, wards, and operating theatre (OT). Functional separation of the department can be performed into two parts without physically separating them, one catering to Accident and Emergency (A&E) and urgent OPD cases at all hours and the other catering to the needs of inpatients and other OPD cases with appointments. A traffic control chart should be available with appropriate signposting to facilitate internal patient movement in the department to maintain zoning (Table 19B and Figures 19A and 19B).

TABLE 19B: Internal and External Relationships of Medical Imaging Units

Internal Functional Relationships	External Functional Relationships
• Unit should be arranged in functional zones. • Reception entrance with access control. • Support areas such as reporting and processing will be located conveniently to the imaging areas and may be shared.	• Located close to the main entrance of the facility and ideally situated at ground level. Consideration must be given to its proximity to A&E, Outpatient Unit, and Operating Unit for intra-operative imaging and radiotherapy/oncology for regular patient investigations associated with treatment. • Wayfinding should be easy and the unit identifiable by staff and visitors.
The optimum internal relationships include the following: (a) Reception at the entrance providing access control, with waiting and amenities. (b) Imaging areas arranged into zones including general x-ray, fluoroscopy, CT scanning, angiography, and MRI. (c) Patient areas including bed bays and recovery should be centrally located and convenient to interventional and scanning rooms for sharing between imaging modalities. (d) Support areas should be located centrally to imaging rooms and adjacent to areas of need for staff and patient convenience. (e) Staff areas should be located in a discreet zone at the unit perimeter.	*The optimum external relationships include:* (a) Visitor access from the main circulation corridor with a relationship to the main entrance. (b) Separate entry and access for inpatients, critical care units, and Medical Imaging Unit. (c) Access for service units such as supply and housekeeping via a service corridor.

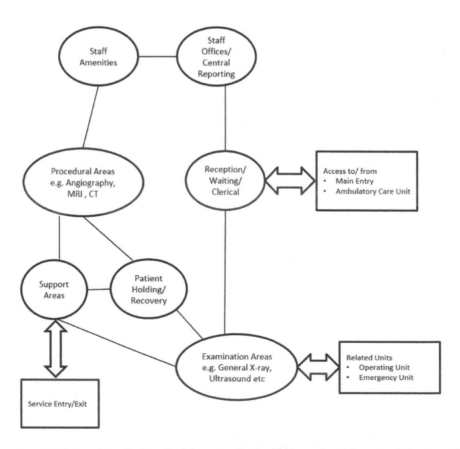

FIGURE 19A Functional Relationship of a Medical Imaging Unit with Procedural Imaging (Courtesy: https://aushfg-prod-com-au.s3.amazonaws.com/%5BB-0440%5D%20Medical%20Imaging%20Unit.pdf).

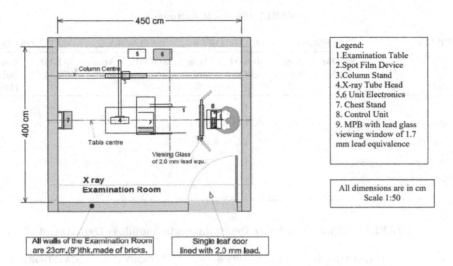

FIGURE 19B Model Layout of an X-Ray Installation (Courtesy: www.aerb.gov.in/images/PDF/DiagnosticRadiology/Model-Layout---X-ray-Radiography-Installation.pdf).

Major Space Determinants and Unit Size

TABLE 19C (a): Major Space Determinants and Medical Imaging Unit Size

S No.	FACILITY	CATEGORY A		CATEGORY B		CATEGORY C		CATEGORY D		CATEGORY E	
		ROOM (NO.)	Area (m²)	ROOM (NO.)	Area (m²)	ROOM (NO.)	Area (m²)	ROOM (NO.)	Area (m²)	ROOM (NO.)	Area (m²)
(1)	(2)	(3)	(4)	(5)	(6)	(7)	(8)	(9)	(10)	(11)	(12)
FUNCTIONAL AREAS											
(a)	X-ray room (spl. Studies) with toilet			1	36						
(b)	X-ray room std. including chest stands			1	27						
(c)	MRI Room			1	45						
(d)	CT scan room			1	45						
(e)	Mammography room			1	27						
(f)	Bone densitometery room			1	27						
(g)	Ultrasound room attached with toilet			1	18						
(h)	Ultrasound room std.			1	18						
(i)	Control room for MRI scanner			1	9						
(j)	Control room for CT scanner			1	9						
(k)	Control room for x-ray			1	9						
(I)	Examination room scanner			1	9						
m)	Dressing booth			15	4.5						
(n)	Dark room			1	9						
(o)	Film viewing room			1	18						
(p)	Machine room			1	9						
(q)	Patient preparation area			1	9						
SUPPORT AREAS											
(a)	Reception and business office			1	9						
(b)	Record room			1	18						

(Continued)

TABLE 19C (a): (Continued)

S No.	FACILITY	CATEGORY A		CATEGORY B		CATEGORY C		CATEGORY D		CATEGORY E	
		ROOM (NO.)	Area (m²)	ROOM (NO.)	Area (m²)	ROOM (NO.)	Area (m²)	ROOM (NO.)	Area (m²)	ROOM (NO.)	Area (m²)
(1)	(2)	(3)	(4)	(5)	(6)	(7)	(8)	(9)	(10)	(11)	(12)
(c)	Waiting room			1	9						
(d)	Consultant office			1	13.5						
(e)	Chief technician office			1	27						
(f)	Secretaries' room			1	13.5						
(g)	Locker changing room for staff			1	13.5						

TABLE 19C (b): Major Space Determinants in Radiology Department

S No.	FACILITY	CATEGORY A		CATEGORY B		CATEGORY C		CATEGORY D		CATEGORY E	
		ROOM (NO.)	Area (m²)	ROOM (NO.)	Area (m²)	ROOM (NO.)	Area (m²)	ROOM (NO.)	Area (m²)	ROOM (NO.)	Area (m²)
(1)	(2)	(3)	(4)	(5)	(6)	(7)	(8)	(9)	(10)	(11)	(12)
RADIO DIAGNOSTIC UNIT											
(a)	Reception registration with waiting area and toilet	—		—		1	10.5	1	14	1	14
(b)	Radiography and fluoroscopy (x-ray rooms) with waiting area, toilet, and dressing facility 17.5 m² per x-ray room: 100 mA Units 200 mA Units 500 mA Units 700 mA Units	1	28	1	28	1	28	1	28	2	28
		—			—	1	42	1	24	2	42
		—			—	—		1	56	1	56
			—	—		—		1	70	1	70
(c)	Film developing and processing area (common for two x-ray rooms)	1	10.5	1	10.5	1	10.5	2	10.5	3	10.5
(d)	Film drying room	—			—	1	10.5	1	10.5	2	10.5
(e)	Contrast studies and preparation room	—			—	1	10.5	1	10.5	2	10.5
(f)	Stores I) Film storage II) Chemical store		—	1	10.5	1	17.5	1	10.5	1	14
(g)	X-ray record room	—		1	14	1	21	1	28	1	35
(h)	Radiologist office with toilet	—		1	17.5	1	17.5	1	17.5	2	17.5
(l)	Technician room with toilet	—				1	14	1	14	1	17.5
(j)	Nurses' room with toilets	—				1	14	1	14	1	17.5
(k)	Film viewing room	—			—	1	10.5	1	10.5	1	14
	Office		—		—	1	10.5	1	14	1	17.5

(Continued)

TABLE 19C (b): (Continued)

S No.	FACILITY	CATEGORY A		CATEGORY B		CATEGORY C		CATEGORY D		CATEGORY E	
		ROOM (NO.)	Area (m²)	ROOM (NO.)	Area (m²)	ROOM (NO.)	Area (m²)	ROOM (NO.)	Area (m²)	ROOM (NO.)	Area (m²)
(1)	(2)	(3)	(4)	(5)	(6)	(7)	(8)	(9)	(10)	(11)	(12)
(l)	Trolley bay	—		—		1	10.5	1	10.5	1	10.5
(m)	Switch room	—		1	7.0	1	10.5	1	17.5	1	21
(n)	Janitor's closet	—		1	3.5	1	3.5	1	3.5	1	3.5
RADIO THERAPY UNIT											
(a)	Contact therapy (45 kV)	1	14	1	14	1	14	1	14	1	14
(b)	Superficial therapy (100 kV)	—		—		1	14	1	14	1	14
(c)	Intermediary therapy with dressing cubicles and control desk 3.5 m² each	—		—		1	14	1	14	1	14
(d)	Deep therapy (200 kV)	—		—		—		1	28	1	35
RADIO DIAGNOSTIC UNIT											
(a)	Cobalt therapy with dressing cubicle 3.5 m² and control room 7 m². Room height to be 4.5 m² including thickness		—	—			—	1	70	1	70
(b)	Megavoltage therapy (12 Mev) with dressing cubicle 3.5 m² and control room 7 m² and transformer room wherever required. Room height to be 4.5 m including thickness		—	—			—	1	91	2	91
(c)	Radiotherapist room with examination room and toilet facility	—			—		—	1	28	1	28
(d)	Physicist room with laboratory and toilet		—	—		1	21	1	42	1	42
(e)	Mould room	—		—			—	1	21	1	21
(f)	Simulator room with control room 7 m² and waiting area 14 m²	—		—			—	1	35	1	35
(g)	Treatment planning system (TPS) room	—		—			—	1	17.5	1	17.5
(h)	CT Scanner control room with computer 10.5 m²	—		—			—	1	7	1	7
(i)	Transformer room	—		—		1	14	1	14	1	17.5
(j)	Dressing room/ preparation room with darkroom facility	—		—			—	1	10.5	1	10.5
(k)	Records room	—		—			—	1	42	1	42
(l)	Reception and waiting with toilet	—		—	—	1	21	1	56	1	56

19.5 Layout & Zoning

The model layout for x-ray and CT scan installation are shown in Figures 19B to 19H and Tables 19D and 19E.

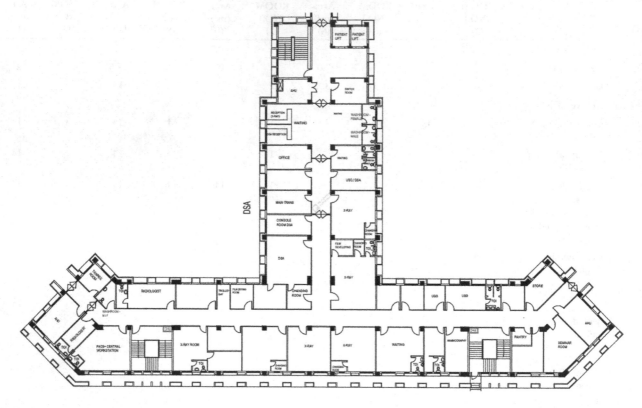

FIGURE 19C   X-Ray Sample Layout.

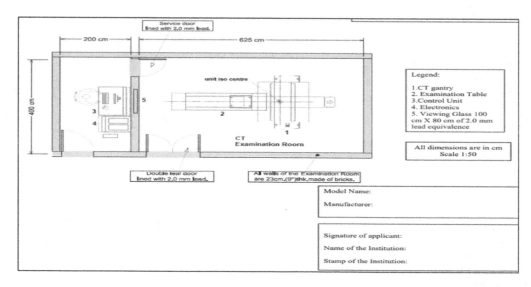

FIGURE 19D   Model Layout of a CT Installation (Courtesy: www.aerb.gov.in/images/PDF/DiagnosticRadiology/Model-Layout-CT-Scan.pdf).

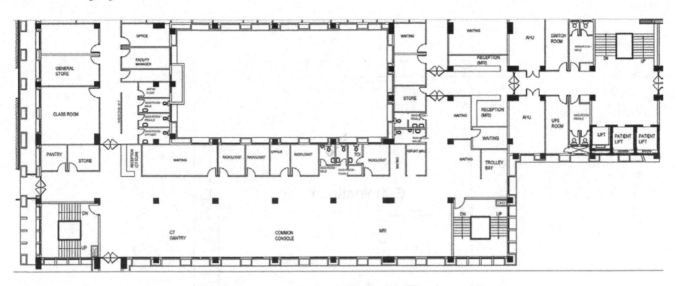

FIGURE 19E   CT and MRI Sample Layout.

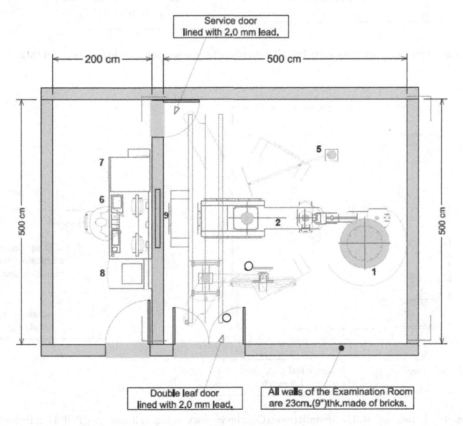

FIGURE 19F Model Layout of Interventional Radiology Installation (Courtesy: www.aerb.gov.in/images/PDF/DiagnosticRadiology/Model-Layout---Interventional-Radiology-Installation.pdf).

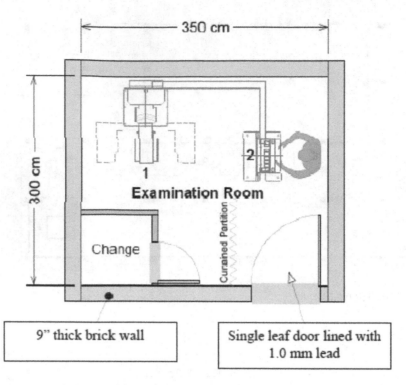

FIGURE 19G   Model Layout of Mammography Installation (Courtesy: www.aerb.gov.in/images/PDF/Mammo.pdf).

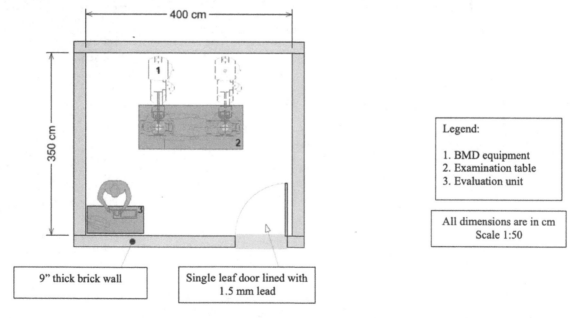

FIGURE 19H   Model Layout of BMD Installation (Courtesy: www.aerb.gov.in/images/PDF/DiagnosticRadiology/Model-Layout---BMD-Installation.pdf).

TABLE 19D: Basic Layout Requirements for X-Ray Installation

- Diagram depicts that the wall thickness of the x-ray installation room should be at least 23 cms and made of bricks.
- Single-leaf door lined with 2-mm lead.
- Separate entrances for procedure room and control console.
- Minimum space requirement of the procedure room is 450 cm × 400 cm.
- Alignment of equipment with respect to entrance door.
- No waiting area should be planned adjacent to the wall facing direct radiation exposure.

TABLE 19E: Basic Layout Requirements for CT Installation

- The control console should be installed in a separate room located outside but adjoining the CT room provided with appropriate shielding, a direct viewing window, and communication facilities between the operator and the patient.
- The gantry and couch should be placed such that they enable the operator to have a complete view of the patient from the control room viewing window.
- The interventional radiology equipment room should have an adjoining control room with appropriate facilities for shielding, a direct viewing window, and communication facilities.
- A chest stand should be located in the x-ray room such that no significant stray radiation reaches the control console/entrance door/areas of full-time occupancy.
- A permanent radiation warning symbol, illustrating the radiation hazard to pregnant women and others, and instructions should be pasted on the entrance door of the x-ray installation.

Built Environment: General Considerations

TABLE 19F: General Considerations for Built Environment for a Medical Imaging Unit

Construction Standards	(a) Structural support for equipment including equipment mounted to ceilings. (b) Level floor for equipment positioning and safe patient movement. (c) Provision for cable support trays, ducts, or conduits may be made in floors, walls, and ceilings, and the impact on room space of large diameter electrical cable trays (on floors or surface-mounted on walls), equipment ventilation, clocks, task lighting/dimming, and room blackout should be determined, as required. (d) Ceiling height should suit the equipment to be installed but should not be less than 3,000 mm. For ceiling tube mount installation, the ceiling may be higher if required. (e) Flooring in radiography rooms should be of insulating material such as rubber, linoleum, and asbestos vinyl tiles. (f) As the department deals with high voltages and seepage in walls, the floor and ceiling should be avoided, and all equipment should be effectively earthed.
Standards and Codes	Radiological facilities are to comply with relevant local legislation, regulations, and statutory requirements. (a) The employer is the owner of the hospital/board, and the licensee is the radiologist who will be performing the investigations. (b) No diagnostic x-ray equipment such as a USG machine should be operated for patient diagnosis unless the license for operation is obtained from the Atomic Energy Regulatory Board.
Acoustics	(a) Acoustic privacy should be provided in all imaging rooms, interview rooms, and particularly in reporting areas.
Natural Light/Lighting	(a) Natural light is desirable for patient waiting areas, offices, and staff recreation areas to provide a sense of well-being for patients and staff.
Privacy	Doors to imaging and screening rooms should be located to avoid patient exposure to circulation areas.
Interior Décor	Colours should be used in combination with lighting to ensure that they do not mask skin colours in procedure and scanning rooms where clinical observation takes place.
Accessibility	(a) Wheelchair access is required in all patient areas including waiting, consult, and imaging rooms.
Doors	Doors through which trolleys and beds must pass should be a minimum of 1,200 mm wide.
Safety and Security	Access control of the reception zone within the unit should allow patients to access the intended areas and prevent patients and visitors entering unrelated areas.
Finishes	Finishes should be selected with consideration of the following: (a) Infection control and ease of cleaning. (b) Acoustic properties of the materials. (c) Durability. (d) Fire safety. (e) Wall protection should be provided where bed or equipment movement occurs including corridors, bed bays, and imaging rooms.
Communications	The Medical Imaging Unit requires reliable and effective IT/Communications service for efficient operation of the service. The IT design should address (a) Booking, appointment, and queuing systems. (b) Patient/clinical information systems and electronic records. (c) Telephones including cordless and mobile phones. (d) Computers, laptops, and hand-held devices. (e) Duress alarms for staff and emergencies. (f) Wireless and hospital network requirements; high capacity and speed for digital equipment. (g) Video-conferencing and tele-conferencing requirements, including connection to imaging rooms for educational purposed. (h) Communications and server room/s. (i) Reporting and recording systems that may include dictation or voice recognition and include printing of reports. (j) Picture Archiving Communications Systems (PACS).

(Continued)

TABLE 19F: (Continued)

Heating, Ventilation, and Air Conditioning (HVAC)	(a) The Medical Imaging Unit should be air conditioned to provide a comfortable working environment for staff and visitors. (b) Interventional imaging rooms may require air conditioning equivalent to operating room conditions, that is, filtered and positive-pressured (refer Chapter 34). (c) Rooms with heat-generating equipment may require special air conditioning. (d) The local or country-specific mechanical provision requirements should be consulted (National Building Code).
Medical Gases	Medical gases will be included in general and interventional imaging rooms in accordance with standards, components, or project-specific requirements.
Radiation Shielding	(a) All rooms that use x-ray/radiation for imaging require radiation shielding as per AERB guidelines.
Infection Control	(b) Route for inpatients should be separated from outpatients as far as possible. (c) Consideration should be given to separate clean and dirty workflows in all imaging/procedure, preparation, and clean-up rooms.

TABLE 19G: Specific Room and Functional Requirements for Built Environment for Medical Imaging Units

Entry/Reception/Waiting Areas	(a) The waiting areas should be designed for compliance with accessibility standards with provisions for prams and a play area for children. (b) Bed waiting areas should be separated from the ambulatory patient waiting areas for patient privacy.
General X-Ray and Fluoroscopy	(a) General x-ray rooms can be clustered with fluoroscopy screening rooms in order to share support facilities. (b) The general x-ray room equipment will generally include an upright bucky stand for chest films. (c) OPG and mammography imaging equipment may be included in a general x-ray room where imaging equipment is not fully utilized. Additional equipment will require a slightly larger room.
Orthopantomography (OPG)	This equipment may be incorporated into a general x-ray room, a separate bay, or within the Dental Unit.
Computerized Tomography (CT)	(a) The room should have an associated control room and computer equipment room. A control room may service two rooms. (b) The room should include services for general anaesthesia and be sized for interventional procedures. (c) A bed/trolley bay adjacent to each room is required for staff observation of waiting patients.
Angiography/Digital Subtraction Angiography (DSA) Endoscopic Retrograde Choleopancreatography (ERCP)	Equipped with a crash cart and monitoring equipment. The patient's heart rate and blood oxygenation are monitored continuously, while blood pressure is measured intermittently via a self-inflating cuff.

Magnetic Resonance Imaging (MRI)
Image of MRI zoning to be added
	(a) Specifically, the MRI should be located with good external access for installing and servicing the equipment; this may be achieved through an accessible side panel distant to any moving metal objects that may cause interference, such as lifts, passing cars, and construction equipment.
	(b) The MRI should not be located below a helipad or next to a substation.
	(c) Recommended exclusion zones are divided into four stages including
	   (i) Zone 1: Entrance, which may be shared with general radiology
	   (ii) Zone 2: Reception, waiting, which may be shared, with patient screening, toilet, and change room
	   (iii) Zone 3: MRI Waiting, patient preparation, recovery, control, and equipment rooms
	   (iv) Zone 4: MRI Scanning room.
	(d) Equipment and fittings in the room including emergency equipment, such as fire extinguishers and gas bottles, need to be constructed of non-ferrous material.

Ultrasound	(a) Ultrasound rooms should require close access to drinking water and a toilet for particular scanning procedures.
Preparation Room	(a) A preparation room is provided for preparation of contrast media solutions and storage of medications and sterile supplies. (b) The preparation room, if conveniently located, can serve several imaging rooms.
Film Storage	(a) For digital imaging applications, there will need to be an area for the PACS (Picture Archiving and Communications System) servers. The PACS server room should be located with ready access to the imaging rooms. (b) Film storage areas must provide a suitable environment to protect films from deterioration and damage.

19.6 Summary

A Medical Imaging Unit is an equipment-heavy unit and is preferably located on the ground floor of a hospital. This specialized facility is essential for conducting various diagnostic imaging procedures, such as X-rays, MRIs, CT scans, and ultrasounds. Adequate space for advanced imaging equipment, control rooms, and waiting areas must be allocated. Additionally, stringent infection control measures and radiation shielding are paramount. Adherence to and licensing by AERB, clustering of various imaging modalities, and electrical back up are important considerations while planning a Medical Imaging Unit in a hospital.

20 MEDICAL LABORATORY UNIT

20.1 Introduction

Medical laboratory (lab) services form an essential component of hospital diagnostics. It is of utmost importance to know the process of sample collection and sample processing and subsequently perform appropriate tests to obtain accurate results. Systematic quality management in a medical laboratory is important. The lab must have adequate space for all the equipment and staff required for the services. The Medical Laboratory Unit provides facilities and equipment for the examination of body tissues and fluids that involves receiving patient specimens, testing them, and issuing reports. The Medical Laboratory Unit can be divided into specialist disciplines as mentioned in Table 20A.

20.2 Medical Laboratory Unit and Wider Hospital Context: Location & Access

(a) **Location:** The unit must be in a service zone of the health care facility with consideration of travel distances, the amount of time taken to receive specimens and for staff travelling between various key departments, and ease of access for patients attending the unit for specimen collection. Location criteria are as follows:

(i) It is preferable to have the hospital laboratory on the ground floor.

(ii) Accessibility of patients should be limited to collection centres only. In case of query, telephonic access should be provided.

(iii) Easy access to biomedical waste facility.

(iv) Other activities of the laboratory should be situated in such a way so that they are away from patients' view but within the control of the person in charge of the laboratory.

With automated delivery methods such as pneumatic tube systems and satellite specimen collection zones within the facility, the location of the unit becomes less critical.

20.3 Medical Laboratory Unit: Configuration and Process Flow

The Medical Laboratory Unit may be planned as a series of modular laboratories, providing flexibility for change of function and equipment as necessary. Each module may be sized to accommodate a specific specialty and the equipment required, with the ability to adapt and reconfigure modules. The process flow of the medical laboratory unit is shown in Figure 20A.

20.4 Classification of a Medical Laboratory Unit

The National Fire Protection Association, USA (NFPA) codes classify laboratories based upon the amount of inflammable/combustible chemicals that are stored in them (Table 20B).

The National Accreditation Board for Testing and Calibration Laboratories classify medical laboratories as follows.

(a) **Small laboratory**: A laboratory receiving samples of up to 100 subjects per day.

TABLE 20A: Specialist Disciplines in a Medical Laboratory

Specialist Disciplines	Details of the Specialist Disciplines
General Pathology	It involves a mixture of anatomical and clinical pathology specialties in one unit.
Anatomical Pathology	It involves diagnosis of disease based upon the microscopic, chemical, immunologic, and molecular examination of organs, tissues, and whole bodies (autopsy).
Clinical/Chemical Pathology	It involves diagnosis of disease through the laboratory analysis of blood and bodily fluids and/or tissues by using the tools of chemistry, microbiology, haematology, and molecular pathology.
Haematology	It is concerned with diagnosing haematological disorders/diseases.
Microbiology	It involves diagnosis of diseases caused by microorganisms such as bacteria, viruses, fungi, and parasites; clinical aspects involve prevention and control of infectious diseases and infections in the health care facility.
Genetics/Clinical Cytogenetics	It is a branch of genetics concerned with studying the structure and function of the cell, particularly the microscopic analysis of chromosomal abnormalities; molecular genetics uses DNA technology to analyse genetic mutations.
Immunology	It is a broad discipline that deals with the physiological functioning of the immune system and malfunctions of the immune system such as autoimmune diseases, hypersensitivities, immune deficiency, transplant rejection, etc.

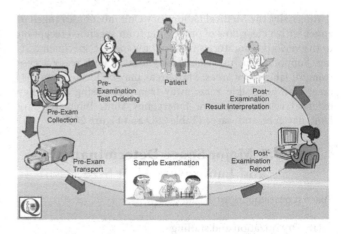

FIGURE 20A Process Flow of the Medical Laboratory Unit (Courtesy: www.medicallaboratoryquality.com/2017/04/revising-laboratory-path-of-workflow.html).

DOI: 10.1201/9780367460884-21

TABLE 20B: NFPA Classification of Laboratories

Sl. No.	Class of Laboratory	Level of Hazard	Amount of Inflammable/Combustible Liquids Allowed to Be Stored
01.	Class A	High	10 to 20 gallons
02.	Class B	Intermediate	5 to 10 gallons
03.	Class C	Low	2 to 4 gallons

(b) **Medium laboratory**: A laboratory receiving samples of up to 101–400 subjects per day.
(c) **Large laboratory**: A laboratory receiving samples of up to 400–1,000 subjects per day.
(d) **Very large laboratory**: A laboratory receiving samples of more than 1,000 subjects per day.
(e) **Multiple locations**: A laboratory with more than one location in the same district with the same legal identity.

The Centers for Disease Control and Prevention (CDC) and the National Institutes of Health (NIH) have categorized medical laboratories based upon biosafety levels:

(a) **BSL 1** — Infectious agents not known to cause disease in healthy adults
(b) **BSL 2** — Infectious agents associated with human disease; ability to infect through autoinoculation, ingestion, and mucous membrane exposure
(c) **BSL 3** — Infectious agents with potential for aerosol transmission. Effects may be serious or lethal
(d) **BSL 4** — Infectious agents that pose high risk of life-threatening disease, aerosol transmitted lab infections, or agents with unknown risk of transmission

20.5 Key Result Areas & Quality Indicators for a Medical Laboratory Unit

Important key result areas and quality indicators for a Medical Laboratory Unit are given in Table 20C.

20.6 Internal & External Functional Relationships

Internally, the Medical Laboratory Unit must be arranged in zones with a clear flow of processing from specimen reception to the various laboratories required for specific specimen testing. Support areas must be ideally located with ready access from all laboratory areas. Staff areas may be located in a discreet staff-accessible zone, away from processing areas. Key external relationships are Emergency Unit, Intensive Care Unit, day care, and wards (Table 20D and Figure 20B).

20.7 Major Space Determinants and Laboratory Unit Size

Space requirements are based on

(a) Organization and staffing
(b) Functions performed
(c) Workload
(d) Equipment used
(e) Containment requirements
(f) Waste management requirements

Primary Space: Space utilized by technical staff for carrying out professional work. It is also known as Laboratory Space Units/Laboratory Module.

(a) **Laboratory Module or Laboratory Surface Unit:**
 (i) Space occupied by professional or technical staff
 (ii) Basic building block
 (iii) Contains all standard requirements to support lab operations
 (iv) Recommended size of the module: 6 m × 3 m = 18 sq m (WHO)
(b) **Module Width is Based On:**
 (i) Standard depth for benches: 75 cm
 (ii) Laboratory bench dimensions per technician: 0.80 m (H) × 0.60 m (W) × 2.00 m (L)
 (iii) Required clearance in front of bench: 75 cm
 (iv) Dado: 1.20 m high glazed (ceramic tiles) in all laboratories and in the areas with work benches. It must be 0.5 m above the workbench.

Secondary Space

(a) Space utilized for all supportive activities.
(b) Administrative space, that is, offices for the pathologist and others, restrooms and locker rooms, staff toilets, etc., should be considered separate from secondary space.

TABLE 20C: Key Result Areas and Quality Indicators for a Medical Laboratory Unit

Key Result Areas

- Service in scope should have appropriate diagnostic backup
- Adequate and appropriate infrastructure and human resources
- Turnaround time for the analysis of samples
- Reporting of critical results (including outsourced investigations)
- Uptime of the equipment
- Calibration of equipment including point of care equipment
- Uptime of Laboratory Management Information System (LMIS)
- Maintenance and storage of records
- Storage of reagents and hazardous chemicals with MSDS
- Prevention and control of infections
- Use of appropriate PPE
- Cleaning and disinfection of equipment
- Biomedical waste management
- Fire safety in laboratory
- Quality assurance and quality control

Quality Indicators

- Number of reporting errors per 1,000 investigations
- Percentage of adherence to safety precautions by staff working in lab
- Hand hygiene compliance rate
- Rate of re-do
- Percentage of reports correlating with clinical diagnosis
- Equipment downtime
- Waiting time for diagnostics

TABLE 20D: Internal and External Relationships of a Medical Laboratory Unit

Internal Functional Relationships	External Functional Relationships
Specimen reception area at the entrance	Emergency Unit
Controlled access at entry points to staff and laboratory areas	Intensive Care Unit/Coronary Care Unit
A specimen workflow from specimen reception to sorting/initial processing and then to laboratories	Operating Unit and Day Surgery/Procedures Units
Support areas must be located centrally to laboratories at the point of use and at the perimeter for supplies and shared areas	Birthing Unit and neonatal nurseries
	Inpatient Units
	Outpatient Units
Staff areas including offices and meeting room must be located in a staff zone and be accessible without traversing sample handling and processing areas in the laboratory	Oncology Units including radiotherapy and chemotherapy
	Day Patient Units such as the Renal Dialysis Unit and Medical Day Chairs
Staff changing areas located near the entrance and exit of the unit for staff to don the PPE on entry and doff the PPE at the exit	Access from Outpatient and Day Patient Units to specimen collection through a public corridor
	Specimen collection area may be located adjacent to laboratories or in a remote location
	Indirect relationships between Laboratory Unit and all inpatient and critical care areas through public corridors; specimen transit may be automated
	Access through a staff/service corridor for supplies and housekeeping including waste disposal

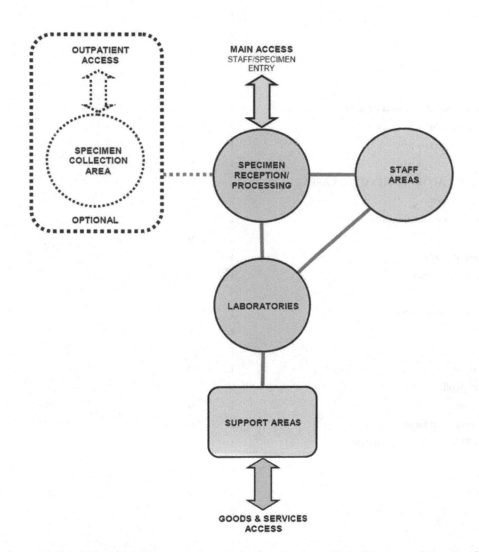

FIGURE 20B Functional Relationship Diagram of a Medical Laboratory Unit (Courtesy: https://aushfg-prod-com-au. s3.amazonaws.com/HPU_B.0550_6_SOA%20Extract%202.pdf).

20.8 Space Requirements

The extent of automation and type of technology used are the main space determinants in a Medical Laboratory Unit (Table 20E). The space requirements for a Medical Laboratory Unit are given in the following.

1. The U.S. Public Health Service (USPHS) has specified the area required for the hospital lab as follows:
   (a) 50-bed hospital = 25 sq m
   (b) 100-bed hospital = 60 sq m
   (c) 200-bed hospital = 103 sq m
2. Area required can be calculated based on the number of beds: 0.7–0.8 m/bed or 5–7.5 sq ft/bed

TABLE 20E: Space Requirements for a Medical Laboratory Unit

S No.	FACILITY	CATEGORY A		CATEGORY B		CATEGORY C		CATEGORY D		CATEGORY E	
		ROOM (NO.)	Area (m²)	ROOM (NO.)	Area (m²)	ROOM (NO.)	Area (m²)	ROOM (NO.)	Area (m²)	ROOM (NO.)	Area (m²)
(1)	(2)	(3)	(4)	(5)	(6)	(7)	(8)	(9)	(10)	(11)	(12)
FUNCTIONAL AREAS											
(a)	Stat lab			1	9						
(b)	Clinical pathology lab			1	9						
(c)	Haemotology and coagulation area			1	9						
(d)	Biochemistry lab			1	9						
CLINICAL MICROBIOLOGY LAB											
(a)	Media kitchen			1	4.5						
(b)	Autoclave area			1	4 5						
(c)	Incubation area			1	9						
(d)	Staining area			1	9						
(e)	Microscopy area			1	9						
HISTOPATHOLOGY LAB											
(a)	Preservation, grossing & preparation area			1	9						
(b)	Section and staining area			1	13.5						
(c)	Microscopy area			1	13.5						
(d)	Slide store			1	9						
SPECIAL ANALYTICAL LABORATORIES OTHER AREAS											
(a)	Sample collection area			1	18						
(b)	FNAC room-cum-examination area			1	9						
(c)	Sample receiving area			1	9						
(d)	Glassware cleaning area			1	9						
(e)	Terminal sterilization area			1	9						
SUPPORT AREAS											
(a)	Reception and business office			1	9						
(b)	Record room			1	9						
(c)	Waiting room			1	9						
	Consultant office			1	9						
(e)	Chief technician office			1	9						
(f)	Secretaries room			1	9						
(g)	Locker changing room for staff			5	9						
(h)	Record office library and documentation office			1	9						
(i)	General store			1	9						
(j)	Janitor's closet			1	9						
(k)	Staff toilet			2	9						
(l)	Public toilets			1	9						
(m)	Electric room			1	9						

TABLE 20F: Major Space Determinants for Pathology Department

S No. (1)	FACILITY (2)	CATEGORY A		CATEGORY B		CATEGORY C		CATEGORY D		CATEGORY E	
		ROOM (NO.) (3)	Area (m²) (4)	ROOM (NO.) (5)	Area (m²) (6)	ROOM (NO.) (7)	Area (m²) (8)	ROOM (NO.) (9)	Area (m²) (10)	ROOM (NO.) (11)	Area (m²) (12)
FUNCTIONAL AREAS											
(a)	Reception and specimen collection/distribution	—		1	21	1	28	1	35	1	42
(b)	Patient waiting area with toilet	—		1	21	1	28	1	35	1	42
(c)	Pathologist laboratory with toilet	—		2	17.5	3	175	4	17.5	4	17.5
	Office and records	—		1	17.5	1	14	1	14	1	21
(e)	Technician room with toilet	—				1	14	1	14	1	21
(f)	Stores	—		2	10.5	3	10.5	4	10.5	4	14
(g)	Biochemistry	—		1	21	1	28	1	35	1	42
(h)	Microbiology with incubator	—		1	17.5	1	28	1	35	1	42
(i)	Media room	—		1	10.5	1	14	1	14	2	14
(j)	Clinical pathology and haematology	1	14	1	17.5	1	28	1	35	2	28
(k)	Photometry and other electronic equipment room	—		—		—		—		1	14
(I)	Histology and cytology	—		—		1	14	1	21	1	28
(m)	Microphotography	—		—		—		—		1	14
(n)	Washing and sterilizing area	—		1	10.5	1	14	1	14	1	21
(o)	Serology laboratory	—		—		1	10.5	1	14	1	21
(p)	Animal room with washing, weighing, and feeding facilities	—		—		1	17.5	1	21	1	28
(q)	Janitor's closet	—		1	3.5	1	3.5	1	3.5	1	3.5
(r)	Specimen disposal and sluice room	—		1	7.0	1	7.0	1	10.5	1	10.5

Layout & Zoning (Figure 20C)

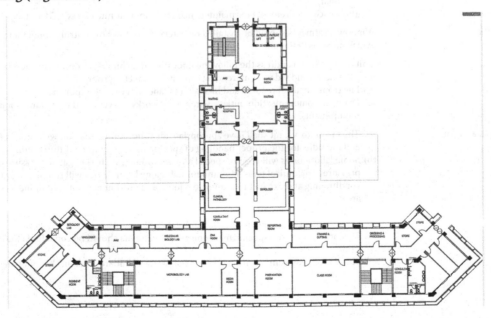

FIGURE 20C Sample Layout of Medical Laboratory Unit.

Built Environment: General Considerations

TABLE 20G: General Considerations for Built Environment

Environmental Considerations

Natural Light/Lighting	(a) Internal and task lighting must be sufficient for safe operation of equipment and use of computer screens and provide good visibility for digital displays on equipment.
	(b) The lighting requirements in a Medical Laboratory Unit are given as follows:
	  (i) Reception areas and stores: 300 lux
	  (ii) Offices: 400 lux
	  (iii) Working places: 600 lux (1 Lux = 11 lumen/m)
	  (iv) Colour Rendering Index of all the luminaires must be > 85.

Interior Décor	The décor and design of the unit should create a pleasant, professional atmosphere without appearing institutional or industrial.
Accessibility	Reception, offices, meeting rooms, waiting areas, and specimen collection areas should be designed to provide access for people in wheelchairs who may include staff or visitors.
Doors	Doors to enclosed laboratories must be adequately sized to accommodate equipment located in the laboratory, such as fume hoods and automated processing analysers.
Ergonomics	Chemical agents used in analysers and cleaning/decontamination processes and flammable liquids that involve specific chemical handling requirements (refer to local regulations), electrical and fire hazards related to equipment in use, and biological hazards of contaminated material undergoing processing require stringent infection control management.
Safety and Security	(a) Access control system should be installed to prevent unauthorized entry into the laboratory to ensure security for staff working in the unit after working hours particularly if the unit is located in an isolated area within the facility. (b) Emergency shower with eye-flushing device must be accessible from laboratory and specimen reception areas. (c) Chemicals and reagents including flammable liquids used in the unit should be stored safely in a separate room that is dark, and it must be accessed by authorized personnel only. (d) Safe storage, handling, and disposal of radioactive and cytotoxic materials including reagents and patient specimens, depending on the service provided. (e) Suitable non-slip floor finishes must be installed where water and chemicals are in use. (f) Equipment safety to prevent spills and accidents must be ensured.
Finishes	Finishes should be selected with consideration of the following: (a) Infection control and ease of cleaning (b) Fire safety (c) Durability (d) Acoustic properties (e) Floors should be water- and chemical-resistant, sealed, and coved at the edges (f) Work surfaces should be smooth, impervious to moisture and chemical-resistant
Fixtures, Fittings, and Equipment	(ii) Structural assessment may be required for large equipment such as automated laboratory analysers. (iii) Space requirements for maintenance of equipment must be considered.
Window Treatments	Window treatments should be installed on external windows to control sunlight and glare into the working areas of the unit.
Communications	Unit design should address the following information technology/communications issues: (a) Telephones and video-conferencing capacity for meeting rooms. (b) Electronic medical records and inclusion of laboratory result reporting. (c) Data and communication outlets, wireless networks, servers, and communication room requirements.
Heating, Ventilation, and Air Conditioning	(a) The Laboratory Unit shall have appropriate air conditioning that allows control of temperature and humidity for the proper handling of specimens and equipment functioning. (b) Some laboratories will require special air conditioning such as negative pressure or positive pressure. Anatomical pathology and microbiology laboratories will require negative pressure air conditioning and exhaust to minimize odours and prevent aerosol contamination of adjacent areas. (c) Offices, open-plan workstation areas, meeting rooms, and staff rooms should be air conditioned for the benefit of visitors to the unit and staff. (d) The local or country-specific mechanical requirements should be consulted (National Building Code). (e) The HVAC requirements for a Medical Laboratory Unit are given in the following.

(Continued)

TABLE 20G: (Continued)

Temp.	Humidity	Air-changes / Hrs, Fresh Air-F, Recirculated-R	Pressure Relation Ship to Adjacent Areas	Bio. Med. Eqpt. Load
22°±2°C	Up to 60%	6-8/h – R	Histology, Microbiology, Virology, Mycology Mobid Anatomy- N	20000 W

Pneumatic Tube Systems	The Laboratory Unit may include a pneumatic tube station, connecting key clinical units with the main support units as determined by the facility operational policy. If provided, the station should be located in the specimen reception under direct staff supervision.
Infection Control	(a) Personnel working in the medical laboratory must adhere to the standard precautions. Therefore, PPEs must be available at an appropriate location, near the working/processing areas.
	(b) It is recommended that in addition to handwashing basins, medicated handwash soap and alcohol-based hand rub dispensers be located strategically at appropriate areas within the Medical Laboratory Unit.
	(c) It is recommended that at least one emergency shower and eyewash station should be available in each laboratory.
	(d) These emergency showers and eyewash stations should be tapped to the laboratory water supply. When installing showers, the pull handle should be located in direct proximity to the shower head. Safety showers should be no more than 25 ft from the chemical fume hood or other area where corrosive chemicals are used.
	(e) An eyewash station must be readily available in all Biosafety Level 2 (BSL-2) laboratories. When a tissue culture room is located within a main lab room, the eyewash station should be installed next to the handwashing sink located inside the tissue culture room.

TABLE 20H: Specific Room and Functional Requirements for Built Environment

High Volume Analyser	(a) The Processor should be located with convenient access to specimen reception for efficient sample processing.
	(b) The equipment is automated and will require a temperature-controlled environment along with services and data connections as per the manufacturer's specifications.
Physical Containment Laboratory	(a) The physical containment laboratory is a fully enclosed, negative pressured, HEPA-filtered laboratory with entry via a dedicated airlock.
	(b) The airlock is moderately negative pressured with airflow towards the laboratory. Doors between the airlock and laboratory are interlocking—only one can be opened at a time.
	(c) The physical containment laboratory is used for handling infective organisms; therefore, a sample is processed in a biosafety cabinet as per the biosafety level.
	(i) Walls, floors, and ceiling finishes should be smooth, impervious to water, chemical resistant, and easy to clean.
	(ii) A fail-safe communication system within the laboratory.
Pneumatic Tube Station	(a) The pneumatic tube station should be located at the specimen reception under the direct supervision of staff. The location should not be accessible to any unauthorized personnel or visitor.
Sorting and Processing Area	Located adjacent to the specimen receiving area with easy access to the laboratories.
	(a) The sorting and processing area will require
	(i) Workstations for data entry
	(ii) Holding areas for specimens awaiting transit to specialist internal laboratories or remote laboratories
	(iii) Scanning equipment
	(iv) Refrigerators and freezers in close proximity
	(v) Incubator for microbiology samples
	(vi) Handwashing basin within the processing area
	(vii) BMW bins and a temporary storage area for Biomedical Waste

20.9 Future Trends

Laboratory practice is rapidly changing with advances in technology that affect service delivery. Future trends that will have a direct influence on the type of services being offered and the amount of space required in laboratories include the following:

(a) Increase in testing speed and degree of automation due to improvement in software capability resulting in a reduced turnaround time
(b) Total laboratory automation
(c) Analysers with specimen storage and retrieval capabilities
(d) Increase used of genetic testing and biopsy testing
(e) Increased use and accuracy of point of care devices
(f) Use of AI in laboratory

20.10 Summary

A medical laboratory is a critical process that requires meticulous attention to detail and careful consideration of various factors. The successful establishment of a well-designed Medical Laboratory Unit is essential for ensuring accurate diagnostic testing, efficient workflow, and optimal patient care. Key considerations in the planning and designing process include adequate space allocation, proper ventilation and environmental control, efficient workflow design, appropriate placement of equipment and storage areas, adherence to safety and regulatory requirements, integration of advanced technologies, and provision for future expansion.

21 BLOOD BANK

21.1 Introduction

The Blood Bank provides licensed facilities for the collection, storage, processing, and distribution of human blood and blood components, in accordance with the National Blood Policy, 2002, under the administration of the Central Drugs Standard Control Organisation (CDSCO) India.

The range of services provided by the Blood Bank include

- Collection from donors and donor management; this can include
  - Autologous blood—collection from a patient for transfusion to themselves at a later date.
  - Apheresis, which involves donation of plasma only or blood elements such as platelets only while the other blood elements are transfused back into the patient at the time of collection.
- Blood storage.
- Blood grouping and compatibility testing or cross-matching.
- Testing for transmissible diseases.

21.2 Blood Bank and Wider Hospital Context: Location & Access

The Blood Bank must not be located close to open drains, sewage, public toilets, animal houses, or any unhygienic surroundings. The facility must prevent the entry of flies, insects, and rodents; mesh screens can be provided as necessary. The Blood Bank Unit shall have a minimum floor area of 100 m² and an additional 50 m² for preparation of blood products. The unit should be sized according to the level of service provided (National AIDS Control Organization guidelines).

21.3 Operational Models and Hours of Operation

Blood Bank services may be provided according to the following models and will depend on the role delineation and the operational policy of the facility:

- A dedicated unit within a hospital.
- A unit collocated with a Pathology Laboratory Unit.
- A stand-alone facility, providing services to regional facilities and hospitals.

The Blood Bank is either provided within a hospital or free-standing. It generally operates during business hours for collection and routine laboratory services but offers a 24-hour service for deliveries.

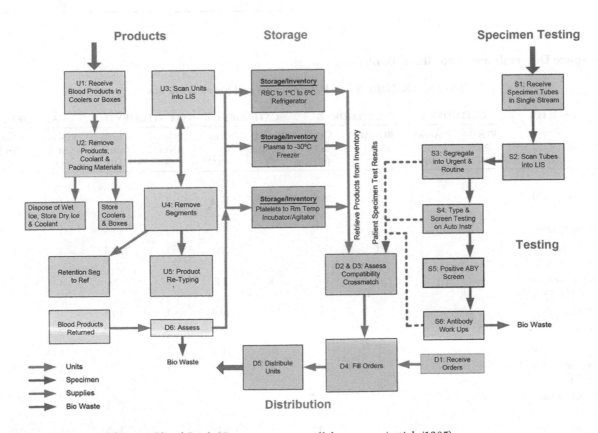

FIGURE 21A   Process Flows in Blood Bank (Courtesy: www.medlabmag.com/article/1305).

DOI: 10.1201/9780367460884-22

TABLE 21A: Key Result Areas and Quality Indicators for a Blood Bank

Key Result Areas

- Valid blood bank license
- Policies for rational use and transfusion of blood and blood products
- Informed consent for donation and transfusion
- Turnaround time of availability of blood
- Process for availability and transfusion in emergency
- Transfusion reactions analysis
- Adherence to infection prevention and control practices
- Availability of adequate and appropriate hygiene facility
- Instructions for handwashing displayed at appropriate locations
- Use of PPE
- Equipment cleaning and disinfection
- Housekeeping
- Safe injection practices
- Segregation of biomedical waste
- Fire safety
- Documented policies and procedures
- Periodic training of staff
- Safe exit plan in case of fire and non-fire emergencies
- Maintenance plan for facility and furniture
- All equipment is inventoried and log maintained/calibrated
- PM labels on equipment/calibration records/refrigerator
- Patient and staff interview

Quality Indicators

- Percentage of transfusion reactions
- Hand hygiene compliance rate
- Wastage against percentage of issue of blood and blood products
- TAT

21.4 Internal and External Functional Relationships

The Blood Bank located within a hospital facility will require good functional relationships with units that need frequent deliveries of blood such as the Operating Unit and Intensive Care Units. A stand-alone Blood Bank will require good access for donors and rapid access to transport services for blood deliveries to hospital facilities.

Ser No.	Facilities	Up to 399 Beds	400 Beds & Above
1.	Reception, registration-cum-waiting room	14.00	14.00
2.	Blood donation room	17.50	21.00
3.	Donor recovery/rest and refreshment room	10.50	10.50
4.	Med exam or counselling room	10.50	10.50
5.	Blood bank laboratory and blood storage room	17.50	17.50
6.	Blood screening laboratory	10.50	10.50
7.	Washing/cleaning/autoclaving room	07.00	07.00
8.	MO's room	10.50	10.50
9.	Records and stores	07.00	07.00
10.	Centrifugation, thawing, and blood component storage room	—	24.50
11.	Plasma/components separation room	—	14.00
12.	Office-cum-documentation-cum-change over room	—	10.50
13.	Toilet (Common for Ser Nos. 2, 3, 4, and 5)	2 × 03.50	2 × 03.50
	Total	117.75	164.50

Floor area in square meters

Major Space Determinants and Blood Bank Size

TABLE 21B: Major Space Determinants and Blood Bank Size

S No. (1)	FACILITY (2)	CATEGORY A ROOM (NO.) (3)	Area (m²) (4)	CATEGORY B ROOM (NO.) (5)	Area (m²) (6)	CATEGORY C ROOM (NO.) (7)	Area (m²) (8)	CATEGORY D ROOM (NO.) (9)	Area (m²) (10)	CATEGORY E ROOM (NO.) (11)	Area (m²) (12)
GENERAL											
(a)	Reception and waiting	—		1	10.5	1	17.5	1	21	1	28
(b)	Bleeding area	—						1	17.5	1	17.5
(c)	Donor restroom with kitchenette			1	17.5	1	21	1	17.5	1	17.5
(d)	Laboratory and blood storage area	—		1	14	1	21	1	28	1	28
(e)	Office			—	—	1	10.5	1	10.5	1	10.5
(f)	Stores			—	—	1	10.5	2	10.5	2	10.5
(g)	Bottle washing area	—		—	—	1	10.5	1	14	1	17.5
(h)	Doctor room with toilet	—		1	17.5	1	17.5	1	17.5	1	17.5
(i)	Social worker room	—									
(j)	Lavatory	—		1	7.0	1	7.0	1	10.5	1	10.5
(k)	Janitor's closet	—		—	—	1	3.5	1	3.5	1	3.5

Layout & Zoning (Figure 21B)

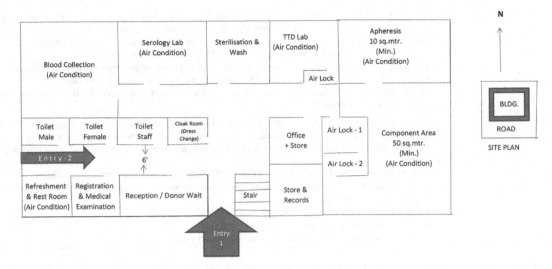

FIGURE 21B Built Environment: General Considerations (Table 21C).

TABLE 21C: General Considerations for Built Environment in a Blood Bank

Building	• The building (s) used for operation of a blood bank/blood centre and/or preparation of blood components shall be constructed in such a manner to permit the operation of the blood bank/blood centre and preparation of blood components under hygienic conditions and shall avoid entry of insects, rodents, and flies. • It should be well-lighted, ventilated, and screened (mesh) whenever necessary. • The walls and floors of the rooms where collection of blood or preparation of blood components or blood products is carried out should be smooth, washable, and capable of being kept clean. • Drains should be of adequate size and where connected directly to a sewer, should be equipped with traps to prevent back-siphoning.
Environment Control	• The blood bank/blood centre should have a process to minimize and respond to environmentally related risks to the health and safety of employees (including immunization), donors, volunteers, patient/recipients, and visitors. • Suitable environment and equipment should be available to maintain a safe environment.
Biological, Chemical, and Radiation Safety	• The Blood Bank/Blood Centre should have a policy and procedure for monitoring adherence to biological, chemical, and radiation safety standards and regulations, as applicable. • The Blood Bank/Blood Centre should monitor, control, and record environmental conditions, as required by relevant specifications or where they may influence the procedures and quality of the results (MoHFW, DGHS, Manual on Blood Bank). • Attention should be given to sterility, dust, electromagnetic interference, radiation, humidity, electrical supply, temperature, and sound and vibration levels as appropriate to the technical activities concerned.
Internal Communication Systems	Communication systems within the Blood Bank/Blood Centre should be appropriate to the size and complexity of the facility for the efficient transfer of information.
Finishes	All floors and walls in processing areas must be smooth, impervious to fluids, and easily cleaned.
Fixtures and Fittings	• The Blood Bank laboratory areas will include special equipment with installation and services provided including power, data, and water to comply with government regulations and manufacturer's specifications. • Blood refrigerators and freezers will require continuous temperature monitoring to maintain desired temperatures and alarms when the temperature is not reached or exceeded. Alarms should be automatically recorded.
Air Conditioning	• Blood collection, preparation and laboratory areas should be air conditioned with the ability to maintain air temperature between 20⁰ Centigrade to 25⁰ Centigrade. • Sterile manufacturing areas will require a HEPA-filtered, positive pressure air supply in accordance with licensing regulations.
Hydraulic Services	Drains must be sized appropriately and where connected to a sewer, must have traps installed to prevent back flow.
Electrical Services	Blood storage equipment must be provided with a 24-hour essential power supply. A back-up generator will be required. Laboratory areas will require effective lighting in work areas.

(Continued)

TABLE 21C: (Continued)

Building	• The building (s) used for operation of a blood bank/blood centre and/or preparation of blood components shall be constructed in such a manner to permit the operation of the blood bank/blood centre and preparation of blood components under hygienic conditions and shall avoid entry of insects, rodents, and flies. • It should be well-lighted, ventilated, and screened (mesh) whenever necessary. • The walls and floors of the rooms where collection of blood or preparation of blood components or blood products is carried out should be smooth, washable, and capable of being kept clean. • Drains should be of adequate size and where connected directly to a sewer, should be equipped with traps to prevent back-siphoning.

Infection Control	• Infection control is important in this unit. Strict infection control measures are required within the unit to protect laboratory staff from potentially contaminated body fluids (blood, plasma) and to ensure an aseptic environment for manufacture and packaging of blood products to prevent cross infection.
	• Measures will include
	   • Hand basins for staff handwashing in patient donor areas and processing laboratories.
	   • Use of laboratory clothing and laminar flow biosafety cabinets in laboratories; processing and filling areas must be separate.
	   • Separate area for handling of contaminated samples.
	   • Proper handling of contaminated waste.
	   • Sharps containers and clinical waste collection and removal.

TABLE 21D: Specific Room and Functional Requirements for Built Environment in a Blood Bank

Preparation and Processing Laboratory Areas

Description and Function	• Processing and laboratory areas include serology, infectious serology, plasma apheresis.
	• In these areas, the following procedures are undertaken:
	   • Pre-transfusion testing of samples for general serology and infectious diseases such as Hepatitis B and C, HIV, and malarial parasites.
	   • Blood grouping.
	   • Cross matching or compatibility testing.
	   • Apheresis, plasmapheresis, platelet pheresis, and leucopheresis procedures, according to the operational policies and scope of service of the unit.
	   • Quality control testing procedures.
	• Manufacturing of blood products requires separate enclosed areas with airlocks at the entry, in accordance with licensing regulations.
	• A separate testing area is required for infectious samples.
	• Manufacturing laboratories will be HEPA-filtered and positive pressured clean environments.

Location and Relationships	Preparation, processing, and manufacturing areas should be located with ready access to blood storage and wash up areas.
Considerations	• Separate storage refrigerators are required for tested and untested blood within the preparation and laboratory areas. • Processing, manufacturing, and packaging of blood will require a laminar air flow bench or unit in a clean environment. • Laboratory areas should have restricted access for authorized staff only.

Blood Storage

Description and Function	The blood store provides for the secure, temperature-controlled storage of blood and blood components in refrigerators or freezers for access by authorized staff only.
Location and Relationships	Within the Blood Bank, the blood store should be located with ready access to the blood collection and processing areas. Externally, ready access is required to Pathology Unit, Emergency Unit, Operating Unit and critical care areas. Consideration should be given to blood storage location in relation to external after-hours access and security.
Considerations	The blood storage refrigerators shall be secured, accessed by authorized staff only, and equipped with temperature monitoring and alarm signals. Alarms and controls should be located to ensure easy staff control. The blood refrigerators/freezers will require an essential power supply.

21.5 Summary

No other fluid can totally substitute for blood in the human body. Blood contains nutrients along with oxygen in adequate quantities and helps in maintaining a balanced temperature in the body. In many cases, transfusion of blood or blood components becomes necessary to save the life of an individual. Therefore, we need to have a network of Blood Banks/Blood Centres. The blood stored in Blood Banks/Blood Centres must be safe and free from contamination. The collection and storage of blood/blood components is performed by Blood Banks/Blood Centres attached to hospitals. Voluntary agencies and private sector blood Banks/Blood Centres also provide this service. The process is controlled through regulation, which to great extent is responsible to ensure the purity of blood and blood products.

22 REHABILITATION UNIT

22.1 Introduction

The Rehabilitation Unit provides multi-disciplinary rehabilitation service care in which the clinical intent or treatment goal is to improve the functional status of a patient with an impairment, disability, or handicap. Facilities for physiotherapy and occupational therapy will vary greatly, ranging from large, purpose-designed, central facilities for inpatients and/or outpatients to basic on-ward or bedside services. Extent, design, and location of facilities will be affected by the presence or otherwise of the following services (not inclusive):

♦ Rehabilitation medicine
♦ Aged care
♦ Spinal cord injury service
♦ Orthopaedic services
♦ Neurosciences—(strokes, multiple sclerosis, traumatic brain injuries, etc.)
♦ Amputees
♦ Hand surgery/plastic services
♦ Speech pathology

(a) **Patient Characteristics:** All ages from children to the elderly may be treated. Almost all patients attending physiotherapy are physically incapacitated to some extent, and many use wheelchairs or walking aids and—increasingly—motorized chairs that have implications for parking and recharging. Many patients may be disfigured (burns, throat surgery, etc.) and require a non-threatening, private environment. Patients may require access to interpreter services.

(b) **Specific Needs in Inpatient Units:** To avoid unnecessary transport to and from the main unit, space, and facilities for ward-based therapy could be considered, including but not confined to
- 10 m corridor length for walking tests.
- Storage for equipment and mobility aids.
- Ward-based treatment space larger than the area around a patient's bed.
- Access to stairs for practicing crutches.
- Access to write-up area and storage of resource material.

22.2 Rehabilitation Unit and Wider Hospital Context: Location & Access

(a) **External:** If the unit is on the ground floor with its own entry, then an undercover set-down bay should be provided at the entrance for outpatients who arrive by bus or car and for return of loan equipment, with parking for people with disabilities.

(b) **Internal:** The unit should be accessible from inside the hospital's main entrance. Wheelchair access is required for all patient-accessed areas of the unit.

22.3 Models of Care

Traditionally, the model of care has been one-to-one, specifically, therapist to patient. Increasingly, an educative model is

DOI: 10.1201/9780367460884-23

TABLE 22A: Key Result Areas and Quality Indicators for a Rehabilitation Unit

Key Result Areas

- Adequate space and equipment
- Multidisciplinary team approach
- Functional assessment scales
- Care of vulnerable patients
- Safe and secure environment
- Safety of patients
- Maintenance plan for facility and furniture

Quality Indicators

- Patient fall rates
- Equipment downtime

being used that assumes a staff-to-patient ratio of 1:4 or more and incorporates:

- Group sessions for peer support;
- Group exercise classes;
- Involvement of caregivers so that they can learn how much activity the patients can safely tolerate at home and how best to support them; and
- Education programs.

There may need to be separate areas for respiratory and cardiac rehabilitation and general rehabilitation as the patients have differing needs and sometimes equipment. However, this will depend on the number of sessions, and every opportunity should be made to share areas between programs.

22.4 Functional Relationships and Flow in a Rehabilitation Unit (Figures 22A to 22C)

The most critical relationship in circumstances where rehabilitation medicine is an established service is with its own Inpatient Unit/s. The unit should have ready access to allied health units such as speech pathology, social work. Physiotherapy areas will also require ready access to orthopaedic clinics.

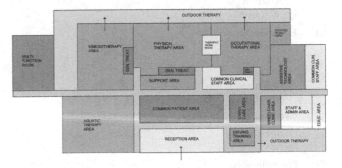

FIGURE 22A Functional Relationships and Flow in a Large Rehabilitation Unit (Courtesy: www.wbdg.org/FFC/VA/VADEGUID/dg_pmrs.pdf).

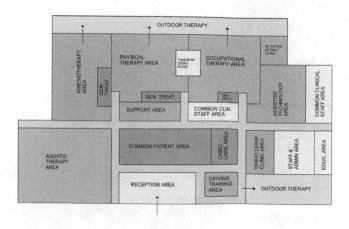

FIGURE 22B Functional Relationships and Flow in a Medium-Sized Rehabilitation Unit (Courtesy: www.wbdg.org/FFC/VA/VADEGUID/dg_pmrs.pdf).

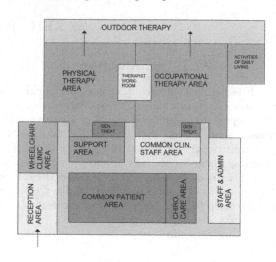

FIGURE 22C Functional Relationships and Flow in a Small Rehabilitation Unit (Courtesy: www.wbdg.org/FFC/VA/VADEGUID/dg_pmrs.pdf).

Major Space Determinants & Rehabilitation Unit Size

TABLE 22B: Major Space Determinants and Rehabilitation Unit Size

S No.	FACILITY	CATEGORY A		CATEGORY B		CATEGORY C		CATEGORY D		CATEGORY E	
		ROOM (NO.)	Area (m²)	ROOM (NO.)	Area (m²)	ROOM (NO.)	Area (m²)	ROOM (NO.)	Area (m²)	ROOM (NO.)	Area (m²)
(1)	(2)	(3)	(4)	(5)	(6)	(7)	(8)	(9)	(10)	(11)	(12)
FUNCTIONAL AREAS											
(a)	Reception with waiting area and toilets	—		1	21	1	28	1	35	1	42
(b)	Physical and electric therapy										
	(a) Diathermy			1	10.5	1	10.5	1	10.5	1	10.5
	(b) Ultraviolet	—									
	(c) Infrared	2	7.0	2	7.0	3	7.0	3	7.0	6	7.0
	(d) Radiant heat	—		1	10.5	1	10.5	1	10.5	1	10.5
	(e) Selective/ Combined treatment										
	(f) Traction	—			—	1	10.5	1	10.5	1	10.5
	(g) Wax bath	—			—	—		1	10.5	1	10.5
(c)	Hydrotherapy comprising of a tank, shower, and dressing cubicles	—			—	1	28	1	35	1	35
(d)	Gymnasium	1	21	1	28	1	42	1	63	1	91
(e)	Occupational therapy			—	—		—	1	35	1	42
(f)	Physiotherapist office including toilet of 3.5 m²	—		1	17.5	1	17.5	1	21	1	21
(g)	Store	—		1	14	1	21	1	28	1	28

Layout & Zoning (Figure 22D)

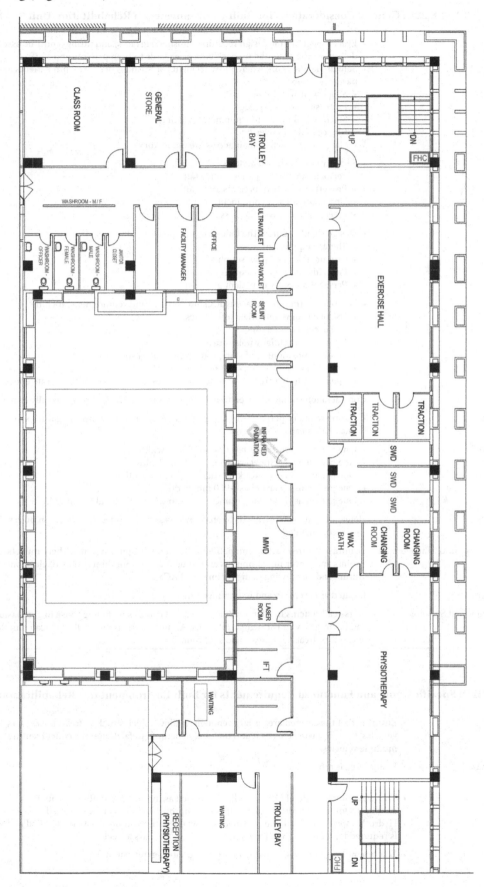

FIGURE 22D   Sample Layout of a Rehabilitation Unit.

Built Environment: General Considerations

TABLE 22C: General Considerations for Built Environment in a Rehabilitation Unit

Safety	• Every aspect of unit design regarding finishes, surfaces, and fittings must be assessed to determine the potential for accidents or hazards to both patients and staff.
	• Sanitary facilities are where most accidents or mishaps occur to both patients and staff. In particular, consider
	  • Slippery or wet floors
	  • Protrusions or sharp edges
	  • Stability and height of equipment or fittings
	  • Choice of floor covering
	  • Handrails and wheelchair access are mandatory

Security	• Security design should address
	  • Personal security of patients and staff
	  • Property security of patients and staff
	  • Unit premises and equipment
	  • Emergency access and egress

Storage	• Design should address the following storage requirements:
	  • Therapy equipment
	  • Consumables and pool supplies
	  • Pool aids and exercise equipment
	  • Personal property of patient and staff

Acoustics	• Solutions to the various acoustic characteristics and requirements include
	  • Use of curtains and other soft fabrics
	  • Use of solid core doors
	  • Co-locate potentially noisy areas
	  • Strategic positioning of storage areas to create a sound buffer
	  • Carpet in patient areas is not recommended
	  • Speech pathology rooms have specific requirements in order to operate effectively

Lighting	Consideration should be given to lighting levels for patients who are visually impaired.
Climate Control	• It is therefore imperative that the gymnasium is air conditioned. Regardless of orientation, there must be a means of sun control.
Average Circulation Space Sizes	• One person using a walking stick—750 mm width • One person using elbow crutches—900 mm width • One person using two walking sticks—800 mm width • One person using crutches—950 mm width • One person using walking frame—900 mm width (National Building Code)
Fixtures and Fittings	Height of light switches needs to abide by accessibility codes. Handrails on both sides of corridors are recommended.
Information Technology and Management	IT infrastructure must be compatible with overall hospital systems. There must be sufficient data points and power for computers and student laptops for direct entry of electronic records in the future and for viewing of digital images (PACS).
Duress Alarm System	Located at Reception and in treatment areas
Nurse and Emergency Call Systems	Nurse call systems in all individual rooms and cubicles including those in gymnasiums. Staff assist and emergency call at regular intervals. Annunciators (non-scrolling) located in Reception, corridors, treatment areas, and staff room.

TABLE 22D: Specific Room and Functional Requirements for Built Environment in a Rehabilitation Unit

Entry Areas	• Ensuring that the covered area is large enough to allow vehicles such as taxis, buses, cars, and emergency vehicles to manoeuvre beneath it and that it is structured to facilitate free concurrent traffic flow for multiple vehicles.
Patient Lounge Areas	A lounge area is required for therapeutic and social purposes, such as reading, writing, and watching television or videos.
Hydrotherapy	• The need for a pool should be carefully considered as the cost per unit of treatment is high, and conditions for which hydrotherapy is the only appropriate treatment are limited. • Hydrotherapy pools should be provided only where patient numbers can be justified and where the pool is required for a minimum of four hours each days, five days a week.
Gait Analysis Laboratory	• Equipment for gait analysis can be incorporated into a gymnasium.

(Continued)

TABLE 22D: (Continued)

Patient Lifting/Transfers	Patient handling measures may include ceiling hoist systems for transfers from wheelchair to plinth or mobile lifters. Mobile patient lifters will require bays with power for recharging. The gymnasium should include additional space for holding lifting devices.
Recharging of Electrical Wheelchairs Wheelchair Parking	• An area should be provided near the entrance for parking wheelchairs and electric scooters.

Occupational Therapy/Workshop Rooms	• The rooms area will be sized according to the number of patients to be accommodated and the activities to be undertaken and will depend on the operational policy and service demand.
	• The occupational therapy area can be located adjacent to rehabilitation therapy areas, with ready access to waiting and amenities areas.
	• Fittings and equipment required in this area may include
	  • Benches with an inset sink, wheelchair accessible.
	  • Shelving for storage of equipment or tools.
	  • Tables of adjustable height.
	  • Chairs of adjustable height.
	  • Handwashing basin with liquid soap and paper towel fittings.
	  • Pin board and whiteboard for displays.
	• Workshop areas will require suitable air extraction and exhaust for woodwork activities.

22.5 Summary

If you are in the hospital recovering from surgery, healing from an injury, or being treated for a disabling health problem, then physical rehabilitation may be an important part of your treatment. Physical medicine and rehabilitation, or simply rehab, is a branch of medicine called physiatry. Design of a Rehabilitation Unit focuses on heavy equipment, patient and staff safety, and special finishing, lighting, and accessibility requirements.

23 DAY SURGERY/PROCEDURE UNIT

23.1 Introduction

A Day Surgery/Procedure Unit is where operative procedures are performed and admission, procedure, and discharge occur on the same date. The unit will have access to or include one or more operating rooms, with provision to deliver anaesthesia and accommodation for the immediate post-operative recovery of day patients. The range of procedures that can be undertaken in a Day Surgery/Procedure Unit may include the following:

- Surgical procedures, particularly ENT, dental, plastic surgery, and ophthalmology
- Endoscopy—gastrointestinal, respiratory, and urology
- Electroconvulsive therapy (ECT) for mental health inpatients
- Day medical procedures including intravenous infusions and minor treatments

23.2 Operational Models

The range of options for a Day Surgery/Procedure Unit may include

- A stand-alone centre, fully self-contained
- A dedicated, fully self-contained unit within a hospital
- A unit collocated with a specialist clinical service such as gastroenterology or respiratory medicine, within an acute hospital
- A unit collocated with the Operating Unit with shared facilities

TABLE 23A: Key Result Areas and Quality Indicators for a Day Surgery/Procedure Unit

Key Result Areas

- Documentation for initial assessment
- Informed consent for moderate sedation
- Informed consent for procedures
- Monitoring for at least two hours after the procedure
- Procedures documented in the patient record
- Informed consent for anaesthesia
- Type of anaesthesia and medications documented
- Informed consent for surgery
- Documented policies to prevent the wrong site, wrong patient, and wrong surgery
- Surgery anaesthesia, medication notes and post-op care plan documented

Quality Indicators

- Time taken for initial assessment of patients
- Percentage of unplanned returns to OT
- Percentage of surgeries where organization's procedure to prevent adverse drug events such as wrong site, wrong patient, and wrong surgery have been adhered to
- Percentage of cases who received appropriate prophylactic antibiotics within the specified timeframe
- Percentage of rescheduling of surgeries

Functional Relationship & Patient Flow (Table 23B and Figure 23A)

TABLE 23B: Functional Relationship of a Day Surgery/Procedure Unit

Internal Functional Relationships	External Functional Relationships
Within the unit, key functional relationships will include	*The Day Surgery/Procedure Unit will have functional relationships with the following units*
• Unidirectional patient flow from arrival at Reception, through holding, procedure rooms, recovery rooms, then to the Peri-Operative Unit or Inpatient Unit or lounge areas and then discharged to home	• Operating suite • Pre-admission clinic • Transit lounge
• Separation of clean and dirty traffic flows	
• Staff visibility of patient areas for patient supervision and safety	

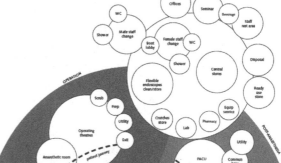
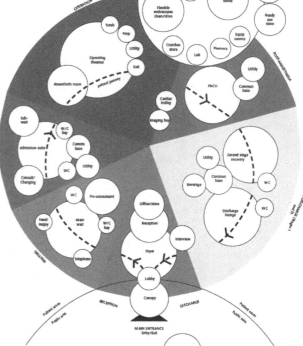

FIGURE 23A Functional Relationship and Patient Flow in a Day Surgery/Procedure Unit (Courtesy: HBN 10–02).

DOI: 10.1201/9780367460884-24

Major Space Determinants & Day Care Size

A unit of 10 beds each, in addition to the overall authorization of beds (in a hospital), is to be provided with ward ancillary accommodation for hospitals of 100–399 beds, and two such units of 10 beds each for hospitals of 400 beds and above. The unit will be sited near the operating theatre, casualty, OPD, radiology, and laboratory.

TABLE 23C: Major Space Determinants for a Day Care Centre

Description	Quantity	Area (m²)	Total Area (m²)
Entrance Reception & Waiting Facilities			
Vehicle drop-off point	–	–	–
Car parking spaces	–	–	–
Car parking spaces for people with disabilities	–	–	–
Main entrance draught lobby	1	11.0	11.0
Foyer/concourse area	1	–	–
Reception: two staff	1	10.0	10.0
Waiting area: 30 persons including wheelchair users	1	49.5	49.5
Infant feeding room	1	5.5	5.5
Nappy changing room with handwash	1	4.0	4.0
Public telephone: single booth	1	1.5	1.5
Public telephone: single booth, accessible	1	2.0	2.0
Parking bay: 3 wheelchairs	1	2.0	2.0
WC & handwash: accessible, wheelchair	1	4.5	4.5
WC & handwash: semi ambulant	4	2.5	10.0
Secondary entrance	1	–	–
Pre-Assessment Facilities			
Consulting/examination room: both sides couch access	2	16.5	33.0
Admissions Suite Facilities			
Admission & examination room	6	13.5	
Patient changing room: accessible, wheelchair: 1 person	6	6.0	
Waiting area: individual bay, 2 person	6	5.0	
WC & handwash: accessible, wheelchair assisted	1	4.5	
Staff base: 2 staff	1	6.0	
Parking bay: 3 wheelchairs	1	2.0	
WC & handwash: specimen, accessible, wheelchair	1	4.5	
Dirty utility: urine test	1	9.0	
Operating Theatre Suite Facilities			
Anaesthetic room	4	19.0	
Scrub-up & gowning room: 3 places	4	11.0	
Preparation room	4	12.0	
Operating theatre: day surgery	4	55.0	
Exit/parking bay: theatre, 1 bed/trolley	4	12.0	
Store: equipment, local to theatre	4	1.0	
Dirty utility: serving 1 theatre	4	12.0	
Recovery Unit or Post-Anaesthetic Care Unit (PACU) Facilities			
Recovery bay: post-anaesthetic. 1 place		9	13.S
Staff & communications base: enclosed: 2 staff		1	11.0
Clean utility with blood bank		1	17.0

(Continued)

TABLE 23C: (Continued)

Description	Quantity	Area (m²)	Total Area (m²)
Dirty utility bedpan disposal & urine test	1		12.0
Waiting area: 5 persons including 1 wheelchair user	1		9.0
Recovery bay: second stage	16		6.0
Staff & communications base: enclosed: 2 staff	1		11.0
Beverage & snack preparation bay	1		6.0
Discharge lounge: 8 places	1		20.0
Interview & counselling room: 5 places	1		9.99.0.00
WC & handwash: accessible, wheelchair	1		4.5
Store: patients clothing	1		4.0
WC & handwash: accessible, wheelchair	2		4.5
Support Facilities			
Office: medical reporting: 2 staff	1		13.0
Near patient testing/status laboratory	1		8.5
Service room equipment	1		12.0
Parking bay mobile x-ray & ultrasound unit	1		5.0
Parking bay: resuscitation trolley	1		1.0
Parking bay: fibre optic bronchoscope light source trolley	1		1.0
Utility cleaning room, flexible endoscope	1		15.0
Store: dean flexible endoscopes	1		6.0
Store: satellite pharmacy	1		6.0
Store: bulk supplies	1		80.0
Store: clinical equipment	1		30.0
Store: linen	2		3.0
Store: ready to use medical gas cylinders	1		4.0
Store: crutches and splints	1		2.0
Hold: disposal	1		15.0
Cleaners (housekeeping) room	4		7.0
Switchgear room	1		4.0
UPS & IT hub room	1		9.00.0

Layout & Zoning (Figure 23B)

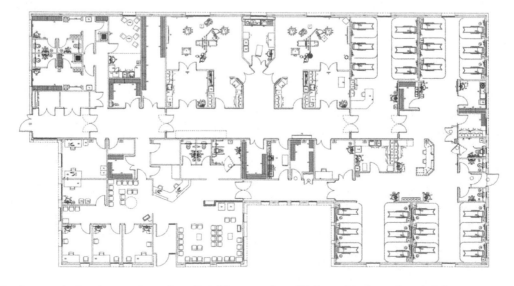

FIGURE 23B Layout of a Day Surgery/Procedure Unit (Courtesy: http://dcfw.org/singleton-hospital-day-surgery-unit-swansea/).

Built Environment: General Considerations

TABLE 23D: General Considerations for Built Environment in a Day Surgery/Procedure Unit

Acoustics	• Acoustic privacy treatment will be required for
	  • Consulting/interview rooms.
	  • Preparation rooms where patient pre-treatments can be undertaken.
	  • Operating/procedure rooms.

Natural Light	• Care must be taken to minimize glare and ensure that privacy is not compromised. Sun penetration should be controlled to exclude glare and heat gain or loss. • In operating and procedure rooms, the provision of a controlled level of lighting during procedures should be considered.

Privacy	• Staff observation of patients and patient privacy must be well-balanced within the unit. The following features should be integrated into the design of the unit:
	  • Doors and windows are to be located appropriately to ensure patient privacy and not comprise staff security.
	  • Discreet spaces to enable confidentiality of discussions related to a patient and storage of patient medical records.
	  • Privacy screening on bed and chair bays.
	  • Consultation, interview, and preparation rooms should not be visible from public or waiting areas; examination couches should not face the door.
	  • Location of patient changing areas to provide direct access to waiting areas to prevent patients in gowns from travelling through public areas when changing before and after procedures.
	  • Separation of male, female, and paediatric changing rooms and waiting areas.

Finishes	• The following additional factors should be considered in the selection of finishes:
	  • Acoustic properties.
	  • Durability.
	  • Ease of cleaning.
	  • Infection control.
	  • Fire safety.
	  • For movement of equipment, floor finishes should be resistant to marring and shearing by wheeled equipment.
	• In all areas where patient observation is critical, colours should be chosen that do not alter the observer's perception of skin colour.
	• Wall protection should be provided where bed or trolley movement occurs, such as corridors, patient bedrooms, equipment and linen storage, and treatment areas.

Safety and Security	• A high standard of security through grouping functions, controlling access and egress from the unit, and providing optimum observation for staff.
Radiation Shielding	• Radiation protection requirements must be incorporated into the final specifications and building plans.
Information Technology (IT) and Communications	It is vital to provide reliable and effective IT/communications service for efficient operation of the unit. The following items relating to IT/communications should be addressed in the design: • Appointment systems. • Patient Administration System (PAS) including clinical records and pathology results through Picture Archiving Communications Systems (PACS). • Scheduling systems to manage procedures or operating room sessions. • Procedure recording and printing of reports within the procedure room. • Materials management including bar coding for supplies, x-rays, and records. • Management and statistical information required for administration and quality assurance. • Education and training utilization of video and camera equipment.
Nurse/Emergency Call	• Nurse call and emergency call facilities must be provided in all patient areas (e.g., bed/chair spaces, toilets, and showers) and procedure areas for patients and staff to request urgent assistance.
Infection Control	• Separation of clean and dirty workflows in treatment and clean-up areas and separation of patient care areas and contaminated spaces and equipment are critical to the function of the unit and to prevent cross infection. • Standard precautions must be taken for all clients regardless of their diagnosis or presumed infectious status. • Staff handwashing facilities, including disposable paper towels, must be readily available.

TABLE 23E: Specific Room and Functional Requirements for Built Environment in a Day Surgery/Procedure Unit

Entry/Reception/Administration and Waiting Areas	• A covered entrance for dropping off and collection of patients after surgery should be provided. The entry may be a shared facility and should include
	  • Reception and information counter or desk.
	  • Waiting areas that allow for the separation of paediatric and adult patients.
	  • Convenient access to wheelchair storage.
	  • Convenient access to public toilet facilities.
	  • Convenient access to public telephones.

(Continued)

TABLE 23E: (Continued)

Ambulance Access	A discreet pick-up point, preferably under cover, should be provided for the transfer of patients to and from the Day Surgery/Procedure Unit.
Car Parking	Adequate car parking facilities with convenient access need to be provided.
Administration Areas	General and individual offices should be provided as required for business transactions, records, and administrative and professional staff.
Consult/Examination Rooms	The number of rooms will be determined by the service plan and operational policy of the unit.
Patient Changing Areas	The patient changing areas should include waiting rooms and lockers.
Holding Area	A pre-operative holding area should be provided with the following minimum requirements as appropriate to the proposed service: • A patient trolley or patient seating. • Privacy screening. • Hand basins with liquid soap and paper towel fittings. • Patient nurse call/emergency call buttons with pendant handsets and indicators. • Medical gases including oxygen and suction and power outlets to each bed.
Preparation Room	A preparation room can be required for patients undergoing certain procedures such as endoscopy or ophthalmology. If included, the preparation room should include • Hand basin—clinical. • Bench and cupboards for setting up procedures. • Adequate space for procedure equipment trolleys. • Examination couch. • Patient privacy screening.
Operating/Procedure Rooms	The design of the operating/procedure rooms must allow for adequate space, ready access, free movement, and demarcation of sterile and non-sterile zones.

Operating Room/s for Endoscopy	• The number and operation of operating rooms for endoscopy should be as determined by the service plan. Room size may vary, depending upon
	  • The use of video equipment.
	  • Electrosurgical laser treatment.
	  • Fluoroscopy equipment installed.
	  • Multiple endoscope activity.
	  • Multiple observers.
	  • The use of x-rays (image intensifying).
	• Where basic endoscopy is to be performed, the room size should be no smaller than 36 m².
	• Where video equipment is used, the room size should be 42 m².
	• Larger sizes, where possible, are recommended for flexibility and future developments.
	• The ceiling height should be 3,000 mm.
	• Operating rooms for endoscopy should be outfitted as a minor operating room; for example, it will be suitable for general anaesthetic with appropriate medical gases, power, lighting, air conditioning, and ventilation.
	• Staff assistance call should be provided. Consideration should also be given to the special requirements of laser equipment.
	• A clinical scrub-up basin should be provided outside the entrance to the operating room/s for endoscopy.
	• Direct access to the clean-up room is recommended.
	• Impervious wall, floor, and ceiling treatments are essential for ease of cleaning.

Recovery Areas	• In larger facilities, it is often considered desirable to have a three-stage recovery area. • The first stage involves intensive supervision, the second stage has flexible facilities in more casual surroundings, and in the third stage, the patient is fully mobile and is awaiting discharge. • Supervision of the patient is vital at each stage. • If paediatric surgery is part of the function, the recovery room should provide for the needs of parents/attendants.
Peri-Operative Area	• Where day procedures (day-only surgical service) are provided within the same area as inpatient acute surgery (shared facility), the design should consider the need to separate the two distinct functions at the incoming side. • The design should also preclude unrelated traffic from the Day Procedures Unit and the Operating Unit. • Provide patient accommodation to comply with standard components.

23.3 Summary

Day care centres adopt a customer-centric or patient-friendly approach to treatments and therapies that do not require overnight hospitalization. They are a win-win model for both the patient and the hospital. Patients and family members save a lot of time and hassle, while the hospital can maximize its returns on the health care infrastructure. Above all, day care hospitals have a transformative effect on society, as they help many patients receive super-specialty treatment without increasing the out-of-pocket health care expenditure.

24 PHARMACY UNIT

24.1 Introduction

The purpose of the Pharmacy Unit is to provide all inpatient and outpatient pharmacy services including dispensing of non-sterile and sterile commodities as required, reporting on adverse drug reactions, and providing drug information and education. The size and type of service to be provided in the Pharmacy Unit will depend upon the type of drug distribution system used, the number of patients to be served, and the extent of shared or purchased services.

24.2 Operational Models

A pharmacy may extend its service from a single health care facility to outlying facilities. Specific design requirements for packing, storage, and dispatch of goods should be considered for different operational models.

(a) **Unit Dose Systems**: The unit dosage system involves the packaging of each dose of each medication for patients in a blister pack to provide easy and uniform medication dispensing. For a unit dosage system, the pharmacy must include additional space and equipment for supplies, packaging, labeling, and storage.

(b) **Private Pharmacy**: If a private pharmacy is also to be provided within the hospital's retail area, the hospital's operational policy should determine the type of prescription drugs to be supplied by the private pharmacy. It should also study the impact that it has on the main pharmacy in relation to outpatient dispensing.

24.3 Planning Models

(a) **Dedicated Outpatient Pharmacy**: In facilities where the main pharmacy cannot be located in a position readily accessible to the outpatient areas due to site constraints, then a separate outpatient pharmacy can be provided. This arrangement may result in duplication of services, equipment, and support facilities.

(b) **Satellite Pharmacy Units**: Satellite Pharmacy Units refer to a series of rooms/suites in a hospital that is remotely positioned from the main pharmacy and yet managed by the staff of the main pharmacy. This may include, for example, a dedicated Cytotoxic Unit within a Cancer Day Care Unit or an after-hours drugstore.

(c) **Unit/Department-Based Pharmacy Areas**: This refers to medication areas located within an Inpatient Unit and may include automated dispensing. Unit-based facilities may be located within the clean utility or dedicated medication rooms in Inpatient Units. Facilities will include secured drug storage, refrigerated drug storage, space for medication trolleys, and computer access for pharmacy personnel.

Process Flow for Medication Request (Figure 24A)

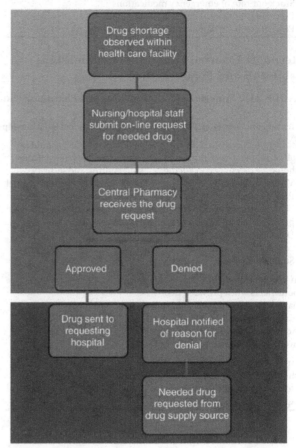

FIGURE 24A Process Flow for Medication Request (Courtesy: Holm M, Rudis M, Wilson J. Pharmaceutical supply chain management through implementation of a hospital Pharmacy Computerized Inventory Program (PCIP) in Haiti. Annals of Global Health. 2015 Mar 12;81(1)).

TABLE 24A: Key Result Areas and Quality Indicators for a Pharmacy Unit

Key Result Areas

- Documented policies and procedures on medication procurement, storage, formulation, prescription, dispensing, administration, monitoring, etc.
- Separate D and C Act license for each of the pharmacies
- Procedure to obtain medications when the pharmacy is closed
- Re-order levels, vendor evaluation, and generation of purchase order
- Policies and procedures for storage of medicines and consumables
- Inventory control practices such as FIFO
- Precautions against theft
- Identification and storage of LASA drugs
- List of emergency medications is defined and stored uniformly
- Medication recall procedure
- Verification of high-risk medication orders before dispensing

---

(Continued)

DOI: 10.1201/9780367460884-25

TABLE 24A: (Continued)

Quality Indicators

- Stock out rate of emergency medications
- Percentage of drugs/consumables rejected
- Percentage of variations from the procurement process

Internal & External Functional Relationships (Table 24B and Figure 24B)

TABLE 24B: Functional Relationships of a Pharmacy Unit

Internal Functional Relationships	External Functional Relationships
Access points provided for the following personnel/purpose should be carefully considered: • Visitors to the unit • Pharmacy staff • Non-pharmacy staff to collect prescriptions and medications • Delivery and prescription collection for outpatients • Supply delivery An interview room for outpatients when provided shall have dual access separate entries from public area and staff area. Access shall be controlled from inside of the pharmacy. Corridors and door openings should provide sufficient clearance for large items and equipment from bulk stores.	The Pharmacy Unit should be located for convenient access, staff control, and security. Direct access to the loading dock and bulk storage is required if not located within the main Pharmacy Unit.

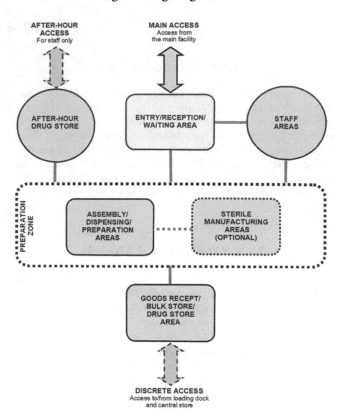

FIGURE 24B Functional Relationship of a Pharmacy Unit (Courtesy: https://aushfg-prod-com-au.s3.amazonaws.com/%5BB-0560%5D%20Pharmacy%20Unit.pdf).

Major Space Determinants and Pharmacy Unit Size

TABLE 24C: Major Space Determinants and Pharmacy Unit Size

S No.	FACILITY	CATEGORY A		CATEGORY B		CATEGORY C		CATEGORY D		CATEGORY E	
		ROOM (NO.)	Area (m²)	ROOM (NO.)	Area (m²)	ROOM (NO.)	Area (m²)	ROOM (NO.)	Area (m²)	ROOM (NO.)	Area (m²)
(1)	(2)	(3)	(4)	(5)	(6)	(7)	(8)	(9)	(10)	(11)	(12)
PHARMACY											
(a)	Office with toilet			—		1	10.5	1	14	1	17.5
(b)	Dispensing area with issuing counter					1	21	1	28	1	17.5
(c)	Preparation and compounding area	1	17.5	1	28	1	17.5	1	14	1	17.5
(d)	Bottle washing area							1	10.5	1	14
(e)	Queuing area			—		Adequate		Adequate		Adequate	
(f)	Pharmacist room with toilet			1	14	1	14	1	17.5	1	17.5
(g)	Pre-packaging area			1	14	2	14	1	14	1	17.5
(h)	Stores							2	14	2	17.5
(i)	Janitor's closet			—		1	3.5	1	3.5	1	3.5
(j)	Trolley bay			—		1	10.5	1	10.5	1	14

Layout & Zoning (Figure 24C)

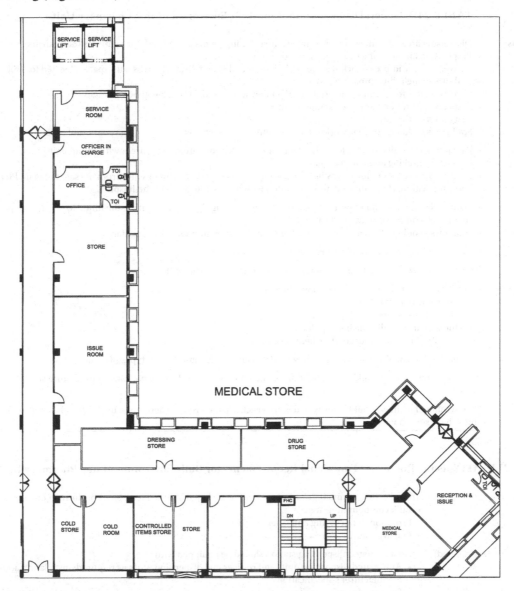

FIGURE 24C Sample Layout of a Pharmacy Unit.

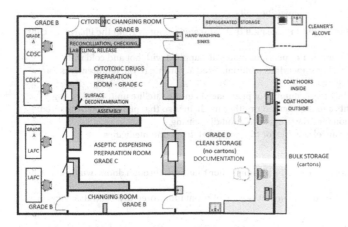

FIGURE 24D Layout of an Aseptic Production Suite Combining Conventional and Containment (Courtesy: https://aushfg-prod-com-au.s3.amazonaws.com/%5BB-0560%5D%20Pharmacy%20Unit.pdf).

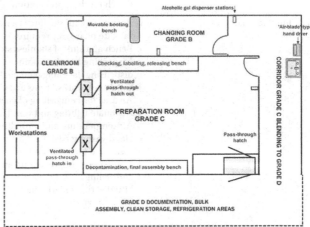

FIGURE 24E Layout of an Aseptic Production Suite (Courtesy: https://aushfg-prod-com-au.s3.amazonaws.com/%5BB-0560%5D%20Pharmacy%20Unit.pdf).

Built Environment: General Considerations

TABLE 24D: General Considerations for Built Environment in a Pharmacy Unit

Restricted Areas	• Dispensing areas that may include separate areas for inpatients and ambulatory patients (outpatients). • Preparation and manufacturing areas of non-sterile goods. • Active store for imprest stock storage, including assembly and dispatch areas with space allocated for trolley parking. • Bulk stores including unpacking area. • Secured stores for accountable drugs, refrigerated stores, and flammable goods storage. • Dispatch area for deliveries to Inpatient Units. • Drug information areas. • Staff areas including offices, workstations, meeting rooms, staff room, changing rooms, and toilets.
Accessible Areas	• Reception and waiting areas for outpatients; it is possible to share waiting areas with an adjoining unit. • Patient counselling and consult areas. • After-hours drug store for access only by authorized personnel and direct entry from outside the main Pharmacy Unit if located within; this room can also be located within a 24-hour zone of the hospital.
Natural Light	• Natural light and windows permitting outside views are highly desirable within the unit. However, such provisions should not compromise the security of the unit. • Windows should not permit casual viewing from any adjacent public thoroughfare.
Privacy	Privacy should be considered in patient consultation areas.
Acoustics	Patient interview and counselling rooms will require acoustic treatment.

Safety and Security	• Security measures for consideration will include
	  • Electronic door controls.
	  • Movement sensors.
	  • Duress alarms at dispensing counters.
	  • Security glazing or shutters at dispensing counters.

Finishes	Wall protection should be installed to prevent damage to walls caused by all types of trolleys.
HVAC	All drug storage areas should have temperature and humidity controls; internal room temperature should be kept below 25°C.
Infection Control	Handwashing facilities should be provided within each separate room where open medication is handled. Sterile suites must have scrub facilities.

TABLE 24E: Specific Room and Functional Requirements for Built Environment in a Pharmacy Unit

Manufacturing Area	The following minimum elements should be included if manufacturing is performed on-site: • Bulk compounding area. • Provision of packaging and labelling area. • Quality control area.

Dispensing Stations (Automated)	• An automated dispensing station should be equipped with
	  • Automated dispensing units and refrigerated dispensing units as required; installation according to manufacturer's specifications.
	  • Shelving for reference texts.
	  • Lighting level adequate for drug preparation areas.
	  • Handwashing facilities in close proximity.
	  • Bench for drug preparation adjacent to dispensing units.

Satellite Pharmacy	• A Pharmacy Unit satellite is a room or unit in a hospital that is located remotely from the Pharmacy Unit.
	• A satellite pharmacy requires
	  • Bench and sink of stainless steel or other impervious material, supplied with hot and cold water.
	  • Dispensing bench of stainless steel or impervious material; sized according to the requirements for dispensing, labelling, and packaging.
	  • Computer workstations according to the number of pharmacists in the satellite unit.
	  • An area for counselling of clients about dispensed or other medicines so that privacy can be assured.
	  • Adequate lighting and ventilation for drug preparation and dispensing.
	  • Air temperature and humidity control suitable for the storage of drugs and medicines.
	  • Handwashing basin and fittings.
	• The satellite pharmacy must be
	  • Constructed to prevent unauthorized access by persons other than staff through doors, windows, walls, and ceilings.
	  • Fitted with a security intrusion detector alarm that is control room monitored to a central agency on a 24-hour basis.

(Continued)

TABLE 24E: (Continued)

Storage	• The following minimum elements, in the form of cabinets, shelves, and/or separate rooms or closets, should be included as required:
	  • Bulk storage.
	  • Active storage.
	  • Refrigerated storage.
	  • Volatile fluids and alcohol storage with construction as required by the relevant regulations for the substances involved.
	  • Secure storage for narcotics and controlled drugs.
	  • Storage for general supplies and equipment not in use.
	  • Storage for prescriptions and any documents required by relevant legislation.

Clinical Trial Dispensing	• The clinical trial dispensing area will include storage, dispensing, packaging, labelling, and records holding for clinical trial drugs. The clinical trial facilities will be a separate area within the main pharmacy.
	• Clinical trial storage, preparation, and dispensing will be located in a separate area within the pharmacy and will have ready access to patient interview and consultation rooms.
	• Clinical trial drugs/medications area will require the following considerations:
	  • Workspace with computer for pharmacist.
	  • Preparation bench and sink.
	  • Lockable storage for clinical trial drugs, separate from other pharmacy supplies.
	  • Lockable records storage.
	  • Staff handwashing basin should be located in close proximity.

Aseptic Room (Sterile Manufacturing)/Cytotoxic Room (Cytotoxic Manufacturing) (Figures 24D, 24E)	• The aseptic room and the cytotoxic room are clean rooms for the manufacturing of medications in a sterile environment.
	• The room will contain laminar flow cabinets and/or isolators for sterile manufacturing.
	• The room will be positive pressured and accessed via an anteroom.
	• It should be located on the perimeter of the facility with an external outlook and access via an anteroom.
	• The following features should be considered while designing sterile manufacturing facility:
	  • Electronic door management system to prevent the opening of both doors in the anteroom at the same time.
	  • Handwashing facilities should be provided immediately outside the aseptic (clean) rooms in an adjoining anteroom; hand basins are not to be located within the aseptic (clean) rooms.
	  • An intercom system should be provided between aseptic (clean) rooms and an anteroom.
	  • High-resolution CCTV cameras for remote monitoring.
	  • Comply with room requirements according to relevant international clean room standards for sterile and cytotoxic manufacturing.

Store—Refrigeration	• This can be a room/bay that consists of multiple refrigerators for storing specific medications.
	• Alternatively, a commercial grade cool room can also be used.
	• This should be located in proximity to assembly/preparation area and other storage areas within the unit.
	• Refrigerated storage areas in the pharmacy will require the following considerations:
	  • All access doors (either to room or refrigerators) should be lockable.
	  • Temperature monitoring system installed and connected to a centralized alarm/warning system.

24.4 Summary

The primary mission of a hospital pharmacy is to manage the use of medications in hospitals and other medical centres. Goals include the selection, prescription, procuration, delivery, administration, and review of medications to optimize patient outcomes. It is important to ensure that the right patient, dose, route of administration, time, drug, information, and documentation are respected when any medication is used.

25 CENTRAL STERILE SUPPLY DEPARTMENT (CSSD)

The Sterile Supply Unit's role is to clean, decontaminate, and store reusable equipment and medical devices to ensure patient safety, compliance, efficiency, and economy. Where viable, centralized units minimize duplication and facilitate effective auditing while delivering a one-way flow of items between soiled and clean areas. Service planning models will determine the size of each department. Where a full service is unavailable, external suppliers will be relied upon to maintain stock levels.

25.1 CSSD and Wider Hospital Context: Location & Access

To minimize the distance for transportation and to save time, CSSD should be located as near the main user areas as possible such as operating theatres, intensive care areas, etc. Therefore, CSSD should be on the same floor or the floor immediately above or below. While planning the location, a supply location, such as a linen store, laundry, and general store, can be planned in the vicinity of CSSD.

25.2 Operational Models

The size and role of the sterile goods supply service should be clearly defined in the operational policy statement. Operational policies will be drafted on a project-specific basis by users and staff of the Sterile Supply Unit, the Operating Unit, and all other relevant staff associated with this service. If the service model permits, a 24-hour service is desirable.

25.3 Size of the Unit

The size of the SSU will be depend on

- The number of operating rooms, procedure rooms, and clinical areas.
- The clinical specialties of surgery performed, for example, orthopaedic surgery or microsurgery.
- The projected workload according to the operating caseload and the specialty types.
- The amount of sterile stock storage required within the unit or decentralized to clinical units.
- The amount of commercially supplied pre-sterilized stock in use.
- The provision of outsourced supplies of linen required for processing.
- The number and type of cleaning/decontamination equipment, sterilizers, and dryers, either single-sided or pass-through models.
- The ability to share areas such as changing rooms and staff rooms with an adjacent Operating Unit.

These aspects will be determined by the hospital's service plan and operational policies.

25.4 Process Flow in CSSD

The process flow in CSSD is shown in Figure 25A.

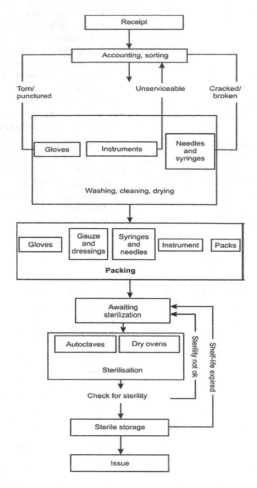

FIGURE 25A Process Flow in CSSD (CSSD; http://mainai-sakyuhoon.blogspot.com/2015/07/central-sterile-supply-department-cssd.html).

TABLE 25A: Key Result Areas and Quality Indicators for CSSD

Key Result Areas

Equipment cleaning, disinfection, and sterilization practices
- Space and zoning for sterilization activities
- Layout—unidirectional flow and segregation of areas
- Documented policies and procedures on cleaning, packing, disinfection, and/or sterilization, storing, and issue of items
- Reprocessing of instruments and equipment through policies and procedures
- Shelf life of sets
- Regular validation testing for sterilization carried out and documented
- Recall procedure when breakdown in sterilization system
- ETO chimney
- Re-use of medical devices policy
- Qualified and trained personnel operate and maintain equipment
- Operational and maintenance (preventive and breakdown) plan of equipment
- Procedure for equipment replacement and disposal

DOI: 10.1201/9780367460884-26

25.5 Internal and External Functional Relationships

General: Design solutions must ensure the separation of clean and dirty products, avoiding routes and cross-flows that potentially could re-contaminate processed items or adversely affect the microbiology of raw materials. There must be a unidirectional workflow from contaminated to clean and sterile areas. Adequate circulating space to accommodate trolleys and containers demanded by the departmental workload is required to ensure effective demarcation of clean and dirty areas (Table 25B).

TABLE 25B: Functional Relationships of CSSD

Internal Functional Relationships	External Functional Relationships
A unidirectional flow for instrument processing from contaminated or dirty areas to clean and sterile areas is critical to the functioning of the unit.	The Sterile Supply Unit (SSU) should be located with direct or close access to the Operating Unit and Day Surgery Units. This may be achieved with the use of lifts.

Internal Functional Relationships

The following represents the correct relationships in the processing from dirty to clean:

- Goods arrive from clinical areas to the cleaning/decontamination area (dirty) via lifts or service corridors to a holding area.
- Trolleys and instruments are processed through the cleaning/decontamination area and trolley wash and move to the sorting/packing area—a clean zone.
- There is a separation between dirty and clean areas with controlled entries and no back-flow; airlocks may be required to maintain the air pressurization of the separate zones.
- Goods then flow from clean packing areas to the sterile areas and are then delivered to clinical units.
- Incoming clean goods are taken directly to a neutral or clean zone including non-sterile supplies and loan equipment.
- There is a separate entry for staff who can enter clean areas only through a controlled entry.
- Staff leaving the dirty zone re-enter via changing rooms.

External Functional Relationships

The SSU should have ready access to

- Service units of the hospital including the Supply Unit, Linen Handling Unit, and loading dock for delivery of supplies.
- Hospital units requiring return and delivery of sterilized items including Critical Care Units and Inpatient Units.
- Access to the SSU should be restricted to authorized personnel only.

TABLE 25C: Major Space Determinants and CSSD Size

S No.	FACILITY	CATEGORY A		CATEGORY B		CATEGORY C		CATEGORY D		CATEGORY E	
		ROOM (NO.)	Area (m²)	ROOM (NO.)	Area (m²)	ROOM (NO.)	Area (m²)	ROOM (NO.)	Area (m²)	ROOM (NO.)	Area (m²)
(1)	(2)	(3)	(4)	(5)	(6)	(7)	(8)	(9)	(10)	(11)	(12)
GENERAL											
(a)	Bulk storage	—		—		1	10.5	3	14	3	17.5
(b)	Officer-in-charge with toilet	—		—		1	17.5	1	21	1	17.5
(c)	Technician room with toilet	—		—		—		1	14	1	17.5
(d)	Receipt counter							1	10.5	1	10.5
(e)	Dissembling and decontamination			1	28	1	28	1	14	1	10.5
(f)	Washing and cleaning	1	21					1	14	1	10.5
(g)	Assembly and set packing room							1	21	1	28
(h)	Gloves preparation room and gauze cutting area					1	21	1	14	1	17.5
(i)	Autoclave area	1	14	1	17.5	1	21	1	28	1	28
(j)	Hot air oven room	—		1	7.0	1	10.5	1	10.5	1	10.5
(k)	Sterile store	1	14	1	17.5	1	28	1	28	1	35
(l)	Issue counter							1	10.5	1	17.5
(m)	Class IV room	—		—		1	10.5	1	10.5	1	10.5
(n)	Trolley bay	—		—		1	10.5	1	10.5	1	10.5
(o)	Switch room	—		—		1	7.0	1	7.0	1	10.5

Layout & Zoning (Figure 25B)

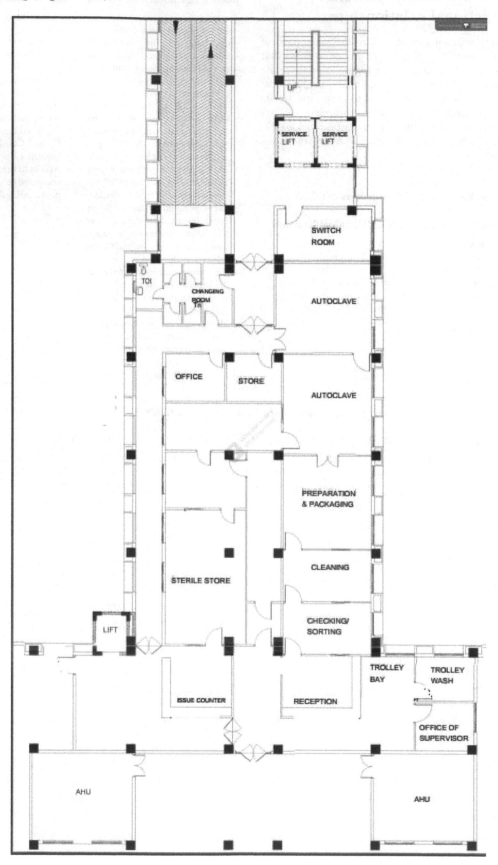

FIGURE 25B   Sample Layout of CSSD.

Built Environment: General Considerations

TABLE 25D: General Considerations for Built Environment in CSSD

Acoustics	• Provide acoustic treatment for noise-generating equipment including washer/decontaminators, sterilizers, and dryers located in cleaning/decontamination and sterilizing areas.
Natural Light/Lighting	• Natural lighting aids visual inspection and has positive morale on staff. Where natural lighting is not possible, glazed panels should be considered. • Task lighting, including magnification inspection lights, is desirable for instrument inspection. • Light levels should not be less than 400 lux on the working surface.
Ergonomics	• Benches, sinks, and packing workstations should be provided as suitable working heights. • Adjustable-height equipment is recommended.
Safety and Security	• Controlled access should discourage unauthorized entry and isolate the area from general hospital traffic.
Finishes	• All finishes should withstand frequent cleaning and be tolerant of surface cleaning agents.
Floors	Floor finishes should be hard-wearing, non-slip, easy to clean, of a uniform level, and suitable for heavy trolley traffic. Flooring should have integrated coved skirting continuous with the floor. Floor scrubbing equipment is not appropriate for SSUs.
Walls	Hollow wall constructions are vulnerable to trolley damage and risk of pest infestation. Solid, rendered, and smooth walls, either epoxy-coated or spray-painted, withstand heavy treatment and allow ease of repair.
Ceilings	Ceilings should prohibit the ingress of airborne particles or contaminants and be resistant to humidity. Ceiling should be flush, sealed against walls, and easily cleaned.
Fixtures, Fittings and Equipment	• Shelving systems installed should be constructed of non-porous materials, dust-resistant, and easily cleaned and avoid inaccessible corners.
Communications	• Management information systems (MIS) require adequate data points and electrical points for the tracking and tracing of products and quality assurance records passing through the decontamination process including wet areas, packing areas, and sterilizing areas.
Heating, Ventilation and Air Conditioning	• The SSU is a controlled environment, and ventilation should be provided by a treated air supply, with compliant air conditioning systems and HEPA filters. • Positive air pressure differential should be maintained above that of the surrounding areas in clean and sterile zones. • Negative pressure should be maintained in cleaning/decontamination areas. Indicators and alarms systems to alert staff of ventilation system failure should be provided. • Humidification will be required to avoid dehydration and subsequent processing problems associated with absorbent materials. • Washers, disinfectors, and sterilizers emit considerable heat and humidity affecting electronic controls. • Fully insulated pipework and machinery backed up by extract ventilation are essential to ensure tolerable working conditions, conserve energy, and minimize operating costs. • Heat recovery from ventilation systems should be incorporated where appropriate.
Infection Control	Handwashing facilities should be provided at the following locations: • Entry and exit of cleaning/decontamination areas. • Entry/exit of clean and sterile areas. • Hand basins should be located to avoid water splashing on clean and sterile goods.
Disaster Planning	• The SSU should be capable of continued operation during and after a natural disaster, except in instances where a facility sustains primary impact.

TABLE 25E: Specific Room and Functional Requirements for CSSD

Receiving Area	• The trolley holding area is a lobby or holding space provided for the return of used items and trolleys awaiting stripping and cleaning.
	• Trolley holding should be located with ready access to the trolley wash, decontamination, and disposal rooms.
	• The receiving area is a wet area and will include a trolley dismantling area where trolleys are stripped. Dirty linen and waste are dispatched to the disposal room.
	• Used instruments are delivered to cleaning/decontamination area.
	• The receiving area will require
	  • Benches and sinks with parking space for trolleys
	  • Hot and cold water outlets to sinks
	  • Smooth, impervious, and easily cleanable surfaces on walls and ceiling
	  • Impervious and wet area non-slip finishes on the floor
	• Staff handwashing basin.

(Continued)

TABLE 25E: (Continued)

Decontamination Area
- The decontamination area is a wet area where used instruments are sorted and processed.
- In the cleaning/decontamination area, instruments are rinsed, ultrasonically cleaned if appropriate, washed/ decontaminated through instrument processing equipment, and dried.
- Special instruments may be handwashed in this area. Instruments may be tracked by using an instrument tracking system.
- The cleaning/decontamination area should contain benches for instrument sorting and sinks and mechanical equipment for cleaning and decontamination of reusable surgical equipment.
- The decontamination area should be located between the receiving area and the sorting/packing area.
- Convenient access to a disposal room for the disposal of used/soiled material will be required.
- The area must include handwashing facilities.
- A trolley/cart washing area will be required for washing and disinfecting trolleys and carts prior to re-loading carts with clean and sterilized equipment for return.
- Automated trolley washing equipment can be installed in larger units.

- The decontamination area will require the following finishes:
  - Walls and ceiling that are smooth, impervious, and easily cleanable.
  - Impervious and wet area non-slip finishes to the floor.
  - Fittings, fixtures, and equipment located in this area will include the following:
- Stainless steel benches and deep bowl sinks with air and suction outlets for tube cleaning and additional water outlets for water pistols.
- Instrument and tubing washers/decontaminators, according to service requirements; these may be single sided, pass-through, or index tunnel washers.
- Ultrasonic cleaner, built-in, with consideration for the working height of instrument baskets.
- Instrument and tubing dryers, as required by the service plan.
- Staff handwashing basin.
- Exhaust air extraction will be required over sinks and heat/moisture-generating equipment.
- The trolley washing area will require hot and cold water outlets for manual washing.
- An automated trolley wash unit can be used.

Endoscope Processing
- Endoscopes, both flexible and non-flexible, undergo a process of disinfection by using chemical cleaning agents through manual washing or automated reprocessing machines.
- The process requires large sinks and tanks of disinfecting solution or automated machines. Instruments are leak tested, then manually pre-cleaned in an enzyme solution, followed by high-level disinfection with an approved disinfectant solution in a fume cabinet or enclosed automated machine.
- Compressed filtered air is required for the drying process. An ultrasonic machine is required for cleaning of accessory instruments.
- Endoscope processing machines require services including electrical and mechanical ventilation and hydraulics services with filtered water supply and drainage.
- Disinfected endoscopes are stored in endoscope cabinets that are HEPA-filtered and ventilated.

Sorting and Packing
- The sorting/packing area is a clean room where cleaned and dried instruments are removed from the decontaminating/drying equipment, sorted, assembled into sets, and packaged, ready for sterilizing.
- Instruments in this area may be tracked by using an instrument tracking system.
- The sorting/packing area will be located between the cleaning/decontamination area and the sterilizing area, with a unidirectional workflow from contaminated to clean areas.

- The sorting/packing area will require the following finishes:
  - Walls and ceiling that are smooth, impervious, and easily cleanable.
  - Impervious, non-slip finishes to the floor.
- Requirements in this area will include the following:
  - Packing tables complete with wrapping materials and tracking systems that are ergonomically designed to avoid staff fatigue; adjustable-height stations are recommended.
  - Sealing equipment.
  - Trolleys for holding wrapped sets ready for sterilizing.
  - Staff handwashing basin at the entry/exit, located to avoid water splashing on clean, wrapped sets.
  - Positive pressure HEPA-filtered air conditioning with filtration for lint.

Sterilizing and Cooling
- This is a sterile area and includes high and low temperature sterilizers with space for loading/unloading and a cooling area for packed trolleys removed from sterilizers.
- Sterilizing/cooling is located between sorting/packing and sterile stock stores with a one-way flow.
- The sterilizing/cooling area will require the following finishes:
  - Walls and ceiling that are smooth, impervious, and easily cleanable.
  - Impervious, non-slip finishes to the floor.
- High-temperature sterilizers may be single-sided or pass-through. Sterilizer plant equipment should ideally have external access for maintenance to avoid access to the unit.
- A workstation can be located in this area for quality assurance documentation and instrument tracking.
- The air handling requirements of this area include
  - Positive pressure with HEPA filtration
  - Efficient exhaust for heat/steam generating equipment
  - Filtration for lint

(Continued)

TABLE 25E: (Continued)

Dispatch	• The dispatch area will coordinate the distribution of sterile stock to the required hospital units. It will include a counter or desk and trolley holding space for packed trolleys awaiting delivery. • The dispatch area will require external access for hospital units to collect urgent stock with restricted access to the internal departmental areas. • An after-hours cupboard may be provided in this area for staff to collect urgent supplies, preferably a pass-through cabinet with internal access for re-stocking.
Support Areas	• Support areas include cleaner rooms, disposal rooms, and storerooms for chemicals and sterile stock. • Cleaners' rooms should be provided separately in clean and dirty areas of the unit. • The disposal room should be located with access to an external corridor for ease of waste removal, without accessing the unit.
Administrative and Staff Areas	• Changing areas for staff will include toilets, showers, hand basins, and lockers with facilities for clean linen holding.

25.6 Summary

Planning and designing the CSSD in a hospital is a critical process that ensures the safe and efficient management of medical instruments, equipment, and supplies. The CSSD plays a vital role in infection control, sterilization processes, and maintaining the overall cleanliness and hygiene of the health care facility. Key considerations in the planning and designing process include appropriate space allocation, an efficient workflow design, incorporation of state-of-the-art sterilization technologies, adherence to regulatory guidelines and standards, proper storage and distribution systems, and staff training on sterilization protocols. By prioritizing these factors and engaging experts in CSSD design, hospitals can establish a well-designed department that facilitates effective sterilization practices, reduces the risk of infections, and enhances patient safety.

26 MEDICAL GAS PIPELINE SYSTEM

26.1 Introduction

A medical gas pipeline system (MGPS) is installed to provide a safe, convenient, and cost-effective system for the provision of medical gases to the clinical and nursing staff at the point of use (Figure 26A). It reduces the problems associated with the use of gas cylinders such as safety, porterage, storage, and noise. In most hospitals, MGPS is used for the supply of

- Oxygen
- Medical air (4 Bar)
- Surgical air (7 Bar)
- Nitrous oxide
- Carbon dioxide
- Vacuum/suction
- Anaesthetic gas scavenging system
- Heliox (helium + oxygen)
- Nitrogen
- Entonox (nitrous oxide + oxygen) (Refer to Tables 26K and 26L for details)

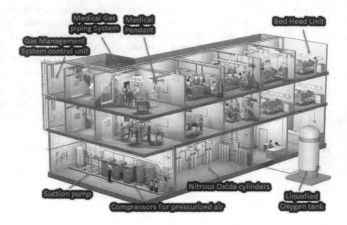

FIGURE 26A Medical Gas Pipeline System (Courtesy: CPWD).

TABLE 26A: Gas Cylinder Manifold System

Primary Supply	Secondary Supply	Reserve Supply
Fully automatic manifold. Number of cylinders based on system design.	• Manual emergency reserve manifold. • To come online automatically via a nonreturn valve. • Number of cylinders based on ability to provide 4 hours of supply at average use.	Automatic/manual manifold supplying via non-interchangeable screw thread (NIST) connectors or locally based integral valved cylinders with regulators/flowmeters attached.

TABLE 26B: Vacuum Insulated Evaporator (VIE) System

Primary Supply	Secondary Supply	Reserve Supply
Simplex VIE vessel system	Automatic manifold system. To come online in the event of plant failure.	Automatic manifold system. May be sited to support high-dependency areas or whole site or Locally based integral valved cylinders with regulators/flowmeters attached.
One vessel of a duplex VIE vessel system (on same plinth).	Second vessel of a duplex VIE system.	Automatic manifold system. May be sited to support high-dependency areas or whole site.
One vessel of a duplex VIE vessel system (on separate plinths).	Second vessel of a duplex VIE system (on separate plinths). (NB: Split-site systems are intended primarily for systems where the risk assessment has identified that the site for the primary supply is limited in size or presents too high of a risk by having both tanks at the same site. These supply systems should be fitted with appropriate non-return valve connections to prevent gas loss in the event of one tank/system failing.)	Type and capacity of supply to be determined by risk assessment. May not be required when a ring main or other dual supply to a pipeline distribution system is provided.

TABLE 26C: Liquid Oxygen Cylinder System

Primary Supply	Secondary Supply	Reserve Supply
Liquid cylinder manifold system. (NB: This is NOT a change over manifold. All cylinders are online simultaneously.)	Automatic manifold system. To come online in the event of plant failure.	Automatic manifold system. May be sited to support high-dependency areas or whole site or Locally based integral valved cylinders with regulators/flowmeters attached.

TABLE 26D: Oxygen Generation Plant (PSA Plant)

Primary Supply	Secondary Supply	Reserve Supply
Multiplex compressors and columns (adsorbers). Subject to design	Automatic manifold system. To come online in the event of plant failure. May be fitted with third-party cylinders or filled from compressor of main plant. Number of cylinders based on ability to provide 4 hours of supply at average use. Locally filled cylinders or gas suppliers' cylinders can be used.	Type and capacity of supply to be determined by risk assessment.

Recommendation: The secondary supply should be filled from the primary supply. This will provide an indication to the hospital operator when the primary supply fails and ensures that the secondary supply serving the health care departments is always filled.

DOI: 10.1201/9780367460884-27

TABLE 26E: Medical Air Supply

Primary Supply	Secondary Supply	Reserve Supply
Duplex compressor system.	Automatic manifold system. To come online automatically in the event of plant failure. Number of cylinders based on ability to provide 4 hours of supply at average use.	Automatic manifold system. May be sited to support high-dependency areas or whole site or Locally based integral valved cylinders with regulators/flowmeters attached.
Two compressors of a triplex compressor system.	Third compressor of a triplex system.	Automatic manifold system. To support whole site.
Two compressors of a quadruplex system.	Other two compressors of a quadruplex system.	Automatic manifold system. To support whole site.

TABLE 26F: Liquid Gas Mixer (Oxygen + Nitrous Oxide) Plant

Primary Supply	Secondary Supply	Reserve Supply
Primary oxygen and nitrogen VIE vessels and mixer unit.	Secondary oxygen and nitrogen VIE vessels and mixer unit.	Type and capacity of supply to be determined by risk assessment.

Recommendation: For the primary and secondary units, depending on the specialty and size of the facility, a cylinder system may be sufficient, but this will need to be confirmed by a risk assessment.

TABLE 26G: Combined Medical and Surgical Air Plant

Primary Supply	Secondary Supply	Reserve Supply
Duplex compressor system.	Two automatic manifold systems: • One dedicated to support medical air (MA) system • One dedicated to support surgical air (SA) system To come online automatically in the event of plant failure. Number of cylinders based on ability to provide 4 hours of supply at average use.	Automatic manifold system. May be sited to support high-dependency areas or whole site or Locally based integral valved cylinders with regulators/flowmeters attached.
Two compressors of a triplex compressor system.	Third compressor of a triplex system.	Automatic manifold system. To support whole site.
Two compressors of a quadruplex system.	Other two compressors of a quadruplex system.	Automatic manifold system. To support whole site.

Recommendation: Each compressor/pump is sized to cope with half the system design flow.

TABLE 26H: Surgical Air Supply

Primary Supply	Secondary Supply	Reserve Supply
Simplex compressor system.	Automatic manifold system. To come online automatically in the event of plant failure. Number of cylinders based on ability to provide 4 hours of supply at average use.	Locally based integral valved cylinders with regulators/flowmeters attached.
One compressor of a duplex compressor system.	Second compressor of a duplex compressor system.	Automatic manifold system.

TABLE 26I: Central Medical Vacuum System

Primary Supply	Secondary Supply	Reserve Supply
Two compressors of a triplex pump system.	Third pump of a triplex system.	Portable suction equipment.
Two pumps of a quadruplex system.	Other two pumps of a quadruplex system.	Portable suction equipment.

Recommendation: Each compressor/pump is sized to cope with half the system design flow.

Important Note: In the event of power failure, cylinder- or medical gas-system-powered vacuum generators can be used, but the use of venturi-type vacuum generators is recommended only for emergency use, as these units are generally driven from the medical oxygen system and use large amounts of gas. This can lead to oxygen enrichment, present a potential fire hazard, and may result in the emission of pathological material.

TABLE 26J: Anaesthetic Gas Scavenging System (AGSS)

Primary Exhaust	Reserve Exhaust
Simplex compressor system.	Simplex compressor system or manual change over.
One compressor of a duplex system.	Second compressor of a duplex system.

For operating theatres and other critical clinical spaces (Grade A), the number of AGSS plant depends on the number of Air Handling Units to these areas. For example, for each operating theatre having its own dedicated Air Handling Unit, a Simplex AGSS plant should then be provided for each operating theatre. The reserve provision should be a Simplex AGSS unit that can serve up to 6 No. Areas. If there are 12 areas, then 2 No. Simplex units should be spare if all 12 areas are being served by 12 No. Simplex AGSS Units.

Important Note: For operating theatres and other critical clinical spaces (Grade A), where more than two areas are being served by a single Air Handling Unit, then a Duplex AGSS plant is to be provided with an automatic change over to the spare pump.

TABLE 26K: Quality of Medical Gases

Gas & Source	Oil	Water	CO (Carbon Monoxide)	CO$_2$ (Carbon Dioxide)	NO (Nitric Oxide) & No$_2$ (Nitrogen Oxide)	SO$_2$ (Sulphur Dioxide)	Odour/ Taste
Oxygen from Bulk Liquid Storage	–	≤67 vpm ≤0.05 mg/L, atmosphere dewpoint of –46°C)	≤ 5 mg/m^3, ≤ ppm v/v	≤ 300 ppm v/v	–	–	None
Oxygen from PSA Plant (Oxygen Generation)	0.1 mg/m^3	≤67 vpm ≤0.05 mg/L, atmosphere dewpoint of –46°C)	≤ 5 mg/m^3, ≤ ppm v/v	≤ 300 ppm v/v	≤ 2 ppm v/v	&	None
Nitrous Oxide	–	≤67 vpm ≤0.05 mg/L, atmosphere dewpoint of –46°C)	≤ 5 mg/m^3, ≤ ppm v/v	≤ 300 ppm v/v	≤ 2 ppm v/v		N/A
Nitrous Oxide/Oxygen Mixture	–	≤67 vpm ≤0.05 mg/L, atmosphere dewpoint of –46°C)	≤ 5 mg/m^3, ≤ ppm v/v	≤ 300 ppm v/v	≤ 2 ppm v/v		N/A
Medical & Surgical Air	0.1 mg/m^3	≤67 vpm ≤0.05 mg/L, atmosphere dewpoint of –46°C)	≤ 5 mg/m^3, ≤ ppm v/v	≤900 mg/m^3 ≤500 ppm v/v	≤ 2 ppm v/v		None
Synthetic Air	–	≤67 vpm ≤0.05 mg/L, atmosphere dewpoint of –46°C)	–	–	–	–	None
Helium/Oxygen O$_2$< 30%		≤67 vpm ≤0.05 mg/L, atmosphere dewpoint of –46°C)	≤ 5 mg/m^3, ≤ ppm v/v	≤ 300 ppm v/v	≤ 2 ppm v/v	–	None

Table 26L: Safety Distance Compliance for Medical Gas Plant

Safety Distances from Exposure to Vessel/Point Where Oxygen Leakage or Spillage Can Occur	Up to 20 Tons (Distance in m)	Over 20 Tons (Distance in m)
Areas where open flames/smoking are permitted	5	8
Places of public assembly	10	15
Offices, canteens, and areas of occupancy	5	8
Pits, ducts, surface water drains (un-trapped)	5	8
Openings to underground systems	5	8
Building footprint	5	8
Public roads	5	8
Railways	10	15
Vehicle parking areas (other than authorized)	5	8
Large wooden structures	15	15
Small stocks of combustible materials, site huts, etc.	5	8
Process equipment (not part of installation)	5	8
Continuous sections of flammable gas pipelines	3	3
Flanges in flammable gas pipelines (over 50 mm)	15	15
Fuel gas vent pipes	5	8
Compressor/ventilator air intakes	5	8
Fuel gas cylinders (up to 70 m^3)	5	5
LPG storage vessels (up to 4 tons)	7.5	7.5
LPG storage vessels (up to 60 tons)	15	15
Bulk flammable liquid storage vessels (up to 7.8 m^3)	7.5	7.5
Bulk flammable liquid storage vessels (up to 117 m^3)	15	15
MV or HV electrical substation	5	8

26.2 Medical Gas Pipeline System and Wider Hospital Context: Location & Access

The manifold should be in a dedicated room on an outside wall near a loading dock and have adequate ventilation and service convenience. The cylinder gas/liquid supply systems should not be in the same room as medical air compressors and vacuum plant. Access to the manifold room should be from the open air, not from corridors or other rooms. Normal commercial lorry access for cylinder delivery vehicles should be ensured. Provision of a raised level loading bay to reduce cylinder handling hazards is recommended.

26.3 Medical Gas Pipeline System: Sources of Supply

Medical gas services within the medical system in a health care facility operate based on a redundancy and resiliency provision of the service to ensure patient safety and maintain the operation of the health care facilities. All medical gas supplies should come from three sources of supply identified as "primary", "secondary", and "reserve", although the latter is more commonly referred to as the third means of supply. Tables 26A through 26J describe the various options for gas supply. For each, the primary, secondary, and reserve sources are identified.

TABLE 26M: General, Specific, and Functional Requirements for Medical Gas Pipeline Systems

Design Criteria	• Safe and effective method of delivering quality medical gas service to the terminals. • Some areas will require gas scavenging disposal systems to control the exposure to nitrous oxide. • Medical gas service should not be provided for non-clinical areas such as workshops (except for biomedical workshops) and pathology departments. These areas shall be provided by 11 Bar compressed air. • The purity of the medical gases should be as the European pharmacopoeia requirements table as shown in Table 26K. • Particulate level tests are to be provided with medical gas purity requirements. • To maintain the sterile services of the medical gas service throughout the health care facility, the quality in terms of particulate content, dryness, and concentration of impurities should comply with the requirements for maximum concentrations given in Table 26K. • Bacteria filters are to be included in medical and surgical compressor systems to reduce the risk of delivering spores of infectious material to vulnerable patients. • The medical gas service connected to the bacteria filter must be a dry service. This is to ensure that any microorganisms are prevented from bypassing the bacteria filter. • Microorganisms can penetrate a bacteria filter if the material is wet. The filter is to be checked every 12 weeks of hospital operation. • Medical gas purity tests are to be checked by the health care operator every 6 months for new builds and refurbished/retrofit facilities.
Basic Sizing of Medical Gas Cylinder Sources	The sizing of the cylinders and major systems such as a VIE system will need to be carried out via risk assessment based on the following parameters: • Health care operating hours. • Distance from supplier. • Traffic data. • Supplier operating hours. • Supplier response time in peak working hours of the day. • Supplier response time in slow night operating hours. • Cylinder delivery and re-stocking history (if known).
Manifold Room (Figure 26B)	• The manifold room must be located on the ground floor. • The medical gas compressors and vacuum can be located in the basement of a facility, provided that the area is ventilated. • In hot climates, the medical gas plant rooms (including the cylinder rooms) need to be air conditioned to provide an air temperature of less than 40°C. • Medical gas cylinder storerooms should be well-ventilated, and cylinders of these gases (especially mixture gases) should be kept above 10°C for 24 hours before use; arrangements should be in place to ensure that cylinders collected from a cold store are not used immediately for patient treatment. • Medical gas cylinders should not be subjected to extremes temperature. Cylinders should be kept away from sources of heat (this includes hot water service pipes, steam pipes, hot air emitters, and direct sun exposure). • No other chemicals, flammable material, or rubbish should be stored within the medical gas plant room. • All cylinders should stand vertically even during storage. • Cylinders should be chained during use and standby. • Each port should be connected to a cylinder by flexible pigtail connections, a header bar, and an outlet port. • Safety distance compliance of medical gas plants is given in Table 26L.
Pipeline Details	
Pipeline Nomenclature (Figure 26C)	• **Main hospital supply pipeline or gas service-specific trunk pipeline**: From manifold to building. • **Feeder pipeline**: Horizontal and vertical up to the distribution pipeline. It also includes risers. • **Distribution pipeline or branch pipeline**: Serves one floor or a part of a floor. • **Drop pipe**: Distribution to terminal units.

(Continued)

TABLE 26M: (Continued)

Pipeline Material (Figure 26D)	• Medical grade copper, which is phosphorus de-oxidized non-arsenical copper conforming to BS EN 1412:1996 grade CW024A (CuDHP), should be used for pipeline. • The material should be seamless, round, and solid drawn with sizes conforming to BS EN 13348. • The material should be suitable for installing vertically or horizontally without sagging or distortion. • The material temper shall be 　• For tailpipe: R220. 　• For pipe of nominal outside diameter (OD) 12 mm—54 mm: R250 (half hard). 　• For pipe of OD 76 mm and above: R290 (hard).
Pipeline Installation	• All tubing, valves, and fittings should be thoroughly checked for any grease, oil, or combustible material prior to installation. • During the brazing of pipe connections, the interior of the pipe should be purged continuously with nitrogen. • Flux-less silver brazing alloy should be used (Silver Copper—Phosphorus Brazing Alloy CP 104 conforming to BS EN 1044:1999). • Soft solder or 50/50 solder must NEVER be used on a medical gas system. • MGPS pipeline must be adequately supported at appropriate intervals as per the details given as follows:

Outside Diameter (mm)	Maximum Intervals for Vertical Runs (m)	Maximum Intervals for Horizontal Runs
12	1.2	1.0
15	1.8	1.2
22-28	2.4	1.8
35-42	3.0	2.4
>54	3.0	2.7

	• Where pipes pass through walls, partitions, or floors, they should be fitted with sleeves of copper pipes.
Pipeline Jointing Validation	• Before the wall outlets are installed, the pipes should be blown free of any particulate. • Pressure testing. • Locating leaks. • Cross connection testing.
Pipeline Sizing	• Determined either by the volume of gas to be delivered or by the impact of overall pressure required. • When sizing for medical vacuum with pipes of one size, a higher diameter must be provided to prevent clogging. • No pipe smaller than 12 mm OD should be used anywhere in MGPS installation. • No pipe smaller than 15 mm OD should be used anywhere in the surgical suite including ORs and pre-op and post-op rooms. • No pipe smaller than 15 mm OD should be used anywhere in the installation for medical vacuum.
Pipeline Specifications	• Pipeline specifications as mandated by BS EN 13348 are given in the following.
Colour Coding of Pipelines	• Ground colours are applied throughout the length of pipeline. • Colour bands are applied at 　• Intersection points and change of direction points. 　• Midway of each piping way near valves. 　• For long stretch of piping at 50-m intervals. 　• At start and terminating points of the pipeline. • Details of the colour coding of a MGPS pipeline is given as follows:

Gas	Ground Colour	Colour Band
Oxygen	Canary Yellow	White
Nitrous Oxide	Canary Yellow	French Blue
Compressed Air	Sky Blue	White & Black
Vacuum	Sky Blue	Black
Carbon Dioxide	Yellow	Grey
Helium & Oxygen Mixture	Canary Yellow	White & Light Brown
Nitrogen	Canary Yellow	Black
Carbon Dioxide & Oxygen Mixture	Canary Yellow	White & Light Grey

Valves, AVSU, Terminal Units, NIST & Bed Head Panels

Valves (Figure 26E)	• All valves should be of a lever ball type with flanged O-ring seal connections. • Valves should open and close with 90-degree rotation. • The handle should be in line with the pipeline when open. • All valves should be in the open position in a commissioned MGPS system. • **Main Line Valve:** Should be provided at the outlet of the supply source and must always be accessible to authorized personnel. • **Branch Valve Including Riser Valve:** Should be provided at the base of risers and every major branch and should be placed in a secured location. • **Line Valve Assembly:** Should be provided at the entry and exit of each defined section. • **Zone Valves:** Should be provided at each fire zone. It should be accessible to floor staff and fire staff. It should be marked in the floor evacuation plan.

(Continued)

TABLE 26M: (Continued)

Area Valve Service Units (AVSU) (Figure 26F)	• The AVSU must be located by a nurse station that is continuously occupied during the health care facility operating hours. • The panel is to be a combined panel with valves and an alarm panel. This is not a separate alarm panel in one location and service isolation valve in another. • The installation height requirements of the panel for health care facilities should be approximately 1,000–1,800 mm. This height is based on the comfortable average heights for nurses so that it is easy to operate. • The panel needs to be provided with access requirements to operate the valves if need be. • Access to the panel must be provided via a dedicated key or a break glass hammer. These should be provided only to hospital operational staff (nurses, doctors, and maintenance staff). • The minimum height for AVSU installation should be 1 m for dual circuits. • Dual circuits should be arranged (in two columns) only if the height from the top to bottom of the unit exceeds 1 m. • To avoid using an excessive number of panels, this can be increased to 1.2 m. • The panels located on a wall will need to ensure that there is a minimum clearance of 100 mm behind the unit for the medical gas pipework (175 mm for back-to-back pipes serving the AVSU). • The panels are to be labelled with permanent naming templates and not adhesive labels. • A key is to be provided at the fire command centre for civil defence access.
Terminal Units (Figure 26G)	• The terminal units should be leak-proof and allow the plugging of probes from the front by using a push to insert and press to release mechanism. • The terminal units should have a self-sealing valve upon disengaging the probe, a non-return valve for ease of line servicing, and colour coded gas specific front plate.
Non-Interchangeable Screw Thread Connector (NIST) (Figure 26H)	• It is a gas-specific connector used as a termination for flexible hoses and copper pipe in MGPS. • The dimensions of the male part of the connector, not the outer screw threaded fastening ring, make it gas-specific for the safety prevention of an incorrect connector to the terminal.

Bed Head Panels (Figure 26I)	• These are provided for dispensing gases in wards and patient care areas.
	• Bed head panels also house the following:
	  • Nurse call system.
	  • Flowmeters.
	  • Reading lights.

Ward/Theatre Vacuum Terminal Unit	• Vacuum terminal units are equipped with a regulator for switching on and off the during use. • The bottle is available in sizes ranging from 250 ml to 2 L. • A suction catheter is connected to the ward vacuum unit.

MGPS Fixtures and Fittings (Figures 26B–26I)

Line ball valve assemblies are designed to provide local isolation of individual parts of the central gas and vacuum piping system in hospitals, clinics, laboratory facilities, or anywhere there is piped medical gas. The area valve service unit modules create an independent zone within the gas pipeline system, which can offer up to six different gases. AVSU modules are pre-assembled wall mounted zone units with an optional alarm, pressure switches, and pipe work. The copper tubes and fittings are pipeline solutions for medical installations.

BS EN 13348 degreased medical grade seamless copper tubes are specifically designed for medical gas and vacuum systems, recognizing the special requirements of the medical gas market. A central alarm panel is designed to monitor the status of up to six medical gas source equipment. The alarm panel comes with easy installation, carefree maintenance, security from unauthorized personnel access, and anti-microbial additives. A 6 Local Alarm System is designed to monitor the high and low pressure downstream of any area valve service within a facility. The local alarm can provide real-time pressure monitoring for up to six medical gas services. The economically designed terminal units are manufactured to be gas-specific to prevent interchangeability between different types of gas services. The medical gas terminal units are attached permanently to the medical gas distribution pipeline system via a copper tube or semi-permanently via medical gas hose assembly.

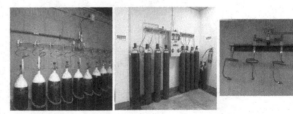

FIGURE 26B Manifold Room (Courtesy: CPWD).

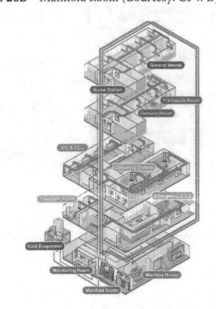

FIGURE 26C Pipeline Nomenclature (Courtesy: CPWD).

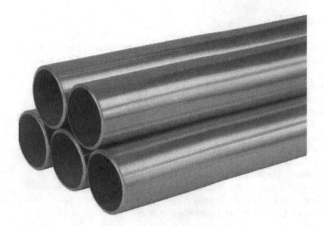

FIGURE 26D   Pipeline Material (Courtesy: CPWD).

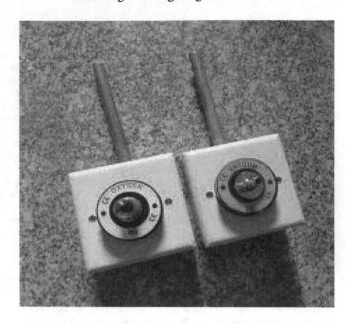

FIGURE 26G   Terminal Unit (Courtesy: CPWD).

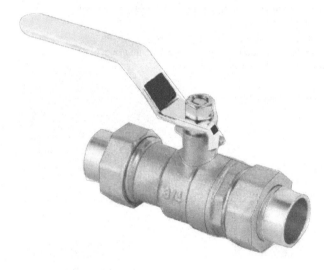

FIGURE 26E   Valve (Courtesy: CPWD).

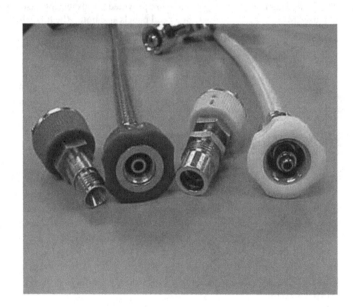

FIGURE 26H   NIST (Courtesy: CPWD).

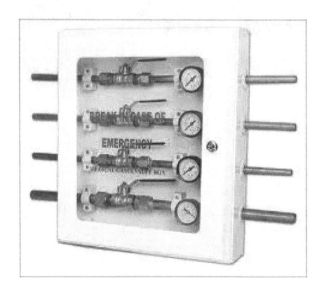

FIGURE 26F   Area Valve Service Unit (Courtesy: CPWD).

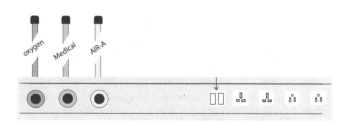

FIGURE 26I   Bed Head Panel (Courtesy: CPWD).

26.4 Summary

Gases can be used through cylinders; however, due to its widespread usage in hospitals and for the purpose of safety, a pipeline system is used for the delivery of medical gases. Each medical gas must be supplied from a separate system, and it is essential that all parts of each system are gas-specific to ensure that there is no possibility of cross-connection between any system.

- During the installation stage, extensive tests are carried out to verify that there is no cross-connection.
- A single MGPS line should not be used to supply the pathology department, dental department, general workshops, or mechanical services.

27 HOSPITAL DIETARY SERVICES

27.1 Introduction

Catering Units, in health care facilities, deliver food to a highly susceptible population who are more likely than other populations to experience foodborne disease as they may be immunocompromised, frail, medically ill, or very young. As a result, providing nutrition is challenging due to the diverse dietary needs of the population. Food must be familiar, tasty, and appealing to patients from all age groups, religious, cultural, and social backgrounds, and those nutritionally vulnerable due to illness.

27.2 Hospital Dietary Services and Wider Hospital Context: Location, Access and Operational Models

(a) Hours of Operation: The Catering Unit will generally operate on a long-day basis, providing a service between 6 am and 9 pm daily for inpatients and covering all meals during the day with preparation and storage of meals for night staff.

(b) Planning Models
   (i) **Location, Configuration:** The Catering Unit may be located on-site within the health facility or off-site, remote from the health facility.
   (ii) **On-Site Preparation:** The Catering Unit may be designed to accommodate a cook-chill or a cook-serve food preparation system.

Cook-Chill refers to the process where food (fresh or frozen) is prepared, cooked, and then chilled for up to five days. Food may be chilled in bulk or cold plated and then chilled. Plated, chilled food is then plated and served. Variations on cook-chill preparation include

- **Extended Shelf-Life Cook-Chill**, where food is processed according to the cook-chill method and stored chilled at a controlled temperature for up to 28 days.
- **Cook-Freeze**, where food is prepared, portioned, or left in bulk form and frozen for up to 12 months; following thawing, food is processed the same way as conventional cook-chill.

Cook-Serve refers to the process where food, fresh or frozen, is prepared, cooked, plated, and served immediately. Variations of the cook-serve process include

- Hot plating, delivery, and serving
- Delivery of hot bulk food, then plating and serving.

   (iii) **Off-Site Preparation:** If food is prepared off-site or in a remote location on the hospital campus, then the following will apply:
   - Briefed requirements under this section (Catering Unit) may be reduced as appropriate.
   - Protection for delivered food must be provided to ensure that it maintains freshness, retains temperature, and avoids contamination.

Workflow Process in Dietary Unit (Figure 27A)

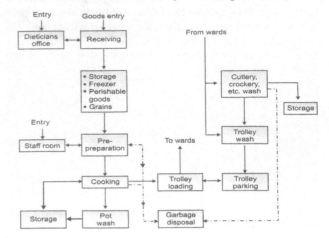

FIGURE 27A Workflow Process in Dietary Unit.

Functional Areas

TABLE 27A: Functional Areas in a Dietary Unit

a)	Entry	• Receipt area for supplies with access to the clean loading dock. • Airlock entry.
b)	Cleaning/Washing Areas	• Trolley return/stripping for returned food delivery trolleys. • Trolley/cart-washing area. • Dishwashing. • Pot washing.
c)	Food Preparation and Distribution Areas	• Separate preparation areas for food types including meat, dairy, vegetables, pastry, special diets, and special requirements such as kosher or halal foods. • Cooking facilities. • Blast chillers for cook-chill processing. • Reheating facilities and/or re-thermalization facilities if cook-chill food is processed. • Plating areas. • Cart-holding area including provision for re-thermalization of pre-plated chilled food for cook-chill service or hot/cold trolleys for fresh-cook service. • Trolley parking for food distribution trolleys.
d)	Storage Areas	• Refrigerator/s, cool rooms, and freezers of adequate size to store perishable foodstuffs. • Storage areas for dry goods. • Fruit/vegetable storage. • Storage for tableware, linen, crockery, and utensils; storage for equipment used in functions—tables and chairs. • Chemicals used in cleaning, dish, and pot washing equipment.

(Continued)

DOI: 10.1201/9780367460884-28

TABLE 27A: (Continued)

e)	Dining Areas	• Servery. • Staff dining room. • Vending machine area (optional).
f)	Staff and Support Areas	• Cleaner's room. • Disposal of waste. • Offices and workstations for manager, dieticians. • Staff changing areas with toilets, showers, and lockers. • Staff toilets in addition to changing areas depending on location of facilities.

TABLE 27B: Key Result Areas and Quality Indicators for a Dietary Unit

Key Result Areas

Food is prepared, handled, stored, and distributed safely
• Storage of raw materials especially pest control, dry storage, and cold storage
• Washing facility
• Unidirectional/non cross-over of flow of activities (clean/dirty)
• Hygiene and cleanliness
• Pest control
• Food handlers use personal protective gear
• Screening for food handlers
• License for canteen
• Any usage of domestic gas cylinders
• Electrical safety practices
• Staff awareness of safety practices
• Maintenance plan of machinery
• Fire safety awareness and firefighting equipment
• Health status of employees—immunization for typhoid and hepatitis A/stool culture and sensitivity

Quality Indicators
• Patient satisfaction with patient food services
• Number of food-related incidents and overall food safety
• Timely patient food delivery
• Patient plate waste
• Number of diets served

Internal & External Functional Relationships (Table 27C and Figure 27B)

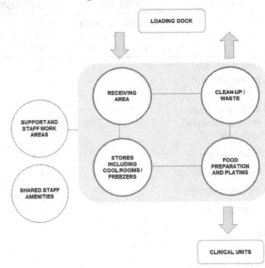

FIGURE 27B Key Internal Functional Relationships (Courtesy: Australasian Health Facility Guidelines).

TABLE 27C: Functional Relationships of a Dietary Unit

Internal Functional Relationships	External Functional Relationships
Flow of food processing from receipt to storage, preparation, cooking, plating, and delivery in one direction.	Entrance for staff and supplies from a staff/service corridor. Entry for supplies from a clean loading dock or external area through an airlock.
Separate entry for supplies and exit for removal of waste demonstrating separation of clean and dirty workflows.	Access to offices and staff areas via a service corridor.
Cooking area is located centrally to the preparation and plating areas.	Access to/from clinical units and areas requiring a catering service via a service corridor with a unidirectional traffic flow from delivery of food trolley/carts to return of soiled food trolley/carts.
Dishwashing and pot washing located conveniently to preparation, cooking, and soiled trolley return.	Access to the dirty loading dock for waste holding via a service corridor.
Support areas located at the perimeter, away from operational areas.	Entry for staff or public to a dining area via the public corridor.
Staff offices and amenities located on a perimeter in a staff-accessible zone.	

TABLE 27D: Major Space Determinants and Dietary Unit Size

S No.	FACILITY	CATEGORY A		CATEGORY B		CATEGORY C		CATEGORY D		CATEGORY E	
		ROOM (NO.)	Area (m²)	ROOM (NO.)	Area (m²)	ROOM (NO.)	Area (m²)	ROOM (NO.)	Area (m²)	ROOM (NO.)	Area (m²)
(1)	(2)	(3)	(4)	(5)	(6)	(7)	(8)	(9)	(10)	(11)	(12)
FUNCTIONAL AREAS											
(a)	Reception area			1	14	1	28	1	35	1	42
(b)	Cooking area	1	28	1	35	1	56	1	70	1	84

(Continued)

TABLE 27D: (Continued)

S No. (1)	FACILITY (2)	CATEGORY A		CATEGORY B		CATEGORY C		CATEGORY D		CATEGORY E	
		ROOM (NO.) (3)	Area (m²) (4)	ROOM (NO.) (5)	Area (m²) (6)	ROOM (NO.) (7)	Area (m²) (8)	ROOM (NO.) (9)	Area (m²) (10)	ROOM (NO.) (11)	Area (m²) (12)
(c)	Therapeutic diet preparation and cooking area			1	10.5	1	10.5	1	14	1	17.5
(d)	Dietitian with toilet stewards and staff with toilet	— —		1	14	1 1	14 14	1 1	17.5 17.5	1 1	17.5 17.5
(e)	Trolley loading	—		1	10.5	1	10.5	1	14	1	14
(f)	Walk-in cold storage	—		1	7.0	1	10.5	1	10.5	1	10.5
(g)	Dry ration storage			1	7.0	1	7.0	1	10.5	1	10.5
(h)	Washing areas a) Pots b) Trolleys c) Dishes			1	28	1	35	1 1 1	10.5 14 14	1 1 1	14 17.5 17.5
(i)	Garbage collection area			1	7.0	1	7.0	1	10.5	1	10.5
(j)	Switch room	—		—		—		1	10.5	1	10.5

Layout of Dietary Unit (Figure 27C)

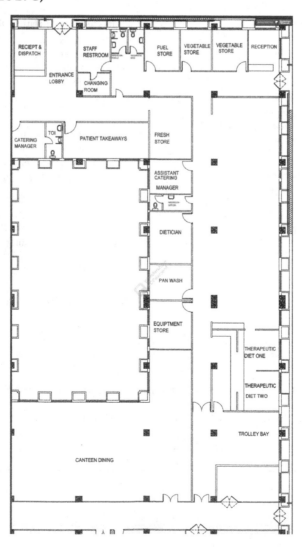

FIGURE 27C   Sample Layout of Dietary Unit.

Built Environment: General Considerations

TABLE 27E: General Considerations for Built Environment in a Dietary Unit

Construction Standards	Food service areas must • Be easy to clean and maintain. • Be provided with potable water, effective sewage disposal, and sufficient light and ventilation for effective operation. • Be protected against entry or harbourage by pests. • Have a unidirectional workflow from receipt of produce and supplies to storage, food preparation, cooking, plating, and food delivery and on to inpatient units and survey areas.

Environmental Considerations

Acoustics	• Provide acoustic treatment to dishwashing areas.
Natural Light/Lighting	• Natural light should be maximized to provide a pleasant work environment where possible. • Artificial lighting should be sufficient to enable people to work, use facilities, and move from place to place safely and without experiencing eye strain.
Accessibility	Dining areas should be designed to provide ease of access for persons in wheelchairs.
Doors	Adequately sized automatic/semi-automatic doors are recommended for ease of passage for food distribution trolleys.
Security	• The Catering Unit will require controlled access to prevent unauthorized entry, and the unit should be isolated from general hospital traffic.
Finishes	All tables, benches, and other surfaces on which food is prepared or handled should be covered in a smooth impervious material.
Ceilings	• A monolithic ceiling should be provided that covers all conduits, piping, duct work, and open construction.
Floors and Walls	• In areas used for food preparation or assembly, floors should be non-slip, water-resistant and greaseproof to comply with relevant standards. • Solid, rendered, smooth walls that are epoxy-coated or spray-painted withstand heavy treatment and allow ease of repair.
Fixtures, Fittings, and Equipment	• Shelving systems installed should be constructed of non-porous materials, dust resistant, easily cleaned, and avoid inaccessible corners. • Equipment installed in the unit including sinks, dishwashing/ware washing equipment, cooking equipment, and exhaust hoods will require mechanical, hydraulics, or electrical services in accordance with manufacturer's recommendations and local regulations.
Heating, Ventilation, and Air Conditioning	• Provide hot water to sinks used for food preparation and dishwashing, ware washing, and pot washing within the catering area. • Provide hot water to all automatic dishwashing and utensil washing machines as specified by the manufacturer. • Under-counter conduits, piping, and drains should be arranged to not interfere with cleaning the equipment or the floor below the counter.

Infection Control

Hand Basins	• Staff handwashing basins should be provided in all clean-up, preparation, cooking, and serving areas of the unit.
Insect Control	• In new hospitals, the kitchen should not open directly to the outside; an airlock should be provided between the kitchen and external areas. • A section of hospital corridor may be used as an airlock. • In existing kitchens being refurbished, any door leading directly from the kitchen to the outside should be fitted with a fly screen door with a self-closer.

TABLE 27F: Specific Room and Functional Requirements for Built Environment in a Dietary Unit

Supplies Receipt Area	• The supplies receipt area should be located with close access to the clean loading dock and with ready access to the Catering Unit entry for prompt deliveries.
	• The receiving area should contain the following:
	  • A control station.
	  • An area for loading, un-crating, and weighing supplies.
	• These areas may be shared with clean dock areas.

Trolley Return/Stripping Area	• The trolley return/stripping area will be located adjacent to the dishwashing and trolley/cart-washing area, with direct access from the entry airlock.
	• There should also be convenient access to the waste disposal area.
	• The trolley return/stripping area will require
	  • Wall and corner protection for trolley impact zones.
	  • A handwashing basin located in close proximity.

Trolley/Cart Washing Area	• The trolley wash area should be located remotely from the food preparation and storage areas with convenient access from the trolley return/stripping area.
Dishwashing & Pot Washing Area	• The dishwashing area should be located in close proximity to trolley/cart stripping and away from food preparation/cooking areas. • Pot washing sinks or equipment should be located with ready access to preparation and cooking areas and can be co-located with dishwashing areas. • Dish/pot washing equipment and sinks will require • Hot and cold water with a flexible hose spray • Services according to manufacturer's specifications • Provision for automated cleaning chemical dosing. • The dishwashing area requires the following finishes: • Walls and ceiling that are smooth, impervious, and easily cleanable • Floors that are impervious and non-slip.

(Continued)

TABLE 27F: (Continued)

Food Preparation Areas	• Food preparation areas will be located with ready access to storage areas, refrigeration for food supplies, cooking areas, boiling water units, and ice dispensing machines.
	• The areas will include benches, sinks, shelving, and mobile trolleys for utensils.
	• Equipment may include food processors, slicers, mixers, and cutters.
	• Food preparation areas require
	  • A temperature-controlled environment.
	  • A handwashing basin with paper towels and soap fittings.
	  • Surfaces that are smooth, impervious, easily cleaned, and resistant to scratches and cleaning chemicals.

Cooking Areas	• Cooking areas will be located in close proximity to food preparation areas and with convenient access to plating areas. • Cooking equipment must be installed to manufacturer's specifications and may include a range of services including gas, electricity, steam, water, and drainage. • Cooking areas must be properly ventilated with an exhaust hood covering the entire area. • Exhaust hoods must be designed and installed to prevent grease or condensation from collecting on walls and ceilings and from dripping into food or onto food contact surfaces.
Blast Chiller/s (Optional) Area	• Blast chillers will require direct power and temperature monitoring and should be installed according to manufacturer's specifications.

Plating/Tray Preparation Areas	• The plating area will be located with ready access to food delivery trolley/cart holding area for efficient distribution.
	• The plating/tray preparation area will consist of
	  • Plating conveyor or bench for tray preparation and meal serving.
	  • Mobile bulk food serving trolleys for plating.
	  • Supplies of trays, plates, utensils, and items for tray setting.
	• Plating/tray preparation areas will require power to heated/chilled food serving trolleys and food delivery trolley/carts.

Meal Trolley/Cart Holding Area	• Meal trolley/cart holding parking space will be required in the Catering Unit and should be located adjacent to plating/tray preparation area with convenient access to the exit doors. • Cool rooms, refrigerators, and freezers should be located with ready access to food preparation, cooking, and re-thermalization areas.
Dining Areas	

Servery Area	• The servery will be located close to a dining area.
	• The servery will require the following fittings and fixtures:
	  • Workbenches with an impervious top and splashback.
	  • Single or double bowl stainless steel sink set in the bench top supplied with hot and cold reticulated water, lever action, or automatically activated taps.
	  • Heated and chilled food display cabinets and serving with bain-marie.
	  • Provision for plates, food trays, and utensils.
	  • Disposable glove dispenser.
	  • Hand basin, with liquid soap and paper towel dispensers.
	• The servery will require the following finishes:
	  • Walls and ceiling that are smooth, impervious, and easily cleanable.
	  • Floors that are impervious and non-slip.

Staff Dining	• The staff dining room should be located in a staff only, discreet area of the facility with direct access to a circulation corridor.
	• It should have ready access to the Catering Unit.
	• Access to an external dining area is desirable.
	• Acoustic privacy may be required to adjoining areas.
	• The dining room should incorporate the following:
	  • External windows.
	  • Dining tables and chairs.
	  • Telephone within or adjacent to the room for staff use.
	  • Provision for dirty plates and trays for return to cleaning areas.
	  • Food waste and recyclables area.

27.3 Future Trends in Catering for Hospitals

There have been technological advances particularly in software to manage the food production process and cost, quality, and nutritional content. Software can be integrated with the patient's medical records to manage special diets and food allergies. It also can be used to provide room service to patients with flexible, customized menus ordered electronically. Improved cooking and delivery systems can also present flexible meal times for patients. Technology offers improved menu options for patients and faster food processing with a greater use of pre-prepared food products. Moreover, automated robotic delivery systems can be used to transport meal carts to Inpatient Units, reducing manual handling and allowing catering staff more time with patients.

28 LAUNDRY SERVICES

28.1 Introduction

Linen handling involves

- The collection of dirty linen on a regular basis
- Processing of dirty linen including sorting, washing, drying, and folding
- Storage of clean linen and supply to Inpatient and Ambulatory Care Units on a regular basis

Linen processing may be conducted within the hospital facility or off-site in a commercial or shared laundry, depending on the operational policy. At a minimum, each facility should have provisions for storage and exchange of clean and soiled linen for appropriate patient care.

28.2 Linen and Laundry and Wider Hospital Context: Location & Access

The Linen Handling Unit will be located in the service area of the facility with close access to clean and dirty loading dock areas. An on-site laundry facility may be located in the hospital or remotely in a separate building with good connectivity to the hospital.

28.3 Operational Models

Linen processing may be performed on-site in a separate facility or within the hospital. Most commonly, linen processing is outsourced in a commercial arrangement with an external provider and delivered to the facility. The minimum service provided by the hospital will generally be a daily collection of dirty linen and daily delivery of clean linen to patient units.

Activity Flowchart of Laundry (Figure 28A)

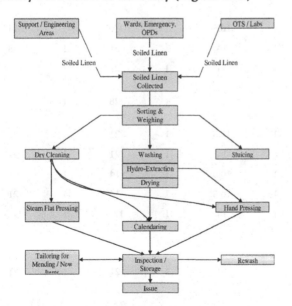

FIGURE 28A Activity Flowchart of Laundry (Courtesy: Singh D, Qadri GJ, Kotwal M, Syed AT, Jan F. Quality control in linen and laundry service at a tertiary care teaching hospital in India. International Journal of Health Sciences. 2009 Jan;3(1):33).

TABLE 28A: Key Result Areas of Laundry

- Laundry and linen management processes
- Policy for change of linen
- Washing protocols for different categories
- Segregation of linen
- Soiled linen management
- Bags and labels
- Quality control system and infection prevention and control
- Electrical safety practices
- Staff awareness of safety practices
- Layout/space
- Maintenance plan of machinery
- Fire safety awareness and firefighting equipment
- Identified hazardous materials
- Documented procedure for sorting, storing, handling, etc.
- Regulatory requirements for radioactive substances

Internal and External Functional Relationships (Table 28B and Figure 28B)

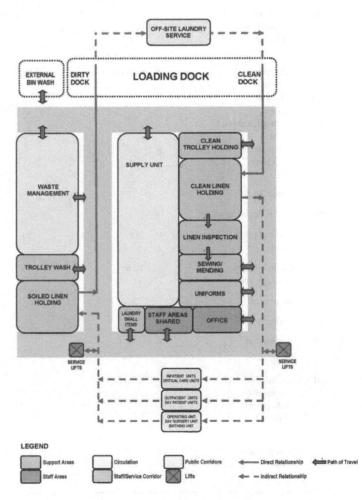

FIGURE 28B Functional Relationship Diagram of Laundry (Courtesy: iHFG).

DOI: 10.1201/9780367460884-29

TABLE 28B: Functional Relationships of Laundry

Internal Functional Relationships

Clean and dirty linen holding areas will generally be separated to prevent the cross-flow of clean and dirty traffic to the loading dock area.

Trolley storage and cleaning areas should be located with convenience for efficient linen handling.

Staff and support areas will generally be shared with other service areas in the hospital.

External Functional Relationships

The service entry and clean loading dock are used for daily deliveries of clean linen on trolleys to the clean linen holding.

Waste management area and dirty loading dock are used for daily collection of dirty linen on trolleys from the dirty linen holding room.

All hospital units are supplied with linen; good connectivity is required to service corridors and service lifts for linen deliveries and collection services.

TABLE 28C: Major Space Determinants and Size

S No.	FACILITY	CATEGORY A		CATEGORY B		CATEGORY C		CATEGORY D		CATEGORY E	
		ROOM (NO.)	Area (m²)	ROOM (NO.)	Area (m²)	ROOM (NO.)	Area (m²)	ROOM (NO.)	Area (m²)	ROOM (NO.)	Area (m²)
(1)	(2)	(3)	(4)	(5)	(6)	(7)	(8)	(9)	(10)	(11)	(12)
(a)	Dirty clothes receiving and sorting area (with weighing facility)	1	10.5	1	14	1	21	1	35	1	42
						1	14	1	21	1	28
(b)	Sluice and autoclaving machine area			1	10.5	1	10.5	1	14	1	14
(c)	Washing area	By use of Dhobi Ghats (Manual washing)				1	28	1	42	1	56
(d)	Hydro extractor area					1	28	1	42	1	56
(e)	Drying tumbler area					1	28	1	42	1	56
(f)	Calendaring machine area					1	17.5	1	28	1	28
(g)	Tailor desk					1	10.5	1	10.5	1	14
(h)	Steam pressing					1	14	1	21	1	28
(i)	Manual press area	1	14	1	21	1	14	1	21	1	28
(j)	Clean clothes storage area	1	10.5	1	14			1	28	1	35
(k)	Issue area					1	17.5	1	21	1	28
(l)	Boiler room					1	14	1	21	1	21
(m)	Trolley bay					1	10.5	1	14	1	14
(n)	Store					1	10.5	1	14	1	21
(o)	Laundry supervisor office with toilet					1	14	1	17.5	1	17.5
(p)	Laundry staff room with toilet					1	14	1	21	1	21
(q)	Switch room					1	3.5	1	3.5	1	7.0

Layout & Zoning (Figure 28C)

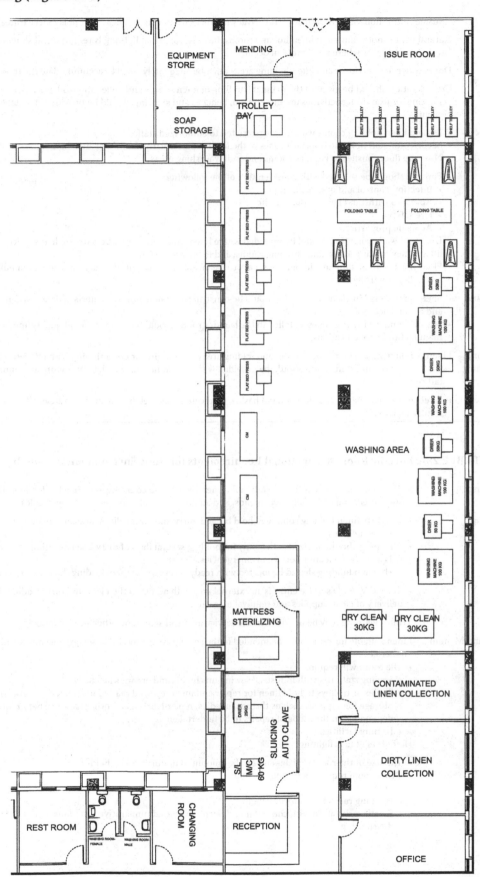

FIGURE 28C Sample Layout of Laundry.

TABLE 28D: General Considerations for Built Environment in Laundry

Acoustics	Consideration should be given to acoustic privacy in offices particularly if located in noisy service areas of the hospital.
Natural Light/ Lighting	Natural light is not required in linen holding rooms; however, artificial lighting is required and should be sufficient to avoid shaded spots where accidents can occur.
Doors	Doors to service corridors and linen holding areas must be adequately sized to accommodate the trolleys in use.
Ergonomics	Consideration should be given to the manual handling of linen supply and collection trolleys. Where linen sorting, counting, or examining activities are undertaken, benches and shelving should be provided at suitable working heights.
Safety and Security	• Locked linen holding rooms with access restricted to authorized staff. • Security for staff in isolated service zones of the facility, particularly if working after hours. • Non-slip floor finishes to laundry rooms and trolley washing areas.

Finishes	• Finishes should be selected with consideration of the following:
	  • Infection control and ease of cleaning.
	  • Ability to withstand heavy trolley traffic.
	  • Fire safety.
	  • Acoustic properties.
	• Door and wall protection should be provided where linen trolley movement occurs such as service corridors, service lifts, trolley parking areas, linen holding rooms, and linen storage bays.
	• Floor finish is to be non-slip, impervious, easy to clean, and durable, with frequent movement of bulky linen supply and collection trolleys.

Fixtures, Fittings, and Equipment	• Shelving installed in clean linen areas should be constructed of non-porous materials, dust resistant, easily cleaned, and avoid inaccessible corners. • Washing and drying machines installed in the laundry room should be of commercial quality and installed to manufacturer's specifications.
Heating, Ventilation, and Air Conditioning	Linen handling areas such as inspection and folding areas will require air conditioning with efficient lint filtration systems. Offices and staff rooms should be provided with air conditioning with temperature and humidity control for staff comfort.
Infection Control	It is recommended that in addition to hand basins, medicated hand gel dispensers be strategically located in staff circulation corridors.

TABLE 28E: Specific Room & Functional Requirements for Built Environment in Laundry

Clean Linen Holding	• The room may include a workstation for linen receipt and counting and shelving for stored items of linen such as curtains, blankets, bedspreads, and additional supplies of general linen articles.
Dirty Linen Holding	• The dirty linen holding room will hold bagged, dirty linen on trolleys awaiting collection and removal to the laundry facilities. • The room should be sized sufficiently for holding several days of dirty linen awaiting collection, allowing for delays in the collection service in emergencies. • Dirty linen holding should be located with ready access to the dirty loading dock area for waste removal.
Service Entry	• The COVERED service entry is an external area with access to the clean and dirty loading dock areas for delivery of clean supplies and removal of waste.
Trolley Washing	Trolley washing may be provided in the service area and shared by other service units.

Linen Inspection and Mending	Linen suitable for repair may be mended in the sewing area, containing sewing machines and patching materials.
	• The room will require
	  • Sewing station/s with industrial sewing machine/s and ergonomic chair/s.
	  • Tables or trolleys to hold linen for repair and linen repaired ready for dispatch to its destination.
	  • Storage for supplies such as threads, needles, repair fabrics, and other haberdashery requirements depending on the scope of repairs to be undertaken.
	  • Ironing facilities.
	High level of task lighting.

Uniform Holding	• The size of the room will depend on the amount of uniforms to be held.
	• Other room requirements may include
	  • Shelving for storage of folded items.
	  • Hanging racks for uniform hanging.
	  • Small workstation with computer and telephone for administrative functions associated with uniform distribution

(Continued)

TABLE 28E: (Continued)

Trolley Washing	• Trolley washing is an area for the manual washing of trolleys including linen handling and may be shared with a number of service units.
	• The trolley wash area should be located in the service area.
	• The trolley washing area will require
	  • Smooth, waterproof, and easily cleanable surfaces of walls and ceiling.
	  • Non-slip, waterproof finishes on the floor.
	  • Hot and cold water outlets with hoses.
	  • Drainage in the floor.
	  • An area for hand drying trolleys and space for holding completed trolleys awaiting transport to clean holding areas.

Staff Registration Bay	• The staff registration bay may include the following:
	  • Staff registration equipment, manual or electronic.
	  • Bench at standing height (optional).
	  • Pin board for display of rosters or other staff information (or computer for computerized rosters).
	  • Computer terminal (optional).
	  • Power and data outlets for computer or electronic staff presence equipment as required.

28.4 Summary

Laundry service is responsible for providing an adequate, clean, and constant supply of linen to all users. The basic tasks include sorting, washing, extracting, drying, ironing, folding, mending, and delivery. A reliable laundry service is of the utmost importance to a hospital. In today's medical care facilities, patients expect linen to be changed daily. An adequate supply of clean linen is sufficient for the comfort and safety of the patient and is thus essential.

29 MEDICAL RECORDS UNIT

29.1 Introduction

The Medical Records Unit provides secure maintenance, storage, and retrieval of confidential clinical records. Provision should be made for 24-hour availability of clinical records either by a computerized or manual system. The functions involved in the development and maintenance of health information systems include the following:

- Collection, assembly, sorting, and circulation of records for all inpatient and outpatient units.
- Transcription/typing service for outpatient letters, discharge summaries, and operation reports.
- Classification of diseases and procedures for inpatient admissions using the International Classification of Diseases, that is, clinical coding.
- Provision of information to management and other authorized staff for purposes such as planning, utilization review, quality assurance, case mix studies, and research.
- Quality assurance of the medical record to ensure that standards are met.
- Storage of current and archived records for the prescribed time period in a secure, moisture-resistant environment.

29.2 Medical Records Unit and Wider Hospital Context

29.2.1 Location

Location will be influenced by the type of records of the system adopted (e.g., paper, EMR) and whether or not a pneumatic or mechanical automated records transport system is to be installed and the departments to which it is linked. The decision to include such a system will strongly influence the external functional relationships of the unit with the outpatient clinic area in particular and may reduce the importance of direct access to the Emergency Unit.

29.3 Operational Models

The Medical Records Unit will generally be provided under the direction and supervision of the Administration Unit.

(a) **Hours of Operation:** The Medical Records Unit typically will operate during business hours, 7 days per week. The unit will organize provision for record retrieval after business hours.

(b) **Service Delivery Models:** The service model depends on a number of operational policies to be addressed in the service plan of the facility as discussed as follows:

   (i) **Operational Policies:** Operational policies that may have an impact on the planning of the Clinical Information Unit and may require decisions by policy makers include the following:

   - How records are to be managed and identified; essential elements include
     - Provision of a centralized record system for all inpatient, emergency, and outpatient/day patient attendances or decentralized systems; where decentralized systems are in operation, the existence of sub-files will require registration, allowing retrieval of the sub-file for patient care or medicolegal purposes.
     - Provision of a unit numbering system providing a unique identification number for every patient who presents to the hospital, for example, the medical record number (MRN); the MRN issued at the time of first admission or attendance is then used for all subsequent admissions and treatment.
   - Provision of patient administration systems with information relating to patient movements, with electronic updating for rapid record location.
   - The use of terminal digit filing systems in both active storage and secondary storage.
   - Tracking of each medical record leaving the unit by using request forms (which may be electronic); tracking can be facilitated by the use of bar code labels on the record folder.
   - Maintenance of record confidentiality, including authorized access to the record and release of information to other parties.
   - Preparation of medicolegal reports and subpoenas in accordance with the local statutory requirements.
   - Retrieval of medical records from secondary storage within a set time if deemed clinically necessary; the location of secondary storage is to be considered.
   - Provision of a centralized dictating system utilizing the telephone system for clinical staff to compile discharge reports and summaries.
   - Transcription of discharge summaries, medical reports from operations and procedures, and outpatient letters are to be completed in the unit.

The record management system chosen will also require consideration of operational policies and specific details related to implementation of new technologies including

- Cabling and network requirements to all related hospital units
- Integration with existing communications systems
- Location of workstations
- Space and security requirements
- Air conditioning, temperature and humidity control requirements for workstations and paper record storage
- The transition process to be utilized when moving from one system to another

   (ii) **Paper Medical Records:** The traditional paper medical record is gradually being replaced by electronic and digitized records. However, paper medical records still exist and require storage space within the health facility.

   (iii) **Electronic Medical Records:** Electronic medical record (EMRs) are computerized online record that track and detail a patient's care during their time spent in hospital. EMRs enable staff to enter patient data at the point of care and allow authorized clinicians access

DOI: 10.1201/9780367460884-30

to a patient's records from any online location, at any time, to make rapid assessments and coordinate care.

(iv) **Digitized (Scanned) Medical Records:** Records may be scanned to create a digital record and filed on a centralized server. The advantages of records scanning include
  - Improved access to records by staff, particularly for clinical staff completing summaries, for quality assurance and availability of patient admission information as needed.
  - Reduced space for storage of records.

(v) **Storage (Table 29A)**

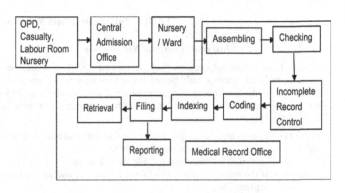

FIGURE 29A Activity Flowchart of Medical Records Unit (Courtesy: Verma S, Midha M, Bhadoria AS. Facts and figures on medical record management from a multi super specialty hospital in Delhi NCR: A descriptive analysis. Journal of Family Medicine and Primary Care. 2020 Jan;9(1):418).

TABLE 29A: Storage Duration for Physical and Electronic Medical Records

Physical Medical Records	Electronic Records
• Inpatient medical record: 3 years. • Medicolegal record: 10 years or until the disposal of the ongoing case in any of the courts related to these records. • OPD record: 3 years.	• All records must compulsorily be preserved and never destroyed during the lifetime of the person. • Upon the demise of the patient where there are no court cases pending, the records can be removed from active status and changed to inactive status. • HSPs are free to decide when to make a record inactive, but it is preferable to follow the "three-year rule" where all records of a deceased are made inactive three years after death. • It is, however, preferred, and HSPs are strongly encouraged to ensure, that the records are never destroyed or removed permanently.
Source: DGHS, MoHFW, GoI, Office Memorandum No. F. No. A.12034/3/2014-MH-II/MH-I dated 28/10/2014.	*Source:* Electronic Health Record Standards for India, 2016 by MoHFW, GoI.

TABLE 29B: Key Result Areas and Quality Indicators for Medical Records Unit

Key Result Areas

- Policies and standard operating procedures (SOPs) implemented for management and control of data and information.
- Ensuring completeness and accuracy of the medical records.
- Maintaining confidentiality, integrity, and security of records.
- Retention of medical records as per the rules established by MCI/state governments.
- Periodic review of medical records.
- Destruction of medical records in accordance with the written guidance.

Quality Indicators

- Percentage of medical records having incomplete and/or improper consent.

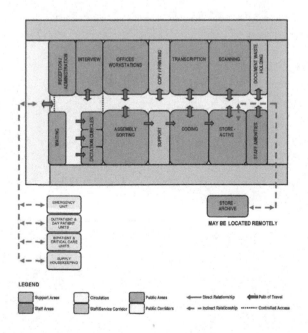

FIGURE 29B Functional Relationship Diagram of Medical Records Unit (Courtesy: iHFG).

TABLE 29C: Functional Relationships of Medical Records Unit

Internal Functional Relationships

A planned and organized workflow is important for efficient functioning of the unit. Internal spaces should be organized from receipt of records to processing, coding, scanning, if appropriate, and storage. Medicolegal and quality assurance areas should be located with convenient access to records and printing areas.

The archival store is ideally located within the Clinical Information Unit but may be located remotely with convenient access.

The optimum internal relationships include the following:
- Reception at the entrance that acts as a receiving point and an interview area in close proximity.
- Access control to the entry and functional areas within the unit to maintain the security of records at all times.
- Dictation cubicles located near the entry to the unit so that medical staff do not need to traverse the unit for reporting or research.
- Support areas located centrally for ease of staff access.
- Staff amenities located at the unit perimeter that may be shared with adjacent units.
- Process of work from assembly/sorting to coding and active storage; transcription and scanning areas are additional to the primary workflow.

External Functional Relationships

In a traditional, paper-based record environment, the critical relationship is with the emergency department for urgent record retrieval. Outpatient Unit/s have an indirect relationship with the Clinical Information Unit where record retrieval can be scheduled to coincide with outpatient sessions.

In a paperless environment, there will probably be no critical relationships except for staff wanting to access records still in hard copy for research purposes, etc.

The ideal external relationships are demonstrated in the following diagram:
- Visitors access from a public circulation corridor.
- Single entry and access for staff and visitors.
- Indirect but important relationship to external units including Emergency, Outpatient, Day Patient, Inpatient, and Critical Care Units.
- Indirect relationship with service units including supply and housekeeping.

Major Space Determinants & Medical Records Unit Size

TABLE 29D: Space Programming for Medical Records

S No.	FACILITY	CATEGORY A		CATEGORY B		CATEGORY C		CATEGORY D		CATEGORY E	
		ROOM (NO.)	Area (m²)	ROOM (NO.)	Area (m²)	ROOM (NO.)	Area (m²)	ROOM (NO.)	Area (m²)	ROOM (NO.)	Area (m²)
(1)	(2)	(3)	(4)	(5)	(6)	(7)	(8)	(9)	(10)	(11)	(12)
MEDICAL RECORDS DEPT.											
	Medical records storage										
	(a) Active (up to 2 years)	—		—		1	28	1	42	1	56
	(b) Inactive (between 2 and 10 years)	—		—		1	84	1	126	1	140
	Medical records office with toilet	—		—		1	21	1	17.5	1	17.5
	Staff office with toilet	—		—				1	17.5	1	17.5
	Medical record processing area	—		—		1	21	1	28	1	35
	Doctor's record completion room	—		—		1	21	1	14	1	14
	Room for various automations	—		—				1	14	1	14
	Printed stationery store	—		—		1	17.5	1	10.5	1	14
	General store	—		—				1	10.5	1	14

Built Environment: General Considerations

TABLE 29E: General Considerations for Built Environment in Medical Records Unit

Acoustics	Acoustic privacy will be required for offices, meeting rooms, interview rooms, dictation cubicles, coding workstations, and all areas where confidential patient information may be discussed.
Natural Light/Lighting	• Wherever possible, the use of natural light is to be maximized for the benefit of staff working in the unit.
Accessibility	Reception, offices, meeting/interview rooms, and waiting areas should be designed to provide access to people in wheelchairs who may include staff or visitors.
Ergonomics	Aspects for consideration will include height of benches and height of equipment in constant use, particularly photocopiers and scanners. Adjustable-height workstations may be considered.

Safety and Security	• Security issues to be addressed include
	  • Adequate security for staff who may be working in an isolated area of the campus
	  • Visitors should only be able to access the department via the reception area
	  • Reception counters should be designed so that they would be difficult/impossible to climb over
	  • Motion sensors in storage areas should be considered to identify unauthorized access
	Security for Scanned and Electronic Records
	• Scanned and electronic medical records including server storage devices will be subject to data security considerations to prevent loss of data and ensure authorized access.

Finishes	• Finishes should be selected with a consideration of the following:
	  • Acoustic properties of the materials; the use of carpet and acoustic panels will assist in absorption of sound
	  • Durability, replacement, and cleaning of materials
	  • Fire safety of the materials
	  • Promote an efficient and pleasant working environment for staff and visitors
	• Provide wall protection to all areas where trolleys are in use.

IT/Communications	The following IT/communications systems may be provided within the Medical Records Unit: • The provision for remote dictating from the administrative and clinical areas to a central dictating unit as required by the operational policy of the unit • Telephones to offices, dictation cubicles, interview rooms, meeting rooms, and records storage areas (active and archive). • Computer networking and servers associated with patient administration systems, electronic records systems, and scanned records • Duress alarm system, to be located at Reception and in meeting rooms
Electrical Services	If an EMR system is implemented, components of the system such as a terminal and servers may require an uninterruptible power supply.
Pneumatic Tube System	The Medical Record Unit may include a pneumatic tube station, connecting key clinical units with the main support units as determined by the facility's operational policy. If provided, the station should be located in close proximity to Reception under direct staff supervision with record security maintained at all times.
Infection Control	Hand hygiene is an essential element, and provision of medicated hand gel dispensers or hand wipes at Reception and in circulation corridors is recommended.
Size of the Unit	• The size of the Clinical Information Unit will depend on the service to be provided by the unit, the type and quantity of physical records to be stored, and the number of staff • In addition to records processing and storage areas, accommodation will be required for • Health information manager • Medicolegal and quality assurance staff • Clinical coders • Medical typists • Administrative staff

TABLE 29F: Specific Considerations for Built Environment in Medical Records Unit

Entry/Reception/Administration	• A small waiting area should be located nearby for visitors • Entry doors should have a buzzer with a key card or electronic access for authorized staff. For units that provide 24-hour service, a peephole in the door and/or a camera/intercom is required for after-hours access

Dictation Cubicles	• The cubicles will provide a single workstation of 3–4 m² and may be partially enclosed with partitions
	• Requirements for each cubicle will include
	  • Acoustic treatment to partitions
	  • Desk or workstation with an ergonomic, adjustable-height chair
	  • Workstation shelf unit
	  • Computer and telephone access with power and data provision

Assembly and Sorting	• Record assembly and sorting involves filing and arranging paper-based documents composing the medical records for outpatient areas, admissions, and discharges and will generally be undertaken in an open plan area • A temporary storage area will also be required for returned files or files awaiting delivery to departments • Note that records awaiting medicolegal attention will generally be stored in the medicolegal office

(Continued)

TABLE 29F: (Continued)

Records Transcription	• This area will provide the medical transcription service. Staff should be located in a quieter area of the unit but within close proximity to the dictating and general assembly/sorting area
	• Requirements include
	  • Workstation with acoustic treatment to partitions
	  • Ergonomic, adjustable-height chair
	  • Dictation system connections
	  • Computer and telephone access with data and power provision

Clinical Coding	Clinical coding of medical records is an activity that involves a high level of attention to avoid errors and is best performed in a quiet area of the unit. Each coder will need a computer workstation and storage for incoming files and coding and reference manuals if these are not available on a centralized server.
Photocopying/ Printing	A dedicated, acoustically treated, and ventilated space is required. This space may also be used for generating bar code labels and stationery storage. It should be located with ready access to the medicolegal office that generates a large amount of photocopying.

Records Scanning	• Scanning of medical records will provide a digital copy of a paper-based record, available on a central server.
	• The records scanning area will require
	  • Benches for checking and organizing each file
	  • Scanning unit/s—bench top or desk top
	  • Quality control workstations of 4–5.5 m²
	  • Storage area for holding the scanned documents prior to destruction

Secure Confidential Waste Holding	• The bay will require
	  • Wall protection to protect from damage
	  • Secure confidential waste holding bins of 240 L; the quantity will depend on the scale of the service and whether scanning and destruction of records is undertaken

Records Storage Area	• Active medical records in constant use are typically stored in open metal shelving units to provide easy access. Standard shelving bays are usually 900-mm wide and 300–400-mm deep • Compact units may be used to store non-active or archived files, which is space-efficient but not recommended for active files where multiple staff may require access to bays at the same time • The number of shelves in each bay should be six or up to a maximum of seven. The highest shelf should not exceed 2,175 mm and should be reachable by staff using a library step stool • The highest shelf for staff reach without a stepstool should not be higher than 1,700 mm. For safety purposes, stepladders should not be used • Aisles between bays of shelving should have a minimum width of 750 mm, but 900 mm is recommended to allow space for records trolleys, library stools, and staff transit • Access aisles used as a thoroughfare should be a minimum of 1,500 mm wide to allow for trolley access and must comply with fire egress requirements • Fire sprinklers should NOT be installed. Records storage areas must be temperature and humidity controlled for preservation of records
Offices	Offices should be located to allow easy access to the unit for the health information manager, staff, and visitors. Offices for medicolegal staff will optimally be located near Reception with dual access from the waiting area and from inside the unit.

29.4 Summary

Planning and designing a Medical Records Unit is a crucial process that requires careful thought and consideration. The efficient organization and management of medical records are essential for maintaining accurate patient information, ensuring seamless communication among health care providers, and safeguarding patient privacy. Key considerations in the planning and designing process include adequate storage space for physical records, secure digital systems, efficient retrieval systems, proper data backup and security measures, compliance with privacy regulations, and integration with electronic health record systems. By prioritizing these factors and involving experts in medical records management, health care organizations can establish a well-designed Medical Records Unit that promotes efficient record-keeping, enhances data accessibility, and contributes to high-quality patient care.

30 MORTUARY SERVICES

30.1 Introduction

The hospital morgue is a facility for the viewing and/or identification of a body and the temporary holding/storage of bodies prior to transfer to a mortuary. The needs of hospital staff, relatives of the deceased, and attendant authorized persons should be considered in the design, layout, and functionality of the unit to provide a safe and private environment. The design must address the following:

- Number of bodies to be stored
- Method of storage, namely, refrigerated cabinets, cool room, and freezing capacity
- Separation of entries for families to view/identify bodies
- Delivery of bodies from inside the hospital and external delivery (if applicable)

It should be noted that the standard hospital morgue facility should not be used for storage of a body associated with a criminal investigation. In this case, the body is evidence, and enhanced security should be provided.

There are two types of morgue cold chambers:

- Positive temperature +2/+4°C (the most common type)
- Negative temperature −15°C/−25°C (used by forensic institutes for the storage of bodies that have not yet been identified)

30.2 Mortuary Services and Wider Hospital Context: Location & Access

The unit should be located in the same building as the main health facility away from any public area or as a stand-alone building (Figures 30A and 30B). It should be located at ground level to allow easy and discrete access to deliver and/or remove bodies via an exit lobby.

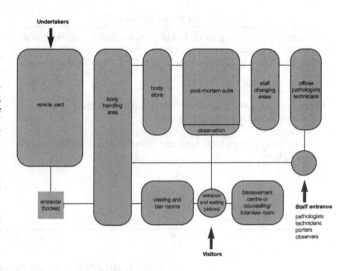

FIGURE 30B Mortuary as Stand-Alone Building (Courtesy: HBN 20).

TABLE 30A: Key Result Areas for a Mortuary

Mortuary Facilities
- Cold storage and back-up power
- Staff safety and personal protective equipment
- Disinfection
- Monitoring of terms quality in case this activity (if outsourced)
- Electrical safety practices
- Staff awareness on safety practices
- Maintenance plan of machinery

Internal & External Functional Relationships (Table 30B and Figure 30C)

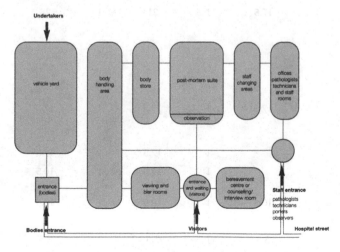

FIGURE 30A Mortuary Attached to the Main Hospital Building (Courtesy: HBN 20).

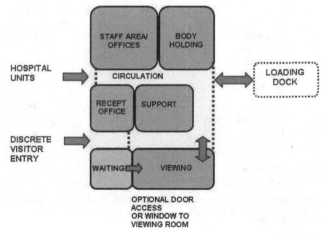

FIGURE 30C Functional Relationship of Mortuary (Courtesy: iHFG).

DOI: 10.1201/9780367460884-31

TABLE 30B: Functional Relationship of a Mortuary

Internal Functional Relationships	External Functional Relationships
The waiting and viewing areas should be collocated, but there should be no access to other sections of the morgue for viewers. The entry lobby, exit lobby, and administrative area form part of a single area.	Mortuary/holding facilities should be accessible through an exterior entrance and located to avoid the need for transporting bodies through public areas. It should also be located in close proximity to anatomical pathology laboratories and relevant clinical areas for transportation of laboratory specimens.
The body holding room is to have direct access to/from • The hospital corridor for use by staff • Viewing room • Discreet access from body hold/cool room to hearse and ambulance parking bays	The morgue is to have separate access as follows: • Direct access from the hospital for delivery of the body • Direct but separate and discreet access for relatives of the deceased from all relevant areas of the hospital to the morgue waiting/viewing area • Adequate access for funeral directors for vehicle parking and discrete, weather-protected facilities for the collection of bodies. • Adequate access for ambulances delivering bodies • Adequate access for police vehicles

TABLE 30C: Major Space Determinants and Mortuary Size

S No.	FACILITY	CATEGORY A		CATEGORY B		CATEGORY C		CATEGORY D		CATEGORY E	
		ROOM (NO.)	Area (m²)	ROOM (NO.)	Area (m²)	ROOM (NO.)	Area (m²)	ROOM (NO.)	Area (m²)	ROOM (NO.)	Area (m²)
(1)	(2)	(3)	(4)	(5)	(6)	(7)	(8)	(9)	(10)	(11)	(12)
FUNCTIONAL AREAS											
(a)	Cold room for body storage	1	10.5	1	10.5	1	14	1	14	1	10.5
		(4 BODIES)		(4 BODIES)		(4 BODIES)		(4 BODIES)		(4 BODIES)	
(b)	Post-mortem area	—		1	14	1	17.5	1	21	1	28
(c)	Autopsy store	—				1	7.0	1	10.5	1	14
(d)	Body wash and prayer room	—		1	10.5	1	14	1	21	1	28
(e)	Relative waiting area with toilet and drinking water facility	1	14	1	14	1	17.5	1	21	1	28
(f)	Doctor's office with toilet	1	14	1	14	1	17.5	1	17.5	1	17.5
(g)	Staff room with toilet							1	17.5	1	17.5
								1	10.5	1	10.5
(h)	Office			1	10.5	1	10.5	1	10.5	1	10.5
(i)	Storage							1	10.5	1	10.5
(j)	Janitor's closet	1	3.5	1	3.5	1	3.5	1	3.5	1	3.5
(k)	Trolley bay	—		—		1	10.5	1	10.5	1	10.5

Layout of Mortuary (Figures 30D to 30I)

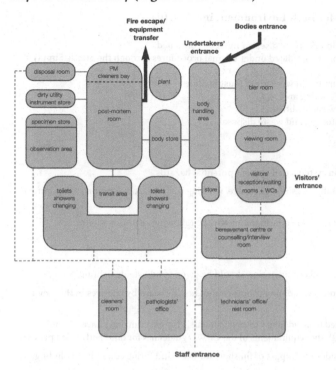

FIGURE 30D Layout of Mortuary (Courtesy: HBN 20).

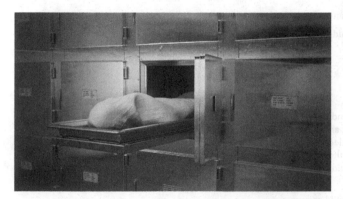

FIGURE 30E Body Holding Area (Courtesy: www.mother-hospitalthrissur.org/mortuary).

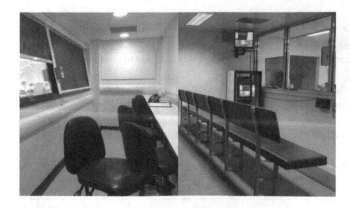

FIGURE 30F Observation Area/Room in Mortuary (Courtesy: Scottish Health Planning Note 16–01).

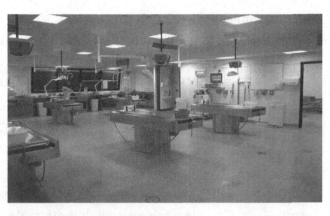

FIGURE 30G Post-Mortem Suite with Observation Room/Area in Mortuary (Courtesy: Scottish Health Planning Note 16–01).

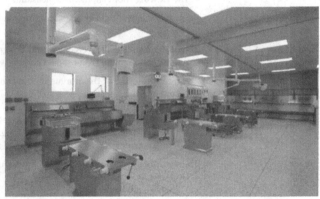

FIGURE 30H Post-Mortem Suite with Observation Room/Area in Mortuary (Courtesy: Scottish Health Planning Note 16–01).

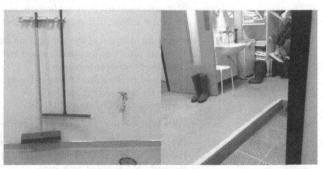

FIGURE 30I Clean-Up Room in Mortuary (Courtesy: Scottish Health Planning Note 16–01).

Built Environment: General Considerations

TABLE 30D: General Considerations for Built Environment in a Mortuary

Infection Control	• Bodies stored in the morgue that may contain infectious diseases must be contained.
	• Cleaned instruments and materials should be re-circulated under normal procedures through the Sterile Supply Unit or autoclaved within the morgue.
	• Layout designed to minimize cross contamination in work areas must include
	  • Provision of a small wash-down/disposal/booting area
	  • Provision of an adequate number of handwash facilities
	  • Provision of appropriate cleaning, waste storage, and waste disposal
	  • Use of suitable materials and finishes
	  • Specimen storage facilities
	  • First aid facilities
	  • Adequate isolation of space and ventilation systems that present potential hazards

General	The morgue needs to be designed to provide staff with sufficient space, working surfaces, and appropriate equipment to safely carry out their duties.
Interior Design	The interior design of the Morgue Unit should have due consideration for the following as primary items of design: • Infection control • Cooling and ventilation • The viewing room should be a pleasant space and consideration should be given to adjustable lighting
Acoustics	Acoustic design should ensure that conversations in adjoining rooms cannot be overheard by relatives in the viewing area.
Ergonomics Access and Mobility	The Morgue Unit shall be ergonomically designed to avoid injury to staff, patients, visitors, or maintenance personnel. Where necessary, the layout should comply with the requirements of the CPWD guidelines for differently abled persons.
Safety	The interior design of the morgue should consider the impact of finishes, surfaces, and fittings on safety including: • Floor covering selection • Adequate drainage • Protection from protrusions or sharp edges • Stability and height of equipment or fittings • Adequate protection against infection and any other hazards
Security	The security aspects of the Morgue Unit should consider the following: • Deceased bodies • Valuables left on the body • Specimens removed during autopsy • Staff personal belongings and security • Access and egress, particularly after-hours
Finishes	• Ceilings must be washable, impermeable, and non-porous. • Floor finishes should be non-slip for all wet areas or areas subject to water. It should be impervious, easy to clean, sealed with coving at the edges, and have adequate drainage. • Drains should be fitted with appropriately filtered traps for ease of hosing down. • Wall surfaces in the body holding area should be washable and/or scrubbable. Wall protection is recommended as the area is subject to damage from trolleys.
Fixtures and Fittings	The equipment layout of the Morgue Unit should ensure • Adequate provision for operation and maintenance • Provision of services as required • Door sized to allow for delivery and removal of the equipment • Design for the required heat loads • Adequate provision for weight loads
Safety Showers/Eyewashes	Provide safety shower and eyewash or eye/face wash equipment.
Heating, Ventilation, and Air Conditioning	• The temperature of the body holding area should be maintained within a comfortable range not exceeding 20–21°C. • The ventilation system should be isolated from other ventilation systems by being designed to minimize the spread of odours and airborne pathogens.
Alarms	The operating temperatures of all cooled and freezing facilities should be continuously monitored and fitted with alarms that are activated when the temperature exceeds a predetermined level. The alarms should be transmitted to a permanently manned station.
Communications	It is recommended that an intercom be provided from the main/exit door to the body preparation room to alert attendants.
Lighting Power Supply	Adequate lighting in all areas should be provided. Protective covers to power supply outlets to protect outlets from wetting and an emergency back-up system for the power supply to the refrigeration, high priority equipment, and illumination should be provided.

Built Environment: Specific Room & Functional Requirements

TABLE 30E: Specific Room and Functional Requirements for Built Environment in a Mortuary

Entry Lobby/Administration/Exit Lobby	The entry and exit lobbies form part of a single space with direct access to the body holding area. The area should include the following: • Hand basin • Workstation for body registration and removal details • Parking space for the transport trolley • Parking space for a hoist/elevating trolley
Body Holding Area (Figure 30E)	The body holding area provides refrigerated space for the temporary storage of bodies. The area should allow for the following: • Separate spaces/cabinets should be allowed for isolation. • Manoeuvring space in front of refrigerated cabinets to insert/withdraw the trays. • 3 sq m is required for a body on a loose tray or trolley in a cool room.
Waiting/Viewing Area	The area should allow for the following: • Discrete entrance away from the main hospital to the waiting area for relatives, police, and others. • Direct visibility into the adjoining viewing area
Storage	The area should allow for the following dedicated areas: • Lockable storage area for the deceased's personal effects • Clean linen area • Cleaning materials and agents • Used linen collection area • Plastic body bags and sealing machine area
Staff Area	The area should allow for the following: • Staff areas comprising offices, workstations, meeting/teaching rooms, and amenities • Office for use by the pathologist and police
Observation Area (Figures 30F,G,H)	This area should be in direct oversight of the autopsy room and have direct access to a staff toilet (in case of physical reaction to the autopsy). An intercom should be installed for the purpose of communication between the autopsy room and observation room. The glass installed should be non-reflective. The floor of the room should be raised to enable view of an autopsy examination.
Clean-Up Room (Figure 30I)	A clean-up room should be provided for the following: • Cleaning and disinfection of instruments • Temporary storage of specimens before delivery to the anatomical pathology laboratory • Temporary storage of waste material and goods and soiled linen • Secure storage of instruments used for dissection and post-mortem examination of bodies • Secure storage of chemicals • Preparation of instrument trolleys • Assembling of equipment items • Removal of soiled gowns, boots, etc • Handwashing • The room should have direct access from autopsy room and changing rooms. • Soiled articles should be returned to this area. A self-flushing cleaning sink should be provided in addition to a separate hand basin. • Mechanical extract ventilation is needed to manage fumes and odours. • A washer/disinfector to clean instruments. • Refrigeration for specimens that require storage at regulated low temperatures. • Storage of disinfectants and tissue fixative—adequate ventilation required for formalin extraction.

30.3 Summary

Planning and designing a hospital mortuary is a crucial process that ensures the respectful and dignified management of deceased individuals. Hospital mortuaries play a vital role in providing appropriate care, storage, and preparation of deceased patients. Key considerations in the planning and designing process include proper space allocation for body storage, specialized equipment for embalming and preservation, adherence to legal and cultural requirements, and maintaining a compassionate and supportive environment for grieving families. By prioritizing these factors and engaging experts in mortuary services and hospital design, health care facilities can establish well-designed mortuaries that uphold ethical standards, respect cultural sensitivities, and provide comfort and solace to grieving families during their time of loss.

31 ADMINISTRATION UNIT

31.1 Introduction

The Administration Unit provides an area of offices, workspaces, and associated facilities for supporting the management of the facility and may include both clinical and non-clinical support staff to oversee the management of a hospital or unit. This may include administrative tasks, interviews, and meetings by a range of executive, medical, nursing, and support personnel.

The level and range of facilities provided for general office and executive administration functions will vary depending on the size and level of the service being delivered in the proposed health facility and as described in the endorsed service plan.

The Administration Unit may include the following administrative positions or services:

- Main Reception and enquiries
- Chief Executive Officer (CEO), senior managers, and support staff
- Nursing executive and senior nurse managers
- Human resources and payroll staff
- Finance and accounting managers and support staff
- Facility management
- Public relations
- Legal services
- Quality management
- Training, education and research, which may be in a separate area in large health care facilities
- Disaster management coordination
- Clinical administration, including medical, clinical, and professional staff with support staff; this may be a separate unit in large health care facilities

31.2 Administration Unit and Wider Hospital Context: Location & Access

The Administration Unit should be located to provide ease of access to visitors arriving from the main entrance of the facility.

A ground-level location is not required. The Administration Unit should be well signposted and easily identifiable by staff and visitors.

The Executive Suite, Nursing Administration, and Finance Units should ideally be located together in one zone to enhance staff communication and collaboration. Clinical administration functions including the Division of Medicine, Division of Surgery, and Clinical Research Units may be located within or near the Administration Unit. Alternatively, these areas may be located close to the relevant clinical area or collocated with the Education Unit, according to the operational policy of the facility.

31.3 Operational Models

Depending on the size of the facility, the Administration Unit may be provided as a single unit for small facilities or as separate functional units grouped according to services (medical, nursing, finance, education, etc.) in multiple locations for larger facilities. The operational model will be determined by the size, operational policies, and service plan of the facility.

The Administration Unit will generally operate during business hours, Monday to Saturday. Some functions such as nursing management, clinical management, and staff allocation may be provided on an extended or 24-hour basis. Meetings and functions being held after hours will require safe and planned access for both staff and visitors.

31.4 Planning Models

The Administration Unit may be located in an area easily accessed by staff in the organization and visitors. It is recommended that a separate secure entry be provided for staff. The Administration Unit may be provided as

- A distinct unit within the health facility
- A unit located in a non-clinical zone of a health facility
- A unit within a separate building on the campus

TABLE 31A: Key Result Areas and Quality Indicators for Administration Unit

Key Result Areas
- Defined and documented roles and responsibilities of personnel identified for governance
- Establishing and communicating organization's vision, mission, and values to relevant stakeholders
- Timely approval of organization's operational plans and annual budget
- Periodically measuring performance of the organization
- Appointing senior leadership with requisite qualifications and experience
- Supporting safety initiatives, quality improvement plans, and ethical management framework of the organization
- Periodically informing relevant stakeholders about quality and performance of services
- Disclosing ownership of the organization
- Portraying affiliations and accreditations of the organization
- Organization complies with the established and applicable legislation, regulations, and notification requirements
- Ensuring effective leadership for each organizational program, service, site, or department
- Reviewing performance of leadership for effectiveness
- Coordinating the functioning with departments and external agencies
- Periodically reviewing functioning of the committees
- Documenting rights and responsibilities of the staff

(Continued)

DOI: 10.1201/9780367460884-32

TABLE 31A: (Continued)

Key Result Areas (continued)
- Documenting measurable service standards
- Change management
- Risk management
- Implanting systems for internal and external reporting of system and process failures
- Outsourcing of services and its management

Quality Indicators
- Patient satisfaction index
- Employee satisfaction index
- Employee absenteeism rate
- Employee attrition rate
- Percentage of employees who are aware of employee rights, responsibilities, and welfare schemes

---

TABLE 31B: External and Internal Functional Relationship of Administration Units

Internal Functional Relationships	**External Functional Relationships**
Optimum internal relationships include	Preferred external functional relationships include
• Reception at the entrance that may act as an access control point and an interview area in close proximity	• Visitors access from a main circulation corridor from the main entrance
• Access to administrative subunits such as public relations, human resources, finance, clinical administration, etc. via internal circulation corridors	• Separate entry and access for staff
• Administration subunits that are more frequently visited, such as public relations and human resources, are located closer to the entry and Reception	• Service corridor access for service units such as supply and housekeeping
• Support areas located centrally for ease of staff access	
• Interview rooms located close to subunits requiring frequent access	

Internal & External Functional Relationships (Figure 31A)

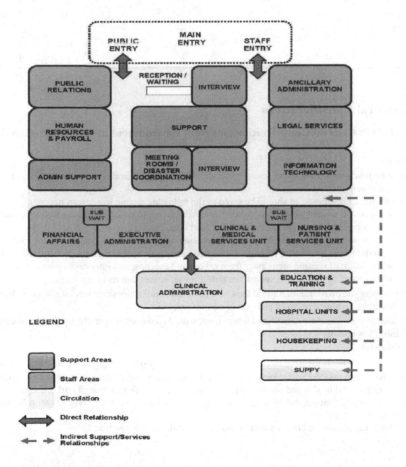

FIGURE 31A   Functional Relationships of Administration Unit (Courtesy: iHFG).

TABLE 31C: Major Space Determinants and Administration Unit Size

S No.	FACILITY	CATEGORY A		CATEGORY B		CATEGORY C		CATEGORY D		CATEGORY E	
		ROOM (NO.)	Area (m²)	ROOM (NO.)	Area (m²)	ROOM (NO.)	Area (m²)	ROOM (NO.)	Area (m²)	ROOM (NO.)	Area (m²)
(1)	(2)	(3)	(4)	(5)	(6)	(7)	(8)	(9)	(10)	(11)	(12)
GENERAL											
(a)	Medical Supdt (M.S) room with toilet	—		—		1	21	1	35	1	42
(b)	Dy/Asstt. Medical Supdt. room with toilet	1	14	1	14	1	17.5	1	21	1	21
(c)	P. S. to Medical Supdt/Dy MS./Asstt. M.S.	1	10.5	1	10.5	1	10.5	1	10.5	1	10.5
(d)	Admn Officer	1	10.5	1	10.5	1	10.5	1	10.5	1	10.5
(e)	Waiting room	—		—		1	10.5	1	10.5	1	10.5
(f)	Library-cum-conference room	—		—		—		1	10.5	1	10.5
(g)	Nursing officer's room with toilet	—		1	14	1	21	1	28	1	28
(h)	Accounts officer	—		—		1	10.5	1	10.5	1	10.5
(i)	Cashier	—		—		1	10.5	1	10.5	1	10.5
(j)	Purchase officer	—		1	7.0	1	10.5	1	10.5	1	10.5
(k)	Clerical staff	—		1	14	1	21	1	28	1	35
(l)	Reception-cum-enquiries	—		1	10.5	1	10.5	1	14	1	17.5
(m)	Welfare/Labour officer	—		—		1	14	1	21	1	21
(n)	Stationery/Records	1	10.5	1	21						
(o)	Security Officer	1	21	1	21	2	21	3	21	4	21
(p)	Lavatory for staff (Separate for males)	—		1	28	1	28	1	35	1	35
MEDICAL RECORDS DEPT.											
	Medical records storage (a) Active (up to 2 years)	—		—		1	28	1	42	1	56
(b)	Inactive (between 2 and 10 years)	—		—		1	84	1	126	1	140
	Medical records officer with toilet	—		—		1	21	1	17.5	1	17.5
	Staff office with toilet	—		—				1	17.5	1	17.5
	Medical records processing area	—		—		1	21	1	28	1	35
	Doctor's record completion room	—		—		1	21	1	14	1	14
	Room for various automations	—		—				1	14	1	14
	Printed stationery store	—		—		1	17.5	1	10.5	1	14
	General store	—		—				1	10.5	1	14

Built Environment: General Considerations

TABLE 31D: General Considerations for Built Environment in Administration Units

Environmental Considerations

Acoustics	• Acoustic performance and sound levels should be designed and documented to meet the function of the spaces being provided.
	• Acoustic consideration should be given to the following during the design process:
	• Acoustic separation of meeting and interview rooms to reduce the noise between rooms, particularly if used for tele-conferencing, video-conferencing, and large meetings.
	• Acoustic separation should be provided among offices, meeting rooms, interview rooms, and adjacent corridors to reduce transfer of noise among rooms, particularly private conversations that should not be audible outside the room.
	• Location of waiting areas away from offices and meeting and interview rooms
	• Location of staff rooms away from public areas, offices and meeting rooms
Natural Light/Lighting	Maximize the provision of natural light to areas where staff offices and workstations are located. Artificial lighting should be arranged to avoid glare on computer screens.
Privacy	Visual privacy must be considered where confidential conversations are likely to take place in offices and meeting and interview rooms.

Space Standards and Components

Accessibility	Reception, offices, meeting rooms, and waiting areas should be designed to provide access for people in wheelchairs.
Ergonomics	• The design process and selection of furniture, fittings, fixtures, and equipment must consider ergonomics and occupational health and safety (OH&S) aspects to avoid injuries to staff and visitors.
	• Particular attention should be given to design of workstations and storage areas. Adjustable-height workstations may be considered.
	• Shelving in storage areas should be placed at suitable reach heights.

(Continued)

TABLE 31D: (Continued)

Size of the Unit	The size of the Administration Unit will depend on the size and level of service of the health facility, as determined by the facility's service plan and operational policies.
Finishes	The Administration Unit décor should be pleasant and professional in character. Finishes should be selected with consideration of the following: • Acoustic properties of the materials; the use of carpet and acoustic panels will assist in absorption of sound. • Durability, replacement, and cleaning of materials. • Fire safety of the materials.
Safety and Security	The Administration Unit should include the following security considerations: • Entry to the Administration Unit, Reception and waiting area may require restricted access such as an electronic card reader, with an intercom/phone, CCTV, and remote door release at Reception. • All offices require lockable doors. • Rooms located on the perimeter of the unit should be locked when they are not in use. • All storerooms for files, records, and equipment should be lockable. • After-hours access that may be required to some offices and meeting rooms and may also involve security personnel.
Infection Control	• Infection control measures applicable to the Administration Unit will involve prevention of cross-infection between staff and visitors. • Hand hygiene is an essential element, and provision of medicated hand gel dispensers or hand wipes at the reception and in circulation corridors is recommended.

Building Service Requirements

Communications	The Administration Unit has a managing role in the facility and requires reliable and effective IT/communications service for efficient operation of the service. The IT design should address • Hospital networking requirements including wireless networks • Video-conferencing and tele-conferencing. • Communications and server room/s. • Telephone systems including cordless and mobile phones. • Computers, mainframes, laptops, and hand-held devices. • Duress alarms and master paging system for staff and emergencies
HVAC	Offices, open plan workstation areas and meeting, interview, and staff rooms should be air conditioned for the benefit of staff and visitors to the unit. The local or country-specific mechanical requirements should be consulted.

TABLE 31E: Specific Room and Functional Requirements for Built Environment in Administration Units

Entry/Reception/Waiting Areas	• Reception is the first point of contact with the Administration Unit for visitors and may act as an access control point to restrict access and direct visitors to the area required. • Waiting areas should be located nearby and be suitable for a range of occupants including those in wheelchairs. • Smaller waiting areas may be provided close to offices as required.

Administration Areas	• Administration areas may be provided as offices and workstations within one unit to promote collaboration between divisions.
	The number of offices provided will be according to the endorsed full-time positions required for the Administration Unit, depending on the size of the facility and the operational policies.
	• Consideration should be given to provision of the following:
	  • Separate offices, shared offices, and workstations where possible for executive, finance, and clinical staff who are required to be situated in the Administration Unit according to the facility's service plan.
	  • Specialized administration functions such as quality management, public relations, etc. as required according to the service plan.
	  • Offices for roster management, staff allocation, and bed allocation staff who may require access after hours.

Support Areas	• Support areas for the Administration Unit, including stores for files and stationery, should be located convenient to staff requiring frequent access. • Secured storage should be provided for confidential records including administration, finance, and human resources records. • Meeting rooms with tele- or video-conferencing facilities provide for meeting flexibility with remote staff. • A large meeting room may be used for disaster management and board meetings. • If multipurpose meeting rooms are provided, then they may be located to enable sharing by several services or units. • Meeting room/s should have access to a pantry for food and beverages as necessary.
Staff Area	Staff room/s and dining areas should include a beverage bay or access to a pantry for use during meal breaks. Staff room/s and toilets may be shared with adjacent units where possible.

31.5 Summary

Planning and designing the Administration Unit of a hospital is a vital process that plays a crucial role in the effective management and coordination of health care services. The Administration Unit serves as the backbone of the hospital, overseeing various functions such as financial management, human resources, scheduling, billing, and overall operations. Key considerations in the planning and designing process include creating an ergonomic and functional workspace, optimizing workflow and communication channels, implementing efficient information management systems, ensuring accessibility and privacy for staff and patients, and incorporating technology solutions for streamlined operations. By prioritizing these factors and engaging experts in health care administration, hospitals can establish a well-designed administration unit that supports efficient processes, enhances productivity, and ultimately contributes to the delivery of high-quality health care services.

32 HOSPITAL ENGINEERING AND MAINTENANCE UNITS

32.1 Hospital Engineering and Maintenance Units and Context

Engineering services are perhaps the most vital of the utility services in a hospital. The efficiency of an entire patient care delivery system of a hospital depends on their efficiency. Even the slightest breakdown of a power supply system, information system, or communication system or malfunctioning of vital equipment can have catastrophic effects.

The scope of engineering services in a hospital comprises civil assets, electricity supply, water supply including plumbing and fittings, steam supply, central medical gases, air and clinical vacuum delivery system, air conditioning and refrigeration, lifts and dumb waiters, public health services, lightening protection, structured cabling, communication system (public address system, telephones, and paging system), TV and piped music system, non-conventional energy devices, horticulture, arboriculture, and landscaping, and workshop facilities for repairs and maintenance.

The scope of services generally includes repair and maintenance of existing facilities to ensure optimum operational reliability, risk reduction, and their safety for the patient, staff, and public. Initial planning and building of civil assets is to be included in the scope of services.

(a) **Objectives of Hospital Engineering and Maintenance Units**
  - To plan and implement a planned preventive maintenance and repair facility for hospitals and medical institutions
  - To ensure that all facilities, systems, and services under the scope of engineering services are in a state of optimum operational efficiency.
  - To provide consultancy service to various department on electromedical equipment in the area of pre-installation and operation of equipment.
  - To conduct training and research in clinical engineering.

(b) **Functions of Hospital Engineering and Maintenance Units**
  - Planning and implementation of a program of planned preventive maintenance in all facilities/services under their responsibility.
  - Ensuring that all facilities, systems, and services under the scope of engineering services are well-maintained and kept in a state of optimum operational efficiency.
  - Maintaining an up-to-date inventory of all the equipment available and their distribution in the hospital.
  - Maintaining an up-to-date history sheet for every single unit of equipment in the hospital.
  - Anticipating the requirements of commonly required spares and arranging for their adequate stocking.
  - Ensuring that break-down maintenance is prompt enough to ensure uninterrupted services. This, however, does not include sophisticated/electronic equipment that should be better handled under the arrangement by suppliers.
  - Ensuring that the facilities/services coming under their scope are safe and hazard-free.
  - Ensuring that the facilities/services under their scope comply with the relevant legal provisions.
  - Ensuring that the facilities/services provided under their scope of responsibility are conductive to efficient and high-quality patient care.
  - Ensuring timely action for renewal of maintenance contracts/insurance cover of the facilities/equipment under their purview.
  - Ensuring that the services under their scope are provided at the minimum possible operating costs.
  - Playing an active role in successful planning and implementation of an equipment audit program.
  - Advising management about the most cost-effective ways of managing the facilities/services under their purview (saving of energy/water and purchase of equipment with low life-cycle cost and high efficiency).
  - A program of continuous training of staff.
  - Planning and implementing a program of quality management of the engineering services department.

32.2 Hospital Engineering and Maintenance Units and Wider Hospital Context: Location & Access

The Engineering and Maintenance Unit should be located on the ground floor to facilitate delivery and dispatch of heavy items of equipment. Access to a loading dock is desirable. The unit will require ready access to all areas of the hospital and in particular, to plant rooms and areas. Depending on the size of the unit and the operational policy, considerable noise and fumes may be generated by the unit, and care should be taken in locating the unit relative to other units such as Inpatient Accommodation Units.

32.3 Functional Areas

The Engineering and Maintenance Unit may consist of the following functional areas depending on the operational policy and service demand:

(a) **Reception areas:** The needs of a reception area are distinctly different from the equipment service area. The reception area will be used to receive the customers and business partners of the clinical engineering department. Comfortable seating in good repair is needed to accommodate these guests. The design of the reception area typically supports the administrative work processes of the department and hence typically includes such things as computers, printers, fax machines, copiers, filing cabinets, and desk furniture. Much of the office equipment can be hidden in well-designed closets that are opened as needed for access. In this manner, the clutter of the workspace is minimized while accommodating convenient access.

DOI: 10.1201/9780367460884-33

(b) **Workshop areas:** A general maintenance workshop should be provided for repair and maintenance. Sufficient space is required for a workbench, drill press, angle grinder, stainless steel trough, tool peg board, and storage cabinets. Floor space is also required for the standing of equipment during repairs. Adequate lighting, power, and ventilation are required. If maintenance services are externally contracted, then a workshop is not required. Maintenance workshops incorporating carpentry, metal fabrication, plumbing, refrigeration, or other noise-generating trades should be acoustically isolated from non-maintenance areas.

(c) **Electronics workshop:** A separate workshop may be provided specifically for the storage, repair, and testing of electronic and other medical equipment. The amount of space and type of utilities will vary with the type of equipment involved and types of service and maintenance contracts used.

(d) **Storage areas:** Storage areas for all specialty services/trades including paint, gardening, and flammable liquids must be provided.

(e) **Office areas for administrative and clerical activities:** Offices are required for full-time management of staff, including engineer/head of department, with file space and provision for protected storage of facility drawings, records, and manuals.

(f) **Staff amenities:** The following, including other amenities, must be provided:
  • Handwashing facilities located close to all workshop areas.
  • Toilet, shower, and lockers, which may be shared with the main hospital.
  • Staff room that may be shared with the main hospital.

(g) Training areas.

(h) Staff amenities, which may be shared.

(i) A refuse room for trash storage located conveniently near a service entrance and one janitor's closet on each floor.

32.4 Key Result Areas and Indicators for Evaluating Quality of Services of Hospital Engineering and Maintenance Units

The important key result areas and indicators for evaluating the quality of services of a Hospital Engineering and Maintenance Unit are given in Table 32A.

TABLE 32A: Key Result Areas and Indicators for Evaluating Quality of Services of Hospital Engineering and Maintenance Units

Key Result Areas
• Service scope to be clearly defined.
• Adequate and appropriate infrastructure and human resources.
• Turnaround time.
• Mechanism to address recall of equipment.
• Documented policies and procedure.
• Quality assurance and quality control.
• Regular training of staff.
• Feedback to stakeholders.
• Safety program documented including usage of safety equipment.
• Maintenance and storage of records.
• Appropriate signage.
• Maintenance plan for facility, furniture, and equipment.
• Waste management.
• Fire safety.

Indicators for Evaluating Quality of Services
• Number of complaints from the patients about lighting, ventilation, air conditioning, water supply (hot/cold), and leaking taps.
• Number of complaints from the departments about slip/trip or fall with or without any injuries.
• Number of complaints from the departments about malfunctioning of equipment or nurse call system.
• Frequency of power failures and time taken for restoration of power (should not be more than 10 seconds).
• Frequency of cancellation of surgical/other procedures due to lack of power supply.
• Incidence of fire/other hazards such as collapse of building/plaster falling off the ceiling/walls, short circuiting, and gaseous explosions.
• Response time for attending to and restoration of operational status.
• Incidence of malfunctioning of equipment during a procedure.
• Observations by the equipment audit committee.
• Incidence of lifts getting stuck and time taken fore rescue of passengers.
• Observations from the regulating authorities about non-compliance with legal provisions.
• Frequency of complaints from OT/cardiac catheter lab/labour room/nursery about faulty temperature/humidity control.
• Critical equipment down time.

Internal & External Functional Relationships (Figure 32A)

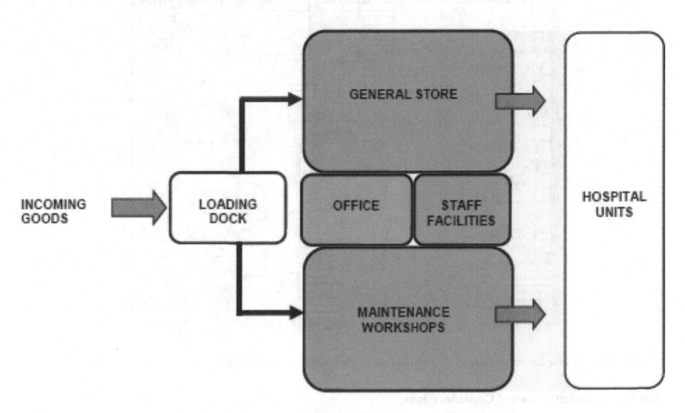

FIGURE 32A   Functional Relationships of Engineering and Maintenance Units (Courtesy: iHFG).

TABLE 32B: Major Space Determinants and Size of Engineering and Maintenance Units

ROOM/SPACE	Standard Component	Level 4 Qty × m²	Remarks
OFFICE—SINGLE PERSON 12 m²	OFF-S12-I	1 × 12	If Engineer on staff
STORE—PLAN FILE	STGN-12–1	1 × 12 Optional	
STORE—FLAMMABLE LIQUID	STFL-I	1 × 9	Or Steel Cupboard
WORKSHOP/STORE— GARDENING	WSS-GAR-I	1 × 12	
PAINTER'S STORE	STFL-I STGN-9–1	1 × 9 optional	Store flammable liquids in appropriate cabinets
WORKSHOP—CARPENTRY	WK-CA-I	1 × 30 optional	Including storage
WORKSHOP—MECHANICAL	WK-MC-I	1 × 30 optional	Including storage
WORKSHOP—PLUMBING	WK-PL-I	1 × 30 optional	Including storage
CIRCULATION ALLOWANCE %		15%	
Shared Areas			
BAY—CLEAN-IP	BCL-1.5-I	1 × 1.5	
STAFF ROOM	SRM-15-I	1 × 15	
TOILET—STAFF	WCST-I	2 × 3	Separate Male/Female where applicable

Layout (Figure 32B)

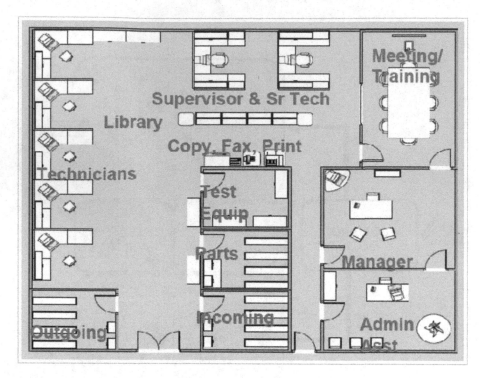

FIGURE 32B   Sample Layout of Engineering and Maintenance Units (Courtesy: iHFG).

Built Environment: General Considerations

TABLE 32C: General Considerations for Built Environment in Engineering and Maintenance Units

HVAC   Air conditioning systems should be provided that can maintain temperature and relative humidity at or between the following ranges:
- Temperature: 23 +2°C.
- Relative Humidity: 50–60%.

Acoustics
- Noise levels should be as defined in the BCA and AS/NZS 2107.
- Acoustic guidelines for hospital engineering and maintenance unit is given as follows.

Room/Space	(dBA)*	RT(sec)*
Assembly/preparation, reception/clerical lounge/activity room	40-50	<0.5
Staff room, staff station	40-45	<0.7
Office staff and technical support	35-45	<0.7

*A-weighted decibels; **Reverberation time

Vibration   Vibration in occupied spaces should be as per the level defined by AS 2670.1. Vibration precautions should include the following:
- Dynamic balancing of machines.
- Isolation of sources of vibration from vibration transmission paths (e.g., machines from pipes, ducts, support structures, etc.).
- Piping being designed to avoid pressure pulse noise or being fitted with effective pulse dampers.
- Structures being isolated from ground transmitted vibrations.
- Equipment being selected and supported to avoid operation at resonant frequencies.

Communications   Voice and telephone communications should be installed within the unit to allow contact with outside personnel and between different areas in the unit.

Data Communications   There should be a data network linking information and computing workstations. The data network should at least involve the following:
- Provide a locked accommodation allocated exclusively to network servers and a main cable distribution hub.
- Have cabling from main to sub-distribution hubs running in dedicated channels in ducts or on trays.
- Have sub-distribution hubs located in locked cupboards where required.
- Except for sub-compartments within compartments required by the building code of Australia (BCA), a hub should not serve more than one fire compartment.
- Have cabling between sub-hubs and data workstations terminating in wall sockets within 2,000 mm of the computing equipment to be connected.

(Continued)

TABLE 32C: (Continued)

Electrical Services	• Provision of normal, vital (30 seconds), instantaneous (1 second), and uninterruptible (no break) electricity supplies. • Switchgear and circuit protection to safely operate and control the supplies. • Distribution arrangements to supply electricity to each end use. • Equipment to transform and condition voltages from supply voltage to end use voltage and within voltage and frequency tolerances. • Equipment to use the electricity for lighting, heating, and motive power. • Where an electrical supply is denoted as being on an "essential supply", then this should be arranged as a vital (30 seconds) supply.
Lighting	• This should take into account the lux requirements of the clinical engineering department. Special precaution for security requirements at entry points, car park, and unattended areas should be considered. • General lighting: 200–300 lux. • Task lighting: 400–500 lux. • Corridors: 100–150 lux. • Natural light and windows permitting outside views are highly desirable within the unit. However, such provisions should not compromise the security of the unit. • Windows should not permit casual viewing from any adjacent public thoroughfare.
Ergonomics/OH&S	• Consideration should be given to the ergonomic functionality in the unit. • Benches, sinks, and packing workstations should be provided at suitable working heights. • Adjustable-height equipment is recommended. • Manual handling of heavy instruments that may require lifting equipment.
Finishes	Wall protection should be installed to prevent damage to walls caused by all types of equipment.
Floors	• Floor finishes should be hard-wearing, non-slip, easy to clean, of a uniform level, and suitable for heavy trolley traffic. • Structural expansion points should be positioned with care in heavy traffic areas particularly where trolleys turn corners. • Flooring should have integrated coved skirting continuous with the floor.
Fire Safety	Fire safety provided must comply with NBC, 2016. Compartmentation of the building(s) into fire and smoke control compartments. • Provision of complying fire egress arrangements. • Provision of fire and smoke alarms. • Storage arrangements for firefighting water. • Firefighting water pressure boosting arrangements. • Provision of smoke-clearing ventilation. • Smoke mode controls for ventilation plant. • Provision of escape route air pressurization. • Provision of emergency warning and information equipment. • Provision of hose reel and hydrant fire extinguishing equipment. • Provision of automatic fire extinguishing systems. • Provision of portable fire extinguishers and fire blankets. • Provision of equipment to aid transportation of disabled persons. • Provision of escape diagrams.

32.5 Summary

The Engineering and Maintenance Unit is responsible for the operation, maintenance, and repair of the hospital's infrastructure, equipment, and systems. Key considerations in the planning and designing process include efficient space allocation for workshops, storage, and equipment, incorporation of safety protocols and regulations, integration of advanced technologies for preventive maintenance and energy efficiency, ensuring accessibility for maintenance staff, and provision for future expansion. By prioritizing these factors and involving experts in engineering and facility management, hospitals can establish a well-designed Engineering and Maintenance Unit that contributes to the reliability, sustainability, and optimal functioning of the health care facility, ultimately supporting the delivery of high-quality patient care.

33 SUPPLY UNIT

33.1 Introduction

The Supply Unit should provide for the following functions:

- Purchase and receipt of equipment and bulk medical supplies
- Storage of bulk dry goods, consumables, intravenous fluids, drugs, and flammable liquids
- Storage of emergency stock for the facility
- Storage of surplus hospital equipment and equipment awaiting repairs
- Deliveries to hospital units for regular re-stocking of unit-based supplies

33.2 Supply Units and Wider Hospital Context: Location, Access, and Functional Relationships

The Supply Unit may be located in a separate building on-site, but the preferred location is within the main building. A portion of the storage may be located off-site. Protection against inclement weather during transfer of supplies should be provided. Fire protection and security are important considerations.

The bulk store is the primary storage area for all delivered supplies and storage prior to distribution to various hospital units. It should be located with ready access to the loading dock area. This area requires security and controlled access.

The bulk store should be located within easy access to a services/goods lift for transportation of materials to the hospital units. The corridor should permit two-way traffic of bulky items, and its access should be restricted to the public. The functional relationships of a Supply Unit is shown in Figure 33A.

33.3 Operational Models

The Supply Unit will generally operate during the day with limited entry provisions after hours.

33.4 Planning Models

The Supply Unit will consist of a number of rooms and areas for storing high volumes of goods, equipment, and furniture as necessary. The rooms may vary in sizes depending on the items to be stored and the frequency of stock delivery. The storage areas may be centrally located within the Supply Unit with satellite storage rooms provided closer to the areas requiring specific stock items.

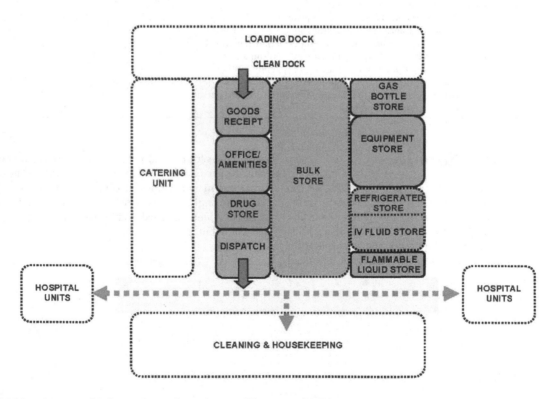

FIGURE 33A   Functional Relationships of Supply Unit (Courtesy: iHFG).

DOI: 10.1201/9780367460884-34

TABLE 33A: Major Space Determinants and Supply Unit Size

ROOM/SPACE	RDL 3 Qty × m²	RDL 4 Qty × m²	RDL 5 Qty × m²	RDL 6 Qty × m²	Remarks
Supply Areas					
Dispatch Area	1 × 3	1 × 12	1 × 20	1 × 20	
Goods Receipt	1 × 3	1 × 8	1 × 12	1 × 20	
Loading Dock—Clean	1 × 0	1 × 0	1 × 0	1 × 0	External space that may be shared with other back-of-house services. Area as required.
Store—Bulk	1 × 50	1 × 100	1 × 100	1 × 150	Size according to requirements.
Store—Drugs	1 × 5	1 × 5	1 × 10	1 × 10	Optional. May be located in the Pharmacy Unit.
Store—Equipment	1 × 25	1 × 25	1 × 50	1 × 50	
Store—Flammable Liquid	1 × 9	1 × 9	1 × 9	1 × 9	
Store—Gas Bottles	2 × 5	2 × 5	2 × 10	2 × 10	Full and empty bottles to be stored separately. May be located externally at a secure location.
Store—IV Fluids	1 × 10	1 × 20	1 × 20	1 × 30	May be located within Store—Bulk.
Store—Refrigerated	1 × 5	1 × 5	1 × 10	1 × 10	Optional. May be located as refrigerator bay within Store—Bulk.
Subtotal	130.0	1940	251.0	319.0	
Circulation %	20	20	20	20	
Area Total	156.0	232.8		382.8	
Support Areas					
Office—Single Person, 12 m²			1 × 12	1 × 12	For Supply Unit manager
Office—Single Person, 9 m²	1 × 9	2 × 9	1 × 9	1 × 9	For Supply Unit manager or purchasing manager
Office—2 Persons Shared			1 × 12	1 × 12	For purchasing officers
Office—Workstation	1 × 5.5	2 × 5.5	2 × 5.5	4 × 12	For purchasing officers or supply personnel
Property Bay—Staff	2 × 2	2 × 2	2 × 6	2 × 6	Separate for male and female
Toilet—Staff (Male/Female)	2 × 3	2 × 3	4 × 3	4 × 3	Separate for male and female
Subtotal	24.5	39.0	68.0	105.0	
Circulation %	20	20	20	20	
Area Total	29.4	46.8	81.6	126.0	
Grand Total	185.4	279.6	382.8	508.8	

Built Environment: General Considerations

TABLE 33B: General Considerations for Built Environment in Supply Units

Natural Light/Lighting	Provide natural light to office and staff areas where possible apart from artificial lighting.
Ergonomics	Consideration should be given to the need for manual handling devices such as dock levellers and lifters. A well-designed and equipped work area will eliminate injuries resulting from manual handling.
Finishes	• Door and wall protection should be installed to prevent damage to walls caused by all types of trolleys, lifting/transport equipment, and movement of large items. • Sturdy wall protection such as rubber or timber wall protection is recommended to withstand impacts from trolleys, pallet jacks, and other bulky transporting equipment. • Solid core door with stainless steel door and door frame protection is recommended to avoid chipping and breakage. • Floor finish is to be non-slip, impervious, easy to clean, and hard-wearing. Movement of large equipment and lifting/transporting equipment are to be considered when choosing an appropriate floor finish.
Safety and Security	• All entrances and exits should be secured. An intercom or call bell should be located at the dock entrance area to announce deliveries when doors are closed. • Where required, concave directional mirrors along corridors and bends should be provided to avoid collision of oversized trolleys, motorised transporters, and staff. • Design of the Supply Unit should ensure that storage areas are free from insects and vermin. • Flammable liquids and items must be stored in a room designed according to relevant national/international regulations. • Exhaust should be provided in rooms for storing and recharging of pallet jacks, motorised transporters, and other equipment depending on battery type to avoid build-up of noxious gases.
Infection Control	• Handwashing facilities should be located in the Supply Unit.
Building Service Requirements	Natural light is not required in storage areas; however, adequate lighting is required in storage areas to avoid shaded spots where accidents can occur.

TABLE 33C: Specific Room and Functional Requirements for Built Environment in Supply Units

Loading Dock	The loading dock should be a covered area for transport access to service units for delivery or collection of goods and should be zoned into clean and dirty areas.
Goods Receipt Area	• A dedicated goods receipt area should be provided for the receipt, checking, sorting, and temporary holding of incoming stock. • The goods receipt area will require off-street unloading facilities. • The goods receipt area should be located adjacent to the loading dock and with ready access to the bulk store. • Security for incoming stock will require consideration. Visual control of the area from the store manager's office is recommended to discourage dumping/leaving of deliveries without proper receiving by stores personnel. • The goods receipt area may include a workstation with a computer.
Dispatch Area	The dispatch area may be used to hold stores that are ready to be delivered to hospital units or stores that are ready to be collected by external contractors such as loaned equipment and incorrect deliveries. It should be located with easy access to the loading dock.
Storage Area (Bulk)	• The size of storage areas will be determined by the type of items to be stored and the frequency of stock delivery. • Stocks are to be stored in heavy-duty shelving or on clean pallets that should elevate the goods off the floor. • Cool room or refrigerators may be required for delivered items that have to be kept at cooler temperatures while awaiting delivery or pick-up to designated units within the facility. • If sterile items are to be stored in the Supply Unit, then it is recommended that they are stored separately from non-sterile items. • Sterile items are recommended to be stored in shelving that is a minimum of 250 mm from the floor and not too close to the ceiling. • IV fluids may be stored in a designated area within the bulk store if the IV fluid storage area is not already provided in the Pharmacy Unit.
Storage Area (Equipment)	• This area is used for the storage of medical equipment and some furniture for use in the facility. • Equipment such as infusion pumps will also be recharged in this room. • Additional storage areas for equipment for loan to patients and outpatients should be provided in an amount not less than 5% of the total area of the outpatient facilities. This may be combined with and in addition to the equipment store or be located in a central area within the Outpatient Unit. This storage requirement is generally for therapy equipment and mobility aids loaned to patients. A portion of this storage area may be provided off-site.

33.5 Summary

Planning and designing a hospital Supply Unit is a critical process that ensures the efficient management and distribution of medical supplies and equipment within a health care facility. The Supply Unit plays a vital role in supporting patient care, maintaining inventory control, and optimizing resource utilization. Key considerations in the planning and designing process include adequate space for storage and organization and integration of technology for inventory management, efficient workflow design, and adherence to infection control protocols. By prioritizing these factors and engaging experts in supply chain management and hospital design, health care facilities can establish well-designed Supply Units that enhance operational efficiency, reduce costs, and ensure the availability of essential supplies for quality patient care.

References

Chapter	Reference
13.	TAHPI. International health facility guidelines; emergency unit. www.healthfacilityguidelines.com/ViewPDF/ViewIndexPDF/iHFG_part_b_emergency_unit
	Office of DGAFMS, Ministry of Defence, Government of India. Scales of accommodation for armed forces hospitals, 2003.
	NHS. HBN 12: Outpatient department. www.england.nhs.uk/wp-content/uploads/2021/05/HBN_12.pdf.
	NHSRC. National Quality Assurance Standards for Public Healthcare Facilities, 2020. http://qi.nhsrcindia.org/cms-detail/revised-national-quality-assurance-standards/MjM3.
	MoHFW, GoI. Clinical establishment (registration and regulation) Act, 2010. Clinical Establishment Act standard for clinic/polyclinic only consultation. https://clinicalestablishments.gov.in/WriteReadData/9361.pdf.
	Directorate General of Health Services, Ministry of Health & Family Welfare, Government of India. IPHS guidelines for district hospitals (101 to 500 bedded), 2021. https://nhm.gov.in/images/pdf/guidelines/iphs/iphs-revised-guidlines-2012/district-hospital.pdf.
14.	TAHPI. International Health Facility Guidelines; Intensive Care Unit. www.healthfacilityguidelines.com/ViewPDF/ViewIndexPDF/iHFG_part_b_intensive_care_unit_general.
	Office of DGAFMS, Ministry of Defence, Government of India. Scales of Accommodation for Armed Forces Hospitals, 2003.
	NHS. HBN 12: Outpatient department, www.england.nhs.uk/wp-content/uploads/2021/05/HBN_12.pdf
	NHSRC. National Quality Assurance Standards for Public Healthcare Facilities, 2020. http://qi.nhsrcindia.org/cms-detail/revised-national-quality-assurance-standards/MjM3.
	MoHFW, GoI. Clinical Establishment (Registration and Regulation) Act, 2010. Clinical Establishment Act Standard for Clinic/Polyclinic only Consultation. https://clinicalestablishments.gov.in/WriteReadData/9361.pdf.
	Directorate General of Health Services, Ministry of Health & Family Welfare, Government of India. IPHS guidelines for district hospitals (101 to 500 bedded), 2021. https://nhm.gov.in/images/pdf/guidelines/iphs/iphs-revised-guidlines-2012/district-hospital.pdf

Ogaji DS, Mezie-Okoye MM. Waiting time and patient satisfaction: Survey of patients seeking care at the general outpatient clinic of the University of Port Harcourt Teaching Hospital. Port Harcourt Medical Journal. 2017;11(3):148.

15.   TAHPI. International Health Facility Guidelines; Intensive Care Unit. www.healthfacilityguidelines.com/ViewPDF/ViewIndexPDF/iHFG_part_b_intensive_care_unit_general.

AHIA. Australasian Health Facility Guidelines; Part B: Health facility briefing and planning; 360: Intensive Care Unit. https://aushfg-prod-com-au.s3.amazonaws.com/HPU_B.0360_7.pdf.

NHS. HBN 04-02: Critical Care Units. www.england.nhs.uk/wp-content/uploads/2021/05/HBN_04-02_Final.pdf.

Rungta N, Zirpe KG, Dixit SB, Mehta Y, Chaudhry D, Govil D, Mishra RC, Sharma J, Amin P, Rao BK, Khilnani GC. Indian society of critical care medicine experts committee consensus statement on ICU planning and designing, 2020. Indian journal of Critical Care Medicine: Peer-Reviewed, Official Publication of Indian Society of Critical Care Medicine. 2020;24(Suppl 1):S43.

Thompson DR, Hamilton DK, Cadenhead CD, Swoboda SM, Schwindel SM, Anderson DC, Schmitz EV, Andre AC, Axon DC, Harrell JW, Harvey MA. Guidelines for intensive care unit design. Critical Care Medicine. 2012;40(5):1586–1600.

Infection Control Directorate, Ministry of Health, State of Kuwait. Guidelines for ICU design, 2008. www.icdkwt.com/pdf/policiesandguidelines/DesignandConstruction/GuidelinesforIntensiveCareUnitsDesign-2008.pdf.

Office of DGAFMS, Ministry of Defence, Government of India. Scales of Accommodation for Armed Forces Hospitals, 2003.

NHSRC. National Quality Assurance Standards for Public Healthcare Facilities, 2020. http://qi.nhsrcindia.org/cms-detail/revised-national-quality-assurance-standards/MjM3.

MoHFW, GoI. Clinical Establishment (Registration and Regulation) Act, 2010. Clinical Establishment Act Standard for Clinic/Polyclinic only Consultation. https://clinicalestablishments.gov.in/WriteReadData/9361.pdf.

Directorate General of Health Services, Ministry of Health & Family Welfare, Government of India. IPHS Guidelines for Sub District Hospital and District Hospital, 2022. https://nhsrcindia.org/sites/default/files/Volume%201_SDH-DH_0.pdf.

16.   NHSRC. National Quality Assurance Standards for Public Healthcare Facilities, 2020. http://qi.nhsrcindia.org/cms-detail/revised-national-quality-assurance-standards/MjM3.

Office of DGAFMS, Ministry of Defence, Government of India. Scales of Accommodation for Armed Forces Hospitals, 2003.

Directorate General of Health Services, Ministry of Health & Family Welfare, Government of India. IPHS Guidelines for District Hospitals (101 to 500 bedded), 2021. https://nhm.gov.in/images/pdf/guidelines/iphs/iphs-revised-guidlines-2012/district-hospital.pdf.

TAHPI. International Health Facility Guidelines; Operating Unit. www.healthfacilityguidelines.com/ViewPDF/ViewIndexPDF/iHFG_part_b_operating_unit.

NHS. HBN 26: Facilities for surgical procedures volume 1. www.england.nhs.uk/wp-content/uploads/2021/05/HBN_26.pdf.

Barach PR, Rostenberg B. Design of cardiac surgery operating rooms and the impact of the built environment. In *Pediatric and Congenital Cardiac Care* (pp. 411–424). Springer, 2015.

Infection Control Directorate, Ministry of Health, State of Kuwait. Guidelines for design of operation theatres, 2007. www.icdkwt.com/pdf/policiesandguidelines/DesignandConstruction/GuidelinesforDesignofOperatingTheater-2007.pdf.

FGI. Hybrid Operating Room Design Basics, 2018. www.fgiguidelines.org/wp-content/uploads/2019/01/FGI-Hybrid-OR-Design-Basics.pdf.

MoHFW, GoI. Clinical Establishment (Registration and Regulation) Act, 2010. Clinical Establishment Act Standard for Hospital (Level 3). http://clinicalestablishments.gov.in/WriteReadData/776.pdf.

17.   NHSRC. National Quality Assurance Standards for Public Healthcare Facilities, 2020. http://qi.nhsrcindia.org/cms-detail/revised-national-quality-assurance-standards/MjM3.

Office of DGAFMS, Ministry of Defence, Government of India. Scales of Accommodation for Armed Forces Hospitals, 2003.

Directorate General of Health Services, Ministry of Health & Family Welfare, Government of India. IPHS Guidelines for District Hospitals (101 to 500 bedded), 2021. https://nhm.gov.in/images/pdf/guidelines/iphs/iphs-revised-guidlines-2012/district-hospital.pdf.

MoHFW, GoI. Clinical Establishment (Registration and Regulation) Act, 2010. Clinical Establishment Act Standard for Hospital (Level 3). http://clinicalestablishments.gov.in/WriteReadData/776.pdf.

TAHPI. International Health Facility Guidelines; Maternity Unit. www.healthfacilityguidelines.com/ViewPDF/ViewIndexPDF/iHFG_part_b_maternity_unit.

NHS. HBN 09-02: Maternity Care Facilities. www.england.nhs.uk/wp-content/uploads/2021/05/HBN_09-02_Final.pdf.

NHM, MoHFW, GoI. LAQSHYA. Labour room quality improvement initiative, 2017. https://nhm.gov.in/New_Updates_2018/NHM_Components/RMNCH_MH_Guidelines/LaQshya-Guidelines.pdf.

Griffin J, Xia S, Peng S, Keskinocak P. Improving patient flow in an obstetric unit. Health Care Management Science. 2012;15(1):1–4.

18.   TAHPI. International Health Facility Guidelines. In Patient Unit. www.healthfacilityguidelines.com/ViewPDF/ViewIndexPDF/iHFG_part_b_inpatient_unit_general.

Office of DGAFMS, Ministry of Defence, Government of India. Scales of Accommodation for Armed Forces Hospitals, 2003.

NHS. HBN 04-01: Adult in-patient facilities. www.england.nhs.uk/wp-content/uploads/2021/05/HBN_04-01_Final.pdf.

NHSRC. National Quality Assurance Standards for Public Healthcare Facilities, 2020. http://qi.nhsrcindia.org/cms-detail/revised-national-quality-assurance-standards/MjM3.

Directorate General of Health Services, Ministry of Health & Family Welfare, Government of India. IPHS Guidelines for Sub District Hospital and District Hospital, 2022. https://nhsrcindia.org/sites/default/files/Volume%201_SDH-DH_0.pdf.

MoHFW, GoI. Clinical Establishment (Registration and Regulation) Act, 2010. Clinical Establishment Act Standard for Hospital (Level 3). http://clinicalestablishments.gov.in/WriteReadData/776.pdf.

19.   TAHPI. International Health Facility Guidelines; Medical Imaging Unit. www.healthfacilityguidelines.com/ViewPDF/ViewIndexPDF/iHFG_part_b_medical_imaging_general.

Office of DGAFMS, Ministry of Defence, Government of India. Scales of Accommodation for Armed Forces Hospitals, 2003.

NHS. HBN 06: Facilities for Diagnostic Imaging and Interventional Radiology. www.england.nhs.uk/wp-content/uploads/2021/05/HBN_6_V1_DSSA.pdf.

AHIA. Australasian Health Facility Guidelines. Part B—Health Facility Briefing and Planning; 440—Medical Imaging Unit. https://aushfg-prod-com-au.s3.amazonaws.com/%5BB-0440%5D%20Medical%20Imaging%20Unit.pdf.

AERB. Regulatory Requirements for Diagnostic Radiology Facilities. www.aerb.gov.in/images/PDF/DiagnosticRadiology/3.4.1-Regulatory-requirements-for-diagnostic-radiology-facilities.pdf.

AERB. Guidelines for Shielding of X-Ray Installations. www.aerb.gov.in/images/PDF/layout_guidelines.pdf.

AERB. Sample Layout Plan for Radiography Facility. www.aerb.gov.in/images/PDF/DiagnosticRadiology/Model-Layout---X-ray-Radiography-Installation.pdf.

AERB. Sample Layout Plan for CT. www.aerb.gov.in/images/PDF/DiagnosticRadiology/Model-Layout-CT-Scan.pdf.

AERB. Sample Layout Plan for Interventional Radiology Facility. www.aerb.gov.in/images/PDF/DiagnosticRadiology/Model-Layout---Interventional-Radiology-Installation.pdf.

AERB. Sample Layout Plan for Mammography. www.aerb.gov.in/images/PDF/Mammo.pdf.

AERB. Sample Layout Plan for BMD. www.aerb.gov.in/english/regulatory-facilities/radiation-facilities/application-in-medicine/diagnostic-radiology.

NHSRC. National Quality Assurance Standards for Public Healthcare Facilities, 2020. http://qi.nhsrcindia.org/cms-detail/revised-national-quality-assurance-standards/MjM3.

MoHFW, GoI. Clinical Establishment (Registration and Regulation) Act, 2010. Clinical Establishment Act Standard for Clinic/Polyclinic only Consultation. https://clinicalestablishments.gov.in/WriteReadData/9361.pdf.

Directorate General of Health Services, Ministry of Health & Family Welfare, Government of India. IPHS Guidelines for Sub District Hospital and District Hospital, 2022. https://nhsrcindia.org/sites/default/files/Volume%201_SDH-DH_0.pdf.

20.   TAHPI. International Health Facility Guidelines; Laboratory Unit. www.healthfacilityguidelines.com/ViewPDF/ViewIndexPDF/iHFG_part_b_laboratory_unit.

Office of DGAFMS, Ministry of Defence, Government of India. Scales of Accommodation for Armed Forces Hospitals, 2003.

NHS. HBN 15: Facilities for Pathology Services. www.england.nhs.uk/wp-content/uploads/2021/05/HBN_15.pdf.

AHIA. Australasian Health Facility Guidelines. Part B—Health Facility Briefing and Planning; 0550—Pathology Unit. https://aushfg-prod-com-au.s3.amazonaws.com/HPU_B.0550_6_SOA%20Extract%202.pdf.

Making Medical Lab Quality Relevant: Revising the Laboratory Path of Workflow. www.medicallaboratoryquality.com/2017/04/revising-laboratory-path-of-workflow.html.

NFPA. NFPA 45: Standard on Fire Protection for Laboratories using Chemicals. https://catalog.nfpa.org/NFPA-45-Standard-on-Fire-Protection-for-Laboratories-Using-Chemicals-P1177.aspx?icid=D729.

NABL. Specific Criteria for Accreditation of Medical Laboratories. www.nabl-india.org/wp-content/uploads/2019/02/NABL-112_Issue-No.-04.pdf.

U.S. Department of Health and Human Resources. Biosafety in Microbiological and Biomedical Laboratories. www.cdc.gov/labs/pdf/CDC-BiosafetymicrobiologicalBiomedicalLaboratories-2009-P.pdf.

NHSRC. National Quality Assurance Standards for Public Healthcare Facilities, 2020. http://qi.nhsrcindia.org/cms-detail/revised-national-quality-assurance-standards/MjM3.

MoHFW, GoI. Clinical Establishment (Registration and Regulation) Act, 2010. Clinical Establishment Act Standard for Clinic/Polyclinic only Consultation. https://clinicalestablishments.gov.in/WriteReadData/9361.pdf.

Directorate General of Health Services, Ministry of Health & Family Welfare, Government of India. IPHS Guidelines for Sub District Hospital and District Hospital, 2022. https://nhsrcindia.org/sites/default/files/Volume%201_SDH-DH_0.pdf.

CPWD, Ministry of Housing & Urban Affairs, GoI. Compendium of Norms for Designing of Hospitals & Medical Institutions. https://cpwd.gov.in/Publication/Compendium_of_Norms_for_Designing_of_Hospitals_and_Medical_Institutions.pdf.

21.   TAHPI. International Health Facility Guidelines; Blood Bank. https://healthfacilityguidelines.com/india-v1.2/Full_Index/part_b_blood_bank.pdf.

AHIA. Australasian Health Facility Guidelines; Part B: Health Facility Briefing and Planning; 0550: Pathology Unit. https://aushfg-prod-com-au.s3.amazonaws.com/HPU_B.0550_7.pdf.

NHS. HBN 15: Facilities for Pathology Services. www.england.nhs.uk/wp-content/uploads/2021/05/HBN_15.pdf.

Medical Lab Management. Planning and Designing a Hospital Transfusion Service. www.medlabmag.com/article/1305.

Office of DGAFMS, Ministry of Defence, Government of India. Scales of Accommodation for Armed Forces Hospitals, 2003.

NHSRC. National Quality Assurance Standards for Public Healthcare Facilities, 2020. http://qi.nhsrcindia.org/cms-detail/revised-national-quality-assurance-standards/MjM3.

MoHFW, GoI. Clinical Establishment (Registration and Regulation) Act, 2010. Clinical Establishment Act Standard for Clinic/Polyclinic only Consultation. https://clinicalestablishments.gov.in/WriteReadData/9361.pdf.

Directorate General of Health Services, Ministry of Health & Family Welfare, Government of India. IPHS Guidelines for Sub District Hospital and District Hospital, 2022. https://nhsrcindia.org/sites/default/files/Volume%201_SDH-DH_0.pdf.

22.   TAHPI. International Health Facility Guidelines; Rehabilitation—Allied Health Unit. www.healthfacilityguidelines.com/ViewPDF/ViewIndexPDF/iHFG_part_b_rehabilitation_allied_health.

AHIA. Australasian Health Facility Guidelines; Part B: Health Facility Briefing and Planning; 0140: Allied Health Therapy Unit. https://aushfg-prod-com-au.s3.amazonaws.com/HPU_B.0140_6_0.pdf.

NHS. HBN 8: Facilities for Rehabilitation Services. www.wales.nhs.uk/sites3/documents/254/HBN%2008%20Rehab2000.pdf.

U.S. Department of Veteran Affairs. Physical Medicine and Rehabilitation Service Design Guide. www.wbdg.org/FFC/VA/VADEGUID/dg_pmrs.pdf.

Office of DGAFMS, Ministry of Defence, Government of India. Scales of Accommodation for Armed Forces Hospitals, 2003

NHSRC. National Quality Assurance Standards for Public Healthcare Facilities, 2020. http://qi.nhsrcindia.org/cms-detail/revised-national-quality-assurance-standards/MjM3.

MoHFW, GoI. Clinical Establishment (Registration and Regulation) Act, 2010. Clinical Establishment Act Standard for Clinic/Polyclinic only Consultation. https://clinicalestablishments.gov.in/WriteReadData/9361.pdf.

Directorate General of Health Services, Ministry of Health & Family Welfare, Government of India. IPHS Guidelines for Sub District Hospital and District Hospital, 2022. https://nhsrcindia.org/sites/default/files/Volume%201_SDH-DH_0.pdf.

23. TAHPI. International Health Facility Guidelines; Day Surgery/Procedure Unit. www.healthfacilityguidelines.com/ViewPDF/ViewIndexPDF/iHFG_part_b_day_surgery-procedure_unit.

AHIA. Australasian Health Facility Guidelines; Part B: Health Facility Briefing and Planning; 0270: Day Surgery/Procedure Unit. https://aushfg-prod-com-au.s3.amazonaws.com/HPU_B.0270_6_2.pdf.

NHS. HBN 10-02: Day Surgery Facilities. www.england.nhs.uk/wp-content/uploads/2021/05/HBN_10-02.pdf.

Design Commission for Wales. Singleton Hospital Day Surgery Unit, Swansea. http://dcfw.org/singleton-hospital-day-surgery-unit-swansea/.

Office of DGAFMS, Ministry of Defence, Government of India. Scales of Accommodation for Armed Forces Hospitals, 2003.

NHSRC. National Quality Assurance Standards for Public Healthcare Facilities, 2020. http://qi.nhsrcindia.org/cms-detail/revised-national-quality-assurance-standards/MjM3.

MoHFW, GoI. Clinical Establishment (Registration and Regulation) Act, 2010. Clinical Establishment Act Standard for Clinic/Polyclinic only Consultation. https://clinicalestablishments.gov.in/WriteReadData/9361.pdf.

Directorate General of Health Services, Ministry of Health & Family Welfare, Government of India. IPHS Guidelines for Sub District Hospital and District Hospital, 2022. https://nhsrcindia.org/sites/default/files/Volume%201_SDH-DH_0.pdf.

24. TAHPI. International Health Facility Guidelines; Pharmacy Unit. www.healthfacilityguidelines.com/ViewPDF/ViewIndexPDF/iHFG_part_b_pharmacy_unit.

AHIA. Australasian Health Facility Guidelines; Part B: Health Facility Briefing and Planning; 560: Pharmacy Unit. https://aushfg-prod-com-au.s3.amazonaws.com/%5BB-0560%5D%20Pharmacy%20Unit.pdf.

NHS. HBN 14-01: Pharmacy and Radio Pharmacy Facilities. www.england.nhs.uk/wp-content/uploads/2021/05/HBN_14-01_Final.pdf.

Office of DGAFMS, Ministry of Defence, Government of India. Scales of Accommodation for Armed Forces Hospitals, 2003.

NHSRC. National Quality Assurance Standards for Public Healthcare Facilities, 2020. http://qi.nhsrcindia.org/cms-detail/revised-national-quality-assurance-standards/MjM3.

MoHFW, GoI. Clinical Establishment (Registration and Regulation) Act, 2010. Clinical Establishment Act Standard for Clinic/Polyclinic only Consultation. https://clinicalestablishments.gov.in/WriteReadData/9361.pdf.

Directorate General of Health Services, Ministry of Health & Family Welfare, Government of India. IPHS Guidelines for Sub District Hospital and District Hospital, 2022. https://nhsrcindia.org/sites/default/files/Volume%201_SDH-DH_0.pdf.

25. TAHPI. International Health Facility Guidelines; Sterile Supply Unit. https://iheem.healthfacilityguidelines.com/ViewPDF/ViewIndexPDF/iHFG_part_b_sterile_supply.

Office of DGAFMS, Ministry of Defence, Government of India. Scales of Accommodation for Armed Forces Hospitals, 2003.

NHS. HBN 13: Sterile Services Department. www.england.nhs.uk/wp-content/uploads/2021/05/HBN_13.pdf.

NHSRC. National Quality Assurance Standards for Public Healthcare Facilities, 2020. http://qi.nhsrcindia.org/cms-detail/revised-national-quality-assurance-standards/MjM3.

MoHFW, GoI. Clinical Establishment (Registration and Regulation) Act, 2010. Clinical Establishment Act Standard for Clinic/Polyclinic only Consultation. https://clinicalestablishments.gov.in/WriteReadData/9361.pdf.

Directorate General of Health Services, Ministry of Health & Family Welfare, Government of India. IPHS Guidelines for Sub District Hospital and District Hospital, 2022. https://nhsrcindia.org/sites/default/files/Volume%201_SDH-DH_0.pdf.

26. TAHPI. International Health Facility Guidelines; Medical Gas System Design. https://india.healthfacilityguidelines.com/Guidelines/ViewPDF/iHFG/Public_Health_Medical_Gas_System_Design_MGS.

Office of DGAFMS, Ministry of Defence, Government of India. Scales of Accommodation for Armed Forces Hospitals, 2003.

NHS. HTM 02-01: Medical Gas Pipeline Systems; Part A: Design, Installation, Validation and Verification. www.england.nhs.uk/wp-content/uploads/2021/05/HTM_02-01_Part_A.pdf.

CPWD. Medical Gas Pipeline System. https://cpwd.gov.in/images/AzadikaAmrit/MGPS290921.pdf.

BIS. IS 2379:1990. Pipeline Identification Colour Code. https://law.resource.org/pub/in/bis/S08/is.2379.1990.pdf.

NHSRC. National Quality Assurance Standards for Public Healthcare Facilities, 2020. http://qi.nhsrcindia.org/cms-detail/revised-national-quality-assurance-standards/MjM3.

MoHFW, GoI. Clinical Establishment (Registration and Regulation) Act, 2010. Clinical Establishment Act Standard for Clinic/Polyclinic only Consultation. https://clinicalestablishments.gov.in/WriteReadData/9361.pdf.

Directorate General of Health Services, Ministry of Health & Family Welfare, Government of India. IPHS Guidelines for Sub District Hospital and District Hospital, 2022. https://nhsrcindia.org/sites/default/files/Volume%201_SDH-DH_0.pdf.

27. TAHPI. International Health Facility Guidelines; Catering Unit. www.healthfacilityguidelines.com/ViewPDF/ViewIndexPDF/iHFG_part_b_catering_unit.

Office of DGAFMS, Ministry of Defence, Government of India. Scales of Accommodation for Armed Forces Hospitals, 2003.

NHS. HBN 10: Catering Department. www.wales.nhs.uk/sites3/documents/254/HBN%2010.pdf.

AHIA. Australasian Health Facility Guidelines; Part B: Health Facility Briefing and Planning; 0700: Logistics/Back of House Services. https://aushfg-prod-com-au.s3.amazonaws.com/HPU_B.0700_1.pdf.

NHSRC. National Quality Assurance Standards for Public Healthcare Facilities, 2020. http://qi.nhsrcindia.org/cms-detail/revised-national-quality-assurance-standards/MjM3.

MoHFW, GoI. Clinical Establishment (Registration and Regulation) Act, 2010. Clinical Establishment Act Standard for Clinic/Polyclinic only Consultation. https://clinicalestablishments.gov.in/WriteReadData/9361.pdf.

Directorate General of Health Services, Ministry of Health & Family Welfare, Government of India. IPHS Guidelines for Sub District Hospital and District Hospital, 2022. https://nhsrcindia.org/sites/default/files/Volume%201_SDH-DH_0.pdf.

28.   TAHPI. International Health Facility Guidelines; Linen Handling Unit. www.healthfacilityguidelines.com/ViewPDF/ViewIndexPDF/
          iHFG_part_b_linen_handling_unit.

          Office of DGAFMS, Ministry of Defence, Government of India. Scales of Accommodation for Armed Forces Hospitals, 2003.

          NHS. HBN 25: Laundry. www.wales.nhs.uk/sites3/Documents/254/HBN%2025%20Arch2004.pdf.

          Singh D, Qadri GJ, Kotwal M, Syed AT, Jan F. Quality control in linen and laundry service at a tertiary care teaching hospital in India.
          International Journal of Health Sciences. 2009;3(1):33.

          AHIA. Australasian Health Facility Guidelines; Part B: Health Facility Briefing and Planning; 0700: Logistics/Back of House
          Services. https://aushfg-prod-com-au.s3.amazonaws.com/HPU_B.0700_1.pdf.

          NHSRC. National Quality Assurance Standards for Public Healthcare Facilities, 2020. http://qi.nhsrcindia.org/cms-detail/
          revised-national-quality-assurance-standards/MjM3.

          MoHFW, GoI. Clinical Establishment (Registration and Regulation) Act, 2010. Clinical Establishment Act Standard for Clinic/
          Polyclinic only Consultation. https://clinicalestablishments.gov.in/WriteReadData/9361.pdf.

          NABH. NABH Accreditation Standards for Hospitals, April 2020. www.nabh.co/images/Standards/NABH%205%20STD%20
          April%202020.pdf.

          Directorate General of Health Services, Ministry of Health & Family Welfare, Government of India. IPHS Guidelines for Sub District
          Hospital and District Hospital, 2022. https://nhsrcindia.org/sites/default/files/Volume%201_SDH-DH_0.pdf.

29.   TAHPI. International Health Facility Guidelines; Clinical Information Unit. https://india.healthfacilityguidelines.com/Guidelines/
          ViewPDF/iHFG/iHFG_part_b_clinical_information_unit.

          AHIA. Australasian Health Facility Guidelines; Part B: Health Facility Briefing and Planning; 0240: Health Information Unit.
          https://aushfg-prod-com-au.s3.amazonaws.com/HPU_B.0240_6_0.pdf.

          MoHFW, GoI. Medical Records Unit. https://main.mohfw.gov.in/sites/default/files/12%20Ch.%20XII%20Meical%20Record.pdf.

          MoHFW, GoI. Electronic Health Record Standards for India. https://main.mohfw.gov.in/sites/default/files/17739294021483341357.
          pdf.

          DGHS, MoHFW, GoI, Office Memorandum No. F. No. A.12034/3/2014-MH-II/MH-I dated 28/10/2014.

          Verma S, Midha M, Bhadoria AS. Facts and figures on medical record management from a multi super specialty hospital in Delhi
          NCR: A descriptive analysis. Journal of Family Medicine and Primary Care. 2020;9(1):418.

          Office of DGAFMS, Ministry of Defence, Government of India. Scales of Accommodation for Armed Forces Hospitals, 2003.

          NHSRC. National Quality Assurance Standards for Public Healthcare Facilities, 2020. http://qi.nhsrcindia.org/cms-detail/
          revised-national-quality-assurance-standards/MjM3.

          MoHFW, GoI. Clinical Establishment (Registration and Regulation) Act, 2010. Clinical Establishment Act Standard for Clinic/
          Polyclinic only Consultation. https://clinicalestablishments.gov.in/WriteReadData/9361.pdf.

          Directorate General of Health Services, Ministry of Health & Family Welfare, Government of India. IPHS Guidelines for
          Sub District Hospital and District Hospital, 2022. https://nhsrcindia.org/sites/default/files/Volume%201_SDH-
          DH_0.pdf.

30.   TAHPI. International Health Facility Guidelines; Mortuary. www.healthfacilityguidelines.com/ViewPDF/ViewIndexPDF/
          iHFG_part_b_mortuary_general

          Office of DGAFMS, Ministry of Defence, Government of India. Scales of Accommodation for Armed Forces Hospitals, 2003.

          NHS. HBN 20: Facilities for Mortuary and Post Mortem Room Services. www.wales.nhs.uk/sites3/documents/254/hbn%2020%20
          3rded%202005.pdf.

          AHIA. Australasian Health Facility Guidelines; Part B: Health Facility Briefing and Planning; 490: Hospital Mortuary/Autopsy Unit.
          https://aushfg-prod-com-au.s3.amazonaws.com/%5BB-0490%5D%20Hospital%20Mortuary%20Autopsy%20Unit.pdf.

          NSS Health Facilities Scotland. Scottish Health Planning Note 16-01: Mortuary and Post Mortem Facilities Design and Briefing
          Guidance. www.nss.nhs.scot/media/1974/shpn-16-01-v2-nov-2017.pdf.

          Mortuary. www.motherhospitalthrissur.org/mortuary.

          NHSRC. National Quality Assurance Standards for Public Healthcare Facilities, 2020. http://qi.nhsrcindia.org/cms-detail/
          revised-national-quality-assurance-standards/MjM3.

          MoHFW, GoI. Clinical Establishment (Registration and Regulation) Act, 2010. Clinical Establishment Act Standard for Clinic/
          Polyclinic only Consultation. https://clinicalestablishments.gov.in/WriteReadData/9361.pdf.

          NABH. NABH Accreditation Standards for Hospitals, April 2020. www.nabh.co/images/Standards/NABH%205%20STD%20
          April%202020.pdf.

          Directorate General of Health Services, Ministry of Health & Family Welfare, Government of India. IPHS Guidelines for Sub District
          Hospital and District Hospital, 2022. https://nhsrcindia.org/sites/default/files/Volume%201_SDH-DH_0.pdf.

31.   TAHPI. International Health Facility Guidelines; Administration Unit. www.healthfacilityguidelines.com/ViewPDF/ViewIndexPDF/
          iHFG_part_b_administration.

          Office of DGAFMS, Ministry of Defence, Government of India. Scales of Accommodation for Armed Forces Hospitals, 2003.

          NHS. HBN 00-01: General Design Principles. https://assets.publishing.service.gov.uk/government/uploads/system/uploads/attach-
          ment_data/file/147842/HBN_00-01_Final.pdf.

          AHIA. Australasian Health Facility Guidelines; Part B: Health Facility Briefing and Planning; 0120: Administration Unit. https://
          aushfg-prod-com-au.s3.amazonaws.com/HPU_B.0120_5_0.pdf.

          NHSRC. National Quality Assurance Standards for Public Healthcare Facilities, 2020. http://qi.nhsrcindia.org/cms-detail/
          revised-national-quality-assurance-standards/MjM3.

          MoHFW, GoI. Clinical Establishment (Registration and Regulation) Act, 2010. Clinical Establishment Act Standard for Clinic/
          Polyclinic only Consultation. https://clinicalestablishments.gov.in/WriteReadData/9361.pdf.

          Directorate General of Health Services, Ministry of Health & Family Welfare, Government of India. IPHS Guidelines for Sub District
          Hospital and District Hospital, 2022. https://nhsrcindia.org/sites/default/files/Volume%201_SDH-DH_0.pdf.

32.   TAHPI. International Health Facility Guidelines; Engineering and Maintenance Unit. www.healthfacilityguidelines.com/ViewPDF/ViewIndexPDF/iHFG_part_b_engineering-maintenance_unit.

Office of DGAFMS, Ministry of Defence, Government of India. Scales of Accommodation for Armed Forces Hospitals, 2003.

NHSRC. National Quality Assurance Standards for Public Healthcare Facilities, 2020. http://qi.nhsrcindia.org/cms-detail/revised-national-quality-assurance-standards/MjM3.

MoHFW, GoI. Clinical Establishment (Registration and Regulation) Act, 2010. Clinical Establishment Act Standard for Clinic/Polyclinic only Consultation. https://clinicalestablishments.gov.in/WriteReadData/9361.pdf.

Directorate General of Health Services, Ministry of Health & Family Welfare, Government of India. IPHS Guidelines for Sub District Hospital and District Hospital, 2022. https://nhsrcindia.org/sites/default/files/Volume%201_SDH-DH_0.pdf.

33.   TAHPI. International Health Facility Guidelines; Supply Unit. www.healthfacilityguidelines.com/ViewPDF/ViewIndexPDF/iHFG_part_b_supply_unit.

AHIA. Australasian Health Facility Guidelines; Part B: Health Facility Briefing and Planning; 0070: Logistics/ Back of House Services. https://aushfg-prod-com-au.s3.amazonaws.com/HPU_B.0700_1.pdf.

Office of DGAFMS, Ministry of Defence, Government of India. Scales of Accommodation for Armed Forces Hospitals, 2003.

NHSRC. National Quality Assurance Standards for Public Healthcare Facilities, 2020. http://qi.nhsrcindia.org/cms-detail/revised-national-quality-assurance-standards/MjM3.

MoHFW, GoI. Clinical Establishment (Registration and Regulation) Act, 2010. Clinical Establishment Act Standard for Clinic/Polyclinic only Consultation. https://clinicalestablishments.gov.in/WriteReadData/9361.pdf.

Directorate General of Health Services, Ministry of Health & Family Welfare, Government of India. IPHS Guidelines for Sub District Hospital and District Hospital, 2022. https://nhsrcindia.org/sites/default/files/Volume%201_SDH-DH_0.pdf.

Unit 3
Planning & Designing of Mechanical, Electrical, and Plumbing (MEP) Services

34 HEATING, VENTILATION, AND AIR CONDITIONING (HVAC)

34.1 Introduction

The HVAC (heating, ventilation, air conditioning) system in a hospital is significantly more intricate compared to those in typical commercial buildings. Its functionality in a hospital setting extends beyond mere thermal comfort, encompassing a myriad of critical roles. In this environment, the HVAC system is tasked with ensuring not only the comfort of patients and staff but also maintaining a sterile, germ-free atmosphere to curb the transmission of diseases. Moreover, the operational integrity of sensitive medical equipment hinges on precise control of temperature and humidity levels, making meticulous air management imperative during system design.

Designing HVAC systems for hospitals demands particular attention due to the diverse functionalities required within different areas of the facility. Varied room uses contribute to the intricacy of the HVAC blueprint. Clear delineation and categorization of spaces are essential, considering that certain rooms need to isolate patients with contagious illnesses, while others must cater to immunocompromised individuals. Hospitals inherently harbour a higher concentration of microorganisms and pathogens compared to commercial buildings, some of which may travel through the air.

Specific hospital zones such as intensive care units (ICUs), neonatal units, and operating rooms (ORs) demand stringent pathogen control to prevent their entry and proliferation. Hence, the air conditioning system must possess high sensitivity in accumulating and filtering out these potentially harmful elements. A flawlessly designed HVAC system can safeguard patients, staff, and visitors by minimizing exposure to such microorganisms and pathogens.

Equally vital is the inclusion of extensive air filtration provisions, especially for the external air introduced into the system for fresh air and circulation. This rigorous filtration helps impede the growth, dissemination, and accumulation of micro-particles and pathogens, fortifying the hospital's air quality and safety standards.

The HVAC systems should be designed to achieve the following key objectives.

- Mechanical services that deliver the anticipated levels of comfort and functionality
- A zero-tolerance approach to patient safety and infection control
- Compliance with the applicable codes and standards.
- Appropriate pressure differentials between adjacent spaces and departments in clinical facilities.
- Adherence to air changes per hour requirements, per code
- Reliable operation at the extreme outside design temperatures
- Reducing operating and maintenance costs shall be a key component in all new constructions
- Flexibility for future modification and expansion
- Energy efficiency and appropriate local or international green building code, such as LEED, BREAM, Green Star, etc.
- An appropriate level of consistency across facilities, recognizing the specific demands of each facility and clinical specialty.

34.2 HVAC and Infection Control

It's crucial to underscore the distinct functions expected from HVAC systems catering to health care facilities, especially when compared to those designed solely for maintaining thermal comfort in other building types.

Infectious diseases can spread through various avenues, including airborne transmission. Illnesses like tuberculosis, influenza, the common cold, and others disseminate through the air. The efficacy of HVAC systems in slowing down or controlling this spread is significant. Designers must conscientiously consider these factors and perceive it as an ethical obligation to adhere to relevant codes and standards.

Within health care settings, HVAC systems assume a pivotal role in mitigating airborne infections by executing specific functions:

- Adjusting air change rates to minimize the duration particles linger in the air
- Employing filtration mechanisms to eliminate microbes
- Implementing ultraviolet germicidal irradiation (UVGI) to deactivate viable agents and impede their growth
- Establishing differential pressurization in spaces to facilitate air movement from clean to less clean or contaminated areas
- Regulating temperature and humidity levels to limit pathogen propagation
- Enforcing 100% exhaust from designated high-risk areas to expel particles effectively
- Ensuring proper air distribution to curtail particle deposition and offer a designed exit path
- Implementing building-wide pressurization strategies to reduce external air infiltration

These measures collectively serve to fortify the health care facility's defences against airborne contaminants, reflecting a crucial aspect of responsible health care infrastructure design.

34.3 HVAC and Life Safety

- Installation of fire dampers, smoke dampers, and a combination of fire and smoke dampers should align with local codes and adhere to fire and life safety drawings, clearly depicted in the design plans.
- Mechanical smoke management systems must be integrated for atriums, corridors, and open-circulation spaces to ensure effective fire control measures.
- Implementing mechanical pressurization is essential for egress stairs, lift hoist ways, and lift lobbies designated for fire lifts to maintain safety during emergencies.
- When utilizing air-handling units' return ducting for smoke control, careful zoning alignment with smoke, fire alarm, and fire sprinkler zones is crucial. Compliance with duct construction standards, fan ratings, fire ratings for ductwork, and extract fan requirements is mandatory.
- To streamline control and operational sequences, especially for typical inpatient floors, it's advisable to install dedicated extract air ducts.

DOI: 10.1201/9780367460884-36

34.4 HVAC: Service Reliability

Reliability of an HVAC system is the quality of the system components, installation, commissioning, and facility maintenance. It is encouraged that owners and facility operators get involved early in the design process and provide feedback on the system components and operational aspects of the design. For future health care projects, HVAC equipment manufacturers that have a strong local presence and full-service support shall be selected. All applicable components should be tested at the local laboratories or other equivalent facilities worldwide and test certificates provided for record. Witness testing is encouraged for all major HVAC system components.

34.5 HVAC: Redundancy

In simple terms, redundancy can be thought of the amount of standby equipment that is available to cover a system or component in the event of a partial system failure. Standby equipment requirement should always be aligned with the owner's facility operation plan. Key system components in health care facilities must be configured in N+1 configuration (Table 34A).

TABLE 34A: HVAC Redundancy Requirements for Health Care Facilities

System Component	Desired Optimal Redundancy Level	Alternate Allowed
Water-Cooled Chillers	N+1	Deviation allowed for smaller hospitals and clinics if the loss of one chiller does not affect critical cooling.
Air-Cooled Chillers	N+1	Deviation allowed for smaller hospitals and clinics if the loss of one chiller does not affect critical cooling.
Central Steam Boilers	N+1	Deviation allowed for smaller hospitals and clinics if the loss of one boiler does not affect critical cooling.
Hydronic Heat Exchangers	N+1	
Chilled-Water and Hot-Water Pumps	N+1	
Operation Theatre Air-Handling Units	N+1	AHUs with dual fans each. Sized at 100% of the airflow or fan arrays with one additional fan are allowed as an alternate to N+1 AHUs.
Air-Side Equipment–Hygienic Air-Handling Units (Critical Care, LDR, Emergency, Diagnostic Imaging, Laboratory, Oncology, In-patient pharmacy, Radiotherapy, Renal Unit, CSSD, Surgical Suite, Isolation Rooms)	N+1 (fans) Each sized at 100% airflow and critical cooling	Fan coil units can be used for emergency, imaging, oncology, in-patient pharmacy, radiotherapy, and renal departments but their use is highly discouraged.
Server Room	N+1	N+1 precision control units or single indoor units with dual coils and dual fans backed up by independent heat rejection equipment.
Critical Rooms—Dedicated Exhaust Fans (Isolation Rooms, Bronchoscopy, Nuclear Medicine Hot Labs, Emergency and Radiology Waiting Rooms, Lab Fume Hoods, CSSD Sterilizers and Washers, Pharmacy Hazardous-Drug Exhausted Enclosures)	N+1	
Fire and Life Safety / Smoke Control System / Pressurization System Fans	N	Per local fire and life safety code requirement.

34.6 HVAC: Resiliency

The resilience of an HVAC system refers to its ability to sustain operation even when faced with failures within its components. This resilience holds particular significance for public hospitals, ensuring continuity during disaster management, and for private hospital operators, preventing revenue losses due to system failures.

Embedding resilience into the design process should commence during the initial concept phase. Consultants ought to assess risks linked to potential system component failures, engaging in constructive dialogue with the client, owner, or operator to devise effective strategies for risk mitigation.

- Evaluation of external risks stemming from climatic conditions (e.g. sand/snow/hailstorms and heavy rainfall) should guide the positioning and sizing of intake and exhaust louvres to withstand extreme events.
- Scrutiny of major equipment placed below grade is essential to assess the risk of flash floods.
- Considering the operating weights of equipment is crucial in structural design, especially for critical loads like absorption chillers, ensuring the structure can support the HVAC equipment loadings.
- Regular operation and testing of redundant systems through Building Management Systems (BMS) at design conditions are imperative.
- Mitigating major equipment risks as outlined in the previous section on redundancy is crucial. Additionally, configuring distribution systems like ductwork and pipework to eliminate single points of failure is essential.
- Adopting measures such as ring mains, multiple risers, dual connections to larger AHU coils, bypass setups over major control valves with appropriate isolation, individual variable frequency drives (VFDs) per fan, VFD bypasses, and manifolded air-handling unit configurations can significantly enhance system resilience.

These measures collectively contribute to fortifying the HVAC system's resilience, ensuring robust functionality even under adverse circumstances, and minimizing disruptions to critical health care operations.

34.7 HVAC: Zoning and Emergency Operation

34.7.1 HVAC System Zoning

HVAC systems designed for clinical buildings should ideally align with the smoke control compartments within the structure. This alignment strategy aims to minimize the impact in the event of a zone shutdown. In cases where following this approach results in an excessive number of air-handling units, designers can merge multiple zones while incorporating fire and smoke dampers to segregate them. To ensure functionality during a fire alarm condition, designers should plan the distribution ductwork strategically, allowing only a portion of the system to be deactivated.

Zoning the HVAC system in accordance with smoke control compartments typically restricts the capacity of a single air-handling unit to 16,500 L/s (60,000 m³/hr). Should this threshold be exceeded, designers are advised to consider splitting the air volume between two air-handling units. Consultants are encouraged to create zoning diagrams during the concept design phase, offering clear demarcation of HVAC zones for effective coordination and clarity in the system's layout. This proactive approach streamlines the design process, ensuring a well-coordinated and efficient HVAC system tailored to the clinical building's specific needs.

34.7.2 HVAC Systems Emergency Operation

Emergency generators play a crucial role in providing backup power to the HVAC systems within buildings during instances of grid power supply failures. The determination of generator capacity follows a risk classification process outlined in the electrical section. Collaborative efforts between the HVAC designer and the building's electrical designer are essential to identify which HVAC systems require emergency power. The outcomes of this assessment also influence how these systems are delineated into zones.

At a minimum, all critical areas as defined in ASHRAE 170 (such as SSU[CSSD]), surgical suite, labour and delivery suite/birthing unit, recovery, emergency, intensive care, nursery, and inpatient rooms) necessitate backup cooling/heating supported by emergency power. Maintaining space ventilation and pressure relationships for critical areas like isolation rooms and operating rooms, including caesarean sections, is vital and should be upheld using backup power. Detailed requirements for various risk categories within the hospital can be found in the electrical section.

It's recommended that the mechanical consultant clearly specify the electrical power requirements (normal power or emergency power) within the mechanical equipment schedules. This initiative ensures transparency and clarity for the electrical engineer, facilitating seamless coordination between the mechanical and electrical aspects of the building's infrastructure.

34.8 HVAC: Acoustic Requirements

The HVAC system design must adhere to HTM 08–01: Acoustics as a fundamental standard, although other comparable standards are also deemed acceptable. Specific guidelines for HVAC system components can be referenced from ASHRAE HVAC Applications Handbook, Chapter 49: Noise and Vibration Control.

- In health care facilities, lining of ductwork post final filtration is prohibited, per ASHRAE 170, except in terminal units, sound attenuators, and air distribution devices like plenum boxes. Any such lining should possess an impervious cover or certifications confirming no vapor absorption, meeting local civil defence requirements. Constant air volume (CAV) or variable air volume (VAV) boxes unable to meet acoustic requirements should incorporate downstream attenuators in critical areas.
- If backup power generators are located within hospital premises, they should be equipped with critical hospital-grade silencers.
- Sound attenuators should be integrated into car park exhaust and make-up air fans to diminish operational noise levels.
- Accurate specifications for acoustic ratings concerning plant room doors should be meticulously detailed, requiring comprehensive coordination among different trades.

Careful adherence to these acoustical standards and guidelines ensures that the HVAC systems in health care facilities maintain suitable noise levels, essential for patient well-being and the overall comfort of the health care environment.

34.9 HVAC: Future Proofing and Spare Capacities

Owing to the dynamic nature of medical facilities, alterations in internal layouts and upgrades to medical equipment frequently occur, leading to fluctuations in HVAC cooling and heating loads. To address these changes, the designer must establish effective communication with the owner or operator to determine the necessary allowances for future expansions, retrofits, and modifications within various departments.

As a significant guideline, it's strongly advised to allocate an additional 20% usable area for mechanical shafts. This extra space facilitates the accommodation of supplementary pipework and ductwork necessitated by structural alterations or equipment upgrades. Moreover, for medium to large hospitals, it's recommended that mechanical air-handling unit (AHU) rooms allot space for an extra AHU for every set of 10 units. Additionally, mechanical pump rooms should be designed with provisions for an additional pump for both primary and secondary systems. This strategic allocation of space anticipates and accommodates future requirements, ensuring smoother adaptation to evolving needs within the medical facility.

34.10 HVAC System Selection: Distribution

TABLE 34B: HVAC System Selection: Distribution

Variable Air Volume with Terminal Reheat	This distribution system is acceptable in all facilities and is considered as the preferred solution for general clinical areas. • VAV terminal units shall be in a pressure independent configuration to maintain airflow under fluctuating upstream duct pressures as system flow changes. • Supply air VAV terminals shall be provided with integral hot-water reheat coil or electrical reheat coil for areas with permanent occupancy as deemed necessary through heat load calculations. • Supply air temperature differential to room temperature shall not exceed 10°C in heating mode to prevent stratification. • Terminal units shall be equipped with sound attenuators as necessary to meet acoustic requirements. • Supply air temperatures shall be reset based on demand to minimize cooling and reheat loads. • VAV terminal units shall be provided for both supply and return/exhaust air systems for areas where mandated pressure control is required, per ASHRAE 170. • Terminal humidification is discouraged expect in operating theatres. • Minimum air volumes for VAV boxes shall be in accordance with the room air change rate specified in ASHRAE 170. This will generally be higher than the typical 30% minimum for a conventional commercial VAV system. The tender drawings and specs should indicate minimum value for each VAV box.
Fan Coil Units	• Chilled-water-based fan coil units (FCUs) are an acceptable solution for administration and support areas as well as clinical areas where ASHRAE 170 does not prohibit recirculation by room units. • For larger facilities, use of FCU is discouraged due to higher energy consumption, maintenance issues, and the need to access clinical spaces to replace components, such as filters, fan motors, and control valves. • In specific cases FCUs may also be used in circulation spaces, if there are high sensible cooling loads from heat gain through the building envelope or in spaces where there are localized heat gain from electro-mechanical equipment's, such as plant rooms, electrical and telecom rooms. Care must be taken to place FCUs outside of the electrical/telecom rooms to avoid chilled-water piping within the room. • FCUs shall not be used to dehumidify the outdoor air as outdoor air has a high moisture fraction. A dehumidified outdoor air supply should be ducted to the FCUs through a dedicated 100% outdoor AHU, utilizing energy recovery. • DX- or VRF-based FCUs are also acceptable where there is no centralized source of chilled water for smaller installations.
Displacement Ventilation	• Displacement ventilation is an acceptable solution for non-clinical areas only. It is not recommended in clinical areas due to the restrictions created by the fixed location of the supply diffusers. Where displacement ventilation is used, the designer shall coordinate locations of terminals carefully with the interior design proposals to ensure thermal comfort is achieved and future flexibility is not compromised. • Displacement ventilation can be particularly effective in spaces with lofty ceilings, such as entrance areas atriums, or spaces with high occupancy levels, such as lecture halls. • If utilizing displacement ventilation, the designer shall refer to the ASHRAE standards and handbooks with consideration for space temperature gradients.
Natural Ventilation	• Natural ventilation is not prohibited but ducted mechanical ventilation will still be required to ensure adequate number of air changes, even if natural ventilation is available. • Depending on climatic conditions, temperature, humidity, risks of natural disasters, natural ventilation constituting of operable windows is not a preferred option anymore. Furthermore, this leads to unfiltered outside air which due to increasing urbanization is under continuous degradation with major cities around the world having poor outside air quality. Thus, hospitals and health care facilities are encouraged to duct in outside air through mechanical ventilation.

34.11 HVAC System Design Criteria

34.11.1 External Design Criteria

The external design conditions can be obtained from ASHRAE climatic database or other local data sources. The design conditions should be carefully vetted, especially the wet bulb temperature for worse-case air intake for outside air. ASHRAE's 20-year projected DB and WB conditions are encouraged to be used for air-cooled chillers and cooling towers, respectively.

34.11.2 Envelope Design Criteria

TABLE 34C: Envelope Design Criteria

Component	Recommendations (U-W/m²·K)
Roof	U-0.3 (insulation entirely above the slab) Solar reflectance index (SRI) > 78
External Wall	U-0.4 (mass walls)
Floors	Per project requirements
Doors	Swinging U-0.74 Non-swinging U-1.45
Vertical Fenestration (Full Assembly)	Window-to-wall ratio 40% (max) Thermal transmittance U-1.9 (or lower) Solar heat gain coefficient 0.25 (max) Light transmittance 0.15 (min)

34.11.3 Internal Design Criteria

34.11.3.1 Non-Clinical Spaces

TABLE 34D: Internal Design Criteria for Non-Clinical Spaces

Criteria	Requirements
Temperature	The internal temperature requirement for non-clinical spaces shall be set at 24°C DB.
Relative Humidity	General non-clinical spaces would not be provided with active relative humidity control, unless it is a requirement related to specialist equipment within the space. The designer to ensure that maximum relative humidity is kept within 60% by employing BMS control algorithms.
Electrical Lighting	Lighting loads shall be based on an average watts/m² figure for each type of room based on a representative lighting layout. General guidance can be obtained from ASHRAE 90.1.2016 Lighting Power Density.
Electrical Small Power	Where there are specific equipment rooms, the heat loads shall be based on the worst-case values from the potential range of suppliers. Where are there no specific equipment layouts, allowances for small power loads shall be made on an average watts/m² basis as appropriate for the space type. Refer to ASHRAE Handbook Fundamentals 2017 Chapter 18 Non-Residential Cooling and Heating Load Calculations.
Occupancy	The design shall be based on the furniture layout or ASHRAE 62.1, whichever is the more onerous.
Infiltration	The building should be designed to be at positive pressure with respect to the atmosphere, always. Infiltration load should only be considered for high rise.
Ventilation	The minimum requirements for ventilation shall be as specified in the ASHRAE Standard 62.1.2016.
Acoustic Requirements	The design for HVAC system should follow the acoustic requirements listed out in HTM 08–01.

34.11.3.2 Clinical Spaces

TABLE 34E: Internal Design Criteria for Clinical Spaces

Criteria	Requirements
Temperature	Internal design temperatures shall generally be in accordance with ASHRAE Standard 170 & HVAC room design segment in this document. If there is an equipment specific space temperature requirement listed in the Room Data Sheets (RDS), it will supersede ASHRAE requirements.
Relative Humidity	Internal relative humidity shall generally be in accordance with ASHRAE Standard 170. If there is an equipment specific temperature requirement listed in the Room Data Sheets (RDS), it will supersede ASHRAE requirements.
Electrical Lighting	Lighting loads shall be based on an average watts/m² figure for each type of room based on a representative lighting layout. General guidance can be obtained from ASHRAE 90.1.2016 Lighting Power Density.
Electrical Load due to Medical Equipment	Medical equipment heat dissipation loads shall be based on the Room Data Sheets (RDS) listed values. RDS values should represent actual equipment heat dissipation values using worst-case manufacturer's published data from the range of potential suppliers.
Occupancy	Design occupancy for each space shall be as specified on the room data sheets. If no occupancy is provided, the design shall be based on the furniture layout or ASHRAE 62.1, whichever is the more onerous.
Infiltration	The building should be designed to be at positive pressure with respect to the atmosphere, always. Infiltration load should only be considered for high rise.
Ventilation	The minimum requirements for ventilation shall be as specified in the ASHRAE Standard 170.2017. For spaces not listed under ASHRAE 170, utilize ASHRAE 62.1.
Acoustic Requirements	The design for HVAC system should follow the acoustic requirements listed out in HTM 08–01.

34.11.3.3 Air Intake and Exhaust

Careful planning of air intake and exhaust louvres/vents is vital in health care facilities to prevent air recirculation and ensure compliance with ASHRAE 62.1's stipulated minimum separation distances. ASHRAE 170 delineates specific requirements for outdoor air intakes and exhaust discharges, which this guideline upholds.

Adverse climatic conditions necessitate special considerations for air intake louvres. At a minimum, outdoor air intake should pass through sand trap louvres sized at 1 m/s across the louvre face area, providing an 80% or higher filtration efficiency at coarse sand grain size (355–425 microns).

For larger health care facilities utilizing a central air intake for 100% outside air energy recovery AHUs, employing a self-cleaning inertial air cleaner is recommended. This air cleaner ensures 99% efficiency at sand grain sizes of 10 to 100 microns, overcoming limitations associated with standard sand trap louvres due to high intake velocities.

In cases where washable aluminium filters are provided behind sand trap louvres, ensuring proper maintenance access is crucial. If access for maintenance cannot be guaranteed without shutting down the AHU, filters should not be installed to prevent clogging, which can lead to increased pressure drop and reduced air volume.

Determining ambient acoustic levels through a site survey conducted by a professional acoustic consultant aids in determining the need for sound attenuators for outdoor air intake and exhaust. Buildings should maintain positive pressurization (5–10% net positive), adjusting for tighter buildings eligible for reduced net pressurization. Designers must ensure adequate outside air supply for proper pressurization and consider undertaking blower door testing as part of the testing and commissioning process to assess facility integrity.

34.11.3.4 Filtration

Mechanical filtration stands as a critical element ensuring that hospitals maintain top-tier care standards and remain fit for occupancy. It's a cornerstone of health care HVAC design, holding paramount importance in preserving air quality and controlling infections.

All AHUs directly servicing spaces and outside AHUs catering to downstream terminal units must feature a first-stage filtration of no lower than MERV 8/ePM10 60% rating. Additionally, a final filter, no less than MERV 14/ePM1 70% rating, should be placed downstream of all wet-air cooling coils and supply fans.

ASHRAE 170's Tables 7.1 and 8.1 outlines health care spaces that prohibit recirculation through room units, primarily critical departments like critical care, operating theatres, NICU, procedure rooms, and others. These stringent measures are

necessary due to cleaning challenges and the potential for contamination build-up in these sensitive areas.

Ultraviolet (UV-C) disinfection, or ultraviolet germicidal irradiation (UVGI), is employed to deactivate microorganisms, particularly recommended for cooling coil surfaces to prevent fungal proliferation. The effective wavelength range for microorganism inactivation falls near 254 nm. Implementing upper air UV in critical care or isolation rooms is encouraged to mitigate viral spread.

Alternative filtration methods such as electronic filters and air cleaners using photocatalytic oxidation (PCO) are discouraged due to health risks associated with ozone exposure and its by-products. Their usage demands substantial technical evidence validated by international agencies and engineering bodies like ASHRAE and CIBSE. If employed, these methods should not replace mechanical filtration but rather complement it to enhance indoor air quality. For comprehensive guidelines, refer to ASHRAE's position document on Filtration and Air Cleaning from 2015.

34.11.3.5 Materials

TABLE 34F: Reference Standards for Material Required for HVAC

Subject	Document	Edition
Ductwork	DSP DW/144 Specification for sheet metal ductwork. Third edition	2016
	DSP DW/172 Specifications for kitchen ventilation systems	2018
	SMACNA HVAC Systems Duct Design	2006
	SMACNA HVAC Duct Construction Standards-Metal & Flexible	2005
Pipework	ASME B31.9 Building Services Piping	2014
	ASTM A53 Pipe, Steel, Black and Hot-Dipped, Zinc Coated (Galvanized), Welded and Seamless.	—
	ASME B31.5 — Refrigeration Piping	2016
Filter Standards	ASHRAE 52.2 — Method of Testing General Ventilation Air-Cleaning Devices for Removal Efficiency by Particle Size	2017
	ISO Standard 16890 Air Filters for General Application	2016
HEPA Filter Standard	EN 1822 High efficiency air filters (EPA, HEPA and ULPA). Aerosol production, measuring equipment, particle counting statistics	2009
	ISO 29463 High efficiency filters and filter media for removing particles from air	2017
Fan Coil Units and Package Units	Eurovent RS 6/C/002–2017 Rating Standard for Certification of Non-Ducted Fan Coil Units	2017
	Eurovent RS 6/C/002A-2017 Rating Standard for Certification of Ducted Fan Coil Units	2017
	AHRI 340/360 Performance Rating of Commercial and Industrial Unitary Air-Conditioning and Heat Pump Equipment	2015
	AHRI 310/380 Standard for package terminal AC and Heat Pump	2017
	AHRI 410 Forced-Circulation Air-Cooling and Air-Heating Coils	2001
	AHRI 440 Performance Rating of Room Fan-Coils	2008
	ANSI/AHRI 1230 Performance Rating of VRF Multi Split AC & Heat Pump Equipment	2010
Standard Air-Handling Unit Construction	Eurovent RS 6/C/005–2017 Rating Standard for Certification of Air-Handling Units	2016
	AHRI 1350 Mechanical Performance Rating of Central Station Air-handling Unit Casings	2014
	AHRI 430 Performance Rating of Central Station Air-handling Unit Supply Fans	2014
Hygienic Air-Handling Unit Construction	VDI 6022 — Ventilation and indoor-air quality—Hygiene requirements for ventilation and air-conditioning systems and units	2011
	DIN 1946-4 — Ventilation and air conditioning—Part 4: Ventilation in buildings and rooms of health care	2008
	Eurovent RS 6/C/011–2017 Rating Standard for Certification of Hygienic Air-Handling Units	2017
Boilers and Chillers	ANSI/AHRI 1500 Performance Rating of commercial Space Heating Boilers	2015
	ARI 550/590 Performance Rating of Water Chilling Packages Using the Vapor Compression Cycle	2017
Cooling Towers	CTI (Cooling Technology Institute) STD-201 Certified	2013
Ventilation Equipment	AMCA 210 Laboratory Methods of Testing Fans for Certified Aerodynamic Performance Rating	2016
	AMCA 300 Reverberant Room Methods for Sound Testing of Fans	2014
	AMCA 301 Methods for Calculating Fan Sound Ratings from Laboratory Test Data	2014

34.11.3.6 Hydronic System Design

Hydronics involves the application of water for heating or cooling purposes. Open systems are exposed to the atmosphere at specific points like cooling towers, while closed systems remain isolated from the atmosphere. Piping systems can adopt direct or reverse return distribution schemes. With the introduction of pressure-independent control valves (PICV), the advantages offered by direct return systems, in terms of cost-effectiveness and system simplification, outweigh those of reverse return systems. Therefore, direct return systems are recommended for new health care facilities.

Innovative hydronic cooling or heating systems in new facilities should integrate pressure independent two-way control valves. Hydronic piping distribution schemes should focus on constant primary/variable secondary pumping or variable primary pumping. In variable primary flow systems, chillers must be equipped with automatic isolation valves, and the decoupler line should include a control bypass regulated by a flowmetre

to ensure guaranteed minimum flow through the chiller. Adequate attention is necessary in sizing expansion tanks and air separators, particularly for heating hydronic systems.

Variable primary flow pumping systems stand as the preferred choice for future medium to large health care projects due to their advantages:

- Lower installation costs
- Reduced mechanical room space requirements
- Higher system efficiency
- Better response to low delta-T syndrome

Constant primary/variable secondary systems are also acceptable. Pumps should be configured in a headered layout and placed within controlled environments. Illustrative examples of various distribution schemes can be found in Figures 34 A–C. When it comes to pipe material, Black Steel Schedule 40 with welded or grooved joints is recommended for use.

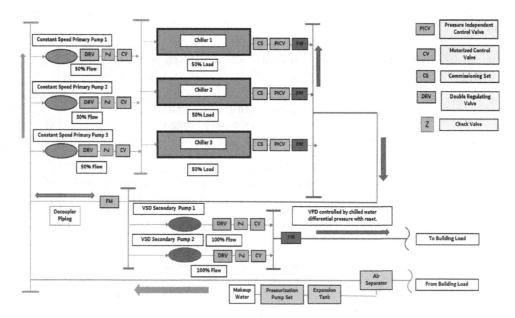

FIGURE 34A   Chilled-Water Production and Distribution—Primary Secondary System (Courtesy iHFG).

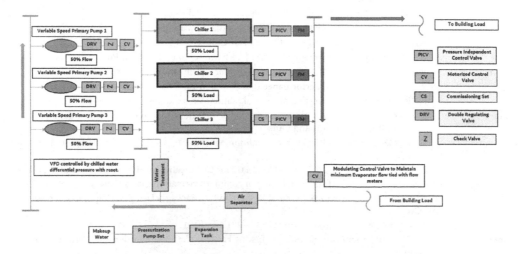

FIGURE 34B   Chilled-Water Production and Distribution—Variable Primary System (Courtesy iHFG).

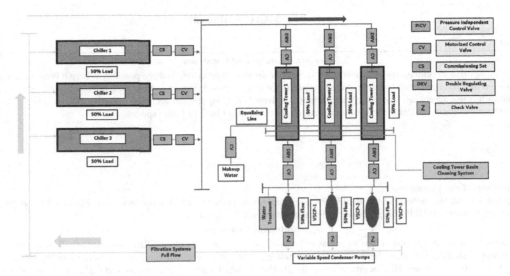

FIGURE 34C Cooling Tower System—Condenser Water Piping System (Courtesy iHFG).

34.11.3.7 HVAC Insulation Requirements
All insulation should be rated to DIN EN 13501 A1, A2, B, C with S1 or S2 smoke performance and D0 droplet performance. ASTM E-84/UL 723 is only applicability should be checked as per material type. The system rating shall be based on insulation, jacket, adhesives, coatings, fittings, and cements. Any treatment of jackets or facings to impede flame and/or smoke shall be permanent. Thermal performance, vapor permeability, and environmental performance should follow local regulations. Anti-microbial requirements should follow VDI 6022 or ASTM G21 or an approved equal standard.

34.12 HVAC Systems: Location, Access, and Maintenance

TABLE 34G: HVAC Systems: Location, Access, and Maintenance

Major Equipment

Location	All significant HVAC equipment, such as FAHUs, AHUs shall be located in enclosed mechanical plant rooms. The only HVAC equipment which may be located externally is the following: • Exhaust fans • Heat rejection equipment (e.g. air-cooled chillers, air-cooled condensers, cooling towers, etc.) • Staircase and lift core pressurization fans • Smoke management fans Rooftop/exposed AHUs are not recommended in high humidity/hot conditions. Mechanical rooms shall be provided with air conditioning and ventilation. In temperate/cold climates, AHUs can be located on rooftop/exposed.
Access	• Mechanical rooms and roofs with mechanical equipment shall be provided with staircase and preferably lift access to facilitate maintenance and equipment replacement. • Access to mechanical rooms and roof mechanical areas shall be directly from cores or main corridors. It is not acceptable for the access to mechanical rooms to be through treatment or patient care areas. • Clear access routes through mechanical rooms and roof areas shall be provided from the lifts and staircases. Routes shall be clearly and permanently marked on the mechanical room floor. • The minimum clear height for access routes shall be 2000mm or higher if dictated by the dimensions of equipment. • Steps on access routes are not acceptable. If changes of level are needed, or if services must be run at low level across an access route, a ramp must be provided.

Service Shafts

Location	• Service shafts shall be strategically located to provide rational and flexible services installations and minimize the size of the distribution ductwork and pipework on each floor. It is recommended that main ductwork shafts are located away from stair cores and elevator shafts to allow ducts to enter and leave the shaft on all sides. • Pipework shafts are most suited to locations adjacent to structural cores. • In clinical facilities, shafts shall not be located inside surgery suites or critical care areas. If the designer encounters a specific situation where a shaft is needed in one these spaces it should be discussed and agreed with AHJ during the schematic designs stage, through architectural design submission.
Access	• Pipework shafts shall be provided with access doors at each floor level to allow for inspection and maintenance and installation of additional pipework in the future. Removable floor gratings are recommended to be provided where clear openings exceed 450 mm × 450 mm. • Ductwork shafts shall be provided with access doors as needed to enable cleaning. It is anticipated that installation of additional ductwork would require the removal and replacement of wall finishes

(Continued)

TABLE 34G: (Continued)

Major Equipment

Terminal Equipment Locations

• Locating HVAC equipment in ceilings above patient, staff, and public areas shall be avoided where possible. Where it is necessary, its location shall be carefully selected to minimize the disturbance during maintenance and limit the infection control measures which are required to access it.
• In clinical facilities it is not acceptable under any circumstances to have HVAC equipment accessed from the space in any of the following areas. Terminal units should be located outside the rooms in corridor spaces or other back of house spaces.
  • Surgical suit/zone
  • Treatment room
  • All critical care areas
  • Patient rooms
  • Sterile store
  • Fire escape horizontal exit passageway
• The only exception is room side accessible terminal HEPA filters and fan filter units (FFUs), where access is obtained through special housing's allowing quick replacement. All HEPA filters should be located at terminal locations.

Maintenance Strategy

It is strongly suggested that the designer develops an access and maintenance strategy document. This document shall clearly describe the access and maintenance strategy for all mechanical systems, including HVAC, plumbing, and medical gas. Document shall be made available during the 90% stage inspection stage. The document must identify the strategy for plant maintenance and replacement including the following considerations:
  • Locations with accessible ceilings for terminal units (VAV, FCU, etc.)
  • Access and maintenance clearances for major equipment
  • Major plant removal routes with mechanical rooms
  • Infection control and patient safety implications.

34.13 HVAC Equipment Design Considerations

TABLE 34H: HVAC Equipment Design Considerations

Central Chilled-Water Plant	• Select cost-effective and optimum central chilled-water plants and/or small chilled-water systems to meet the project-specific requirements. Each installation shall consist of multiple (minimum two) chillers.
	• For central plants and small systems, it is recommended to conduct a comprehensive study to evaluate and define the lowest life-cycle cost performance of the chilled-water system. The study shall address both CAPEX and OPEX.
	• Chillers shall be rated and certified per AHRI conditions.
	• Where a central plant serves more than one air-handling system, the capacity of the central plant shall be calculated based on the peak simultaneous load, not the sum of the individual loads. In addition, the following diversity factors are reasonable when calculating central cooling plant capacity. The actual calculated central plant capacity shall be specific to the nature and size of the system(s), however, and should be determined via computer simulation.
	   • Lighting 0.9
	   • Equipment 0.85
	   • People 0.8
	• For air-cooled chiller in noise-sensitive locations, include chiller manufacturer's standard acoustic options in the design.
	• Imaging systems, such as MRIs, PET, CT scanners, and LINAC, require chilled water for equipment process cooling. Central plants should be sized to cover process loads, if use of plant central chilled-water use is approved by the imaging equipment manufacturer; otherwise, a dedicated chiller plant must be provided. Typically, the chiller, buffer tanks, and pumps for these applications are provided by the manufacturer of the imaging equipment for installation by others.
	• Potable water cooling should be provided per the hydraulics engineering section of this report.
	• Adequate space should be provided for equipment removal and maintenance. Replacement routes should be marked on the design drawings. Design for non-disruptive access to all chillers, pumps, cooling towers, and cooling tower components without the need to disassemble or remove other equipment or systems and/or building components, such as piping, doors, walls etc.
	• Higher delta T should be utilized to obtain energy savings by lowering pumping costs.
	• Consider VFD driven equipment for further energy savings for any pump consuming over 7.5 kW.
	• Arrange piping, especially piping in hydraulic decoupler, to ensure that all water flowmeters have ideal flow conditions for accurate measurement. Follow worse case flowmeter recommendations.
	• Cooling towers should be provided with an automatic basin cleaning system, which helps in mitigating risks associated with natural calamities and the risk of *Legionella* associated with manual cleaning.
	• Cleaner environment-friendly refrigerants should be utilized. ODP value should be 0, and GWP value should be less than 2500. HFOs are being developed which have much lower GWP values <10 and are encouraged for use.

Central Hot-Water Plant	• Select cost-effective and optimum central hot-water plants and/or small hot-water systems to meet the project-specific requirements. Each installation shall consist of multiple (minimum two) boilers/calorifiers. • For central plants and small systems, conduct a comprehensive study to evaluate and define the lowest life-cycle cost performance of the hot-water system. The study shall address both CAPEX and OPEX. • Adequate space should be provided for equipment removal and maintenance. Replacement routes should be marked on the design drawings. • Higher delta T should be utilized to obtain energy savings. • VFD-driven equipment should be utilized, for further energy savings.
Energy Benchmarking	Medium- to large-scale health care projects are encouraged to apply the principles mentioned in ASHRAE 189.3 Construction, and Operation of Sustainable High-Performance Health Care Facilities. In addition, LEED v4 for health care guiding principles are also encouraged to be utilized for a sustainable health care building.

(Continued)

TABLE 34H: (Continued)

Water-Cooled Chillers	• Water-cooled chillers can be centrifugal/screw or absorption type. Most common water-cooled chillers utilized are centrifugal chillers with single compressor or dual compressors based on the tonnage. • Chillers should be in air conditioning environment, with adequate clearance space for maintenance. • Consultant is encouraged to undertake an LCC study for VFD chillers vs. standards chillers and also for the type of chillers used. • Refrigerants with 0 ODP and less than 2500 GWP should be utilized for future health care projects. • Provide emergency chilled-water flanged piping connections covered with blind flanges and isolation valves for emergency chilled-water service where redundant chillers are not installed. • Chillers should adhere to the performance metrics listed in ASHRAE 90.1 or equivalent.
Air-Cooled Chillers	• Air-cooled chillers shall be screw type for tonnage over 100 tons. Scroll type chillers can be utilized for smaller installations. Reciprocating chillers are not allowed to be installed in future health care projects. • Consultant is encouraged to undertake an LCC study for VFD chillers vs. standards chillers. • Provide emergency chilled-water flanged piping connections covered with blind flanges and isolation valves for emergency chilled-water service where redundant chillers are not installed. • Chillers should adhere to the performance metrics listed in ASHRAE 90.1 or equivalent.
Cooling Towers	• Induced draft-type, counter-flow, factory-fabricated, and factory-test cooling towers are preferred choice for new construction and major renovation projects. The cooling towers shall be certified by the Cooling Tower Institute (CTI) and shall meet OSHA safety requirements. • It is recommended that the cooling tower structure should be stainless steel, with FRP removable • louvres and an FRP or Stainless-Steel basin. • Consultant is encouraged to undertake an LCC study for VFD cooling tower fan motors vs. standard motors. • Cooling towers should be provided with a Basin cleaning system. • Legionnaires disease: When a new hospital building is constructed, place cooling tower(s) in such way that the tower drift is directed away from the hospital's air-intake system and design the cooling towers such that the volume of aerosol drift is minimized.
Heat Exchangers	• Heat exchangers used for HVAC applications for district cooling systems should comply with the regulations from the relevant district cooling provider. • For potable water pre-conditioning and other applications, plate-and-frame-type heat exchangers should be utilized. It is recommended that two heat exchangers as a minimum are provided, each sized at 50% of the load. • For low-temperature hot-water circuit for heating, heat exchangers can either be plate-and-frame type or shell-and-tube type. It is recommended that two heat exchangers as a minimum are provided, each sized at 50% of the load.
Outside Air Energy Recovery Air-Handling Units	Outside air units should employ means of energy recovery. Approved methods include: • Air-to-air plate-type heat exchangers. Preferred choice for areas where no cross-contamination is permitted, such as ORs. • Heat pipes. Allowed for all areas but offer lower energy savings. • Total energy recovery wheels. Allowed and encouraged for all areas, except ORs. Must have a cross-contamination limit of less than 0.04% by particulate count and have a purging section. • Run-around coils. Allowed for all areas but offer lower energy savings. Outside air energy recovery should not be employed for the following air streams. These should be directly exhaust to ambient with dedicated exhaust. • Exhaust from all fume hoods and bio-safety cabinets • Kitchen exhaust (range hood and wet exhaust) • Autopsy exhaust • Isolation room exhaust • Wet exhaust from cage and cart washers • ETO—ethylene oxide sterilizers exhaust

Air-Handling Units	• The capacity of a single AHU shall not exceed 50,000 m³/hr (16,500 L/s).
	• AHUs shall be AHRI or Eurovent certified, factory-fabricated, and the standard product of one manufacturer. All AHUs shall be constructed in modular and draw-through configuration. Use of blow-through AHUs are not permitted, as fully saturated air leaving the cooling coil causes damage to the downstream filters and sound attenuators.
	• AHUs serving clinical areas should be hygienic-type units. Refer to the materials section for required certifications and standards.
	• To prevent cross-contamination, separate AHUs should be provided as a minimum for the following spaces.
	  • Operating theatres
	  • Mortuary
	  • Main kitchen
	• Each AHU shall be installed as a standalone entity without any physical interface with another AHU. Selection of stacked (one on the top of another) air-handling units is not permitted. Use of a common return air fan for two or more AHUs is also not permitted.
	• Use of a single or multiple plenum fan (fan array) is permitted and encouraged over housed, air-foil centrifugal fans. Fan motors shall be premium efficiency.
	• Where room air can be returned to the system, provide a dedicated return or relief air fan for each AHU to facilitate room-by-room air balance, economizer cycle, and intended volumetric air balance. Provide a direct digital control (DDC) interlock between the supply and return or relief air fans.
	• Variable frequency drives (VFDs) shall be utilized in all AHUs and rooftop units. Building type (e.g. hospital, outpatient facility, etc.) will determine level of redundancy required for VFDs. VFDs shall include either a bypass switch or be configured in a manner that failure of one VFD does not disable the entire unit. Fan motor shall be high efficiency.
	• Each cooling coil shall not exceed 6 rows and 10 fins per inch (FPI). Design 2 coils in a series arrangement if the cooling coil capacity requirement exceeds the capability of a 6-row, 10-FPI coil. Chilled water shall be piped in series through both coils, and a 42-inch access section shall be provided between the two equally sized coils.

(Continued)

TABLE 34H: (Continued)

	• Maximum cooling coil discharge face velocity shall not exceed 450 fpm. Heating coil discharge face velocity shall not exceed 800 fpm.
	• Ultraviolet (UV) lamps shall be located on the leaving air side of the cooling coil.
	• Access doors (or panels) on the AHU sections shall always open against the positive side of the door and shall not be blocked by internal filter casings or internal equipment components. Micro switches or safety switch interlocks need to be provided at access doors or panels on UV sections to protect maintenance personnel from possible injuries.
Fan Coil Units	• All FCUs must be provided with a source of treated precooled dehumidified fresh air through the DOAS systems. Direct injection of outside air dumped over the ceiling void or ducted to units is not allowed.
	• FCU systems served by chilled water with hot water or electric heating are an attractive solution for areas requiring special control or out of hours operation. Such areas include computer/communication rooms, lift machine rooms, distribution communications and electrical rooms, PABX rooms and administration areas. FCUs are not allowed for areas where ASHRAE 170 prohibits room side recirculation.
	• FCU's usage is highly discouraged for new constructions for areas other than mentioned above, where adequate space for distribution ductwork can be provided.
	• Select FCUs that deliver the required capacity at medium speed.
	• For new construction and major renovation, PICV should be provided for each FCU.
	• FCU shall be located outside of patient occupied spaces/rooms for ease of maintenance.
Terminal Units (VAV, CAV)	• All terminal units shall be pressure-independent type and equipped with DDC controls. All air terminal units (constant volume or variable air volume) serving perimeter or interior spaces with permeant occupancy and mandated ASHRAE 170 air change requirements, shall be equipped with integral reheat coils.
	• The maximum and minimum air volume settings shall be factory-set but field-adjustable. The minimum setting for each space should be dictated by the air change requirement, the ventilation requirement for multi-zone VAVs based on ASHRAE 62.1 and the makeup air requirement for the exhaust. The designer should list out minimum settings for each VAV box in the detailed design drawings.
	• All rooms requiring acoustic treatment according to HTM 08–01 should be provided with terminal sound attenuators.
	• Variable air volume (VAV) boxes shall be located outside of patient occupied spaces for ease of maintenance.

Air Valve Terminals	• If VAV systems are specified, venturi air terminals or air valves with high-speed actuators are highly recommended to be utilized for all new construction and major renovation for the following space types in lieu of VAV boxes due to their higher reliability and stable airflow control.
	  • Operation theatre
	  • Pharmacy clean rooms
	  • Isolation rooms

	• Laboratories with fume hoods (should be equipped with a 3-second or faster response actuator).
	• Additional rooms as identified by the building end user that have strict pressure control requirements due to infection control issues.
	• Venturi air terminal should be programmed as using the variable air volume approach with maximum energy savings. Usage-based controls can also be employed at the facility owner's discretion. Each airflow control device shall be factory characterized on air stations NVLAP accredited.
	• Venturi air valves shall be located outside of patient occupied spaces for ease of maintenance.
	• For an AHU provided with downstream venturi air terminals, it is preferable to utilize all venturis instead of a combination of venturi terminals and VAV/CAV terminals due to varying pressure drops. Low-speed venturis and constant air venturis can be used for non-critical areas, for cost savings.
Humidifiers	• The need for humidification should be ascertained by psychrometric studies. If humidification is required at a large scale, it can be achieved through a clean steam network utilizing steam boilers or electric steam generators.
	• If active humidification is only required for critical areas, such as OT, burns unit, etc., it is better to be achieved by small individual package electric humidifiers.
	• The humidifier should be located prior to the cooling coil and fed with clean steam (steam generated from RO or DI water and piped using stainless steel). Smaller ceiling-mounted electric units should also be fed with RO or DI water.
	• If duct-mounted humidifiers are used, 304 stainless steel ducting should be provided for a minimum of 1.5 m downstream and 0.5 m upstream of the humidifier. Designer team to verify the absorption distance for each application and adjust the length of stainless steel accordingly. Duct sections downstream of steam humidifiers shall be sloped to a low point with drain valve and cap.
Diffusers, Registers, and Grilles	• Diffusers, registers, and grilles should be specified per the project requirements and in alignment with the clinical and interior design. Air diffusion performance index (ADPI) shall conform to selection criteria given in ADPI table of the "Room Air Distribution" chapter of the ASHRAE Handbook—HVAC Applications 2015.
	• Terminal HEPA filters for all spaces other than OTs served by dedicated AHUs should be fan-powered, catering for the entire pressure drop of the filter, allowing for the AHU supply fan to be sized for only the pressure drop of the secondary filtration.
Ductwork	• Rectangular galvanized steel has consistently been shown to be more cost-effective as compared with rigid circular ductwork which is both less efficient in its space requirements and normally more expensive because of the excessive costs of fittings.
	• All clinical areas shall be provided with a fully ducted system. Use of the ceiling void, for air delivery (supply or return) is not allowed, only back-of-house areas and admin areas can use return air plenum but should be provided with appropriate sealing and smoke sensors.
	• Duct sizing is to be based on the recommended velocity and pressure drop ranges in the current version of ASHRAE fundamentals or equivalent.
	• Air-handling duct systems shall be designed to be accessible for duct cleaning, generally by the provision of access panels. Access panels shall be fitted at each reheat coil and fire and smoke damper to allow annual essential services inspection.
	• It is encouraged to provide antimicrobial coating on the internal surface of the duct complying with ASTM 3152 and ASTM G21 or equivalent standard.
	• Commercial dishwasher exhaust, steam sterilizer, and sterile washer exhaust shall be type 304 stainless steel with welded joints.
	• Laboratory hood exhaust ductwork shall be 304 stainless steel with welded joints.
	• Kitchen hood exhaust shall be 16-gauge black steel where concealed and 18-gauge, type 304 stainless steel, welded and polished to a no. 3 finish, where exposed.

34.14 HVAC Services: Instrumentation and Control

HVAC instrumentation and control systems, which are commonly part of the BMS systems, are integral to the proper operation of a health care facility. BMS control systems form the backbone of the operation and maintenance system for HVAC and provide the facility management team with information regarding equipment life and operational performance.

The following points should be kept in mind while designing a BMS system for health care applications:

- The BMS system shall be suitable, compatible, scalable, and flexible to meet the demands imposed by health care facilities. The system shall have spare capacity at field level to allow for departmental changes and equipment changes.
- All actuations shall be electronic.
- Specific requirements related to control actuators, control valves, control dampers, end switches, safeties and safety alarms, control wiring, air flow measuring stations, room temperature and humidity sensors, DDC control systems servers, and tablet displays should be detailed within the project drawings and specifications.
- A detailed input/output point list should be prepared by the consultant in consultation with specialist solution providers and included as part of the project tender documentation.
- BMS systems should be configured to optimize energy usage.
- Control algorithms should be programmed to utilize the data collected and allow for effective energy recovery, air-side filter diagnostics, critical alarms, and sensor calibration checks.
- Ensure system is capable of robust metering. Separate submeters should be allocated for lighting, HVAC plant, HVAC distribution, general power, service water heating, renewables, and whole-building power and water as a minimum. Energy use should be benchmarked every month. Facility managers should be trained on continuous benchmarking.

34.15 HVAC Systems: Commissioning and Handover

The HVAC systems commissioning is an important phase in the project timeline and is critical in confirming that the design parameters are met by the installed system and the system meets the minimum code requirements related to air changes, filtration effectiveness and infection control.

For medium- to large-scale health care projects, an independent commissioning agent (CxA) should be employed the facility owner/client to oversee the commissioning process.

The following points should be kept in mind while preparing for commissioning of HVAC systems for health care facilities.

- Method statements should be provided by the contractor during the commissioning phase for all HVAC equipment.
- Testing and commissioning plan should be developed by the contractor in consultation with the CxA to provide a clear and concise roadmap for the implementation of the commissioning process and to provide a record of the results of the commissioning process.
- The design consultant should engage with the owner and the facility management team and develop the Owner's Project Requirements (OPR). Furthermore, these should

be formulated in a report along with the design narrative, submitted as part of the construction documentation submitted to the contractor.

- Follow ASHRAE Guideline 0–2013 and ASHRAE Guideline 1.1–2007 for HVAC&R systems commissioning.
- It is encouraged to develop monitoring-based procedures and identify points to be measured and evaluated to assess performance of energy and water through advanced meters.
- It is encouraged to perform a building flush-out for IAQ prior to occupancy or conduct testing for IAQ for particulate matter and inorganic gasses to be kept under allowances mentioned in codes and standards.
- As a minimum, a space pressurization report is required for the following spaces:
  - Class N and Class Q—airborne infection isolation rooms
  - Class P—protective environment rooms
  - Bone marrow transplant
  - IVF labs and procedure rooms
  - Operating rooms
  - Interventional imaging rooms
  - Pharmacy clean rooms
  - Laboratory clean spaces
  - Sterile processing rooms
  - Sterile storage rooms
  - Vivarium areas
- Operating rooms and other clean rooms should be tested for particle counts per international standards.
- The commissioning agent (CxA), testing, adjusting, and balancing contractor (TAB), MEP contractor, and controls contractor (BMS contractor) should work together on the commissioning of systems and provide all reports and test results as well as arrange for witness testing for agreed systems for the owner's representative and the supervision consultant.
- Functional testing for all critical systems should be included in the scope of works.
- O&M manuals for all HVAC equipment should be provided by the contractor.
- Training on the systems installed should be conducted by the contractor's team for the owner's facility management team.
- The FM team should keep a record of all O&M activities onsite, preferably through an electronic recordkeeping system.

34.16 Summary

Planning and designing HVAC systems in a hospital is a critical process that ensures a comfortable, healthy, and safe environment for patients, health care professionals, and visitors. HVAC systems play a vital role in maintaining appropriate temperature, humidity, and air quality within health care facilities. Key considerations in the planning and designing process include proper sizing and placement of HVAC equipment, incorporation of energy-efficient technologies, implementation of filtration and ventilation systems to mitigate airborne contaminants, zoning for different areas of the hospital, and compliance with regulatory guidelines. By prioritizing these factors and engaging experts in HVAC engineering and hospital design, health care facilities can establish well-designed HVAC systems that promote patient well-being, prevent the spread of infections, and provide a conducive environment for effective health care delivery.

35 ELECTRICAL SERVICES IN HOSPITALS

35.1 Introduction

Health care premises depend on electrical power supplies not only to maintain a safe and comfortable environment for patients and staff but also to give greater scope for treatment using sophisticated medical equipment at all levels of clinical and surgical care.

Interruptions in electrical power supplies to equipment can seriously disrupt the delivery of health care, with serious consequences for patient well-being. Health care organizations should therefore ensure that their electrical installation provides maximum reliability and integrity of supplies. Every effort must be made to reduce the probability of equipment failure due to loss of power.

Parameters for a quality electric supply are

- Voltage: Steady, variations within permitted limits only
- Frequency
- Absence of harmful harmonics
- Protection against surge/lighting

35.2 Risk Assessment

Electrical power distribution systems are inherently designed to isolate power supplies to parts of the installation where an electrical fault is detected for safety and reliability of electrical distribution in general. In any electrical installation, the power supply may fail at some point, and contingency needs to be in place to mitigate the impact of the power failure by providing redundancy in power source and distribution.

The level of redundancy is to be conducive to the type of health care premises and level of care rendered. A power failure in an outpatient care facility may not have much detrimental effect on patient safety, while a power failure in an acute care facility could have disastrous consequences. Depending on the level of care provided in the health care facility, the stakeholders should carefully consider the risks involved due to a power failure for clinical, non-clinical, and engineering applications and come up with an optimum arrangement that will minimize the risk to patient safety and health care facility operation in general.

The risk assessment can be a simple or complex approach depending on the size and nature of the medical services being provided in the health care facility. This guideline recommends that the risk assessment approach described in the HTM 06–01 2017 edition; chapter 4 be followed for determining the risks; business continuity risks are graded from Grades 1 to 4 (Grade 1 being the highest risk), while clinical risks are graded from Grades A to E (Grade A being the highest risk) (Figures 35A–C).

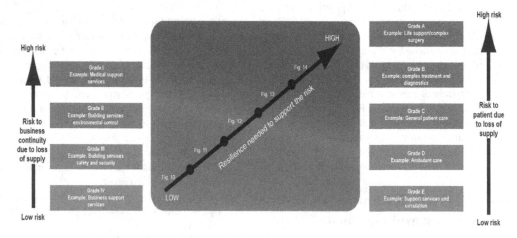

Note: the risk grading system A–E and I–IV is only used as a guide and may differ for each project depending on risk assessment

FIGURE 35A   Grading of Risk in Relation to Loss of Supply (Courtesy: HTM 06–01).

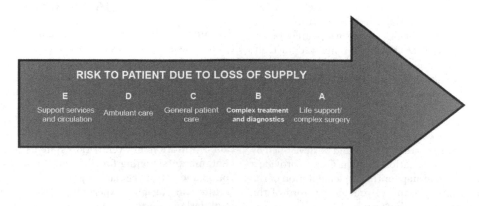

FIGURE 35B   Grading of Patient Risk Regarding Loss of Supply (Courtesy: HTM 06–01).

    DOI: 10.1201/9780367460884-37

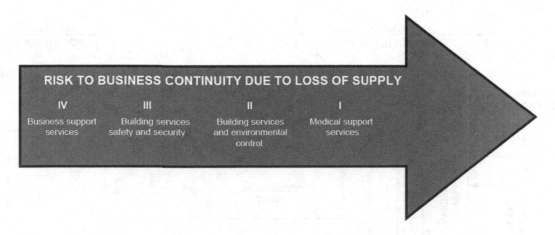

FIGURE 35C   Grading of Business Continuity Risk Regarding Loss of Supply (Courtesy: HTM 06–01).

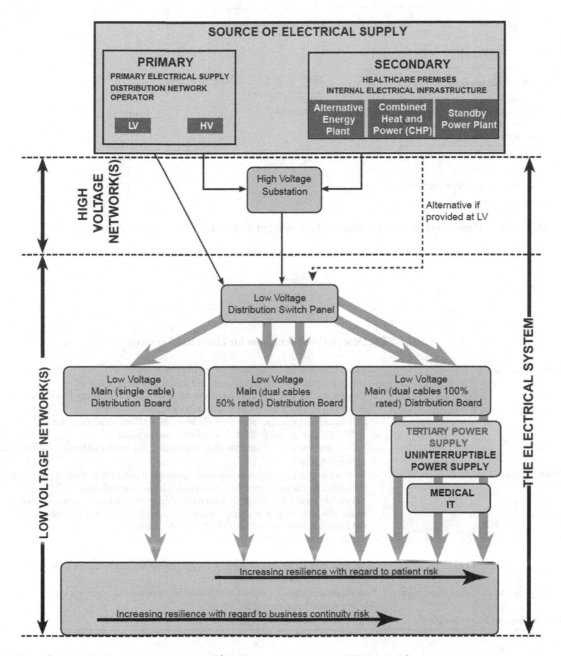

FIGURE 35D   Electrical Infrastructure Generic Flow Diagram (Courtesy: HTM 06–01).

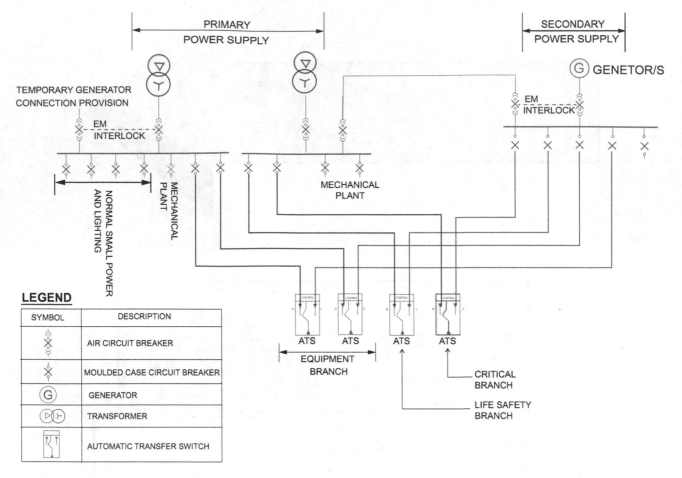

FIGURE 35E   Typical High-Level Power Distribution Arrangement Schematic for a Hospital (Courtesy: iHFG).

TABLE 35A: Design Considerations for Electrical Services

Assess the Load Demand	• For electrical load: 25–40 watts per sq m of built-up area. • Medical equipment/lab equipment: add 25% to the electrical load. • Central AC load: 40 watts per sq m and AC area subject to energy efficient AC. For inefficient AC such as Window/Split AC/VRV, add 20% extra. • DG aggregate capacity: approximately 50–60% of transformer capacity. • UPS aggregate capacity: 20–25% of transformer capacity. • Solar generation: 5–10% of transformer capacity, but more can be provided if land for solar panels is available.
Sources of Power Supply	• Primary power supply: power supplied by the local power distribution company. The power can either be released from the low tension (LT) line or high tension (HT) line. • Secondary power supply (SPS): power supplied by the in-house standby generators. In the event of a primary power supply failure, the secondary power supply should be available to the associated emergency loads in 15 seconds or less. • Tertiary power supply (TPS): power supplied by UPS system (rotary or static), with less than a 0.5-second break.
Quantity and Types of Service Outlets	To be provided in the various medical locations that should be based on the guidance provided as per the room data sheets (RDS).
Non-Medical Equipment in Patient Care Area	Non-medical equipment should not be used in a patient environment unless it meets the electrical safety requirements.
Clinical Risk Grading and Power Supply Types	As per Table 35B.

Electrical disturbances may affect the reliability of high-tech medical equipment.

TABLE 35B: Clinical Risk Grading and Power Supply Types

Clinical Risk Grade (Interpretation of HTM 06–01:2017)	Medical Location (Interpretation of HD 60364–7–710:2015)	Area Description	Power Supply Types
Grade A	Group 2	These are areas where treatment and patient safety will be compromised and endangered by any minor interruption of electrical supply; such areas include but are not limited to operating rooms, anaesthetic induction rooms, recovery bays (stage 1), critical care, angiography and catheter labs, emergency resuscitation bays, IVF procedure rooms, high-dependency units, neo-natal ICUs, brachytherapy rooms, and chemotherapy and embolization rooms.	SPS: Required TPS: Required IPS: Required (Note: PPS is also recommended in these areas to serve power outlets intended for non-clinical applications such as cleaning. Power supply for support systems such as HVAC, hot and cold water, and medical gas alarms should be connected to SPS.)
Grade B	Group 1	These are areas where treatment and patient safety may be compromised (but not endangered) by any minor interruption of electrical supply; such areas include but are not limited to delivery rooms, endoscopy procedure rooms, emergency treatment areas, haemodialysis bays, urology treatment rooms, radiation therapy rooms, imaging equipment and procedure rooms, triage, and staff stations.	SPS: Required TPS: Generally, not required. However, TPS may be required for specific medical equipment. IPS: Not Required (Note: A few power outlets connected from TPS is recommended at nurse stations serving critical care areas. PPS is recommended in these areas to serve power outlets intended for non-clinical applications such as cleaning. Power supply for support systems such as HVAC, hot and cold water, and medical gas alarms should be connected to SPS.) SPS backup for imaging equipment is optional depending upon the level of care provided in the facility. If the health care facility is having interventional procedures, then at least one of each type of imaging system is to be connected to SPS.
Grade C	Group 1	These are areas where treatment and patient safety will not be immediately compromised by an interruption of electrical power; such areas include are but not limited to outpatient treatment rooms, consult/exam rooms, pharmacy, patient bedrooms, recovery—stage II, and observation bays.	PPS: Required SPS: Required TPS: Not Required IPS: Not Required (Note: Power supply for support systems such as HVAC, hot and cold water, and medical gas alarms should be connected to SPS.)
Grade D	Group 0	These are areas where loss of power supply may give rise to disruption, inconvenience, and a reduced environmental quality but would not directly compromise clinical treatment and safety. Such areas include but are not limited to consult rooms, waiting areas, and Sterile Supply Unit (SSU).	PPS: Required SPS: Optional TPS: Not Required IPS: Not Required (Note: SPS for small power outlets in these areas are optional; the designer may provide SPS to mitigate business continuity risk, if required by the end user. It is recommended that 50% of lighting circuits are connected to SPS. SPS backup is highly recommended for at least one of each type of sterilizing and cleaning equipment in the SSU at a minimum.)
Grade E	-	These are areas where loss of the electrical supply does not have an immediate effect on the clinical treatment or safety of patients; such areas include but are not limited to general circulation areas, offices, and other non-clinical areas.	PPS: Required SPS: Optional TPS: Not Required IPS: Not Required (Optional: SPS and TPS for areas such as offices are optional; the designer may provide SPS and TPS to mitigate business continuity risk, if required by the end user.)

35.3 Power Quality: Clinical Risk Grading and Power Supply Types

Electrical disturbances may affect the reliability of high-tech medical equipment. As medical equipment is often connected to vulnerable patients, such a malfunction may result in fatal consequences. Figure 35B presents the clinical risk grading and power supply types of various functional areas in a hospital. To mitigate this problem, careful consideration should be given in terms of the design of the electrical distribution system and selection of electrical distribution equipment. The following approaches should be considered:

- Power supply feeders for sensitive medical equipment, such as x-rays, CT, MRI and Linac scans, etc., should be directly sourced from the main distribution boards (MDBs) rather than from shared sub-distribution panels. Alternatively, a dedicated appropriately sized submain distribution board (SMDB) located in the MDB room to serve a group of imaging equipment will also suffice.
- Providing surge protection devices.
- Providing active harmonic filters: Power system harmonics of the 3rd, 5th, 7th, 9th, 11th, and 15th order can create significant problems such as overcurrent and the overheating of cables, busbars, and transformers. Since it is not practical to accurately estimate the rating of active harmonic filters required for any project in advance, provision such as breakers should be made in the MDBs to install harmonic filters when actual harmonics can be measured at the earliest. Spare breakers designated for this application should be labeled as "For Harmonic Filter Only".
- Harmonics are to be measured once the majority of the mechanical, electrical, and medical equipment are in operation. This guideline recommends that this measurement be made within 6 months following the opening of the facility. Suitably rated harmonic filters should be installed to limit the harmonics stipulated as per IEEE 519 (Recommended Practices and Requirements for Harmonic Control in Electrical Power Systems).
- Power factor correction should meet local authority requirements. Power factor correction equipment can also contribute to the harmonic generation, unless properly designed detuning reactors are incorporated into the design of the power factor correction capacitor banks. Power factor correction capacitor banks should be with detuning reactors. Capacitor banks employing Thyristor-based capacitor switching are recommended.
- It is recommended that the facility display power quality parameters such as THD to be provided in the MDBs.

35.4 Primary Power Supply and Distribution

- Primary power supply shall be sourced from local utility provider based on the standard procedures and approval process mandated by the local power supply authority.
- Main power supply intake rooms (RMU, transformer, and MDB) should be provided as per the regulations of the local authority.
- With fast evolving advancements in the medical treatment field, there is an ever-increasing need for electrical power for health care facilities, and this trend is likely to continue. Considering this spare capacity may be allowed in the power distribution equipment such as transformers.
- Typically, in health care facilities, a large number of small power sockets are provided at patient locations on service panels and pendants for redundancy and convenience rather than simultaneous use. As such, suitable diversity should be worked out by a qualified and experienced designer to avoid ending up with an inappropriately expensive, overdesigned electrical system.
- For critical care facilities, separate, dedicated MDB rooms should be provided for primary and secondary power supplies to segregate primary and secondary MDBs.

35.5 Secondary Power Source and Distribution

- On-site secondary power supply source (diesel generator set) and associated distribution should be provided for health care facilities. Coverage of the secondary power supply should be as per the level of care provided in the facility.
- Location of the generator set should optimize the secondary distribution by reducing the amount of power distribution elements between the critical load and the power source. The location of the generator room should also be protected from general flooding levels.
- It is recommended that diesel generator sets serving health care facilities are not located below the grade level.
- It is recommended that diesel generator sets serving health care facilities are prime rated (ISO 8528–1) and not standby rated.
- Where multiple diesel generator sets form the secondary power supply source and are only supporting critical loads in grades A, B, and C medical locations, N+1 source redundancy should be provided.
- Where the secondary power source is providing power backup for the entire facility, in addition to clinical risk grades A, B, and C locations, N+1 redundancy may not be required. However, in the event of one generator failure, the remaining arrangement should be capable of supporting the entire grades A, B, and C medical locations.
- For health care facilities where the total capacity of the secondary power source requirement is within the limit of a single generator set, it is acceptable to have one diesel generator set.
- This guideline does not recognize an alternate power supply (in addition to PPS) from the local utility company or a solar PV/concentrated plant as a means of secondary power source.
- Special consideration should be given to the choice of starting batteries and battery chargers for diesel generator sets. The diesel generator plant highly depends upon the availability of the batteries for cranking the engine when required. The batteries should be either VRLA or Ni-Cd type; however, Ni-Cd batteries are highly recommended.
- Battery status should be monitored and alarmed though the BMS or any other sperate monitoring system.
- On-site fuel storage should be provided for diesel generator sets. The fuel storage quantity requirements should be carefully determined considering the level of care

provided in the facility; it is recommended that health care facilities providing inpatient and critical care functions are provided with a minimum of 24 hours of fuel storage at a 70% average loading of the respective diesel generator sets. This can be reduced to 4 hours in case of outpatient clinics.

- The diesel fuel storage within the generator room should not exceed 2,400 L.
- Separate, dedicated MDB rooms should be provided for secondary MDBs serving emergency functions of the facility.
- Secondary power supply outlets in clinical areas should be logically grouped in distribution branches with segregated distribution. Automatic change over between PPS and SPS should be as close as practically possible to the point of utilization depending upon the criticality of the application.
- Feeder cables for radiology equipment incorporating high voltage generators that draw pulse currents for a short duration (not exceeding 5 seconds) need not be sized considering the peak current as continuous current. The following general guideline may be followed while determining the demand load and associated feeder cable sizes for medical equipment that draws short duration impulse current.
  - *One unit of imaging equipment:* Demand load and cable size should be designed based on 50% of the short time peak rating of such equipment or 100% of the continuous rating of the equipment, whichever is higher.
  - *Two units of imaging equipment:* Demand load and cable size for an upstream feeder serving two such imaging equipment should be designed based on the sum of (50% of the short time peak rating of the first

equipment or 100% of the continuous rating of the first equipment, whichever is higher) and (50% of the short time peak rating of the second equipment or 100% of the continuous rating of the second equipment, whichever is higher).

  - *More than two units of imaging equipment:* Demand load and cable size for an upstream feeder serving more than two such imaging equipment should be designed based on the sum of the (demand load for the largest of the two-imaging equipment based on "b" stated previously) and 20% of the sum of peak current of the all the remining imaging equipment.
- Note that these criteria are general guidelines for the design stage, and final section of the cable should be verified against the manufacturer's certified requirements once the final selection of the equipment has been made.
- The secondary power supply distribution should be logically organized in separate change over (ATS) and distribution branches. Refer to Table 35C as an example of grouping circuits for secondary power distribution.
- A 100% power supply backup for a chilled water generating plant or hot water generating plant for space cooling/heating is not mandatory but desirable. However, the SPS should have enough capacity to serve chilled water/hot water for space cooling/heating in clinical risk grade areas A and B at a minimum. In cases where the primary cooling/heating for the health care facility is provided by a remote district cooling/heating plant, power backup should be provided for the backup cooling plant.
- SPS backup should be provided for a HVAC air plant such that loss of the PPS will not compromise the pressure differential regime mandated by the HVAC section of this guideline.

TABLE 35D: Illumination/Lighting Levels in Various Areas of the Hospital

Room/Function	Illuminance (Lux)	Colour Rendering Index (%)	Recommended Lighting Control Method*	Lighting Grade (Section 3.16.8,9)
Emergency Unit				
Admissions/Reception	300	80	N	B
Stores	300	80	N/AL	A
Treatment Area	500	80	N	B
Minor Operation	500 (15000/30000 Local)	90	N	B
Triage	500	90	N	A
Plaster Room	500	80	N	B
Procedure Room	500 (15000/30000 Local)	90	N	A
Resuscitation Room/Bay	500	80	N	B
Common and Circulation Areas				
Corridors (General)	200	80	S/AL	B
Entrance Canopy	50 (Min)	80	S/AL	B
Entrance Lobby	200 (Min)	80	S/AL	B
Library	300	80	S/AL	—
Lift Car	150	80	-	—
Lift Lobby	200 (Min)	80	S/AL	B
Loading Bay	100	80	S/AL	—
Reception Area	300	80	S/AL	B
Overnight Stay	150	80	S/AL	—
Lounge	150	80	S/AL	—
Shop/Kiosk	300	80	S/AL	—

(Continued)

TABLE 35D: (Continued)

Room/Function	Illuminance (Lux)	Colour Rendering Index (%)	Recommended Lighting Control Method*	Lighting Grade (Section 3.16.8,9)
Storage (General)	200	80	N/AL	—
Toilets	200	80	N/AL	—
Changing Room, Lockers	100–150	80	N/AL	—
Prayer Rooms	75–100	80	N/AL	—
Tutorial Room	300	80	N/AL	—
Consult/Exam Room	300	80	N	B
Disposal (Clinical, Domestic Waste)	200	80	N/AL	—
Doctor's Office	500	80	N/AL	B
Medication Room	500	80	N/AL	B
General Office	300	80	N/AL	B
Seminar Room	300	80	S/AL	B
Staff Change	100	80	N/AL	—
Staff Room	50/200	90	N/AL	—
Clean Utility	150	80	N	B
Dirty Utility	200	80	N	B
Critical Care				
Critical Care (Night)	5 (Max)	80	N/S	B
Observation/Night Watch	20	80	N/S	B
High-Dependency Unit (HDU)	100	80	N/S	A
Intensive Care Unit (ICU)	100	80	N/S	A
Night Light	5 to 10	80	N	A
Simple Observation/ Examination	300	80	N/S	A
Examination	1000 (Local)	90	N	A
Sterile Supply Unit (SSU)				
Decontamination and Loading	500 (Local)	80	N	A/B
Maintenance (Including Rear of Cleaning Units)	200	80	N	—
Sterile Storage	150	80	N	—
Packing Area	500	80	N	B
Dental Unit				
Laboratories	500	80	N	B
Reception/Administration Areas	300	80	N/S	B
Dental Surgeries	8000 to 20000	90	N/S	A
White Teeth Matching	5000	90	N	B
Laboratory				
Aseptic Laboratory	300	80	N	B
Blood Bank	300	80	N	A
Colour Inspection	1000 (Local)	90	N/V	A
Cold Rooms	200	80	N	B
Inspection	500 (Local)	80	N	A/B
Laboratories	500	80	N	A/B
Relatives' Waiting Room	300	80	N/S	B
Seminar Room	300	80	N/S/V	B
General Treatment Areas				
Dialysis	500	80	N/V	B
General Storage Areas	200	80	N/AL	—
Teaching Areas	300	80	N	—
Administration (Medical Records)	500	80	N	—
Pharmacy	500	80	N	A/B

(Continued)

TABLE 35D: (Continued)

Room/Function	Illuminance (Lux)	Colour Rendering Index (%)	Recommended Lighting Control Method*	Lighting Grade (Section 3.16.8,9)
Morgue				
Autopsy Table	5000	90	N	—
Autopsy Rooms General	500	90	N	—
Body Holding Room	200	80	N	B
General	300	80	Sp	—
Staff Change	100 to 150	80	N	B
Storeroom	150	80	N	—
Viewing Room	50/100	80	S/V	B
Waiting Room	200 (Min)	80	N/S	B
Linen Holding Unit				
Linen Store (Linen Department)	100	80	N	—
Pack and Dispatch	300	80	N	A
Pressing	300	80	N	A
Sewing Room	500 (Local)	80	N	A
Laundry	300	80	N	A
Delivery Unit				
Applying Sutures	1000 (Local)	90	N	A
Circulation Space (Day)	100	80	N	B
Delivery	500	80	N/S	A
Circulation Space (Day)	100	80	N	B
Day	50 to 100	80	N	A
Night	5	80	N	A
Nurseries (Day)	100	80	N	B
Nurseries (Night)	5	80	N	B
Formula Room	300	80	N	B
Special Care Baby Unit	1000 Local	80	N	A
Staff Station				
Day	300	80	N/S	A
Night	30/200	80	N/S	A
Interview	300	80	N	B
Operating Rooms				
Anaesthesia Induction Room	1000 (Local)	80	N	A
Anaesthesia Induction Room	500	80	S	A
Angiography Procedure Room	500	80	s/v	A
Endoscopy Procedure Room	300	80	s/v	B
Operating Room	1000	90	s/v	A
Operating Table/Cavity	10000 to 100000	90	s/v	A
Recovery—Stage 1	500	90	N/S	A
Scrub	500	80	N	B
Clean Utility	100 to 150	80	N	B
Dirty Utility	100 to 150	80	N	B
Allied Health				
Gymnasium	300	80	N/S	—
Hydrotherapy Pool	200	80	N	A
Physiotherapy	200	80	N/S	—
Rehabilitation	200	80	N/S	B
Ophthalmology				
Consult Room	300	80	S/V	B
Examination of Outer Eye	1000 Local	80	N	—

(Continued)

TABLE 35D: (Continued)

Room/Function	Illuminance (Lux)	Colour Rendering Index (%)	Recommended Lighting Control Method*	Lighting Grade (Section 3.16.8,9)
Reading/Colour Vision Test Screen	300	90	N	—
Vision Test Area	100 (Max)	80	S	—
Outpatient Unit				
Consult/Exam Room	300	80	N	B
Treatment Room	500	80	N	B
Medical Imaging/Interventional Cardiology/Nuclear Medicine				
Angiography	300	80	N/V	A
CT/MRI Scanning Rooms	300	80	N/V	A
ECG	300	80	N/S	A
Electro-Medical	300	80	N/S	A
Screening—Fluoroscopy	300	80	N/S	A
Isotope Store	300	80	N/S	B
Radiotherapy	100	80	N/V	A
Ultrasound	300	80	N/S	A
Mammography	500	80	N/V	A
X-Ray	300	80	N/S	B
Inpatient Unit				
Children's Play Area	300	80	N/AL	B
Circulation Space	100	80	N/S	B
Circulation Space (Night)	5	80	N/S	B
Treatment Room	1000 (Local)	90	S/V	A
Treatment Room	500 (General)	80	N/S	B
Staff Station				
Day	300	80	N/S	A
Night	30/200	80	N/S	A
Observation/Night Watch	20	80	N/S	B
Observation/Night	1 to 5	80	N/S	B
Mental Health Units	200	80	N/S	B
Patient Bed	300	80	N	B
Corridors (Day)	200	80	N/S/AL	B
Corridors (Night)	50	80	N/S/AL	B

* LIGHTING CONTROL
- N—Conventional On/Off Switching.
- S—Multilevel switching with ability to control the lighting level in the room by selective on/ off switching of groups of luminaires.
- AL—Automatic lighting control for saving energy.

36 ELV AND ICT SYSTEMS

36.1 Introduction

Extra low voltage (ELV) and information and communications technology (ICT) systems play a key role in the efficient and safe operation of any health care facility. With the advent of a multitude of systems and approaches and rapidly evolving technologies, it is not prudent to mandate specific design criteria in this guideline for ELV and ICT systems.

The local area network (LAN) infrastructure should provide IP connectivity for several services, which may require being isolated from one another from an application point of view while sharing the same physical network. The applications include but are not limited to voice, data, CCTV, video, public address, digital signage, nurse call, central clock, queuing systems, HIS, and PACS. The IT network must be highly dependable and provide sub-second recovery in the event of any component, node, or link failure.

36.2 Medical Grade Networks: Design and Implementation Criteria

High Availability and Resiliency
: Due to the mission-critical nature of many of the systems that will run on the IT network, fault tolerance and resiliency are mandatory requirements in all aspects of design. The solution must be designed with no single points of failure: link redundancy, power redundancy, and core switch redundancy are essential.

Security
: The network design should have capability for virtualizing and segregating users and services in isolated zones over the same physical network. In addition, the proposed solution should be capable of protecting the network from traditional IP hacking and IP exposure.

High Performance
: The network should be able to support latency-sensitive applications by using low-latency switches that can support optimal topologies to reduce the number of hops through the network.

Convergence
: Each virtual network should have its own firewalls to avoid hopping from one virtual network to another.

Scalability
: Scalability is required to guarantee the support for future applications, users, traffic, technologies, etc. without the need for major upgrades or restructuring. Future technologies such as 40G and 100G may be considered.

Simplicity
: Software defined networking (SDN) and configuration of automation technologies should be capable of expanding to the campus and remote sites where users and network devices exist.

Manageability
: Manageability is an essential requirement. All aspects of the solution should provide a method of centralized control via SNMP Management and the normal switches of management features through a console interface and web interface.

Open Standards
: The network design and technology should be based upon open standards and only use IEEE- or IETF-certified protocols to allow interoperability with other vendors supporting the same standards such as HL7 and DICOM. Proprietary protocols and mechanisms are not desirable.

- A fully redundant and resilient converged network is preferred over a number of individual networks supporting different systems. However, high bandwidth systems such as CCTV together with access control may be in a separate network.
- A typical network topology that will provide an enhanced level of availability and network redundancy is illustrated in the following (Figure 36A).
- When public Wi-Fi access is provided in the facility, this should be implemented though captive portals.
- Where cloud storage is considered, it should be compliant with TRA information security policies.

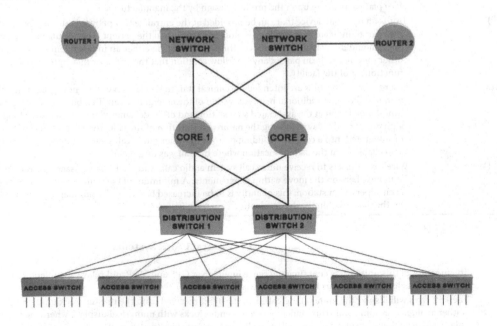

FIGURE 36A Typical IT Network Topology (Courtesy: iHFG).

DOI: 10.1201/9780367460884-38

36.3 Nurse Call Systems

A nurse call system should be provided in all health care facilities to suit the level of care provided in the facility. The components of a nurse call system and its basic functions are given in the following (Table 36A).

36.4 Central Clock Systems

Central clock systems are recommended in critical care and relevant public areas of a hospital for unified time referencing. Due to reliability considerations, it is recommended that clocks are wired type-powered using POE. Where a POE facility is not available, local power supplies or battery cells may be considered. Clocks with additional functions such as elapsed time displays are required in operating theatres. The reset button for these elapsed clock functions are to be located at an accessible height. The system comprises the following components in general (Table 36B and Figure 36B).

TABLE 36A: Components of Nurse Call Systems

Annunciator—Desktop Console (AN-DC)	This unit is intended to be located at the nurse stations for receiving calls and alarms from different patient and staff locations. This unit is recommended to have bi-direction speech capability with patient privacy in mind.
Annunciator—Room Lights (AN-RL)	These are colour-coded lights above or beside each main entrance to the area/room where the nurse calling devise is located to assist the responder to reach the originator of the call quickly and efficiently.
Annunciator—Corridor Display (AN-CD)	Corridor displays, alphanumerically indicating the origin and nature of a call from the patient or other staff member, greatly help in efficiently responding to an emergency call. Depending upon the specific configuration of the clinical department, corridor displays may be required. This can be either dedicated linear LED displays or integrated into strategically positioned IPTV screens if seamless integration of the two systems is implemented.
Patient Call with Handset (PC-H)	These devices should be located in in all patient locations where patients are likely not continuously attended by a staff member. This unit should comprise a fixed unit at the bed head with a staff assist button, speaker, microphone, and emergency call buttons in addition to the jack for plugging in the patient handset. The patient handset should have at a minimum an easily identifiable nurse call button to originate a call to the associate nurse station, speaker, and microphone for bi-directional communication with a nurse and a reading light control. The handset is to be durable, simple, and easy to use and disinfect.
Patient Call without Handset (PC)	These units should be used in areas where all functioning of PC-H (previously) is desired other than the function of the handset. This will be a wall-mounted unit.
Patient Call—En Suite [Toilet] (PC-E)	These units are used to initiate an emergency alarm call from the patient toilets to the associated nurse station. These call buttons are to be easily visible and are recommended to be located at a low level in the patient toilets and reachable from the shower area and from WC. One or two buttons should be provided depending upon the configuration of the toilet. These units should be waterproof and are designed to be located at wet locations. Ceiling-mounted call units with pull cords are not recommended.
Staff Assist Call (SAC)	These devices are intended for staff at a patient location to seek additional help from other staff members. This button may be integrated with a common face plate providing other functions or can be on a separate face plate depending upon the product design by the manufacturer.
Staff Presence (SP)	This is an optional device that can be provided at the entrance to a patient bedroom for activation by a staff member to indicate that someone is already attending to the patient. The annunciator room light above the door should indicate nurse presence. This module can be either an independent button or integrated into other modules to form part of any workflow solution that the end user may optionally include for efficient functioning of the facility.
Emergency Call (EC)	Emergency call buttons are intended for clinical staff to escalate an emergency by alerting other relevant staff members for additional help. Activation of the emergency call (EC) button should generate an audible tone-based alarm at the associated staff station and other designated mobile devises, along with an alphanumeric display indicating the nature and location of the call. The EC button can be a separate unit or integrated into a console including buttons for other nurse call system functions. ECs should only be cancellable from the patient location where the call was originated.
Wireless Handset (WH)	Wireless handsets to receive nurse call system audio calls and alert text messages are recommended for use of staff members on the move within departments. A minimum of two wireless units are recommended at each supervision station; this quantity is to be increased based on the number of anticipated staff members on the move within the department.

TABLE 36B: Components of Central Clock Systems

Master Clock Unit	The function of this unit is to accept time reference inputs over GPS and NTP and relay time reference signals to time display clocks located at various locations in the facility.
Clock Displays	These devises will display the unified time based on the input received from the master clock unit. The clock display can be either analogue or numerical. This guideline recommends clocks with numerical displays where medical procedures take place, while analogue displays are located in public areas (where provided).

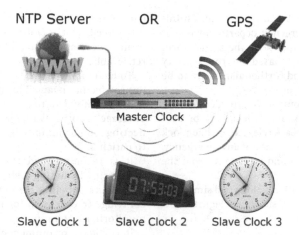

FIGURE 36B Central Clock System (Courtesy: https://sapling-inc.com/wireless-clocks-the-technology-within/).

36.5 CCTV and Access Control

- CCTV system design and installations should meet the requirements of local law enforcement agencies with respect to equipment standards, coverage, monitoring, and data storage requirements.

- Patient privacy is to be considered when deciding the location of CCTV cameras. Cameras should not be installed in areas where patient privacy can be compromised.
- CCTV coverage should include but is not limited to the following:

Inside medication rooms	Outside medication rooms covering the entrance door	Inside laboratories
Inside blood storage rooms	Common corridors	All entry and exits
Emergency room waiting areas and Reception	Pharmacy and medication dispensing areas	Loading dock and receiving areas
Cash counters	Waiting areas	Nursery
Body storage areas	Individual department main entrance doors	Staff/Nurse stations
Staff rooms	Inside enclosed fire exit stairs	Outside public toilet main entrances
Inside hot labs	Nursery	Entrance to technical rooms
Inside main MEP plant rooms	In lift lobbies and inside lifts	Sterile supply unit

- In addition to the CCTV system cameras provided for the general security surveillance, there may be CCTV real-time monitoring required in imaging and radiotherapy areas from the respective treatment control rooms. Such monitoring systems are not required to be connected to the central CCTV system. These monitoring systems are recommended to be provided as part of the medical equipment scope of supply and be positioned as per the respective medical equipment manufacturer's recommendation.

- All security system equipment including cameras should be provided with UPS backup. CCTV cameras may be powered using POE. Associated network switches should be provided with UPS power backup.

Electronic access control is recommended for the areas listed below. However, the exact provisioning of the access control is to be based on the specific security strategy and workflow employed for the project according to the proposed layout of the facility. The following list acts only as a general guide.

Fire exit doors leading to fire exit staircases	Medication rooms	Clean utility
Dirty utility	Electrical, mechanical, and ICT rooms	IT server room/data centre
Imaging rooms	Department entrances	Staff only corridors
All entries and exits to outside	Pharmacy	Cash counters
Entrances to back offices, insurance offices	MRI zones	Radiotherapy areas
Entrances to staff only areas	Medical records	Isolation rooms
Nursery	Airlock area between dirty and clean areas in Sterile Supply Unit (SSU) (with interlock so that only one door can be opened at a time)	

- Discrete panic alarms are to be considered, at a minimum, at cash counters, emergency department reception, and main reception. Expanse of the panic alarm coverage should be reviewed based on the security assessment for the facility, and further alarms are to be provided based on this assessment.
- Where electronic access control is provided in fire escape routes, a suitable failsafe interlock is to be provided to ensure that the locks are released or that a lock overriding facility is available in case of any emergency. Such doors are to be alarmed and monitored from the main security room.
- An example of a CCTV network topology and simplified access control architecture are shown in Figures 36C and 36D.

36.6 Patient/Medical Equipment Monitoring

Much of the medical equipment currently used has the facility to transmit alarms and monitoring data over IP networks for clinical use and for equipment maintenance purposes. For the safe and efficient operation of health care facilities, such monitoring information should be efficiently managed and readily retrievable.

To facilitate this, data outlets are to be provided throughout the facility near all locations where such medical equipment is intended to be used. In addition, wireless LAN coverage is to be available throughout the facility for connecting mobile monitoring equipment likely to be connected to patients.

It is recommended that medical equipment requiring monitoring including fridges and freezers are provided with wired data appoints for connection to a centralized medical fridge/freezer monitoring system rather than a wireless monitoring system.

It is highly recommended that a patient tagging system employing trackable tags (RFID/RTLS) is implemented for psychiatry and geriatric wards. Such system should be interfaced with an access control system to lock down in case of any security breach.

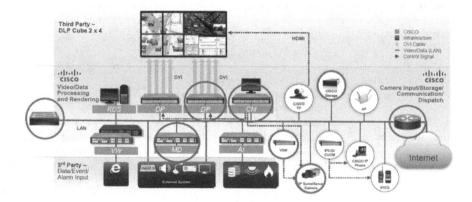

FIGURE 36C   CCTV Network Topology (Falco G, Viswanathan A, Caldera C, Shrobe H. A master attack methodology for an AI-based automated attack planner for smart cities. IEEE Access. 2018 Aug 28;6:48360−73).

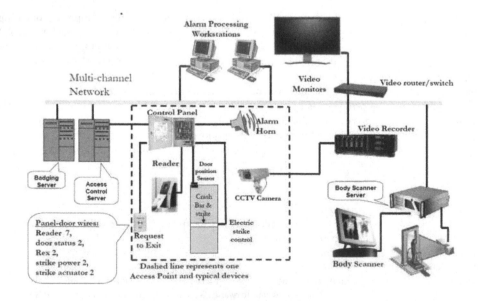

FIGURE 36D   Simplified Access Control Architecture (Courtesy: www.unitedtecgroup.com/access-control-systems.html).

36.7 Intercom Systems

An audio or audio/video intercom system is to be provided as required to suit the workflow and security strategy employed by the designer. IP-based solutions are recommended for better operational flexibility. The intercom functioning in conjunction with the access control system should have the facility to unlock the associated doors (Figure 36E).

Intercoms are recommended for

- Entry doors normally locked by an electronic access control system and required to be occasionally accessible to persons without valid access cards (between the unsecure side and designated door operator).
- Radiotherapy rooms (between control room and patient in a treatment position).
- Computed tomography (CT) rooms (between control room and patient in a treatment position).

- MRI rooms (between control room and patient in a treatment position).
- Isolation rooms (between an outside entry door and patient position).
- Leading locks.
- SSU (Sterile Supply Unit), between the dirty and sterile areas.

36.8 Patient Infotainment Systems

Suitable patient entertainment facilities are recommended in patient bedrooms and at locations that patients are likely to be stationed for an extended time period (Figure 36F).

- The patient infotainment provisions may include but are not limited to a facility to view mainstream television channels, video on demand, patient education videos, hospital department information, dietary menus, and audio/video communication based on the type of facility.

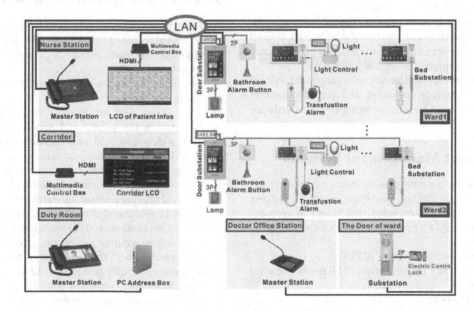

FIGURE 36E   Intercom System Topology (Courtesy: https://saitell.com/healthcare-intercom/semi-digital-intercom-system/).

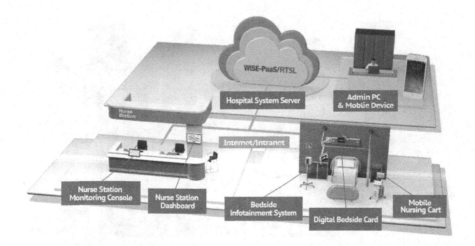

FIGURE 36F   Patient Infotainment System Topology (Courtesy: www.advantech.com/iretail-hospitality/solutions/detail/bedside-infotainment-system-and-digital-bedside-card).

36.9 Queue Management Systems

Queue management systems are recommended to be provided in areas such as outpatient waiting, pharmacy, and other areas where visitors/patients are having to wait their turn. The queue management system should be a consolidated solution integrating different waiting areas of the hospital so that tokens can be transferred from one system to the other. The proposed solution may have the following components and functions (Figure 36G).

- Token dispensing station should be either stand-alone or at suitable location attended by staff members for better and efficient utilization of the system and workflow.
- Waiting area display: This can be suitably sized LED panel screens to display the token number along with the associated counter or room number.
- Counter/room number display: This can be suitably sized displays conveniently placed near individual locations, such as pharmacy counters, to display the counter number and attending token number.
- The system management software should have capabilities such as real-time monitoring of dashboards, overall performance reports, individual employee performance reports, service quality levels, SMS alerts, etc.
- It is recommended that the queue management system also have the facility to accept and record customer experience feedback by incorporating suitable hardware and software.

36.10 Asset Management Systems

- Depending upon the enterprise resource planning (ERP) for the health care facility, electronic means for tagging assets are highly recommended. The asset management system may employ any combination of the following technologies:
  - Real-Time Location System (RTLS)
  - Radio Frequency Identification (RFID)—Active and/or Passive
  - Bluetooth Low Energy (BLE)

- The choice of technology employed largely depends on the type and size of the health care facility. The choice of asset tracking technology is to be decided during the early stage of facility design so that appropriate infrastructure is made available. Although designers are encouraged to embrace modern innovative technologies for improved patient care delivery, it is important to ensure that the selected solution is proven and reliable. Designs should give special attention to ensure that only health care grade-tested solutions are deployed in health care environments.
- Health care facilities having maternity and neo-natal departments should be provided with an infant protection system. This system should be interfaced with the access control system to set off alarms and activate selected door locks.
- An asset management system topology is shown in Figure 36H.

36.11 Health Information Systems (HIS)

- All health information system (HIS) software deployed in health care facilities should follow the Health Information Interoperability Standard issued by the local health authority.
- The objectives of the Interoperability Standard are generally as follows.
  - To serve and establish a cooperative partnership between the public and private sectors to achieve a widely accepted and useful set of standards that will enable and support widespread interoperability among health care software applications in a city-wide eHealth Information Network.
  - To harmonize relevant standards in the health care industry to enable and advance the interoperability of health care applications and the interchange of health care data to assure accurate use, access, privacy, and security, for supporting both the delivery of care and public health.
- Interoperability contributes to enhanced health care delivery that facilitates continuity of care and better decision making while delivering cost savings.

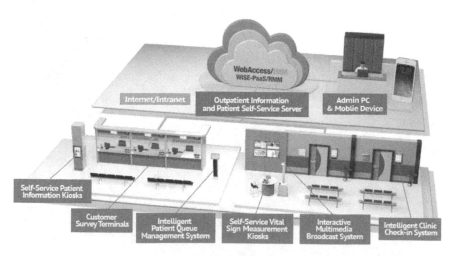

FIGURE 36G Queue Management System Topology (Courtesy: www.advantech.com/iretail-hospitality/solutions/detail/intelligent-patient-queue-management-system).

- Compiling population health data for research, analysis, and improvement measures to enhance the health level of the population.

- The HIS system provided for the health care facilities should be HL7- and DICOM-compliant.
- Electronic medical records of the health care facilities should have the following:

  - Government's data submission requirements shall be fulfilled.
  - Audit trail and role-based access is required.
  - PHI encryption is to be employed.
  - Third-party review.

36.12 Fire Detection and Signalling

Fire detection and signaling are to be provided as per the local civil defence requirement. This includes fire detection and alarm systems comprising detectors, sounders, an alarm speaker, and strobes (Figures 36I and 36J). In addition, the following health care–specific design recommendations should be considered during the design.

- Critical care areas where patients are not normally mobile and are likely to be connected to medical equipment are not required be provided with audible means of alarm sounders or speakers to avoid panic. Such areas should be provided with a discrete means of fire alarm notification at the corresponding nurse stations by providing fire alarm repeater stations at the nurse/supervision stations. In addition, an interface should be provided between the nurse call system and fire detection system to alert staff of any fire alarm incidents.
- Alarm speakers or strobes are not required in operating theatres. An associated nurse station is to be alerted of a fire condition though discrete means.
- Fire alarm and signaling system cables used in health care facilities should be "enhanced" grade, not standard grade.

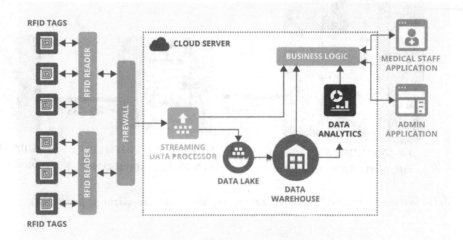

FIGURE 36H   Asset Management System Topology (Courtesy: www.scnsoft.com/healthcare/iot/smart-hospital-asset-tracking).

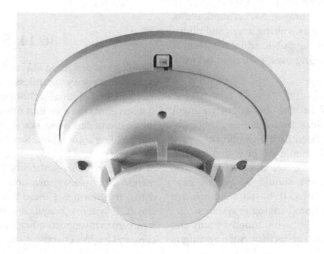

FIGURE 36I   Smoke Detector (Courtesy: https://buildings.honeywell.com/us/en/products/by-category/sensors/smoke-detectors).

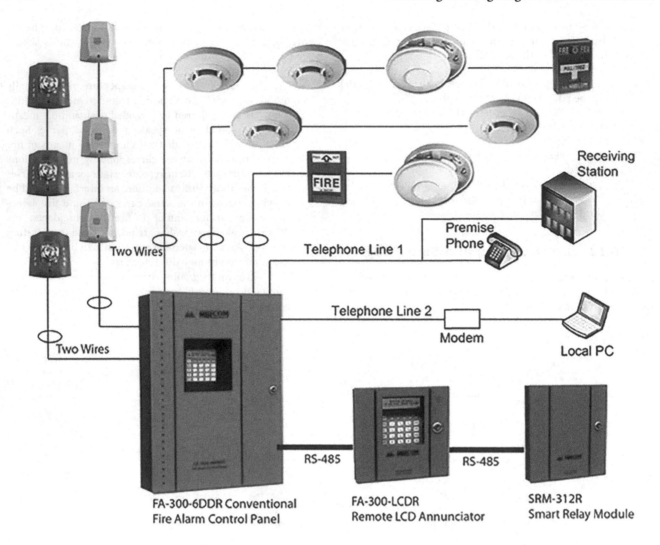

FIGURE 36J Fire Alarm System (Courtesy: https://securityvaultsystems.com/fire-alarm-systems-fas/).

36.13 Public Address Systems

A public address system is recommended in health care facilities for broadcasting calls for prayer, background audio, announcements, etc. in areas such as waiting areas and circulation corridors. Staff paging over the public address system is not encouraged. Discrete staff paging over a wireless network is recommended (Figure 36K).

- Acoustics characteristics of the built environment should be taken into consideration while designing public address systems to ensure audio intelligibility.
- Zone-wise volume control should be provided so that different volume levels can be set depending on the areas. Volume control knobs should be placed near respective supervision stations. IP-based solutions are recommended over conventional analogue systems.
- The public address system is to be zoned to suit the operational requirements of the facility. Such zoning is

to be agreed upon with the stakeholders during the initial phase of design to ensure that cabling is designed to suit.

36.14 Summary

Planning and designing ELV and ICT systems in a hospital is a vital process that ensures seamless communication, efficient data management, and optimal technological infrastructure. ELV and ICT systems encompass various critical components, such as telecommunications, data networks, security systems, audiovisual systems, and building automation. Key considerations in the planning and designing process include proper infrastructure design, integration of diverse systems, scalability for future technological advancements, data security measures, and adherence to industry standards. By prioritizing these factors and engaging experts in ELV and ICT systems, hospitals can establish a well-designed infrastructure that supports efficient communication, enhances patient care, and enables effective management of health care operations.

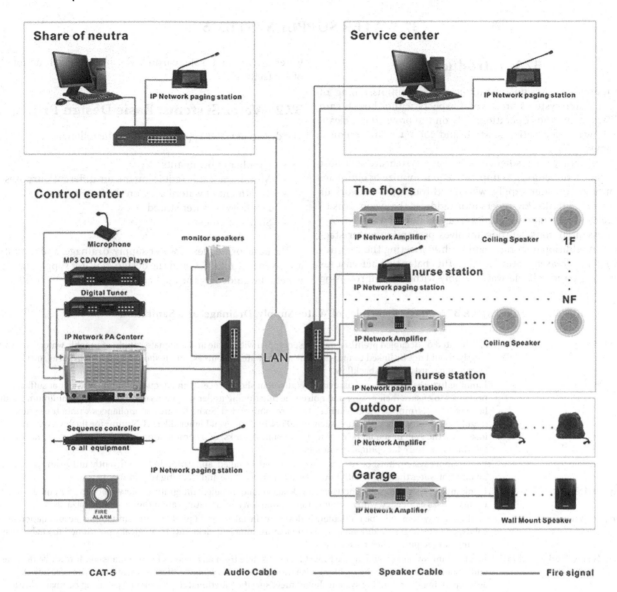

FIGURE 36K   Public Address System Topology (Courtesy: www.dsppatech.com/ip-network-pa-solution-for-hospital.html).

37 WATER SUPPLY SYSTEMS

37.1 Introduction

The meticulous design, installation, and commissioning of potable water systems are pivotal aspects within health care facilities. Numerous operations rely on the provision of clean, treated water for patients, staff, and for operating medical equipment.

The reliability and resilience of the water system are of utmost importance, therefore, it is imperative to minimize or eliminate disruptions in water supply, whether through the network or main storage tanks. Engineers must address these concerns to ensure the continuous and uninterrupted flow of water.

An essential consideration involves preventing water stagnation in additional storage tanks while meeting the requirements for increased water storage. This balancing act ensures a consistent and reliable water supply without compromising water quality and, safeguarding the health and functionality of the facility.

37.2 Water Systems: Basic Design Principles

The design of water supply considers the following:

- Number of occupants
- Minimum water requirements for different purposes
- Treatment of water based on the quality of water
- Quantity of water stored
- Sizing of pipes

The basic principles of water supply, drainage, and sanitation are given in Table 37A, and the design of water supply should in general be guided by the applicable principles.

TABLE 37A: Basic Principles of Water Supply, Drainage, and Sanitation

Potable Water	All inhabited or occupied premises must be equipped with a safe and adequate supply of potable water. This water supply should not be linked to unreliable or unsafe water resources, and it should be safeguarded against potential hazards such as backflow.
Water Provision	Plumbing fixtures, devices, and associated equipment should receive an adequate volume of water at sufficient pressures to ensure their proper and noise-free functioning under regular usage conditions. A minimum residual head of 0.018 N/mm^2 at the consumer's tap is recommended. Some fixtures or appliances within the system might necessitate higher pressure, such as 0.05 N/mm^2 or even higher (like 0.1 N/mm^2 for flush valves). In such instances, the system should be designed with pumps, tanks, or a combination of both to achieve the necessary minimum pressure for optimal operation.
Water Efficiency	The plumbing system must be meticulously designed, installed, and calibrated to efficiently utilize an appropriate quantity of water that aligns with both effective performance and cleaning requirements.
Safety Devices	The plumbing system must be meticulously designed and installed, integrating safety mechanisms and devices to mitigate risks associated with contamination, explosions, overheating, and other potential hazards.
Drainage System	The drainage system must be meticulously designed, installed, and upheld to prevent fouling, accumulation of solids, and blockages. Additionally, it should feature sufficient cleanouts strategically positioned to enable easy cleaning of the pipes when necessary.
Materials and Workmanship	The plumbing system should utilize robust materials, free from any defects in workmanship. It must be designed and installed to provide dependable service throughout its anticipated lifespan. Moreover, the accessories accompanying the plumbing system should meet specific functional requirements, ensuring compatibility to prevent any inconsistencies that might cause leaks and subsequent seepage.
Fixture Traps and Vent Pipes	Each fixture linked directly to the drainage system must contain a liquid seal trap. The purpose of these traps is to uphold trap seals, thereby blocking the entry of sewer gas, harmful fumes, or vermin into the building. Additionally, the drainage system should be meticulously designed to ensure proper air circulation within all pipes. This design should include vent pipes distributed throughout the system, preventing risks associated with siphonage, aspiration, or disruption of trap seals during typical usage conditions.
Foul Air Exhaust	Vent terminals should extend outdoors to prevent clogging and the return of foul air, as they discharge potentially harmful or combustible gases into the atmosphere. It's essential that all vent pipes are equipped with cowls to aid in this process.
Testing	The plumbing system must undergo necessary tests to reveal any leaks or material defects effectively.
Exclusion from Plumbing System	Prohibited substances in the drainage system include those causing clogs, creating explosive mixtures, damaging pipes or joints, or excessively disrupting sewage disposal processes.
Light and Ventilation	Wherever water closet or similar fixture is located in a room or compartment, it should be properly lighted and ventilated.
Individual Sewage Disposal Systems	For buildings without access to a public sewer, provide appropriate methods for treating and disposing of water closets or plumbing fixtures.
Approach for Use and Cleaning	Install plumbing fixtures spaciously for accessibility during use and cleaning. Ensure proper access to doors, windows, and other devices within the toilet area.
Accessibility for Persons with Disabilities	Install doors, windows, and disability-friendly fixtures like WC, urinals, grab bars, washbasins, mirrors, and other accessories with proper accessibility in terms of width, height, space, centrelines, and ease of operation.
Structural Safety	Plumbing system shall be installed with due regard to preservation of the structural members and prevention of damage to walls and other surfaces.
Protection of Ground and Surface Water	Sewage or other waste shall not be discharged into surface or sub-surface water without acceptable form of treatment.

DOI: 10.1201/9780367460884-39

37.3 Water Supply Requirements for Hospital

The daily water demand is determined considering projected occupancy and activities. Designers should locate potential additional water sources to compensate for supply shortages. Assessing available water quality informs treatment decisions for consumption, which vary based on water quality and intended usage.

Projection of population for hospital shall be made on the basis of the following (Table 37B):

- Number of beds + Staff + Patient attendants
- Generally, population density per bed in a secondary care hospital is 5; in tertiary care, 7; and quaternary care, 9.

TABLE 37B: Water Requirements for Hospital, Nursing Homes, and Medical Quarters

Sl. No.	Type of Building	Domestic per Day (L per head)	Flushing per Day (L per head)	Total Consumption per Day (L per head)
1.	Hospital (excluding laundry and kitchen)*			
a.	Number of beds not exceeding 100	230	110	340
b.	Number of beds exceeding 100	300	150	450
c.	Outpatient department (OPD)	10	5	15
2.	Nurses' homes and medical quarters	90	45	135

* The water demand encompasses the needs of patients, attendants, visitors, and staff. Additional water requirements for kitchen, laundry, and clinical purposes shall be calculated based on their specific actual needs.

- Water supply for firefighting purposes: per Part 4, "Fire and Life Safety", of National Building Code, 2016.
- For landscaping needs, water demand is typically estimated at 6 to 8 litres per square meter per day for lawns. However, this value can be significantly reduced for shrubs and trees.
- Health care operators often extend their services, necessitating additional system capacity. Design engineers should allocate a 15% spare water capacity within the system to accommodate the future expansion of the facility.

Source: Source and Quality of Water Supply (Tables 37C and 37D).

TABLE 37C: Sources and Quality of Water Required in Hospitals

Sources of Water	• Connection from the Potable Water Network Supplier • Service Connection for Potable Water Trucks • Underground Water Wells • Bore Hole
TDS/PPM	Depending on the water source the incoming TDS/PPM can vary from 2,000 PPM to 80 PPM. Water must be treated to reach water quality levels of 0–150 PPM.

- Water supplied must meet specific standards, ensuring it is pathogen-free, clear, without taste or odour issues, and non-corrosive and it lacks minerals that might have adverse physiological effects. Adherence to quality standards specified in Table 37D is crucial.
- Non-potable water, when separately supplied for purposes other than drinking, must be entirely free from bacteriological contamination to prevent any health risks to users.
- To mitigate the risk of *Legionella* growth in non-drinking water systems, cold water temperatures should not surpass 20°C, and hot water supplies should maintain a minimum temperature of 55°C across the entire network. This helps ensure absolute safety from bacteriological contamination, safeguarding users' health.

Factor	Standard	Factor	Standard
Turbidity	4 formazin units	Copper	3000 μg/L
Qualitative odour	All odour investigations	Zinc	5000 μg/L
Qualitative taste	All taste investigations	Lead	50 μg/L
Dilution odour and Dilution taste	Dilution no. 3 at 20°C	Silver	10 μg/L
Conductivity	1500 μs/cm at 20°C	Antimony	10 μg/L
Total hardness—alkalinity	Applies only if water is softened	Barium	1000 μg/L
Free chlorine and total Chlorine	Comparison against average	Boron	2000 μg/L
Faecal coliforms	0/ 100 mL	Cyanide	50 μg/L
Clostridia	1 / 20 mL	Cadmium	5 μg/L
Faecal streptococci	0 / 100 mL	Chromium	50 μg/L
Total coliforms	0 / 100 mL (95%)	Mercury	1 μg/L
Colony count: 2-day and colony count: 3-Day	Comparison against average	Nickel	50 μg/L
Oxidizability	5 mg/L	Selenium	10 μg/L
Ammonia	0.5 mg/L	Total organic carbon	Comparisons
Nitrite	0.1 mg/L	Trihalomethanes	100 mg/L
Nitrate	50 mg/L	Tetrachloromethane	3 μg/L

(Continued)

TABLE 37C: (Continued)

Factor	Standard	Factor	Standard
Chloride	400 mg/L	Trichloroethene	30 μg/L
Fluoride	1500 μg/L	Tetrachloroethene	10 μg/L
Phosphorus	2200 μg/L	Fluoranthene 3, 4-benzofluoranthene 11,12-benzofluoranthene 1, 12-benzoperyleneIndeno (1, 2, 3-cd) Pyrene	Individual testing of these substances to provide total
Sulphate	250 mg/L	Total polycyclic aromatic hydrocarbons (PAHS)	0.2 μg/L
Magnesium	50 mg/L	Anionic detergents	200 mg/L
Aluminium	200 μg/L	Pesticides and compounds	5 μg/L total

TABLE 37D: Water Quality Table

Factor	Standard	Factor	Standard
Temperature	20°C	Calcium	250 mg/L
pH	5.5–9.5	Potassium	12 mg/L
Colour	20 Hazen units	Sodium	150 mg/L

37.4 Potable Cold-Water Systems

- In hot climates, incoming and stored water can reach temperatures of 40°C or higher, posing a risk for bacterial growth and contamination. Certain harmful bacteria, like *Legionella*, thrive in such conditions. To mitigate this, potable water-cooling systems are necessary if incoming water temperatures cannot be guaranteed.
- Design considerations should maintain water temperatures within the range of 15–20°C. Achieving this can be facilitated through a plate heat exchanger setup with an N+1 configuration.
- The cooled water should be utilized for wash hand basins, sinks, baths, showers, and hand-held bidets.

37.5 Normal Temperature Potable Cold-Water Systems

- Water that shall not be cooled and shall still be treated to ensure water quality and *Legionella* protection. Potable normal-temperature water service shall only be used in the following:
  - WC flushing system
  - Maintenance areas, workshops, back-of-house areas for services areas
  - Cleaners' sinks
  - Bib tap points
  - Cooling tower makeup water

37.6 Water Storage

Storage capacity calculations consider several key factors:

- Duration of supply at adequate pressure for filling overhead tanks
- Frequency of overhead tank replenishment within 24 hours
- Supply rate and consistency

- Consequences of depleting stored water
- Water storage can be in overhead tanks (OHT) and/or underground tanks (UGT) illustrated in Figures 37 A–D.

Minimum storage tank capacity guidelines are as follows:

- Solely OHT: 33.33 to 50% of daily requirement
- Solely UGT: 50 to 150% of daily requirement
- Combined storage: 66.6% OHT of daily requirement
- For intermittent supply, UGT and OHT capacities may be set at one and a half days and half a day of demand, respectively. If raw and treated water are stored separately in UGTs, the combined storage should meet one and a half days' demand.
- For additional water storage needs for firefighting purposes, consult Part 4, "Fire and Life Safety," of the National Building Code, 2016.

37.7 Protection of Water Supply

- Hospital fixture water supply must safeguard against backflow using reduced-pressure principle backflow assemblies, atmospheric or spill-resistant vacuum breaker assemblies, or air gaps. Vacuum breakers for bed pan washer hoses should be positioned no less than 1525 mm above the floor, while those for hose connections in health care or laboratory areas should be at least 1800 mm above the floor.
- Unless approved backflow prevention assemblies/devices are in place to protect the potable water supply, cross-connections must be prohibited.
- Potable water outlets and combination stop, and waste valves shouldn't be situated underground or below grade. Freeze-proof yard hydrants that drain the riser into the ground are deemed stop and waste valves.
- For non-potable water systems, the piping conveying such water should be distinctly marked using colour

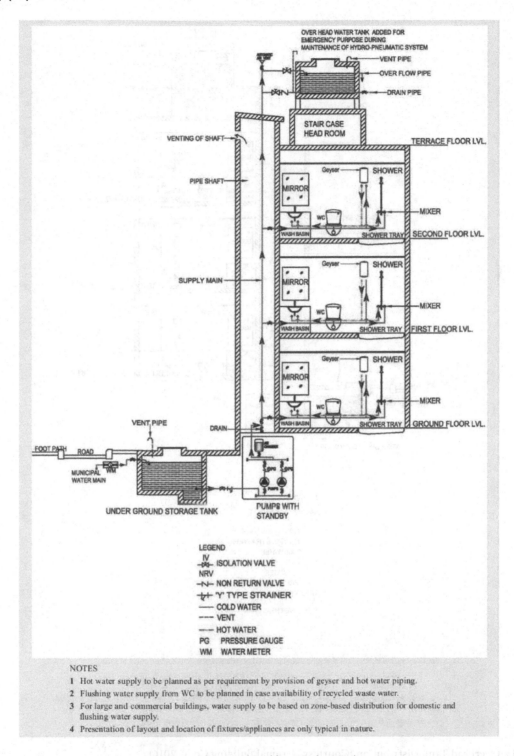

FIGURE 37A   Hydro-Pneumatic System (Courtesy National Building Code, 2016).

codes, metal tags, or tapes per relevant standards and sound engineering practices.

37.8 Materials, Fittings, and Appliances

- All materials, water fittings, and appliances shall conform to Part 5, "Building Materials," of the National Building Code, 2016.

37.9 Water Treatment Systems

- In health care settings, ensuring the safety and microbiological purity of water is crucial to providing a secure and hygienic water supply.
- The degree of water treatment varies based on factors such as water quality, intended usage, and the water source. Identifying the water source—whether from wells, reservoirs, rivers, or lakes—is vital to determining

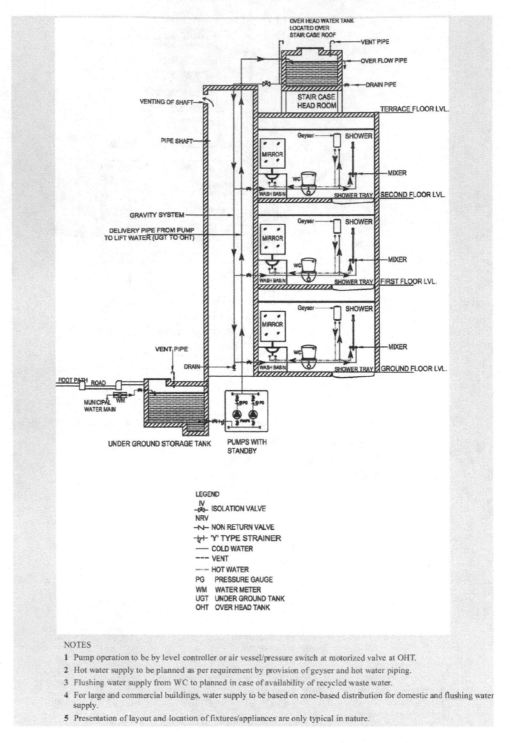

FIGURE 37B   Overhead Tank Distribution (Courtesy National Building Code, 2016).

the appropriate treatment method before its use within the facility.

- Typically, controlling microbiological growth in water systems involves employing temperature, chemical, and mechanical control methods to minimize the risk of contamination. The strategies encompass the following:
  - Pasteurization
  - Chemical treatment (biocides, chlorine, etc.)
  - Silver copper ionization
  - Filtration
- Adapting the water treatment approach based on the health care facility's type and potential future expansions is essential. For instance, in a haemodialysis department, it's crucial to consider a separate mains water supply to ensure that other health care facility areas can be treated without affecting the RO plants.

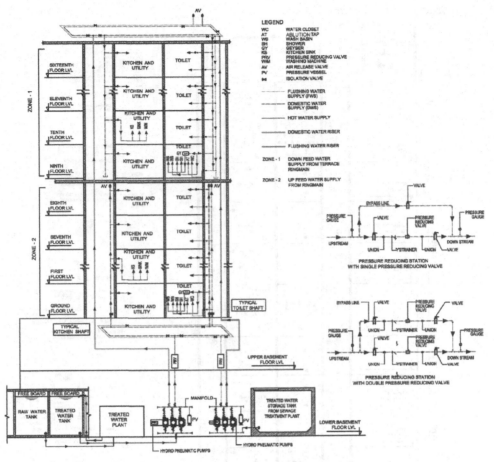

NOTES

1 The given example is for 16 storeyed building with concept of upfeed and down feed ringmains. The choice of ringmain is on designer proposal. For taller building, zones and ringmains shall be planned to meet maximum and minimum pressure requirements. Appurtenance, such as PRV should be planned in main piping network or branch piping, as required, to restrain pressure to upper limits.

2 Requirements for storage and usage fo fire water shall be as per Part 4 'Fire and Life Safety' of the Code.

FIGURE 37C Schematic Diagram Showing the Distribution System in Respect of Hydro-Pneumatic System for a Multi-Storeyed Building (Courtesy National Building Code, 2016).

37.10 Drinking Water

- Some health care facilities opt for a separate water supply specifically designated for drinking water fountains.
- The chemicals employed in treating drinking water must ensure they pose no adverse effects on human health. These chemical products should be sourced from an approved list by the Drinking Water Inspectorate (DWI).
- To prevent water stagnation and mitigate the risk of elevated temperatures (exceeding 20°C, impacting water quality), drinking water should be sourced from a dedicated central chilled water storage tank and pump designed solely for drinking water purposes.
- Installation of drinking water systems without storage prerequisites should be avoided.
- In cases where a central drinking water system isn't available, a bottled water drinking system, typically a water cooler, should be provided.
- Bottled water coolers should offer both chilled and hot water options but must be connected to a dedicated

single water supply exclusively designated for drinking purposes.
- Pantry areas within health care facilities require either above-bench or below-bench hot water boiler/chiller units (per Part B of these Guidelines). These units should receive a standard potable water supply (with internal low-level water treatment).

37.11 Water Booster Pumps

- To comply with the World Health Organization's Infection Control Strategy, health care facilities rely on robust, high-flow water systems for hygienic handwashing. The clinical fixtures should meet specific cold-water pressure and flow requirements:
- Cold-water pressure range at fixtures:
  - Minimum: 1.38 bar (gauge)
  - Maximum: 5.52 bar (gauge)
- Cold-water piping maximum flow velocity:
  - Piping up to 50 mm: 1.5 meters per second (m/s)
  - Piping 65 mm and larger: 1.8 meters per second (m/s)

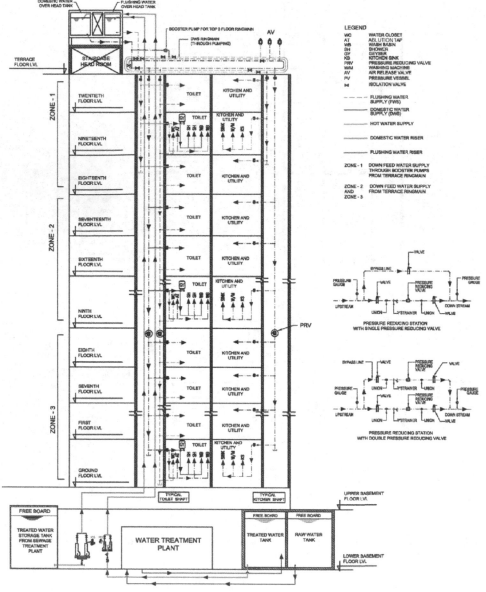

FIGURE 37D Schematic Diagram Showing the Distribution System in Respect of Gravity System for a Multi-Storeyed Building (Courtesy National Building Code, 2016).

- A variable driven speed pump system ensures an adequate water supply across the health care facility. The potable water booster pumps should be multi-stage systems instead of single duty-standby pumps. This approach enhances system longevity, energy efficiency, and provides a wider range of flow rates.
- As a resilience measure for continuous clean water supply in health care facilities, connect booster pumps to emergency power sources. To prevent stagnation, incorporate automatic control in all booster pumps.

- Higher occupant loads on upper floors in health care facilities demand increased pumping. This volume should be regulated using high-level tank sensors. Additionally, install a low-level water alarm to prevent pump dry runs.
- The water pump and storage plant room require waterproof, non-dusty floors, walls, and ceilings. Floors should slope towards designated floor drainage points equipped with trapped gullies, considering potential trap-water seal loss due to evaporation in hot climates. Consider installing a primer valve to prevent such seal loss.

37.12 Hot-Water Systems

- Two distinct hot water supply systems serve health care facilities:
  - Warm water for clinical and general handwash basins
  - Hot water for clinical sterile areas, kitchens, maintenance areas, and cleaners' sinks.
- Design the hot water system in compliance with NBC, 2016, guidelines.
- Treat potable water supplying the hot-water plant with ultraviolet technology before integration into the system.
- Two main types of hot water systems are prevalent:
  - Vented systems, common in older facilities, consist of a cold-water storage above fixtures but are not accepted in new facilities.
  - Unvented systems connect to a boosted main line via valve assemblies, ensuring system efficiency and water quality.
- Four acceptable hot-water system types in health care include the following:
  - Electrical (direct)
  - Fuel burning (indirect; e.g. boiler/steam)
  - Solar (direct, indirect, or both) combined with above methods
  - Heat pump system
- Health care facility systems should include backup water heating, usually electrically, though it can be the primary source too.
- Solar water systems require a duty and standby setup for reliability.

37.13 Steam Systems

There are three types of steam services provided for any health care facility and they are the following:

- Plant Steam—A steam supply service used for health care facilities, laundry, and food and beverages area
- Clean Steam—A steam supply service used for health care laboratories and sterile store units (SSU)
- Pure Steam—A steam supply used for high-grade health care facilities or biotech or pharmaceutical laboratories

In health care facilities, the quality of steam will depend upon the application it will be used for, and this will be known for the health care briefing provided by the health care facility operator. The water quality serving the steam system must be treated (including softened water in some cases to reduce the mineral deposits in the system). Plant steam and clean steam are main types of services that will be used in health care facilities.

There will be two types of sources for the steam system used for health care sterile services, and they are the following:

- Central steam boiler system
- Local or central electric generation steam boiler

Both systems will provide any health care facility with the quality of steam they require, depending on the water quality supply into the system.

Piping must be stainless steel due to the quality of the water and its contents. Stainless steel is a non-reactive metal and can resist corrosion as well as being a hard metal. Other types of metal such as copper are more active metals, and they can leach. Plastic pipes or FRP are not allowed for steam service pipes.

37.14 Maintenance of Water Systems

- In health care facilities, a robust maintenance strategy and a qualified team are essential for system upkeep.
- Tank cleaning occurs weekly; tanks should allow 12-hour operation without incoming water during cleaning.
- Post-treatment tank cleaning, excluding UV-treated tanks, should remove large particles as thoroughly as possible.
- After cleaning, a 24-hour observation period ensures the system's cleanliness, safety, and hygiene.
- Maintenance should involve monthly checks on hot-water heating elements through provided access manholes.
- Proper health care design and maintenance for steam systems prevent wet packs, equipment staining, and chamber scaling.
- The facility's maintenance team needs expertise in water maintenance strategies and the installed equipment.

37.15 Summary

Planning and designing the water supply system in a hospital is a crucial process that ensures the availability of safe and reliable water for various health care purposes. The water supply system in a hospital serves essential functions, such as patient care, sanitation, hygiene, and facility operations. Key considerations in the planning and designing process include water source selection, proper sizing of pipes and storage tanks, implementation of water treatment and purification systems, compliance with quality and safety standards, and integration of backup systems to prevent interruptions in the water supply. By prioritizing these factors and engaging experts in plumbing and water management, hospitals can establish a well-designed water supply system that supports optimal patient care, infection control, and overall operational efficiency.

38 SANITARY DRAINAGE SYSTEMS

38.1 Introduction

The drainage system design should manage the volume of effluent directed into the system, adhering to standard drainage principles in line with municipal requirements, unless specifically outlined differently in these guidelines. Key aspects for the drainage design of health care facilities include the following:

- Geographical location of the health care facility
- Ground surface level at the facility site
- Locations of existing drainage network manholes and primary connection points, if available
- Operational hours of the health care facility and peak load times, if known

- Specific types of drainage discharge (radiation, chemical, grease, etc.)
- Ensuring that the external drainage connection points align with municipal requirements

38.2 Sanitary Drainage Systems: Basic Design Principles

The basic principles of drainage and sanitation are given in Table 38A, and the design of water supply should in general be guided by the applicable principles.

TABLE 38A: Basic Design Principles of Drainage and Sanitation Systems

Potable Water	All human-occupied premises must have potable water supply, free from unsafe sources and protected against backflow hazards.
Water Provision	Plumbing fixtures should receive ample water volume and suitable pressure for quiet and proper functioning. Each tap should have at least 0.018 N/mm² residual head pressure. Some fixtures may need higher pressures, like 0.05 N/mm² or 0.1 N/mm² for flush valves, necessitating pump or tank adjustments
Water Efficiency	Plumbing system should use the ideal water volume for effective performance and cleaning.
Safety Devices	Plumbing system shall be designed and installed with safety devices to safeguard against dangers from contamination, explosion, overheating, etc.
Drainage System	The drainage system must prevent fouling, solid deposits, and clogging. It should have accessible cleanouts for easy cleaning and maintenance.
Materials and Workmanship	The plumbing system must use durable materials, be free from defects, and be designed for a reasonable lifespan. Accessories should meet functional requirements to prevent leaks.
Fixture Traps and Vent Pipes	Each drainage-connected fixture must feature a liquid seal trap to prevent sewer gases and vermin from entering. Vent pipes should ensure proper air circulation and prevent seal breaks during typical use.
Foul Air Exhaust	Vent terminals must extend outdoors to prevent blockages and the return of foul air. Using cowls, install them to avoid potential hazards, conveying harmful gases outside.
Testing	The plumbing system must undergo mandated tests to uncover leaks or defects.
Exclusion from Plumbing System	No substance that will clog or accentuate clogging of pipes, produce explosive mixtures, destroy the pipes or their joints, or interfere unduly with the sewage-disposal process shall be allowed to enter the drainage system.
Light and Ventilation	Adequate lighting and ventilation are necessary in areas with water closets.
Individual Sewage Disposal Systems	If public sewer connection isn't viable, alternate acceptable treatment methods must be arranged.
Approach for Use and Cleaning	Plumbing fixtures should allow easy access for cleaning and use, along with proper door and window placement.
Accessibility for Persons with Disabilities	For users with disabilities, all fixtures and facilities should ensure appropriate access and ease of use.
Structural Safety	Installation of the plumbing system should safeguard structural integrity and prevent surface damage.
Protection of Ground and Surface Water	Discharging waste into surface or sub-surface water bodies requires proper treatment to meet standards.

38.3 Drainage Strategy

The drainage system must primarily rely on gravity for general drainage needs. Any pressure drainage systems should solely serve external or basement areas, connected through sump pumps. Internally applied pressure drainage systems within buildings pose inherent risks of design flaws and potential leaks. System design must prioritize the following aspects:

- Preventing odours through trap maintenance.
- Minimizing blockages.
- Ensuring adequate drainage slope for waste disposal into the main sewer network or central plant.

- Direct connection of sanitary fixtures' drainage discharge to the main drainage runs, avoiding floor traps or other fixtures. Health care facility drainage guidelines specifically pertain to above-ground installations within the health care premises.

38.4 Types of Drainage Systems

In health care facilities, various distinct drainage systems are crucial to maintain separately to uphold infection control

DOI: 10.1201/9780367460884-40

measures and optimize system maintenance. These systems encompass the following:

- **Wastewater Drainage**: Handles discharge from non-contaminated sources like handwash basins, showers, sinks, etc.
- **Soil Water Drainage**: Manages waste-containing systems like WCs, urinals, and other sanitary facilities.
- **Storm Water Drainage**: Addresses external water sources like rain or sprinkler discharge.
- **Chemical Drainage**: Deals with lab-specific drainage that requires neutralization before connecting to the main system.

- **Radiation Drainage**: Pertains to low-level radiation areas within health care facilities, excluding industrial uses.

Integration of certain systems may be necessary to ensure operational efficiency, such as incorporating grease or oil interceptors.

38.5 Sanitary Drainage Requirements for Hospitals (Figures 38 A–C)

Sl No. (1)	Fixtures (2)	Patient Toilets		Staff Toilets	
		Males (3)	Females (4)	Males (5)	Females (6)
i)	Toilet suite comprising one WC and one wash basin and shower stall	Private room with up to 4 patients		For individual doctor's/officer's rooms	
	For General Wards, Hospital Staff and Visitors				
ii)	Water closets	1 per 5 beds or part thereof	1 per 5 beds or part thereof	1 for up to 15 / 2 for 16 to 35	1 for up to 12 / 2 for 13 to 25
iii)	Ablution tap	One in each water closet	One in each water closet	One in each water closet	One in each water closet
		1 water tap with draining arrangements shall be provided for every 50 persons or part thereof in the vicinity of water closets and urinals			
iv)	Urinals	1 per 15 beds	—	Nil up to 6 / 1 for 7 to 20 / 2 for 21 to 45	—
v)	Wash basins	2 for every 30 beds or part thereof. Add 1 per additional 30 beds or part thereof		1 for up to 15 / 2 for 16 to 35	1 for up to 12 / 2 for 13 to 25
vi)	Drinking water fountain	1 per ward		1 per 100 persons or part thereof	
vii)	Cleaner's sink	1 per ward		—	
viii)	Bed pan sink	1 per ward		—	
ix)	Kitchen sink	1 per ward		—	

NOTES
1 Some WCs may be of Indian style, if desired.
2 Male population may be assumed as two-third and female population as one-third.
3 Provision for additional and special hospital fittings where required shall be made.
4 Drinking water fountains are not recommended for hospitals for reasons of infection control. This is to be decided by the health authority recommendations.

FIGURE 38A Sanitary Drainage Requirements for Hospitals with Indoor Patient Wards (Courtesy National Building Code, 2016).

Sl No. (1)	Fixtures (2)	Patient Toilets		Staff Toilets	
		Males (3)	Females (4)	Males (5)	Females (6)
i)	Toilet suite comprising one WC and one wash basin (with optional shower stall if building used for 24 h)	For up to 4 patients		For individual doctor's/officer's rooms	
ii)	Water closets	1 per 100 persons or part thereof	2 per 100 persons or part thereof	1 for up to 15 / 2 for 16 to 35	1 for up to 12 / 2 for 13 to 25
iii)	Ablution tap	One in each water closet	One in each water closet	One in each water closet	One in each water closet
		1 water tap with draining arrangements shall be provided for every 50 persons or part thereof in the vicinity of water closets and urinals			
iv)	Urinals	1 per 50 persons or part thereof	—	Nil up to 6 / 1 for 7 to 20 / 2 for 21 to 45	—
v)	Wash basins	2 per 100 persons of part thereof	2 per 100 persons or part thereof	1 for up to 15 / 2 for 16 to 35	1 for up to 12 / 2 for 13 to 25
vi)	Drinking water fountain	See Note 2		1 per 100 persons or part thereof	

NOTES
1 Some WCs may be Indian style, if desired.
2 Drinking water fountains are not recommended for hospitals for reasons of infection control. This to be decided by the health authority recommendation.
3 The WCs shall be provided keeping in view the location of main OPD waiting hall and sub-waiting halls, floor wise, so as to serve the people effectively. The number of patients shall be calculated floor wise. The OPD population shall include patient attendants @ at least 1 per patient.
4 Male population may be assumed as two-third and female population as one-third.
5 Provision for additional and special hospital fittings where required shall be made.

FIGURE 38B Sanitary Drainage Requirements for Hospitals with OPD (Courtesy National Building Code, 2016).

Sl No. (1)	Fixtures (2)	Staff Toilets Males (3)	Females (4)
i)	Toilet suite comprising one WC, one urinal and one wash basin (with optional shower stall if building used for 24 h)	For individual doctor's/officer's rooms	
ii)	Water closets	1 per 25 persons or part thereof	1 per 15 persons or part thereof
iii)	Ablution tap	One in each water closet	One in each water closet
		1 water tap with draining arrangements shall be provided for every 50 persons or part thereof in the vicinity of water closets and urinals	
iv)	Urinals	1 for 6 to 15	—
		2 for 16 to 50	
v)	Wash basins	1 per 25 persons or part thereof	1 per 25 persons or part thereof
vi)	Drinking water fountain	1 per 100 persons or part thereof (See Note 2)	
vii)	Cleaner's sink	1 per floor, Min	
viii)	Kitchen sink	1 per floor, Min	

NOTES
1 Some WCs may be Indian style, if desired.
2 Drinking water fountains to be provided only when it is a separate block and patients will not use it.

FIGURE 38C Sanitary Drainage Requirements for a Hospital's Administrative Building (Courtesy National Building Code, 2016).

38.6 Vent Pipes

Sanitary drainage systems necessitate venting to the atmosphere through a vent pipe connection at high or near-discharge levels of fixture units. In smaller facilities with only local toilet facilities, a stub stack suffices instead of high-level vent pipes. In compact health care setups, automatic air vents or air admittance valves atop the drainage system are plausible, particularly in single-floor refurbishments within high-rise buildings requiring separate drainage systems.

38.7 Wastewater Drainage

The drainage from sanitary fixture units in the drainage system must be directly connected to the main drainage line (vertical or horizontal main drainage lines). Cleanouts must be located behind the sanitary fixture unit or above ceilings or floor access in service areas.

38.8 Floor Drains

Areas like dirty utilities, SSU, and clean-up zones mandate floor drains. A combined fitting for floor drains and cleanouts with traps is necessary to counter odours. In dry environments, floor drains should connect to a primer valve from the potable water system to replenish trap water lost due to evaporation. Consider using specialized floor drains with seals instead of combining traps and primer valves.

38.9 Soil Water Drainage

- Soil drainage includes discharge from toilets (WCs), dirty utilities, and baby-washing facilities.
- The system can adopt S-trap or P-trap discharge mechanisms, contingent on local limitations.
- Ceiling restrictions, structural constraints, or limited shaft space impact the drainage system's design.
- A P-trap system is recommended to be installed because of its ease of maintenance thus avoiding sensitive health care areas.

- If multiple WCs connect, ensure a minimum 150 mm (160 mm) drainage connection.
- Avoid 90° bends in soil drainage lines prone to blockages.
- Install rodding eye (RE) access doors at bends for unblocking, located in service areas or behind WCs, not clinical areas.

38.10 Soil Water and Wastewater Drainage over Critical Areas

- This is not always possible to route drainage away from sensitive areas like Grade A and B spaces.
- In such cases, use sleeved or double-walled drainage through critical zones, with open ends to non-critical areas to manage leaks.
- Alternatively, implement a double-ceiling system over clinical areas if double-wall piping isn't used.
- For dialysis areas, ensure dedicated clean drainage points below the water supply, allowing easy disconnection between machine and station with no air gaps.

38.11 Rainwater Drainage Systems

- Every health care facility requires a comprehensive rainwater drainage system.
- Health care facility roofs drain into horizontal pipes, connecting to external stormwater networks, on-site tanks, or soakaways, adhering to municipality guidelines.
- Siphonic rainwater systems are suitable for spaces with limited ceiling room or where water seals secure the symphonic process in rainwater gullies.
- Drainage pipe materials must comply with BS EN 12056 or local regulations:—Sanitary Sewer, Stormwater, Vent (Above Grade): uPVC as per BS EN 1329.—HDPE for Force Mains, Gravity Drainage (Below & Above Grade), and kitchen waste.

38.12 Special Drainage Systems

- Special drainage systems are used in laboratory and in special health care departmental areas, such as morgues, incinerators, etc.
- Special drainage systems are the following:

Acid Waste Drainage

- An acid waste drainage system handles liquids with a pH below 7, often in teaching health care facilities where pharmaceuticals are made.
- All acid waste must be neutralized to at least pH 4 before connecting to the external drainage.
- Avoid floor drains in labs; if necessary, cover them with odour-sealed caps and equip them for disinfection.
- Wipe spills with a cloth destined for hazardous waste bins to manage contamination.

Acid Waste Drainage Health and Safety Concerns

- High concentrations of acidic drainage can cause severe harm (to eyes, skin, etc.) to health care workers. Emergency showers, eye wash units, and drench systems must be near exit doors.
- Floor drains prevent flooding during emergencies and connect to a neutralization plant. In case of gas or foggy acid, fog water nozzles can contain the spread.

Acid Waste Drainage Design Considerations

- Install individual traps for each sanitary fixture and ensure vent pipes connect to the atmosphere.
- Connect laboratory drainage to a sole acid neutralization plant, unless mixing chemicals poses risks, requiring additional systems and plants.

Acid Waste Drainage Pipe Material

- The following pipes materials are required for acid waste drainage systems:
  - Polypropylene with electrofusion welding joints
  - Glass with compression joints (encased in plastic for protection)—but not vent pipes
  - High-silicon cast iron with compression gasket joints
- Other materials such as PVC or UPVC or CPVC may be considered but should be avoided as they have a lower chemical compellability and lower temperature rating.
- Polytetrafluoroethylene (PTFE) seal is the only material that is resistive to a wide range of chemicals as well as having the highest temperature rating.
- The pipe for the acid waste drainage systems should be supported through the system to prevent drainage spots in the drainage system that could lead to leaks.

Acid Waste Drainage Treatment

- Health care lab acid drainage must be neutralized between pH 4 and 7 before entering the external drainage. Local regulations might enforce stricter pH requirements, barring discharge to the network.

- Post-neutralization probes ensure correct pH levels for external drainage. If unable to connect to the municipal system, a licensed contractor must empty a holding tank used for a few days.
- Neutralization involves contact with limestone chips, gel, chemical faeces, or equivalent materials in the treatment system, designed for maximum anticipated lab flow rates.
- In smaller facilities, a central neutralization setup may be costly. Instead, individual sinks with acid-neutralizing traps, solely for acid waste discharge, could be installed.

Infectious Contaminated Drainage

- Drainage that will consist of biohazardous material carrying suspended living organisms which risk causing infection to patients, visitors and health care operational staff is considered infectious contaminated drainage.
- The drainage will be from type Q isolation rooms.
- These systems need to be disposed of correctly and safely to ensure the continuity of the facility clean and safe environmental conditions via discharge to a holding tank.
- The holding tank will be connected to all the areas of concern where there is a biohazardous material being discharged.
- The containment is divided into the following parameters:
  - Primary measures—Particular equipment such as the biological safety cabinet, glove boxes, etc.
  - Secondary measures—Measures used to support primary measures.

Types of Biological Safety Levels

- CDC/NIH Guidelines for Biosafety in Microbiological and Biomedical Laboratories have provided biosafety level of contaminates for facilities. The range is from Biosafety Level (BL) BL1 to BL4. In the majority of health care facilities, the safety level is between BL1 and BL2 (BL3 is very rare).

Infectious Contaminated Drainage Treatment

- The holding tank, which is also known as a kill tank, is the when the tank is injected with a chemical that attacks the hazardous organisms.
- Please note that the decontamination process is not an instantaneous process, but the kill tank works in stages for the drainage to be neutralized before connecting to the system.

Infectious Contaminated Drainage System Components

- For health care facilities, the drainage system must be closed system and the floor drains (if provided) are to be sealed.
- Floor drains will need to have valve connections when the system is not in use.
- In many of these areas the HVAC areas (as discussed in section 2 of these guidelines) will have negative air requirement, therefore the floor trap will need to be 90–100 mm deep.

- The floor trap seal will need to be filled with a disinfectant solution that can prevent the spread of organisms.
- The pipe system will be a double wall pipe system with leak detection.

Infectious Contaminated Drainage System Pipe Material

- The proposed drainage materials for such systems are the following:
  - Stainless steel
  - PTFE—for higher-temperature systems
  - PVC, CPVC, PP, or lined FRP pipe—for lower-temperature systems.

Infectious Contaminated Drainage System Vents

- Vents from pipes, fixtures, sealed sump pits, and kill tanks must be filter-sterilized prior to leaving the system using an HEPA (EP1) filter (connected to HVAC system exhaust).

38.13 Radiation Drainage

As per international standards, there is no need for radiation/Contaminated Drainage holding tanks for drainage from toilets coming from patients who have just used iodine-131 or other low-level radioactive isotopes.

If a health care facility would like to provide a radiation tank, they will need to provide the tank external to the building in a location where there is limited to radiation exposure. The level acceptable radiation levels will be determined by the radiation safety officer.

Local municipality may not allow for radiation drainage to be diluted and connected to the external drainage network; therefore, a holding tank shall be provided.

38.13.1 Radiation Drainage Strategy

- Radiation drainage shall be discharged to its own dedicated system. The system may be a diluted type of system or a holding tank system for a licensed contractor to remove the tanks contents.
- A sample access to the system is to be provided for the radiation safety officer to take periodic samples of the system.
- Many facilities may wish to hold radiation drainage confined to glove boxes or protected hoods. Radiation drainage in these areas should be shielded.

38.13.2 Radiation Drainage Holding and Decontamination

- External radiation storage tank shall be a divisional storage tanks to allow for operation and maintenance of the radiation storage tank.
- Depending on the level radiation used, the tank storage capacity can be for 30 to 90 days (it may sometimes be less for an oncology-dedicated facility).
- It is highly recommended a second set of holding tanks should be provided to reduce the risk of health care operations. Depending upon the operational parameters of the oncology department & capability of licenced contractor, a second set of holding tanks are highly recommended.

38.13.3 Radiation Pipe Material

- The pipes used for radiation drainage will depend on the level of radiation being discharged or carried in the drainage system. Per the NRC requirements, the pipe material will need to have the following properties:
  - Pipe must be nonporous.
  - Pipe must be easy to clean and decontaminate.
  - Pipe must be acid-resistant.
  - Pipe must be nonoxidizing as the oxides of the pipe can become radioactive.
  - Pipe joints should not form a crud trap for drainage discharge.
  - Pipe joints should not be by radiation exposure such the weakening of gaskets.
- For health care facilities with low levels of radiation drainage levels some materials such as plastic are not acceptable since there is possibility for certain plastics to react to different types of radiation drainage.
- Stainless-steel pipes (typical 316L) with welded joints is the only pipe that covers these requirements and does not allow crud trap on the pipe joints.
- Stainless-steel press fitting pipe fittings with smooth surfaces may also be used instead of welded joints.
- In bunker areas, where thick concrete is used, the drainage pipe shall be pipe-in-pipe, the pipe, with a duplex stainless-steel pipe to be the exterior pipe that is in contact with concrete.
- Pipe joints are to be outside the concrete cast (unless its unavoidable).

38.14 Condensate Drainage

- All condensate drainage from local air conditioning and HVAC main equipment and plant is to be collected or discharged to foul drainage via a trap (i.e. hepVo trap).
- For water re-use efficiency, condensate should be collected in a single tank and treated prior to use.
- In line with majority of the green building codes, condensate collected shall be used as irrigation purposes.

38.15 Kitchen Grease Drainage

- Where there is a facility for hot food to be cooked, then a grease interceptor is to be provided for all the drainage in that area to be connected to before being discharged to the external drainage network.
- If the health care facility is a small clinic, then a local below the kitchen sink grease interceptor is to be provided.
- In larger facilities the grease interceptor should be provided in an area that is readily accessible by the health care maintenance staff.

38.16 Oil and Fuel Drainage

- Many health care facilities may have main electrical equipment that relies on a fuel source. Any drainage around this area is to be provided with an oil interceptor, per BS EN 858.
- An oil interceptor, per BS EN 858, is to be provided in car park areas where care washing takes place.

- For generator areas where a foam extinguishing system has been activated, the drainage from the discharge shall not be directly discharged into the sewer network.
- Foam systems have a high BOD and therefore will need a storage drainage tank stored below the generator and treated before discharging to the external drainage network via the oil interceptor, per BS EN 858.

38.17 Summary

Planning and designing the sanitary drainage system in a hospital is a critical process that ensures proper waste management, hygiene, and infection control within the health care facility. The sanitary drainage system is responsible for the safe and efficient disposal of waste and wastewater from various hospital areas, including patient rooms, operating theatres, laboratories, and sanitary facilities. Key considerations in the planning and designing process include proper sizing of pipes, appropriate slope for efficient drainage, installation of traps and vents to prevent odours and backflow, compliance with plumbing codes and regulations, and integration of waste management systems. By prioritizing these factors and engaging experts in plumbing and sanitary engineering, hospitals can establish a well-designed sanitary drainage system that promotes cleanliness, prevents contamination, and contributes to the overall health and safety of patients, staff, and visitors.

39 VERTICAL TRANSPORTATION SYSTEMS IN HOSPITALS

39.1 Introduction

Vertical transportation is a phrase used to describe the various means of travelling/transporting people, goods, equipment, etc. between floors in a building. The vertical transportation system is a crucial element in the efficient operation of a building and for the experience and comfort of building occupants.

Hospitals are one of the most complex environments for which to plan vertical transportation for fluent traffic handling. There are several needs for transportation: people, beds with nurses, and goods. In modern hospitals, the transportation of goods, food, linen, supplies, and trash is arranged with automatically guided vehicles by using elevators on their journeys. Consequently, the need for manual labour and transportation devices decreases. There are various types of vertical transportation system in hospitals by which building occupants access specific areas of the building, including internal lifts, stairs, and internal ramps.

39.2 Lifts

Health care facilities greatly depend on lifts to provide a reliable and efficient vertical transport system for the movement of patients, staff, visitors, medical equipment, and associated support services. They also depend on lifts to provide firefighting and evacuation facilities. All lifts should meet the statutory regulations. The lifts in health care buildings are be categorized and provisioned based on the function as follows:

(a) **General passenger lifts:** General traffic lifts should have minimum internal dimensions of 1,600 mm (wide) × 1,400 mm (deep) (Figure 39A). Handrails should be provided on both the side and rear walls of lift cars for general traffic. Consideration should be given to the provision of larger general traffic lifts of 2,000 mm (wide) × 1,400 mm (deep). This size can accommodate any type of wheelchair together with wheelchair attendants and other passengers.

(b) **Lifts for trolley/stretcher movement:** The recommended minimum lift size for patient trolley/stretcher movement is 1,400 mm × 2,400 mm (this will accommodate trolleys up to 800 mm × 2,375 mm) (Figure 39B). A lift of this size will just accommodate an extended standard hospital bed (1,000–1,050 mm × 2,370 mm). However, it is not recommended for moving patients in beds. Where trolley/stretcher lifts are to be used for general traffic, the lift car will require handrails; the internal dimensions of the lift (that is, 1,400 mm × 2,400 mm) will need to be clear of handrails. Where provided, handrails should be limited to one sidewall of the lift car to minimize the potential risk to patients on trolleys; although patient trolleys may fit underneath side

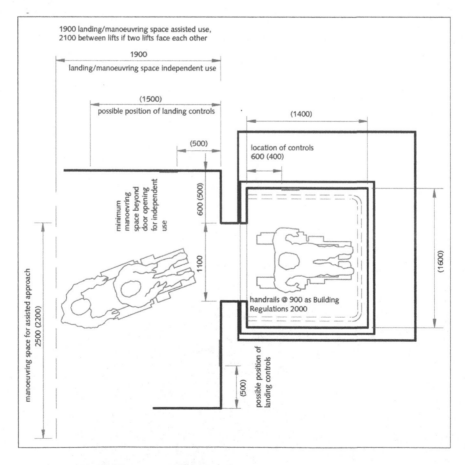

FIGURE 39A General Passenger Lift (Courtesy: HBN 00–04).

DOI: 10.1201/9780367460884-41

handrails, the rail overhang may inconvenience or pose a hazard risk to a patient on a trolley.

(c) **Lifts for bed movement:** The recommended minimum lift size for the movement of patients on beds is 1,800 mm × 2,700 mm. In order to segregate traffic, for operational and infection control reasons, it is not anticipated that lifts for bed movement will be used for general traffic. Where bed lifts are also to be used for general traffic, the lift car will require handrails (Figure 39C).

(d) **Service/goods lift:** These lifts are intended for the movement of items such as furniture, equipment, building materials, equipment maintenance supplies, waste, etc. The service/goods lifts should have a minimum rated load capacity of 2,500 kg, with a minimum clear car dimension of 1600 mm wide × 2,200 mm deep. Clear door-opening width must be not be less than 1,200 mm and 2,200 mm high. Lift car internal height should not be less than 2,500 mm. For smaller health care facilities

(less than 50 beds) smaller goods lifts may be considered based on proper due diligence. However, in facilities where heavier equipment is anticipated to be transported, larger goods/service lift with a wider door opening size is to be provided.

39.3 Design Considerations for Lifts

(a) **Lift landings and lobbies:** Each lift should open onto a landing of 1,800 mm × 1,800 mm, which should be visually contrasting in order not to restrict traffic flow in front of the lift entrance or onto a protected lobby. Lifts should not open directly onto corridors. A protected lobby should be provided where a lift does not open off a hospital street. Figures 39A-C illustrate the minimum space requirements outside lifts. Not only the lift landing/lobby walls and lift door but also the landing floor and lift floor should contrast visually.

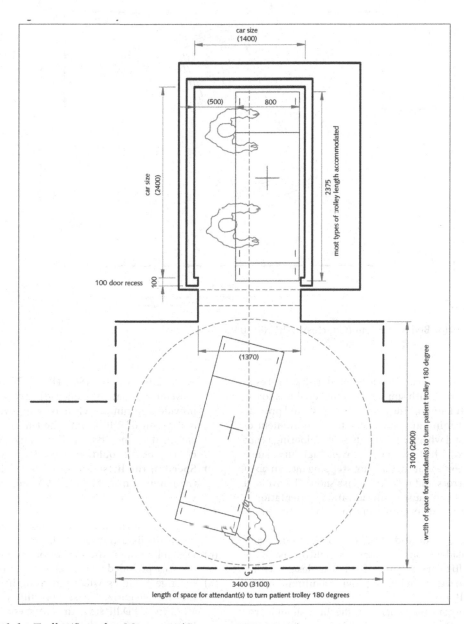

FIGURE 39B   Lift for Trolley/Stretcher Movement (Courtesy: HBN 00–04).

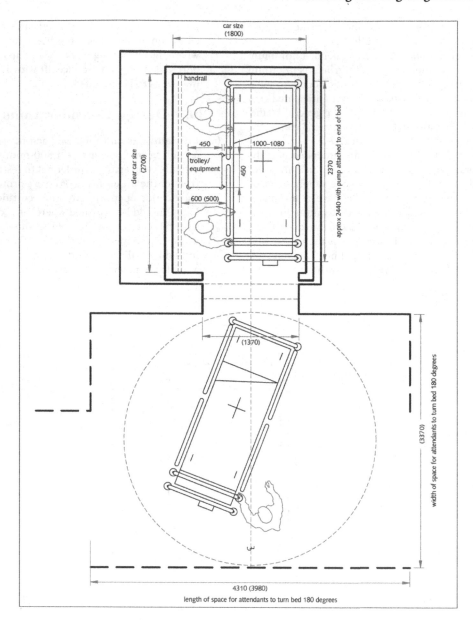

FIGURE 39C   Lifts for Bed Movement (Courtesy: HBN 00–04).

(b) Lift finishes: The lift car should be fitted with a slip-resistant floor covering with similar frictional qualities to the floor of the lift landing. The floor covering should provide good grip but minimum resistance to the movement of wheelchairs and wheeled trolleys (studded flooring is not recommended). The floor should have a high luminance to reassure people that they are not stepping into an open lift shaft. Mirrors and reflective glass should be avoided in lifts, as they can cause confusion and disorientation.

(c) Lighting: Diffused soothing illumination of 100 lux is to be provided in lift cars at floor level. The car should not be widely over or underlit due to patient safety and comfort considerations. Emergency lighting is to be provided in lift cars as part the lift car design with a 3-hour local battery backup to provide a minimum illumination of 10 lux.

(d) Doors: Lift doors for general traffic lifts should provide a clear opening width of 1,100 mm and height of

2,000 mm (see BS ISO 4190–1:2010). Lift doors for movement of patient trolleys/stretchers and beds should provide a minimum clear opening width of 1,370 mm and height of 2,100 mm. The time of an automatically closing door should be a minimum of 5 seconds, and the closing speed should not exceed 0.25 m/second.

(e) Speed of the lifts: The speed of the lift depends upon the building height. Table 39A indicates the suggested values.

(f) Lifts should be located away from sensitive areas in consideration of vibration and acoustics and with respect to magnetic distortion for MRIs.

(g) Depending upon the nature of the facility, firefighting lift/s are provided where called for as per NBC, 2016.

(h) In large facilities with numerous lifts, passenger lifts may be categorized based on different usages such as VIP lifts, OPD lifts, visitor's lifts, etc. Such designation, however, is not mandatory.

TABLE 39A: Speed of the Lifts

Travel Height (m)	Rated Speed (m/s)
18	0.63
30	1.0
48	1.6
75	2.5
100	3.5
120	4.0
150	5.0

(i) It is recommended that as far as possible, the bed lifts and service lifts be identical in design and specifications. This will give the operator maximum flexibility to allocate the lift types for different uses as the need arises and as the operation of the facility changes over time.

(j) Service lifts need to be categorized for different types of use. At a minimum, there should be two groups: dirty lifts and clean lifts.

　(i) Dirty lifts may be used to transport waste bins, dirty linen, diseased patients, infected patients, dirty SSU goods, returned food trolleys, similar goods, and staff.

　(ii) Clean lifts may be used to transport items from the central stores, clean food trolleys, clean SSU goods, medication, occasionally a patient bed (when the bed lift is under maintenance), and staff.

(k) In large facilities, with numerous lifts, the operator should consider designating specific tasks to the service lifts such as food-safe lift, waste lift, clean goods, etc. Apart from clean/dirty, these subdivisions are not mandatory.

(l) In a hospital building, the size, capacity, operational speed, and drive system should be chosen effectively. Some of the main criteria that should be considered are as follows:

　(i) Anticipated number of patients
　(ii) Anticipated number of staff
　(iii) Operation and visiting hours
　(iv) Nature of the departments
　(v) Location of imaging equipment such as MRIs
　(vi) Food deliveries
　(vii) Waste disposal
　(viii) Emergency evacuation
　(ix) Clinical workflows
　(x) Configuration of the building

(m) Centre-opening doors provide better traffic performance than side-opening doors; in consideration of this, only centre-opening doors should be provided for lifts serving patients and clinical staff. Side-opening lifts may be acceptable for goods lifts not intended for clinical staff or patients. The centre-opening doors should be in either a two or four leaves configuration to suit the available lift shaft.

(n) In order to reduce the stress imposed on vulnerable patients, the acceleration of the lift cars used to serve surgical and clinical areas should not exceed 0.6 m/s^2, while rate of change of acceleration or deceleration should not exceed 1.0m/s^3.

(o) During a vertical transportation traffic analysis for health care buildings, lift car occupancy is to be considered lower than the normal 80% of rated capacity used in commercial building traffic calculations to account for the space requirements for wheelchairs, stretchers, equipment, etc.; 25% of the rated capacity is more appropriate for health care buildings.

(p) Lift shafts generally penetrate all floors of a health care building and therefore pose a risk for the transmission of infection across floors. To reduce this risk, the lift shaft wall and ceiling should be sealed and painted.

(q) Lift car doors should be fitted with contact-free passenger/obstruction detection to minimize the risk of car/landing door collisions with persons, beds, or equipment, and should work in conjunction with the automatic door operator.

(r) Lift cars and all landings should indicate the floor number and the direction of travel of the lift car.

(s) When functions of the physically located lifts as a group are similar, such cars should be grouped and controlled in a "collective" method; when the function of each lift in the group is different (such as dirty, clean, staff, etc.), the cars may have to be controlled individually (Simplex).

(t) Depending upon operational workflows and security strategy, electronic card access systems are to be implemented, along with an emergency bed services function. Emergency bed services facilitate the priority lift car call option for patients in critical care and associated staff.

(u) At least one elevator in a bank of lifts is to be fed from the emergency (secondary) branch of power distribution. The power supply for lifts is to be sourced directly (grouped or individually) from the main distribution board (MDB) of the health care building.

39.4 Stairs

Steps and staircases should be intended as an alternative to lift access in buildings and should be of adequate design to allow all persons, with or without a disability, to travel safely and independently.

Dimensions and Orientation

(a) The required staircases and the main circulation staircase in common areas of a building should be constructed with treads of not less than 300 mm in width (measured at the centre of the flight) from the face of one riser to the face of the next riser and with risers of not more than 150 mm in height.

(b) The risers should be built with a vertical or receding face of not more than 15 mm from the vertical, without a projecting nosing.

(c) There should not be more than 11 steps in any flight without the introduction of a landing.

(d) Staircases should be provided on both sides with properly fitted handrails.

(e) Staircases should be provided with non-slip nosing in contrasting colour.

(f) A landing should be provided at the top and bottom of each flight of stairs.

(g) The minimum clear landing depth is 1,200 mm but must equal the clear stair width between handrails.

(h) The top and bottom steps of a flight should not encroach onto the landing area. Doors must open clear of the unobstructed clear landing.

(i) To indicate that there are descending steps ahead, consideration should be given to providing a hazard warning zone on each landing. The zone should use a floor finish that contrasts visually with the general floor finish but has the same slip resistance.

(j) The warning zone should be at least 400 mm from the nosing and a minimum of 800 mm deep and 1,200 mm wide (see Figure 39D).

(k) Risers should not be of the open type, as they are a trip hazard (especially for semi-ambulant people with leg braces and prostheses), disorientating, and may transmit distracting sounds.

Colour contrast: Treads and walls of a staircase should be in contrasting colours.

Edge protection: For steps not adjacent to a wall, a barrier with a minimum height of 100 mm above the level of the treads should be provided for safety reasons (to prevent feet, crutches, and sticks from accidentally slipping off the edge of steps).

Step finishes and type: Stair finishes should not have patterns that may cause step edges to be indistinguishable or cause visual confusion of any kind. Helical and spiral steps, whose treads are often too narrow, should be avoided.

Handrails: Handrails should be provided on both sides of steps. Handrails should be located within the width of the tread of the stairs.

Clear width of steps: Steps should be wide enough to allow people to negotiate them comfortably by holding onto one or both handrails or by being assisted. The width of the steps should reflect the amount of pedestrian traffic. A minimum unobstructed, clear stair width between handrails of 1,000 mm for one person or 1,500 mm for two-way traffic is necessary. The minimum 1,000-mm wide channel ensures that people can use both handrails if they wish.

Tactile warning strip: Tactile warning strips should be provided at landings and at both the bottom and top ends of a staircase, regardless of the number of steps

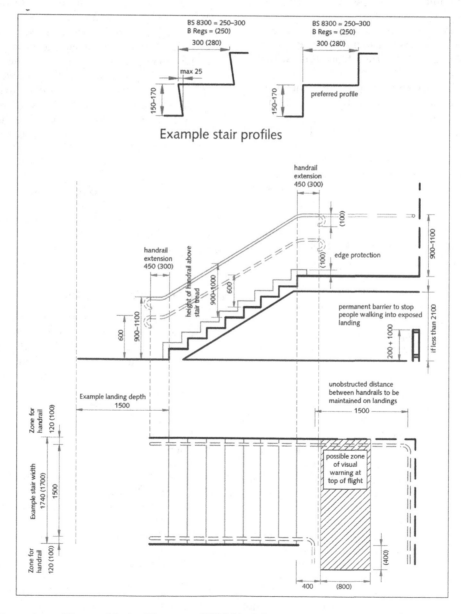

FIGURE 39D Dimensions of Internal Stairs (Courtesy: HBN 00–04).

that it comprises. For landings leading to a floor or those enclosed by wall, railing, or balustrade, tactile warning strips of 300 mm in width should be provided; for those leading to an open space or to the entrance/exit of a building, the tactile warning strips should be 600 mm in width. In this case, Braille and tactile information signs should be provided on the adjacent wall to indicate the presence of an opening. For a staircase with intermediate steps between two flights, the provision of tactile warning strips should follow the arrangement in (Figure 39E).

Avoidance of projection: No appliances, fixtures, or fittings should project beyond 90 mm from the surface of any wall in a staircase below a level of 2,000 mm above the treads of the staircase unless they are unavoidable, in which case they should also be extended downwards to the level of the treads.

Lighting: Stairs and landings should be well-illuminated. The lighting should be designed so that it highlights the differences between risers and treads, the top and bottom steps, and any changes in direction. Lighting that causes glare (for example, poorly located spotlights, floodlights, or low-level light sources) should be avoided.

Mattress evacuation: For mattress evacuation, the number of turning manoeuvres in descending a staircase should be as few as possible. Figure 39F illustrates an example staircase design for mattress evacuation. Figure 39G provides optional/alternative dimensions for the clear width of stairs and landings.

Design Considerations

(a) Where steps or stairs are in an accessible route, complementary ramps, lifts, or escalators should be provided.
(b) All steps should be uniform.
(c) Circular stairs and sloped landings should be avoided.

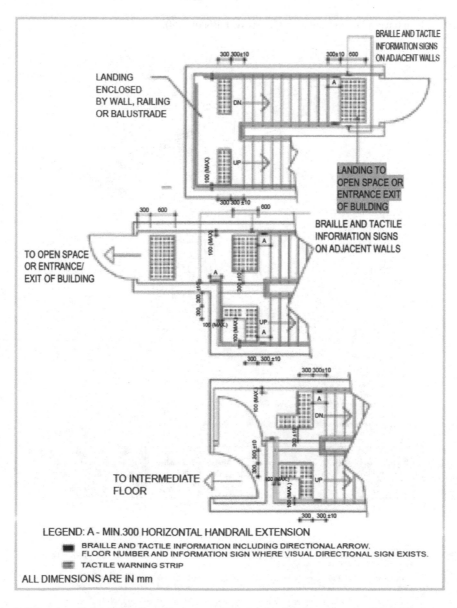

FIGURE 39E Tactile Warning Strip at Landing (Courtesy: CPWD Handbook on Barrier Free and Accessibility; https://cpwd. gov.in/Publication/HandbookonBarrier.pdf).

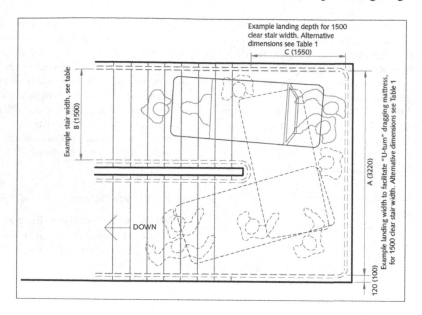

FIGURE 39F   Mattress Evacuation Down Stairway (Courtesy: HBN 00–04).

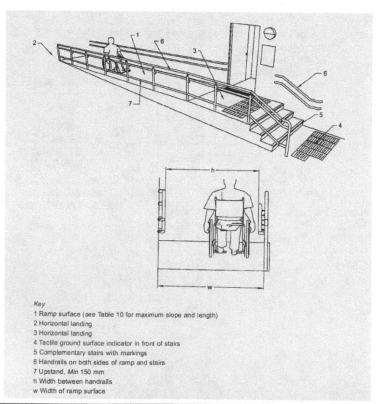

Key
1 Ramp surface (*see* Table 10 for maximum slope and length)
2 Horizontal landing
3 Horizontal landing
4 Tactile ground surface indicator in front of stairs
5 Complementary stairs with markings
6 Handrails on both sides of ramp and stairs
7 Upstand, *Min* 150 mm
h Width between handrails
w Width of ramp surface

A Minimum clear landing width	B Minimum clear stair width	C Minimum clear landing depth	
2800	1100	1950	allows mattress evacuation only
2800	1200	1925	
2800	1300	1850	allows mattress evacuation and restricted ambulant passing
3000	1400	1750	
3220	1500	1550	
3400	1600	1600*	allows mattress evacuation plus ambulant passing
3800	1800	1800*	

* Stair width is not determined by the number of people expected to use the stairs in a fire emergency, but principally by the requirements of mattress manoeuvrability.

For a clear landing width of 3400 mm, the minimum clear landing depth for mattress evacuation is 1450 mm. 1600 mm is recommended to enable ambulant passing and to equal the clear stair width. See BS 8300.

For a clear landing width of 3800 mm, the minimum clear landing depth for mattress evacuation is 1350 mm. 1800 mm is recommended to equal the clear stair width. See BS 8300.

FIGURE 39G   Alternative Stair and Landing Dimensions to Facilitate Mattress Evacuation (Courtesy: HBN 00–04).

(d) It is necessary to provide a safe and well-dimensioned staircase for the comfort of all people, especially those with mobility problems.

(e) When ascending a stair, people who wear callipers or who have stiffness in hip or knee joints are particularly at risk of trapping the toes of their shoes beneath projecting nosings.

(f) Stairs should be designed with more generous dimensions, for example, wider tread and a shorter travel distance is recommended.

(g) Open risers should be avoided.

(h) Unawareness of steps is dangerous to persons with visual impairment. Timely tactile or audible warning of change in level is therefore essential. Warnings should be placed sufficiently in advance of any potential dangers.

(i) The provision of Braille and high luminous contrast signs is recommended. For persons with visual impairment, high luminous contrast, larger font, and a more prominent and well-defined shape of sign/signage are recommended.

(j) Despite the design requirements of tactile guide paths, tactile warning strips would help orientation for persons with visual impairment; they sometimes impose hazards to people with limited mobility, children, and the elderly.

39.5 Internal Ramps

A ramp is a sloping pathway leading from one level to another. Ramps of an appropriate design should be provided at all changes in level other than those served by an accessible lift or accessible lifting mechanism accommodating the specific requirements of persons with disabilities. Ramps allow persons with reduced mobility to move from one level to another. However, many ambulant persons with disabilities negotiate steps more easily and safely. Hence, it is preferable to provide accessibility by both steps and ramps.

Gradient: The gradient should be constant between landings. The minimum specifications for ramp gradients addressing different level differences are given in Table 39B.

Width: A ramp should not be less than 1,800 mm in width.

Surface: Ramps and landing surfaces should be non-glare, smooth, level, even, and slip-resistant even when wet. Outdoor ramps and their surface should be designed to prevent water from accumulating on the walking surfaces. The surface finish should be hard and suitable for the volume of traffic that the ramp is likely to experience.

Landings: An end landing should be provided at the bottom and the top of a sloped path, a stepped path, or a ramp and where the run changes direction. The area of the end landing may be a part of the continuing path (Figures 39F and 39G). The length of an end landing and an intermediate landing should be not less than 1,500 mm. Where the ramp run changes direction, the minimum landing dimensions should be 1,500 mm × 1,500 mm. The area of a landing should be clear of any obstruction including the path of the swing of a door or gate. Landings should also be provided at regular intervals of not more than 9,000 mm of every horizontal run. It should conform to other provisions of this annex if served by a doorway. If the end landing follows or precedes a turn for a pathway or an entrance, the minimum dimension of the landing should be a minimum of 1,500 mm × 1,500 mm. The width of the ramp and consequently the dimension of a landing in the direction perpendicular to the direction of the ramp should also be governed by the provisions of Table 39B.

Handrails: A ramp run with a vertical rise greater than 150 mm should have handrails that should (Figure 39H)

(a) be securely fixed and rigid; the fastenings and the materials should be able to withstand a minimum point load, both vertical and horizontal of 1.7 kN.

TABLE 39B: Minimum Specifications for Ramp Gradients Addressing Different Level Differences

Sl. No.	Level Difference	Maximum Gradient of the Ramp	Ramp Width (mm)	Handrails on Both Sides	Other Requirements
1.	150 mm to 300 mm	1:12	1,200	Yes	—
2.	301 mm to 750 mm	1:12	1,500	Yes	Landings after every 5 m of ramp run
3.	751 mm to 3,000 mm	1:15	1,800	Yes	Landings after every 9 m of ramp run
4.	> 3,000 mm	1:20	1,800	Yes	Landings after every 9 m of ramp run

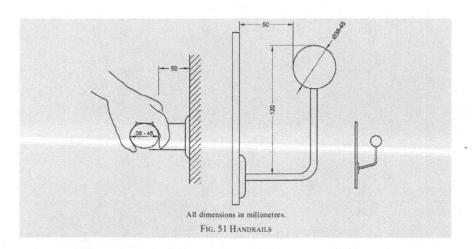

All dimensions in millimetres.
FIG. 51 HANDRAILS

FIGURE 39H Dimensions of a Handrail (Courtesy: NBC, 2016).

(b) be slip resistant with round ends.

(c) have a circular section of 38–45 mm in diameter.

(d) be free of any sharp or abrasive elements.

(e) have continuous gripping surfaces, without interruptions or obstructions that may break a hand hold.

(f) contrast with the wall behind.

(g) be provided with Braille/tactile markings at the beginning and at the end to give information to people with visual impairment.

(h) be provided on both sides.

(i) be continuous, even at the landings.

(j) extend at least 300 mm beyond the first and last nosing. A handrail should not project into a transverse circulation path unless it is continuous and intended to form part of the guidance along this path. The end of the horizontal extension should be turned towards the wall on the closed side of the ramp or stairs or be turned down and terminate at floor or ground level.

(k) have a minimum clear space of 50 mm from the walls.

(l) the height to the top of a handrail should be between 850 mm and 950 mm above the surface of a ramp, the pitch line of a stair, and with a lower profile than the first one. The height to the top of the second handrail should be between 650 mm and 750 mm above the surface of a ramp, the pitch line of a stair, and the surface of a landing. There should be sufficient distance between the two handrails (for example, 200 mm). In case the handrail is enclosed in a recess, the recess should extend at least 450 mm above the top of the rail.

Edge protection along ramps: Ramps and landings not adjacent to a wall should have an edge protection in form of a 75 mm kerb.

Design Considerations

(a) Where there is a change in level, the provision of a ramp is an effective method to ensure largely independent accessibility for persons with a disability and the elderly. Interior ramps are preferred as a means of egress to stairs as they accommodate a wider range of building users, including wheelchair users.

(b) When the slope of a ramp is more gradual (i.e., the less steep it is), people can use it more easily without assistance. Therefore, a slope with the ratio of 1:20 (5%) to 1:15 (6.7%) is preferred. It can take much energy to get up ramp with steep gradient, which also makes speed control difficult when going down. Steep inclines can put a wheelchair in danger of tipping backwards or forwards as many users cannot lean or adjust their balance to accommodate gradients.

(c) A level resting space outside the swing of any door at the top of a ramp should be provided to avoid the possibility of "roll-back" for a wheelchair user when trying to open the door.

(d) A ramp should have handrails on both sides so that it can be used in both directions by people with a mobility problem on one side such as may be the case for stroke sufferers.

(e) A ramp that surmounts a major change in level has to be very long and requires multiple ramp and landing combinations. In such circumstances, other design solutions should be considered.

(f) A curved ramp is not a preferred design solution. Similarly, a cross fall can put a wheelchair user at risk and may adversely affect steering, particularly on a manually propelled chair.

40 PNEUMATIC TUBE SYSTEMS IN HOSPITALS

40.1 Introduction

A pneumatic air tube transport system—which may be either a point-to-point or multi-point system—is a distribution network of tubes through which carriers of various sizes containing small items are driven by airflow. The prime mover is a blower that can alter the direction of the airflow in the tube as required to move the carrier through the system.

In health care facilities, Pneumatic Tube Systems (PTS) transport small materials, documents, laboratory samples, etc. to and from pharmacies, laboratories, blood banks, surgery centres, emergency departments, nurse stations, and other locations throughout health care facilities.

(a) **Point-to-point system:** Point-to-point pneumatic air tube transport systems (Figure 40A) provide two-way transfer via a single continuous tube linking stations up to 1,000 m apart. This system is suitable for use in an application that requires simple operation and a dedicated link between departments, for example, between an operating theatre and the pathology department.

(b) **Multi-point system:** Multi-point pneumatic air tube transport systems (Figure 40B) provide full intercommunication among all points in the system. Where systems are large and traffic is heavy, the network may be split into zones. This allows local transport of carriers in each zone and transfer to another zone when required. This type of system is commonly used in large hospitals, with, for example, the pharmacy and pathology departments being in separate zones.

40.2 Components of Pneumatic Tube Systems

(a) **Blower and Reverse Air Valve:** The blower (PTS compressor system) generates the air that moves the PTS carriers throughout the health care facility via pressure or vacuum suction. The location of the blower will be in the health care facility plant room as per coordination with the health care operator and health planning briefing. As soon as all pending processes are finished, the blower disconnects automatically. Blowers should come fitted as standard with energy-efficient IE2/NEMA motors (according to the destination country) that conform to the IEC 60034–30 standard. Blowers are to be installed in the plant room along with the system control unit and interzone/linear coupler if applicable (Figure 40C).

(b) **Blower Group:** This is a group of PTS blowers that are interconnected that include sending and receiving drivers to allow any single blower to handle the carrier delivery from sending and receiving, and vice versa. These are usually installed in large health care facilities such as a tier 4–6 delineation health care level.

(c) **Carrier:** A PTS reusable plastic container that holds and protects contents (lab specimens, pharmaceuticals, blood products, etc.) sent through a pneumatic tube system. Carriers come in different sizes to cater to the functions or requirements of the facility. All carriers should be equipped with an RFID sensor for easy distribution of carriers to departments by programming the "Home"

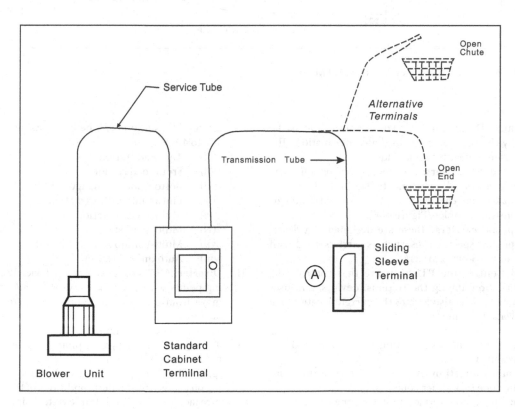

FIGURE 40A Point-to-Point System (Courtesy: HTM 2009).

DOI: 10.1201/9780367460884-42

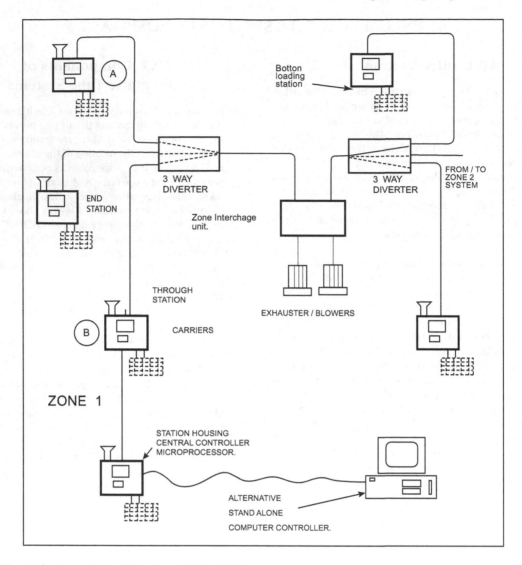

FIGURE 40B   Multi-Point System (Courtesy: HTM 2009).

station and "Destination", which will automatically be guided by the scanner mode or dialed destination. The carriers used in health care include

(i)   **Standard carriers:** For medications or solid particles and small instruments (Figure 40D).

(ii) **Leak-proof carriers:** For transport of liquid or sensitive samples (Figure 40E).

(iii) **Special carriers:** These are designed and developed for specific uses, such as carriers lined with lead or cooling carriers.

(d) **Control Centre:** The PTS software that controls the communication among the stations, devices, and user requirements. This also locates the current location of a carrier via a user interface.

(e) **Database:** A repository of information for each of the PTS carrier movements including a date, time, and station operability.

(f) **Interzone Connection:** A section of tubing that connects one zone to another zone.

(g) **Station:** The user interface unit that may include an interactive touch screen system, a mechanical dialing system, and/or an RFID scanner to send or receive the

carrier. The stations can be of following types (Figures 40F to 40L):

(i)   Top-load station
(ii)   Front-load station
(iii) Bottom-load compact station
(iv)   Linear auto unload station
(v)   Multi-receive station
(vi)   Multi-send station
(vii) Multi-combo station 160 mm
(viii) Auto unload station

(h) **Diverter:** A PTS route switching device used at branching points within a tube network to allow a carrier to move from one path to another. In many health care facilities, this is usually located within riser shafts or above the ceilings (Figure 40M).

(i) **Tubing:** Tubing or system piping is generally provided for 110 mm or 160 mm. The tubes are available in PVC (grey), PVC (transparent), GI, and stainless steel, depending on the environmental conditions of the site. In health care facilities, PVC and stainless steel pipes are preferred over galvanized iron pipe. Health care operators may request a pipe greater than 160 mm to be provided for

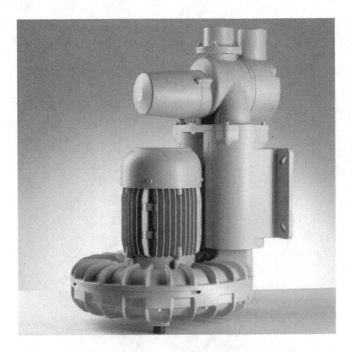

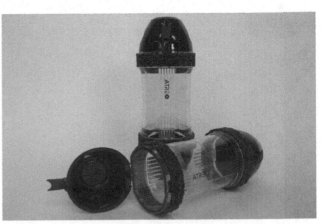

FIGURE 40E Leak-Proof Carrier for a Pneumatic Tube System (Courtesy: www.businesswire.com/news/home/2015 0312006039/en/Atreo-Services-Introduces-6-Inch-Sealed-Pneumatic-Tube-System-Carrier-for-Hospitals).

FIGURE 40C Three-Phase Blower for a Pneumatic Tube System (Courtesy: www.aerocomusa.com/products/three-phase-blower/).

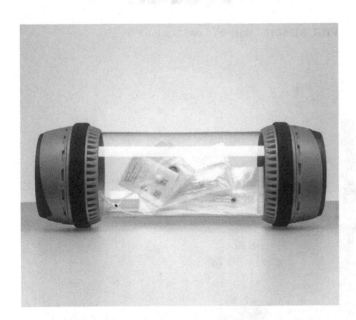

FIGURE 40D Standard Carrier for a Pneumatic Tube System (Courtesy: www.swisslog-healthcare.com/en-sg/products/transport-automation/transponet-pneumatic-tube-system).

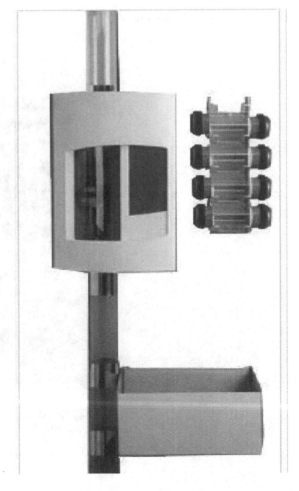

FIGURE 40F Front-Load Station.

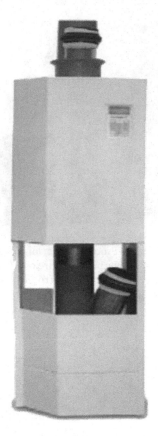

FIGURE 40G   Top-Load Station.

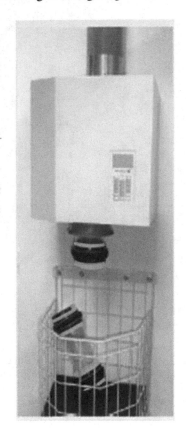

FIGURE 40H   Bottom-Load Station.

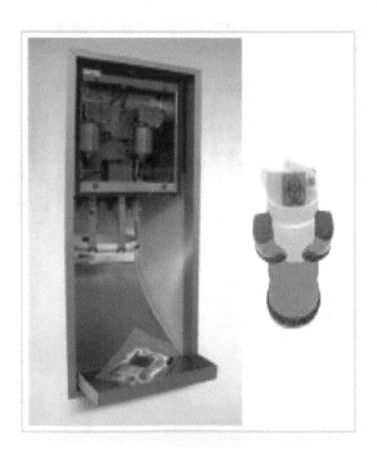

FIGURE 40I   Auto Unload Station.

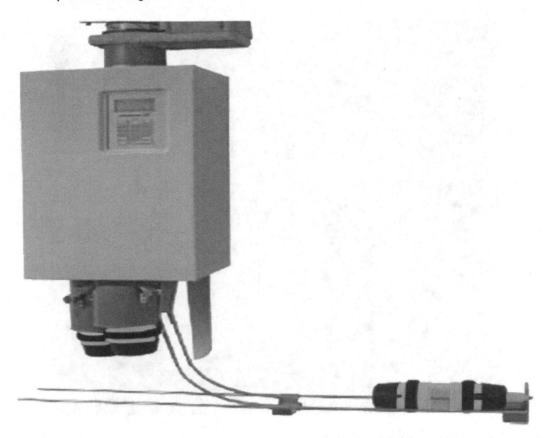

FIGURE 40J Multi-Receive Station.

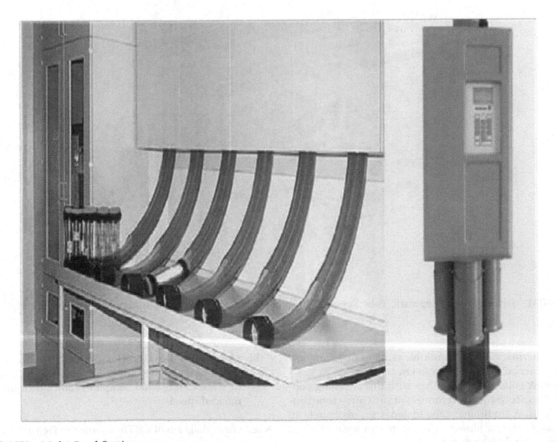

FIGURE 40K Multi-Send Station.

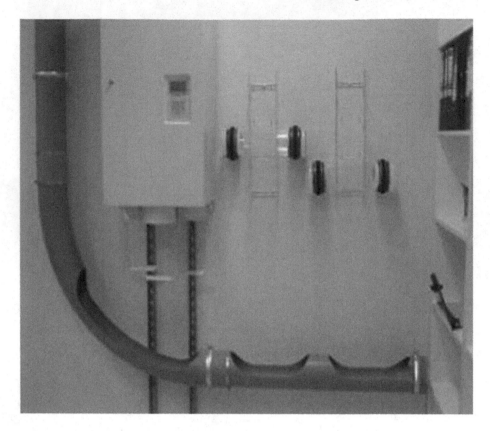

FIGURE 40L   Lab High-Volume Station (Courtesy: CPWD).

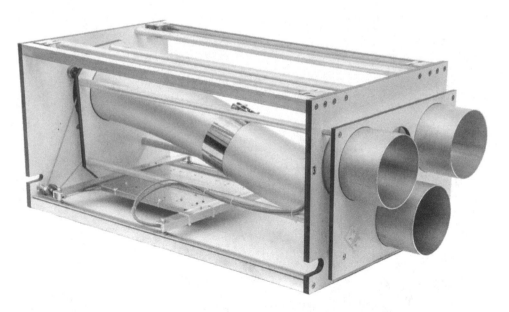

FIGURE 40M   Diverter for a Pneumatic Tube System (Courtesy: www.telecomtubesystems.com/en/products.html).

bulk pharmacy items or multiple samples or documents being carried from one location to another.

(j) **Zone:** A collection of stations with direct tubing connections. Zones are interconnected with inter-zone connections. A traditional zone includes approximately 10 stations, while a blower group zone can support up to approximately 60 stations.

(k) **Slow Speed Device:** This device is used especially in hospitals where certain sensitive goods such as laboratory tests and blood samples require transport with a reduced speed.

A schematic diagram of a PTS is shown in Figure 40N.

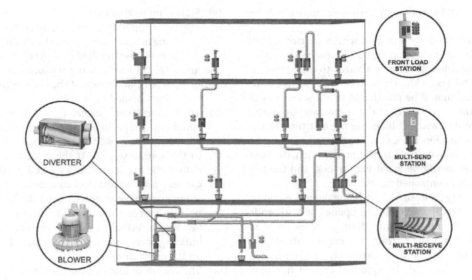

FIGURE 40N   Schematic Diagram of a PTS (Courtesy: CPWD).

40.3 Design Considerations for Pneumatic Tube Systems

(a) The results of the traffic survey will help to identify where stations should be allocated. Stations may be shared between departments to reduce the overall cost of the installation, for example, one station for adjacent wards that are possibly already sharing facilities.

(b) The system should be capable of transferring packages safely and securely between all or only selected stations within the network, which may cover a single hospital or a number of adjacent hospital sites.

(c) A central controller should continuously poll all stations in sequence to initiate the required send/receive sequence for carriers loaded into stations. A system of send/receive priorities for each station ensures that urgent items are handled with minimum delay. A maximum time should be set to ensure carriers are not indefinitely parked in the system.

(d) It should be possible to take manual control of the system to override the central control (with a subset of operations available at all stations) to allow, for example, manual purging of the system in the event of a carrier becoming blocked.

(e) Two separate purging procedures should be provided, namely, system wide and specific to a station to assist in recovering carriers lost in the system by setting the system to pull/push carriers to the specified station.

(f) Printed reports of status/alarms/traffic should be provided by the central controller as required.

(g) For large systems, the network will be faster and more efficient if it is split into zones. This will allow the majority of traffic to be contained within a local zone and will reduce the number of inter-zone transfers. Each zone will have a dedicated, suitably sized blower.

(h) Carriers can be colour-coded for each department. Identification of specific users may be required by the infection control officer. Empty colour-coded carriers can be returned automatically to the relevant station.

(i) The blower should be housed in a clean, dust-free environment isolated from areas in which patients may be sleeping.

(j) A filter may be required in the air intake to the system to protect samples or aseptic areas. Planning teams should seek the advice of the infection control officer.

(k) The station should be located in a secure area preferably only accessible to staff and that can be locked if the area is vacated. If a station is to be shared, then access arrangements should be agreed upon and the security of the station assigned to one department.

(l) Diverters should be located in service areas with good access for maintenance.

(m) Tubing should be routed in ducts and ceiling voids if space is available. The tubing will require large bend radii to avoid blockages. If the tube has to be routed externally or in hostile environments, then it should be protected and insulated to reduce the risk of damage or condensation occurring within the pipework. Access to areas that contain send/receive stations should be secured to prevent unauthorized entry or provided with a lockable basket/cabinet.

(n) Plant rooms containing pneumatic air tube transport systems should be well-illuminated and should permit safe access to all parts of the plant requiring inspection, service, and maintenance.

(o) Blower capacity should be established by the system designer and should be sufficient for transporting the carriers through the local zone at the agreed velocity and if required across to other zones connected in the network.

(p) The average velocity of full carriers between stations should not exceed 6 m per second (m/s). The carrier velocity may sometimes need to be lower to protect the integrity of samples: a velocity of 5 m/s is used at a number of hospital sites. System velocity should be agreed with the pathology and pharmacy department. The system should gradually accelerate and then slow the carrier on arrival at the destination station.

(q) Empty carriers can be transported at 10 m/s if required by the system manager. However, this may cause additional noise, and the majority of systems may operate satisfactorily using a velocity of 5 m/s.

(r) Carrier deceleration on arrival at the destination station should be carried out using the "air column technique" in which an approaching carrier activates a pressure release device and is braked by a still column of air above the station.

(s) Each station should be provided with a carrier arrival basket or cabinet of sufficient size and capacity to accommodate the number of carriers allotted to the appropriate station. The basket should be fixed to the wall or floor under the station and be positioned to allow carriers of an agreed number to arrive at the station and be stored within the basket without blocking the exit tube of the station. If the station is located in an area that may be unmanned or is accessible to the public, then the basket or cabinet should be fitted with a lock, and the key should be under controlled access.

(t) The carriers may be designed with one openable end or alternatively, be capable of being opened at both ends to facilitate loading and unloading of items such as blood bags that fill the carrier. The carrier lids should be designed so that the lid is positively secured before loading the carrier into the system (screwed lids may unscrew from the carrier within the system). The carriers should be transparent to enable the contents to be viewed by the recipient before opening the carrier.

(u) Each station should be provided with a laminated/encapsulated list of instructions, which should be mounted on or adjacent to the station. The label should be easy to clean and securely fixed and should include the following:
  (i)   directory of all available stations
  (ii) clear, step-by-step operating instructions
  (iii) action to be taken in the event of system failure

(v) Each station should be equipped with a visual display unit having at least a two-line, 16-character per line minimum. Normally, a liquid crystal display screen is incorporated in the station housing.

(w) When a carrier is sent from any station, the visual display screen at the station should
  (i)   indicate that the station is ready to accept a carrier
  (ii) request the identification of the destination station
  (iii) request the confirmation of the instruction
  (iv) confirm that the carrier has arrived at the selected destination

(x) Text messages on the visual display screen should be clear and easy to understand.

(y) Station mounting heights
  (i)   For top-side and front-entry stations, the mounting height to the top of the cabinet should be 1.6 m above the finished floor level.
  (ii) For bottom-loading stations, the mounting height from the bottom of the station should be 1.2 m to the finished floor level.

(z) The system should be capable of carrying out an initial automatic purge in an attempt to clear a blockage or sticking carrier, with the sticking carrier being purged to the source station. If the purging operation fails to deliver the carrier to the assigned destination, then the carriers may be diverted to a designated station. If the automatic purge is not successful, then the system will need to be reset manually. In addition, a volt-free contact may be provided to allow connection to the hospital building energy management system (BEMS) to indicate an alarm condition.

(aa) The system should be capable of attempting to automatically clear and eject a blocked carrier in the exit tube at any station by agitating the station's diverter/carrier transfer mechanism.

40.4 Summary

According to a study, only a negligible amount of total spending is spent on automating these facilities. However, it has also recently been revealed that inefficient intra-facility logistics have increased the cost of human resources and other factors such as health care delivery. Moreover, inefficient logistics have also caused several problems in hospitals including increased risks of treatment and have decreased the quality of patient care in the facility.

For these reasons, the optimization of hospital logistics is becoming increasingly more important. There is a growing need for an integrated health care system to provide seamless care to patients, reduce manual work, and improve efficiency. PTS is one such advanced microprocessor-based system of transportation that combines speed with reliability in numerous logistical needs. These are highly complex systems that are used for a variety of small and medium-sized tasks.

41 SIGNAGE AND WAYFINDING IN HOSPITALS

41.1 Introduction

Signage is the design or use of signs and symbols to communicate a message. It is the recognizable physical and visual interpretation of the objectives of the organization that it represents. Hospitals regularly have a large number of footfalls of patients, visitors, staff, and other stakeholders; hence, welcoming this diversity with care, reassurance, and warmth is essential. Floor plans of many hospitals are generally complex and, sometimes, even intimidating. Visitors often get lost in the maze and get anxious and annoyed when they are supposed to feel calm and welcomed. Since today's hospital premise consists of several different buildings housing several different facilities, a carefully planned and well-thought-out health care signage is key. Signage should create a comforting and familiar experience for patients and visitors who visit hospitals.

Types of Signage: Various signage used in health care is enumerated in the following:

(a) **Exterior Façade Signage:** provides preliminary information regarding a hospital (Figure 41A).
(b) **External Directional Signage:** provides general directions to the visitors regarding different areas in the hospital (Figure 41B).
(c) **Internal Maps:** enable patient, staff, visitors, and other stakeholders to orient themselves to different facilities at a particular location in a hospital and help them reach their respective destinations (Figure 41C).
(d) **Regulatory and Cautionary Signage:** include signage for fire as per NBC 2016, radiation hazard as per AERB, prohibition of sex determination as per PCPNDT Act 1994, ensuring silence in and preventing smoking on hospital premises as per BMWM Rules, 2016, etc. (Figure 41D).
(e) **Internal Wayfinding Signage:** ranges from a directory of the facilities to departmental directional signage (Figure 41E).
(f) **Universal Health Symbols/Pictograms:** enable visitors with limited language abilities to find their destinations (Figure 41F).
(g) **Wayfinding Maps:** incorporate limited information about different facilities in hospital and the means to reach them (Figure 41G).
(h) **Touch Screen Technology:** enables the use of IT to effectively guide visitors to their destination (Figure 41H).
(i) **External Totem (Figure 41I)**

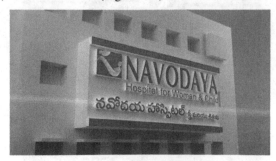

FIGURE 41A Exterior Façade Signage (Courtesy: www.indiamart.com/proddetail/hospital-building-sign-7940139033.html).

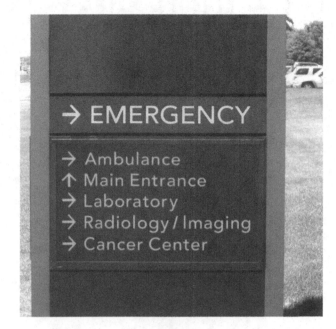

FIGURE 41B External Directional Signage (Courtesy: https://punctualprint.com/signage/exterior-signage/directional-signs/).

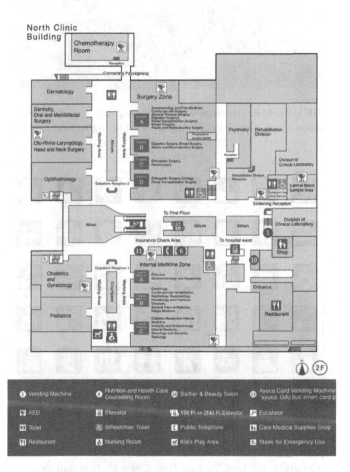

FIGURE 41C Internal Map of a Hospital (Courtesy: www.hosp.gifu-u.ac.jp/eng/map.html).

DOI: 10.1201/9780367460884-43

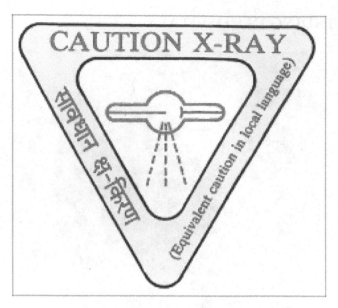

FIGURE 41D Radiation Symbol for X-Ray Radiation Hazard (Courtesy: www.aerb.gov.in/english/radiation-symbol).

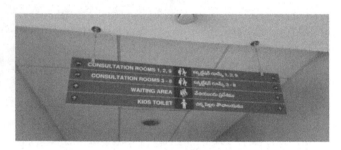

FIGURE 41E Internal Wayfinding Signage (Courtesy: www. aaabusinesssolutions.net/hospital-wayfinding-signage-5/).

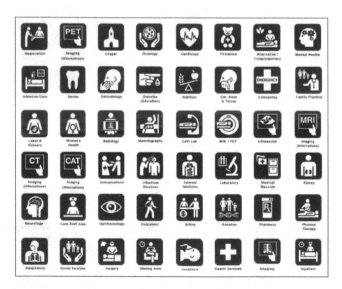

FIGURE 41F Universal Health Symbols/Pictograms (Courtesy: Joy Lo CW, Yien HW, Chen IP. How universal are universal symbols? An estimation of cross-cultural adoption of universal healthcare symbols. HERD: Health Environments Research and Design Journal. 2016 Apr;9(3):116–34).

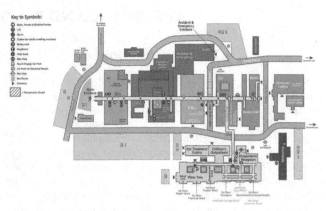

FIGURE 41G Wayfinding Maps (Courtesy: www.yumpu. com/en/document/view/38423461/whipps-cross-hospital-site-map-and-wayfinding-system).

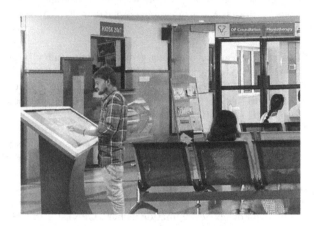

FIGURE 41H Touch Screen Wayfinding Technology (Courtesy: https://firstouchkiosk.com/customized-solutions/healthcare).

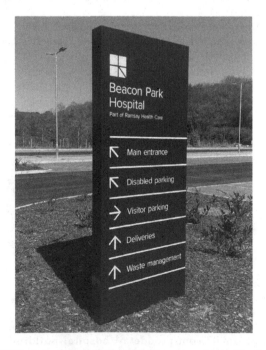

FIGURE 41I External Totem (Courtesy: https://betasigns. co.uk/portfolio/beacon-park-hospital-signage/).

41.2 Key Planning and Design Considerations for Hospital Signage

(a) Due consideration should be given to the simplicity, consistency, flexibility, and visibility of the signage.

(b) Symbols, pictographs, and language used in the signage should be universally accepted and understandable by the users of the facility.

(c) Illuminated or non-illuminated signage may be used as needed.

(d) Shape, form, colour, and dimensions should enable optimal reading. The height of the letters for symbols of access for varying viewing distances should be carefully selected.

(e) Signage should be placed in the natural line of vision.

(f) Displayed content should be concise and unambiguous.

(g) Materials used for signage should resist damage and be easy to replace.

(h) Signage should be placed at major decision points.

(i) Signposting should be appropriate and comprehensive.

(j) Luminance contrast between the lettering and background should be at minimum 30%.

(k) One symbol should be used for one message.

(l) Text should be on a contrasting background.

(m) Signage should not be obstructed to ensure visibility.

(n) Signage for differently abled users should also be placed.

41.3 External Signage: Planning and Design Considerations

(a) Development of an effective external signage program requires the coordination of several interdependent criteria identified as follows:

(i) Character and configuration of the roadway system/highways in proximity to the hospital.

(ii) Roadway system/paths/means currently adopted by the patients and visitors to reach the hospital.

(iii) Parking plan for patients, staff, visitors, and other stakeholders in relation to the hospital.

(iv) Location of buildings in the hospital campus in relation to the roads, parking, and walkways.

(v) Location of the building entrance.

(vi) Weather, especially in relation to events such as wind and snow.

(vii) Location of electricity source and voltage determines use of illuminated external signage.

(viii) Landscaping and marking an area make the signage easily visible.

(ix) Adequate illumination on and around the signage.

(x) Correct placement of signage.

(xi) Avoiding cluttering of signage.

(b) Guidelines for placing signage, to be viewed from an approaching vehicle and for mounting signage for pedestrian viewing, are discussed in the following:

(i) Use of text that is familiar, easy to understand, and comfortable to the viewer.

(ii) Signage must be placed within approaching driver's immediate cone of vision.

(iii) Signage must be perpendicular to the approaching viewer.

(iv) Signage must be placed on the left side of the roadway.

(v) Signage to be read from moving car must have a font size of not less than 3 in in height and should be a minimum of 1.5 in in height for pedestrian viewers.

(vi) Signage must be mounted or placed at eye level. Height of eye level is taken as 1,650 mm for a standing viewer and 1,350 mm for a person driving a car.

(vii) Adequate overhead clearance of 15 m or above for overhead signage must be ensured.

(viii) All the signage must be bilingual with at least one language being the vernacular language of the area/region where hospital is located.

(ix) The message in the signage is to be kept simple and brief.

(x) Use of internationally accepted **Helvetica Medium Bold** font for signage is recommended.

(xi) Background of the signage to be blue or green and letters in white.

(xii) Signage can be illuminated and non-illuminated depending on requirements.

(xiii) Size of text and symbols in signage in relation to patients coming by car or pedestrian is mentioned in Table 41A.

(xiv) Use of distance letter spacing is recommended.

(xv) Paragraph spacing should not be less than the height of the upper-case form.

(xvi) A flush upper-left alignment should be done except in cases of overhead panels, inserts, changeable modules, and listing strips, which should be vertically centred-aligned.

(xvii) The standard position for arrows, in relationship to the text, is either left of the first line of text or immediately above the first line of text.

(xviii) On signs with numerous destinations, a single arrow will be placed adjacent to the first line of text to identify the direction for all destinations grouped together. The arrow size should be 1.5 times the capital letter height.

TABLE 41A: Size of Text and Symbols in Relation to Patients Arriving by Car/Pedestrians

TEXT

Viewing Distance Up To		Letter Height		Application
7.5 m	25'	25 mm	1"	Pedestrian
12 m	40'	40 mm	1.5"	Pedestrian
15 m	50'	50 mm	2"	Pedestrian
24 m	80'	75 mm	3"	Car Driver
33 m	110'	100 mm	4"	Car Driver
48 m	160'	150 mm	6"	Car Driver
75 m	250'	225 mm	9"	Car Driver
97.5 m	325'	300 mm	12"	Car Driver
150 m	500'	450 mm	18"	Car Driver
195 m	650'	600 mm	24"	Car Driver

SYMBOLS

Viewing Distance Up To		Symbol Height	
7.5 m	25'	75 mm	3"
12 m	40'	100 mm	4"
15 m	50'	125 mm	5"
18 m	60'	150 mm	6"
30 m	100'	200 mm	8"
34.5 m	115'	225 mm	9"
39 m	130'	250 mm	10"
45 m	150'	300 mm	12"

41.4 Internal Signage: Planning and Design Considerations

(a) Development of an effective internal signage program requires the coordination of several interdependent criteria described as follows:

    (i) Location of building entrances and modes of vertical transportation.

    (ii) Character and configuration of the corridor system.

    (iii) Desired path of travel within the building for patient, staff, visitors, and other stakeholders.

    (iv) Location of departments and clinics.

    (v) Simple and clear room numbering system that follows a clear, understandable pattern.

    (vi) Identifying appropriate location for placement of signage.

    (vii) Adequate illumination in and around signage.

(b) Guidelines for placing signage to be viewed by patient, staff, visitors, and other stakeholders are identified in the following:

    (i) Directories must be placed in lobbies and elevator landings.

    (ii) Text size on directories should also meet requirements for visually impaired people. The overhead signage requires large lettering, and lettering on directional signage should be larger than the room identification signage (Table 41B and Figure 41J).

    (iii) Directories must be bilingual with at least one language being the vernacular language of the area/region where the hospital is located and incorporate symbols depicting the facility along with direction to the facility.

    (iv) Directories are also to be placed inside elevators.

    (v) More signage is to be placed in intersections with high traffic.

    (vi) Maps, wherever placed, should present information in a simple and understandable form.

    (vii) Maps should be mounted near an identifiable object or structure to facilitate patients/visitors becoming oriented.

    (viii) For internal maps, a perspective "Birds Eye View" graphic of the building layout is more effective than a traditional plain view.

    (ix) Signboard that has to be hung from the ceiling in the corridors should preferably be made of plastic or acrylic sheets.

    (x) Signboard may be self-illuminated; therefore, LED luminaire is to be used.

    (xi) Use of internationally accepted Helvetica Medium Bold font for signage is recommended.

    (xii) Cluttering of signage is to be avoided.

    (xiii) Placement of signage should be conducted in such a manner as to allow clear viewing. Interior lighting, wall colours, and material finishes need to be considered.

    (xiv) Signage should always be placed perpendicular to the viewer. Position signage with a clear line of sight from the viewing point to the sign face.

    (xv) Dimensions and details of interior signage are given in Table 41C.

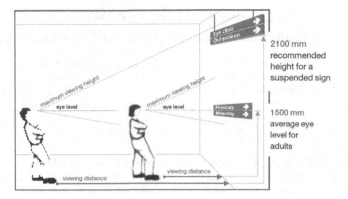

FIGURE 41J Position of Signage (Courtesy: www.england. nhs.uk/wp-content/uploads/2021/05/Wayfinding.pdf).

TABLE 41B: Viewing Distance for the Typeface "Health Alphabet"

X—Height (mm)	Viewing Distance with Normal Vision (6/9 Acuity)	Viewing Distance Registered Partially Sighted (6/60 Acuity)	Suggested Sign Type
15	Up to 7.5 m	No more than 0.5 m	Directories
30	Up to 15 m	No more than 1.0 m	Door Identity Signs
40	Up to 20 m	No more than 1.5 m	Internal Location and Direction Signs
60	Up to 30 m	No more than 2.0 m	Internal and External Signs
90	Up to 45 m	No more than 3.0 m	External Location and Direction Signs
120	Up to 60 m	No more than 4.0 m	Location Signs
200	Up to 100 m	No more than 7.0 m	Fascia Signs

TABLE 41C: Dimensions and Details of Interior Signage

Type of Signage	Dimension (H × W)
Ceiling-mounted identification signage	305 mm × 1,016 mm
Soffit-mounted identification signage	305 mm × 1,016 mm
Small directory of the facility	762 mm × 610 mm
Large directory of the facility	915 mm × 915 mm
Large directory of the facility with maps	762 mm × 1,220–1,524 mm
Large floor directory	762 mm × 610 mm

Signage for the differently abled: It is essential that suitable signs are placed at prominent and required positions inside and outside a building to indicate clearly the exact locations of facilities that are available for use by persons with a disability. To design an effective signage system, the needs of different types of users in a building and the complexity of the building layout must be considered.

(a) **International Symbol of Accessibility:** The international symbol of accessibility should be the wheelchair figure in white on a blue background and is to be provided at conspicuous locations for the purposes of identifying/advertising/signifying (Figure 41K)
  • Accessible entrance to the building.
  • Accessible exit from the building.
  • Reserved car parking facilities for persons with a disability.
  • The location of toilets for persons with a disability.
  • Usable vertical circulation facilities.
  • Usable cloakroom facilities.
  • The availability of special services of information/ service counter and telephones in the building.

(b) **Directional Signage:** Directional arrows and visual information should be provided at conspicuous locations in conjunction with the international symbol for accessibility to guide persons with a disability to the exact locations of the accessible facilities (Figure 41L).

(c) **Size:** The height of signs should not be less than the following:
  • 60 mm for doors
  • 110 mm for corridors
  • 200 mm for external use

(d) **Braille and Tactile Signage:** Braille and tactile signs should be installed on adjacent wall or door of public toilet to indicate whether the toilet is for male, female, or unisex. The sign should be placed at 900 mm to 1,500 mm above the finished floor level. The specification of Braille cells is shown in Figure 41M. If there is no door, then the sign should be provided on the wall in front of the toilets. A Braille and tactile fire exit map should be provided directly above the call button of the accessible lift in its lobby in a building if a fire exit map for the use of the public is provided. The map should be placed at 800 mm to 1,200 mm above the finished floor level.

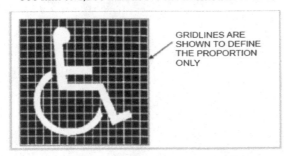

FIGURE 41K International Symbol of Accessibility (Courtesy: https://cpwd.gov.in/Publication/HandbookonBarrier.pdf).

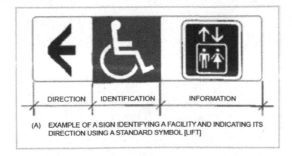

FIGURE 41L Directional Signage (Courtesy: https://cpwd.gov.in/Publication/HandbookonBarrier.pdf).

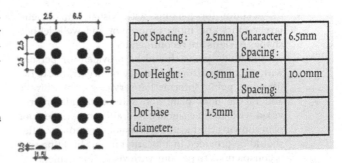

Dot Spacing:	2.5mm	Character Spacing:	6.5mm
Dot Height:	0.5mm	Line Spacing:	10.0mm
Dot base diameter:	1.5mm		

FIGURE 41M Tactile Signage (Courtesy: https://cpwd.gov.in/Publication/HandbookonBarrier.pdf).

(e) **Special Design Requirements to Assist Persons with Visual or Hearing Impairment (Figure 41N):**
  • If a floor plan for the use of the public is provided, then a Braille and tactile floor plan showing the main entrance, public toilet, and major common facilities should be provided in a place in this building that is prominent to persons with visual impairment.
  • A tactile guide path should be installed from a point of access at the lot boundary to the main entrance of the building and from the main entrance to the lift zone, the nearest accessible toilet, public information/service counter, Braille and tactile floor plan, and staircase.
  • If a visual display board (such as LED) is provided, then this should be able to display the essence of the information broadcasted by the public address system in the building.

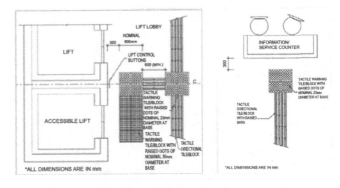

FIGURE 41N Special Design Requirements to Assist Persons with Visual or Hearing Impairment (Courtesy: https://cpwd.gov.in/Publication/HandbookonBarrier.pdf).

(f) **Design Considerations:**
  • Signs should be clear and easy to read and understand in order to assist persons with intellectual, cognitive, and sensory disabilities.
  • Prominent signs with high colour, luminous contrasts, and special shapes are recommended to be used for the elderly.
  • Safety for persons with visual impairment should be considered.
  • Information such as distance to the destination, name of building, etc. should be conveyed to the persons with visual impairment. The suggested provisions are voice messages, Braille, and signs with high luminous contrast.

- To account for persons with visual impairment, larger fonts and more prominent and well-defined shapes of signs are recommended.
- Tactile guide paths should be provided for persons with visual impairment from the main entrance to the lift zone, public information/service counter, Braille and tactile floor plan, and staircase/escalator provided with audible signals. A Braille and tactile floor plan showing the locations of major common facilities should be provided in a location in this building that is conspicuous to persons with visual impairment.
- Braille and tactile building name and address (i.e., street name with number) or a device that when activated will provide the same information in audible form should be provided on both sides of the building entrance at a height of between 900 mm and 1,500 mm above the finished floor level.
- If a public address system is provided to convey information to the public in a building, then a means of conveying the same or equivalent information to persons with hearing impairment should also be provided. If a floor plan for the use of the public is provided, then a Braille and tactile floor plan with an audible device indicating the main entrance, public toilet, and major common facilities should be provided in a place in this building that is conspicuous to persons with visual impairment.
- A visual display board (such as LED) should be provided in public waiting areas and where there is an announcer installed to regularly convey information to the people inside. The visual display board should be able to display the essence of the information so announced.

TABLE 41D: Recommended Materials for Signage

Type of Signage	Recommended Material
External Signage	Acrylic sheets
	Aluminium
	Aluminium composite material/Alumalite
	Vinyl sheets
Internal Signage	Acrylic sheets
	PVC & Polystyrene
	Coroplast
	Fibre-reinforced plastic
	Polycarbonate

41.5 Summary

Planning and designing signage and wayfinding in hospitals is a critical process that ensures clear and efficient navigation for patients, visitors, and staff within the health care facility. Effective signage and wayfinding systems help to reduce confusion, minimize stress, and improve overall patient experience. Key considerations in the planning and designing process include strategic placement of signage, clear and concise messaging, incorporation of universal symbols, legible typography, appropriate colour contrast, and integration with digital technologies for real-time information updates. By prioritizing these factors and engaging experts in environmental design and wayfinding, hospitals can establish a well-designed signage and wayfinding system that promotes seamless navigation, enhances patient satisfaction, and contributes to efficient health care delivery.

42 BIOMEDICAL WASTE MANAGEMENT SYSTEMS

42.1 Introduction

Biomedical waste as the name suggests is the waste generated as a result of various activities and processes in the medical and health care field. It is the major outcome of patient care, treatment, surgical procedures, laboratory testing, and research conducted and related to health care.

The amount of biomedical waste production ranges from 1–2 kg/bed/day in developing countries and is as high as 4.5 kg/bed/day in developed countries, which reflects the biomedical waste load generated around health care facilities. According to the WHO, approximately 85% of hospital waste is non-hazardous, 10% is infective and remaining, and 5% is non-infective but hazardous. Biomedical waste includes all the waste generated from a health care facility that can have any adverse effect on the health of a person or on the environment in general if not disposed properly. All such waste that can adversely harm the environment or health of a person is considered infectious, and such waste has to be managed as per BMWM Rules, 2016 (Figure 42A).

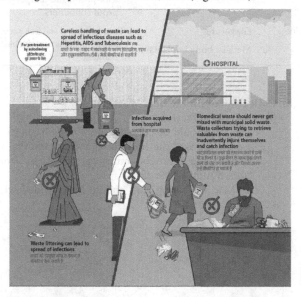

FIGURE 42A Risk to Environment and Health Due to Untreated BMW (Courtesy: CPCB).

Classification of Health Care Waste: The waste generated in hospitals and health care facilities can be classified into (Figure 42B)

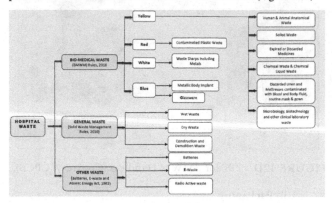

FIGURE 42B Classification of BMW (Courtesy: CPCB).

(a) **Biomedical Waste:** According to Biomedical Waste Management Rules, 2016, biomedical waste is defined as any waste that is generated during the diagnosis, treatment, or immunization of human beings or animals or the research activities pertaining thereto, in the production or testing of biologicals, or in health camps, including the categories mentioned in Schedule I appended to these rules. The Biomedical Waste Management Rules, 2016 categorizes the biomedical waste generated from a health care facility into four categories based on the segregation pathway and colour code.

(b) **General Waste:** General waste consists of all waste other than biomedical waste that has not been in contact with any hazardous, infectious, chemical, or biological secretions and does not include any waste sharps. This waste consists of mainly

   (i)   Newspaper, paper, and card boxes (dry waste)
   (ii)   Plastic water bottles (dry waste)
   (iii)   Aluminium cans of soft drinks (dry waste)
   (iv)   Packaging materials (dry waste)
   (v)   Food containers after emptying residual food (dry waste)
   (vi)   Organic/Bio-degradable waste—mostly food waste (wet waste)
   (vii)   Construction and demolition waste

      This general waste is further classified as dry waste and wet waste and should be collected separately. This quantity of such waste is approximately 85% to 90% of total waste generated from the facility. Such waste is required to be handled as per the Solid Waste Management Rules, 2016 and the Construction and Demolition Waste Management Rules, 2016, as applicable.

(c) **Other Waste:** Other waste consists of used electronic waste, used batteries, radioactive waste that is not covered under biomedical waste but has to be disposed of, and when such waste is generated as per the provisions established under E-Waste (Management) Rules, 2016, Batteries (Management and Handling) Rules, 2001, and Rules/guidelines under Atomic Energy Act, 1962, respectively.

42.2 Steps Involved in Biomedical Waste Management

First, five steps of biomedical waste management (segregation, collection, pre-treatment, intramural transportation, and storage) are the exclusive responsibility of the health care facility. Meanwhile, treatment and disposal is primarily the responsibility of the CBWTF operator except for lab and highly infectious waste, which is required to be pre-treated by the health care facility.

(a) **Segregation of Biomedical Waste:** Biomedical waste generated from a health care facility is required to be segregated at the point of generation as per the colour coding stipulated under Schedule-I of BMWM Rules, 2016 (Table 42A and Figure 42C). The following activities are to be followed to ensure proper waste segregation:

DOI: 10.1201/9780367460884-44

(i)   Waste must be segregated at the **point of generation** of source and not in later stages.

(ii) Adequate number of colour-coded bins/containers and bags should be available at the point of generation of biomedical waste.

(iii) Colour-coded plastic bags should be in line with the Plastic Waste Management Rules, 2016. Specifications for plastic bags and containers are given at Annexure 1 of the BMWM Rules, 2016.

(iv) Provide personnel protective equipment to the biomedical waste handling staff.

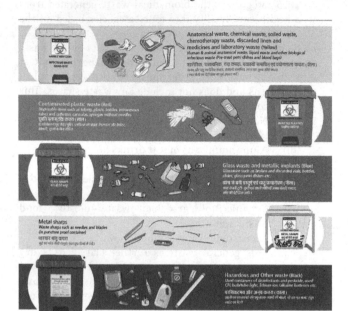

FIGURE 42C   Segregation of BWM (Courtesy: CPCB).

TABLE 42A: Segregation of BMW as per Schedule I of BMWM Rules, 2016 and Amendment Thereof

Category	Type of Waste	Colour and Type of Bag or Container to Be Used
Yellow	Human anatomical waste	Yellow, non-chlorinated plastic bags and containers
	Animal anatomical waste	
	Soiled waste: Items contaminated with blood and body fluids, such as dressings, plaster casts, cotton swabs, etc.	
	Discarded linen including masks, head covers, shoe covers, disposable linen gowns, non-plastic or semiplastic coveralls	
	Chemical waste: Soiled discarded chemicals	Yellow plastic container
	Expired or discarded medicines	Yellow, non-chlorinated plastic bags or container with cytotoxic labels
	Chemical liquid waste: Liquid waste generated due to the use of chemicals and used or discarded disinfectants	Separate collection system leading to ETP

Category	Type of Waste	Colour and Type of Bag or Container to Be Used
Red	Microbiology, biotechnology, other clinical laboratory waste, and PVC BLOOD BAGS	Autoclave safe yellow plastic bags and containers
	Contaminated waste (recyclable): Plastic tubing, bottles, intravenous tubes and sets, catheters, urine, bags, syringes (without needle and fixed needle syringes), vacutainers with their needles cut, gloves, goggles, face shields, splash-proof aprons, plastic coveralls, hazmat suits, pre-treated viral transport media, plastic vials, Eppendorf tubes, etc.	Red, non-chlorinated plastic bags and containers
White	Waste sharps including metals	White, translucent, puncture-proof, leak-proof, and temper-proof containers
Blue	Glassware	Puncture-proof and leak-proof boxes or containers with blue marking
	Metallic body implants	

(b) Collection of Biomedical Waste (BMW)

(i) Time of Collection

- BMW should be collected on a daily basis from each ward of the hospital at a fixed interval of time. There can be multiple collections from wards during the day.
- BMW collecting staff should be provided with PPE (Figure 42D).

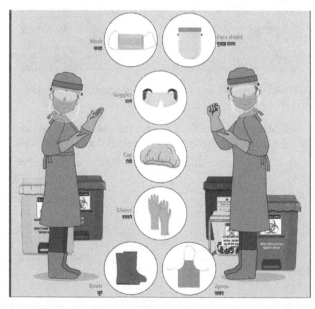

FIGURE 42D   PPE for BMWM Handlers (Courtesy: CPCB).

(ii) Packaging

- Biomedical waste bags and sharps containers should be filled to no more than three-quarter full. Once this level is reached, they should be sealed to be ready for collection.

- Replacement bags or containers should be available at each waste collection location so that full ones can immediately be replaced.

  (iii) Labelling
  - All the bags/containers/bins used for collection and storage of BMW must be labelled with the symbol for biohazard or cytotoxic hazard as the case may be (Figure 42E).
  - BMW bags/containers are required to be provided with bar code labels in accordance with CPCB guidelines (Figure 42F).

  (iv) Interim Storage
  - Interim storage of biomedical waste is discouraged in the wards/different departments of a health care facility.

(c) In-House Transportation of BMW
  (i) In-house transportation of BMW from the site of waste generation/interim storage to a central waste collection centre within the premises of the hospital must be done in closed trolleys/containers preferably fitted with wheels for easy manoeuvrability. The size of such waste transport trolleys should be as per the volume of waste generated from the health care facility (Figure 42G).

(d) Storage of BMW in a Central Waste Collection Room: Each health care facility should ensure that there is a designated central waste collection room situated within its premises for storage of BMW, until the waste is picked up and transported for treatment and disposal at CBWTF. Such room should be under the responsibility of a designated person and should be under lock and key.

(e) Record Keeping
  - Every health care facility needs to maintain the records regarding the category-wise BMW generation and its treatment disposal (either by captive facility or through CBWTF) on a daily basis.
  - Category-wise quantity of waste generated from the facility must be recorded in a BMW register/logbook being maintained at the central waste collection area under the supervision of one designated person.

(f) Treatment and Disposal of BMW
  (i) **Yellow Category Waste (Table 42B and Figure 42H)**
  (ii) **Red Category Waste (Table 42C and Figure 42I)**
  (iii) **White Category Waste (Table 42D and Figure 42J)**
  (iv) **Blue Category Waste (Table 42E and Figure 42K)**

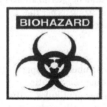

Bio-Hazard Label

Cyto-Toxic Label

FIGURE 42E Biohazard and Cytotoxic Label for BMW Bags/Containers (Courtesy: CPCB).

FIGURE 42F Bar Code/QR Code for BMW Bags/Containers (Courtesy: CPCB).

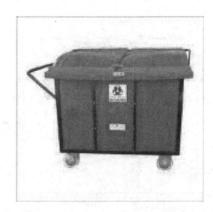

FIGURE 42G Covered Trolley for Transporting BMW (Courtesy: CPCB).

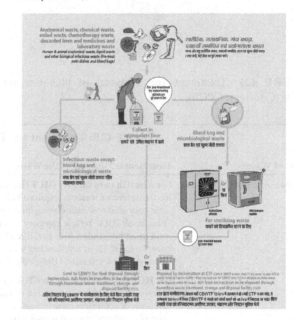

FIGURE 42H Treatment and Disposal of Yellow Category BMW (Courtesy: CPCB).

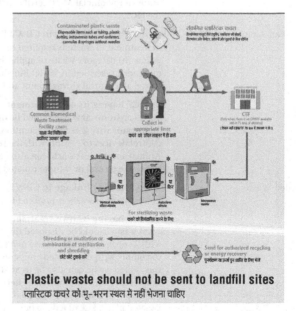

FIGURE 42I Treatment and Disposal of Red Category BMW (Courtesy: CPCB).

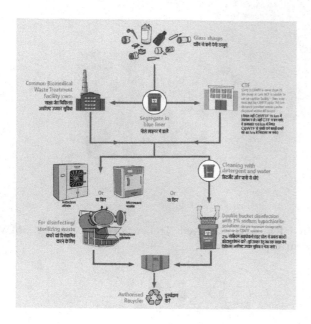

FIGURE 42J Treatment and Disposal of Blue Category BMW (Courtesy: CPCB).

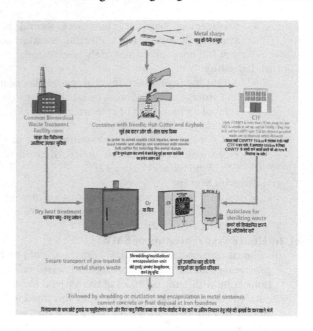

FIGURE 42K Treatment and Disposal of White Category BMW (Courtesy: CPCB).

TABLE 42B: Treatment and Disposal of Yellow Category BMW

Type of Waste	Treatment & Disposal of the Waste
Human Anatomical Waste	**For a health care facility (HCF) having linkage to CBWTF** No treatment of waste is required to be carried out at the HCF except pre-treatment (sterilization) of yellow (h) category waste by autoclaving/microwaving/hydroclaving or sterilizing as per the methods prescribed in WHO Blue book 2014. Yellow category waste along with pre-treated waste should be stored at a central storage point and must be handed over to CBWTF. It is mandatory for each HCF that dead faetus waste should be handed over to CBWTF in a yellow bag with a copy of the official medical termination of pregnancy (MTP) certificate from the obstetrician or the medical superintendent/SMO/CMO of the HCF. **For HCF without linkage to CBWTF** This waste should be disposed of through a plasma pyrolysis unit or twin-chambered compact incinerator with 2 seconds of retention time in a secondary combustion chamber that has adequate air pollution control devices to comply with the revised emission norms prescribed under BMW Management Rules, 2016. Disposal of the waste in a deep burial pit should not be practiced unless the hospital is located in a rural or remote isolated place. Use of a deep burial pit should be as authorized by the respective SPCB/PCC. A copy of the official MTP certificate from the MO I/C for a faetus below the vitality period must be kept with the HCF.
Animal Anatomical Waste	**For HCF having linkage to CBWTF** No treatment of waste is required to be carried out at a veterinary hospital except pre-treatment (sterilization) of yellow (h) category waste (if applicable) by autoclaving/microwaving/hydroclaving or sterilizing as per the methods prescribed in WHO Blue book 2014. Yellow category waste along with pre-treated waste should be stored at a central storage point and must be handed over to CBWTF. **For HCF having its own treatment and disposal facility** Animal anatomical waste should be disposed of through a plasma pyrolysis unit or twin-chambered compact incinerator with 2 seconds retention time in a secondary combustion chamber with adequate air pollution control devices to comply with the revised emission norms prescribed under BMW Management Rules, 2016. Animal anatomical waste can also be disposed of in captive deep burial pits only in case of veterinary hospitals located in a rural or remote isolated place. Use of a deep burial pit should be as authorized by SPCB/PCC.
Soiled Waste	**For HCF having linkage to CBWTF** No treatment of waste is required to be carried out at the HCF. Waste must be handed over to CBWTF. **For HCF having its own treatment and disposal facility** Soiled waste should be disposed through a plasma pyrolysis unit or in a twin-chambered compact incinerator with 2 seconds retention time in a secondary combustion chamber with adequate air pollution control devices to comply with the revised emission norms prescribed under BMW Management Rules, 2016. In the absence of this, soiled waste can also be treated by autoclaving or microwaving/hydroclaving followed by shredding or mutilation or a combination of sterilization and shredding for ultimate disposal through waste to energy plants. Soiled waste can also be disposed in captive deep burial pits only in case of hospitals located in a rural or remote isolated place. Use of a deep burial pit should be as authorized by SPCB/PCC.

(Continued)

TABLE 42B: (Continued)

Type of Waste	Treatment & Disposal of the Waste
Expired and Discarded Medicine	**For HCF having linkage to CBWTF** No treatment of waste is required to be carried out at the HCF. As per the BMW Rules, 2016, all expired and discarded medicine including expired cytotoxic drugs are either returned to the manufacturer or are handed over to the CBWTF to be disposed of through incineration at a temperature > 1,200°C. *For HCFs where there is no established system for returning drugs to the manufacturer, it is recommended that the expired and discarded medicine is handed over only to CBWTF for disposing of through incineration.* **For HCF having its own treatment and disposal facility** Expired and discarded medicine is required to be sent back to the manufacturer or can be disposed of though the nearest common BMW or hazardous waste incinerators with prior intimation to SPCBs/PCCs. This waste can also be disposed of through a twin-chambered captive incinerator with 2 seconds retention time in a secondary combustion chamber that can withstand a temperature of 1,200°C and that has adequate air pollution control devices to comply with emission norms.
Chemical Waste: Soiled Discarded Chemicals (Yellow—e)	**For HCFs having linkage to CBWTF** No treatment is required to be carried out at the facility. The chemical waste (liquid or solid chemicals) should be collected into different yellow plastic containers, whereas empty chemical containers with residual chemicals should be collected in yellow bags and handed over to a CBWTF operator for final disposal by incineration. It is required to specify the name of the chemical on the yellow containers so that it would help the CBWTF operator decide whether to incinerate it or transfer it to a hazardous waste TSDF for final disposal. **For HCF having its own treatment and disposal facility** This waste should be incinerated in a captive incinerator or it can be sent to a nearby hazardous waste TSDF for final disposal.
Chemical Waste: Liquid Waste Generated Due to Use of Chemicals and Used or Discarded Disinfectants	As per the BMWM Rules 2016, the chemical liquid waste of a hospital must be collected through a separate collection system for pre-treatment. Hospitals with large stand-alone labs should install a separate drainage system leading to a pre-treatment unit for further treatment prior to mixing the same with the rest of the wastewater from a hospital. For medium and small HCFs having no system of separate drainage/collection system, the liquid waste is required to be collected on-site in containers for pre-treatment before mixing the same with other wastewater. Silver x-ray film developing fluid should either be given or sold to authorized recyclers for resource recovery or it should be handed over to CBWTF as yellow (e) chemical waste.
Discarded Linen Including Masks, Head Covers, Shoe Covers, Disposable Linen Gowns, Non-Plastic or Semiplastic Coveralls, and Mattresses and Bedding Contaminated with Blood and Body Fluids	**For HCF having linkage to CBWTF** Disinfect the waste linen with non-chlorinated chemical disinfection and hand it over to the CBWTF operator for final disposal by incineration. The waste mattresses should be cut into pieces and disinfected and can be sent to the CBWTF operator for final disposal by incineration. Alternatively, waste mattresses can be cut into pieces and disinfected with non-chlorinated chemicals for disposal as general waste (dry-waste) for energy recovery in cities having waste to energy plants or refuse-derived fuel RDF plants. Waste mattresses should not be sold or auctioned. Used bed sheets that are not soiled and are re-usable can be sold or auctioned only after washing and disinfection. Disposable (single-use non-linen based) masks and gowns after use should be treated as yellow (soiled) waste. **For HCF having its own treatment and disposal facility** The waste mattresses after cutting into pieces and being disinfected with non-chlorinated chemicals can be incinerated in a captive incinerator or can be disposed of as general waste in dry bins in cities having an RDF plant or waste to energy plants.
Microbiology, Biotechnology and Other Clinical Laboratory Waste, PVC BLOOD BAGS (Yellow—h)	**For HCF having linkage to CBWTF** Pre-treatment by disinfection should be performed before handing over the waste to a CBWTF operator. Pre-treatment can be conducted by autoclave/microwave/hydroclave. Pre-treatment can also be performed by using non-chlorinated chemical disinfectants such as aldehydes, lime-based powders or solutions, ozone gas, ammonium salts, and phenolic compounds. The pre-treated waste bags should be handed over to a CBWTF operator on daily basis. **For HCF having its own treatment and disposal facility** Pre-treated waste should be disposed of by an HCF by installing a twin-chambered compact incinerator with 2 seconds retention time in a secondary combustion chamber with adequate air pollution control devices to comply with the revised emission norms prescribed under BMW Management Rules, 2016. Pre-treated waste can be disposed of in captive deep burial pits in case a hospital is located in a remote rural or isolated place. Use of deep burial pit should be as authorized by SPCB/PCC.

TABLE 42C: Treatment and Disposal of Red Category BMW

Type of Waste	Treatment & Disposal of the Waste
Contaminated Waste (Recyclable): Plastic tubing, bottles, intravenous tubes and sets, catheters, urine, bags, syringes (without needle and fixed needle syringes), vacutainers with their needles cut, gloves, goggles, face shields, splash-proof apron, plastic coveralls, hazmat suits, pre-treated viral transport media, plastic vials, Eppendorf tubes, etc.	**For HCF having linkage to CBWTF** Vacutainers/vials with blood samples should be pre-treated by autoclave/microwave/hydroclave and disposed of as yellow—h. No on-site treatment of red category waste is required. All such waste needs to be sent to CBWTF for final treatment and disposal. **For HCF having its own treatment and disposal facility** All the recyclable waste generated from the HCF must be sterilized by using autoclaving/microwaving/hydro-calving followed by shredding or mutilation or a combination of sterilization and shredding. Recyclable waste must never be disposed of along with general waste in a dry stream and is required to be disposed of only through registered or authorized recyclers, as waste to energy plants, as plastics to diesel or fuel oil, or for road making, whichever is possible.

TABLE 42D: Treatment and Disposal of White Category BMW

Type of Waste	Treatment & Disposal of the Waste
Metallic Sharps	**For HCF having linkage to CBWTF** After collection in puncture-proof, leak-proof, and tamper-proof containers, the waste should be handed over to CBWTF without any alteration or on-site treatment. **For HCF having its own treatment and disposal facility** Sharps waste should be disinfected either with autoclaving or dry-heat sterilization or a combination of autoclaving-cum-shredding; for each of these options, the methods for disposal are as follows:

Method of Disinfection	Treatment	Options for Disposal
Autoclaving	Shredding, mutilation, or encapsulation in cement concrete	Concrete pit, sanitary landfill, or steel foundry
Dry heat sterilization	Encapsulation in metal container	
Autoclaving-cum-shredding as a single-unit operation	None	

TABLE 42E: Treatment and Disposal of Blue Category BMW

Type of Waste	Treatment & Disposal of the Waste
Glassware	**For HCFs having linkage to CBWTF** Dispose of the empty glass bottles by handing over to CBWTF without any on-site treatment. The residual chemicals in a glass bottle should be collected as chemical waste in yellow containers/bags and handed over to CBWTF as per yellow (e) waste. **For HCF having its own treatment and disposal facility** The waste glass bottles/broken glass have to be sterilized or disinfected (either by autoclaving, microwaving, hydroclaving, or by sodium hypochlorite solution) followed by soaking and washing with detergent prior to sending it for recycling. Broken glass should also be disinfected, and if the same cannot be given or sold for recycling, it can be disposed of in a sharps pit. The residual chemical in a glass bottle should be collected as chemical waste in yellow coloured containers/bags as yellow (e) waste and given to either a CBWTF or common hazardous waste treatment and disposal facility. Glass vials with positive controls should be pre-treated and disposed of as yellow (h) waste.
Metallic Body Implants	Dispose of the waste by handing over to CBWTF. In case of no access to CBWTF, metallic body implants should be disinfected (either by autoclaving, microwaving, hydroclaving, or by sodium hypochlorite solution) and later washed with detergent prior to sending/sold to metal recyclers.

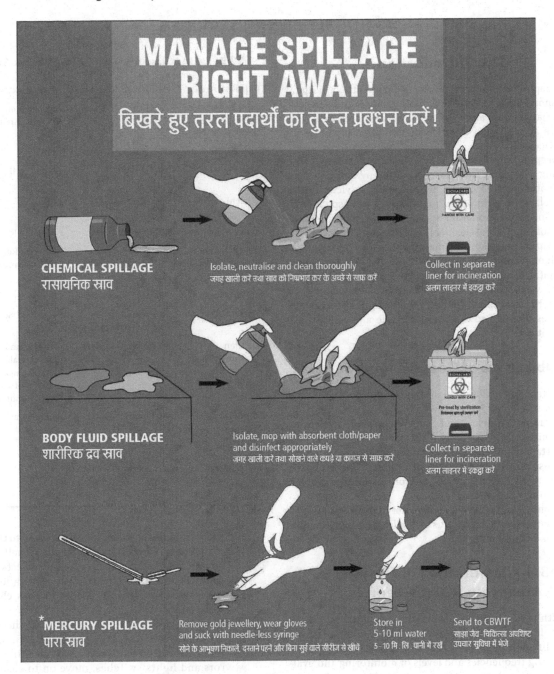

FIGURE 42L   Spill Management Procedures (Courtesy: CPCB).

Spill Management: HCFs have to ensure environmentally sound management of mercury or other chemicals or blood and body fluid spills as shown in Figure 42L given in the following.

42.3 Summary

Planning and designing a BMW management system in a hospital is a crucial process that ensures the safe and proper disposal of hazardous medical waste. The BMW management system is responsible for collecting, segregating, treating, and disposing of various types of waste generated in health care settings. Key considerations in the planning and designing process include designing dedicated waste storage areas, implementing segregation protocols, incorporating appropriate waste treatment technologies, ensuring compliance with regulatory guidelines, and providing staff training on waste management practices. By prioritizing these factors and engaging experts in waste management, hospitals can establish a well-designed biomedical waste management system that protects the environment, prevents the spread of infections, and promotes the overall health and safety of patients, staff, and the community.

43 HOUSEKEEPING SERVICES

43.1 Introduction

Housekeeping is a support service department in a hospital that is responsible for cleanliness, maintenance, and aesthetic upkeep of patient care areas, public areas, and staff areas. It is also known as sanitation department/sanitation section/sanitation services, etc.

Housekeeping services in a hospital are entrusted with maintaining a hygienic and clean hospital environment conducive to patient care. Hospital housekeeping services involve activities related to cleanliness, maintenance of hospital environment, and good sanitation services for keeping premises free from pollution. Housekeeper literally means "keeper of the house". Hospital housekeeping management may be defined as the branch of general management that deals with cleanliness of the hospital, general environmental hygiene, sanitation, and disposal of waste using appropriate methods, equipment, and manpower. Housekeeping services can be summarized as "All the activities directed towards a clean, safe and comfortable environment".

43.2 Objectives of Housekeeping Services

- To attain and maintain high standards of cleanliness and general upkeep.
- To train, control, and supervise staff under its establishment.
- To attain good relations with other departments.
- To ensure safety and security of all staff under its department and to keep superior authorities informed about day-to-day activities.
- To control and issue cleaning materials and equipment.
- To maintain official records on staffing, cleaning materials, and equipment.

43.3 Classification of Hospital Areas into Risk Categories

All health care environments should pose minimal risk to patients, staff, and visitors. However, different functional areas represent different degrees of risk and therefore require different cleaning frequencies and levels of monitoring and evaluation. A functional area refers to any area in a health care facility that requires cleaning. Consequently, all functional areas should be assigned to one of the following three categories (Table 43A).

- **High-risk areas**
- **Moderate-risk areas**
- **Low-risk areas**

43.4 Principles of Housekeeping Services

- **Basic Principles of Cleaning**
  - Work from the highest point in the room to the lowest point in the room. For example, environmental cleaning should start by cleaning any ceiling lights and fans and then moving down to the objects closest to the floor.

TABLE 43A: Classification of Hospital Risk Areas

High-Risk Areas	Moderate-Risk Areas	Low-Risk Areas
Major and Minor OT including Recovery Areas	Medical and Allied Wards	Departmental Areas/ Office Areas
Critical Care Areas	Laboratory Areas	OPD
HDUs	Blood Bank	Non-Sterile Supply Areas
Accident and Emergency	Pharmacies	Library
Labour Room	Dietary Services	Meeting Rooms
Post-Operative Units	Laundry Services	Medical Records Department/ Section
Surgical Wards	Mortuary Services	Stores Section
CSSD/TSSU	Restrooms for Doctors and Nurses	Manifold Services/ Room
Radiation Treatment Areas	Rehabilitation Areas	Telephone Rooms, Electrical, Mechanical, and External Surroundings
Chemotherapy Wards	Psychiatric Wards	Staff Areas
Dialysis Unit		
Burn Unit		
Isolation Wards/ Rooms		

- Work from the outside walls of the room to the centre of the room. For example, clean all the wall-attached objects first before the horizontal objects such as counters and sinks. Then, finish up with items that come into contact with clients such as chairs and exam tables.
- Work from the cleanest surfaces in the room to the dirtiest surfaces in the room. For example, when cleaning a bathroom, start cleaning the mirrors and lights switches, move on to cleaning the sink, and then finish by cleaning the toilet and then the floor.
- Cleaning with water, detergents, and mechanical action leads to removal of dust, soil, and organic material that may include blood, secretions, and microorganisms. Cleaning is achieved by the use of friction to remove microorganisms and debris.
- Dry mopping is always done before damp mopping.
- Cleaning physically removes, rather than kills, microorganisms, thereby reducing the microorganism burden on a surface. Routine cleaning is sufficient in hospitals to achieve this reduction in bioburden. Based on the risk of infection assessment, more frequent cleaning may be required in some areas.
- In hospitals, the practice of "topping up" liquid soap containers is not acceptable as it can result in contamination of infections.

DOI: 10.1201/9780367460884-45

- Cleaning solutions will not be sprayed onto a surface to prevent aerosolization of cleaning chemicals. Spray directly onto cleaning cloth instead.
- **Disinfection**
  - All surfaces that need to be disinfected must be cleaned first. Most disinfectants lose their effectiveness rapidly in the presence of organic matter.
  - Disinfectants must always be used in prescribed dilutions and retained on surfaces for the recommended contact time to be effective.
  - Disinfection will kill most disease-causing microorganisms but may not kill all bacterial spores.
  - Surface disinfection should be performed infrequently, on the advice of the functional unit head and as part of hospital SOP.
  - It should always be conducted after a spilling accident of body fluids.
  - Routine disinfection of equipment to be used on patients should always be performed by the primary caregiver at the point of care. Disinfection of equipment between patients should always be accomplished when the same equipment is used on multiple patients.
- **Sterilization**
  - Sterilization will kill all forms of microorganisms.
  - Sterilization is a special process, and it must result in asepsis. Therefore, this process should *not be done by Housekeeping Staff*.
- **Frequency of Routine Cleaning**
  - The frequency of cleaning and disinfecting individual items or surfaces in any area depends on
    - Whether surfaces are high-touch or low-touch
    - The type of activity taking place in the area

- The risk of infection (e.g., examining room vs. meeting room)
- The vulnerability (immunity status) of patients seen in the area
- If there is an outbreak in the facility or the surrounding community
- The amount of body fluid contamination surfaces in the area

- **Special Precautions for Infection Control Repair/Construction Works to Protect Working Areas**
  - To protect the working of a hospital's high-risk areas (Spaulding's Critical Cleaning Level) from commensal infections, during the previously listed works, all adjacent areas of areas under repair will observe the following.
    - The areas under repair should be completely sealed off, and dust comprehensive control measures should be implemented before construction begins. Seal holes, pipes, conduits, and punctures appropriately. Construct barriers and airlocks for access of any type.
    - Isolate HVAC system and ventilation systems in area where work is being done to prevent contamination of duct system.
    - Use tacky mats.
    - Vacuum work area with filtered vacuum cleaner.
    - Seal all accesses except for one or two to high-risk areas and provide air showers.
    - Wet-mop access to high-risk areas with detergent during works.
    - Contain construction waste before transport in tightly covered and sealed containers.

TABLE 43B: Cleaning Frequency, Level of Cleaning/Disinfection, and Evaluation/Audit Frequency

Functional Area Risk Category	Frequency of Cleaning	Level of Cleaning/ Disinfection	Method of Cleaning/ Disinfection	Evaluation/Auditing Frequency
High-risk areas	Once every two hours and spot cleaning as required	Cleaning and intermediate level disinfection	Cleaning with soap and detergent plus disinfection with alcohol compound, aldehyde compounds (Formaldehyde, glutardehyde), hydrogen peroxide, and phenolics (not feasible in the nurseries)	Weekly or monthly if high standards of cleanliness are maintained as certified by Officer I/C Sanitation and infection control team
Moderate-risk areas	Once every four hours and spot cleaning as required	Cleaning and low-level disinfection	Cleaning with soap and detergent plus disinfection with aldehyde compounds (Formaldehyde, glutardehyde), hydrogen peroxide, and phenolics	Once a month or once every two months if high standards of cleanliness are maintained as certified by Officer I/C Sanitation and infection control team
Low-risk areas	For areas working around the clock, at least once in a shift; in areas having a general shift, at least twice in the shift and spot cleaning as required	Only cleaning	Physical removal of soil, dust, or foreign material followed by cleaning with water and detergent	Once every three months

Housekeeping Department: Planning & Design Considerations (Table 43C and Figure 43A)

TABLE 43C: Planning and Design Considerations for Housekeeping Department

Working Hours	The Housekeeping Unit will generally operate up to 12 hours per day, 7 days per week with some specific cleaning services operating 24 hours a day. Some hospital units may be cleaned at night to avoid disruption to the unit during the day.
Location	The unit will be located in the service area of the facility.
Offices and Meeting Rooms	Provide offices for senior full-time staff such as manager and supervisors.
Meeting Rooms	Meeting rooms are to comply with standard components.
Sign-On Bay	A recessed area may be required for staff to sign-on, check and record rosters. The sign-on bay should be a minimum of four m². The sign-on bay should be located in a discreet area with ready access to staff entry area and circulation corridor. It may also be located close to the unit manager's office. The sign-on bay will require the following fittings and services: • Bench at standing height • Pin board for display of rosters (or computer for computerized rosters) • Computer terminal (optional) • Power and data outlets for computers as required
Storage Areas	• Cleaner's equipment, such as trolleys, buckets, mops, and brooms. • Bulk cleaning materials, consumable supplies including soap, and paper towel supplies for hand basins.
Trolley Wash	An area should be provided for washing trolleys and cleaners' equipment and may be shared with another service unit. The trolley wash area should be located in the service area. The trolley washing area will require • Smooth, impervious, and easily cleanable surfaces to walls and ceiling • Impervious and non-slip finishes to the floor • Hot and cold water outlets
Functional Relationships	The Housekeeping Unit will require ready access to • Waste management area • Loading dock • Laundry/Linen handling areas • Storage areas for cleaning supplies
Equipment	The Housekeeping Unit will require sufficient cleaning equipment for cleaning and maintaining all type of finishes installed in the facility including vinyl, floors, carpeted floors, and other finishes. This may include polishers, scrubbers, vacuum cleaners, and steam carpet cleaners.
Infection Control	Cleaning staff will require ready access to staff handwashing basins. Hand basins may be located within the cleaner's rooms or in adjacent corridor areas.
Safety and Security	All electrical cleaning equipment should have prominent shut off switches for staff safety. Storage areas for equipment and supplies must be locked with access restricted to authorized staff.

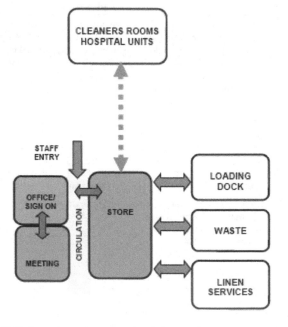

43.5 Summary

Planning and designing housekeeping services in a hospital is a crucial process that ensures a clean, safe, and comfortable environment for patients, staff, and visitors. Effective housekeeping services play a vital role in infection control, maintaining hygiene standards, and creating a positive impression of the health care facility. Key considerations in the planning and designing process include determining optimal staffing levels, defining cleaning protocols, identifying appropriate cleaning equipment and supplies, establishing waste management systems, and incorporating sustainability practices. By prioritizing these factors and engaging experts in facility management, hospitals can establish a well-designed housekeeping system that promotes cleanliness, enhances patient satisfaction, and contributes to a healthy and welcoming atmosphere for all.

FIGURE 43A Functional Relationship Diagram of Housekeeping Department (Courtesy: iHFG).

44 FIRE SAFETY

44.1 Introduction

44.1.1 Scope

The provisions presented in this chapter establish the minimum requirements for a reasonable degree of safety from fire emergencies in hospitals such that the probability of injury and loss of life from the effects of fire are reduced. All health care facilities should be designed, constructed, maintained, and operated to minimize the possibility of a fire emergency requiring the evacuation of occupants, as the safety of hospital occupants cannot be assured adequately by depending on evacuation alone. Hence, measures should be taken to limit the development and spread of a fire by providing appropriate arrangements within the hospital through adequate staffing and careful development of operative and maintenance procedures consisting of

- Design and construction.
- Provision of detection, alarm, and fire extinguishment.
- Fire prevention.
- Planning and training programs for isolation of fire.
- Transfer of occupants to a place of comparative safety or evacuation of the occupants to achieve ultimate safety.

44.1.2 Expected Levels of Fire Safety in Hospitals

Hospitals should ensure provision for two levels of safety within their premises:

(i) **Comparative Safety**: Which is protection against heat and smoke within the hospital premises, where removal of the occupants outside the premises is not feasible and/or possible (Table 44A).

(ii) **Ultimate Safety**: Which is the complete removal of the occupants from the affected area to an assembly point outside the hospital building. Ultimate safety may be achieved through the following (Table 44B).

TABLE 44A: Comparative Safety Requirements

Compartmentation	Automatic Detection System (Figure 44H)
Fire-Resistant Wall Integrated in the Flooring (Figure 44A)	Manual Call Point (Figure 44I)
Fire-Resistant Door of Approved Rating (Figure 44B)	First Aid
Pressurized Lobby, Corridor, and Staircase (Figure 44C)	Firefighting Appliances
Pressurized Shaft (all vertical openings) (Figure 44D)	Fire Alarm System (Figure 44J)
Refuge Area (Figure 44E)	Alternate Power Supply
Independent Ventilation system	Public Address System (Figure 44K)
Fire and Smoke Dampers (Figure 44F)	Signage (Figure 44L)
Automatic Sprinkler System (Figure 44G)	Fire Exit Drills and Orders

TABLE 44B Ultimate Fire Safety Requirements

Compartmentation	Public Address System
Fire-Resistant Door of Approved Rating	Signage
Protected Lobby, Corridor, Staircase, and Shaft	Fire Drills and Orders

44.1.3 Structural Elements of Fire Safety

(i) **Open Spaces (Table 44C)**

(ii) **Basements (Table 44D)**

(iii) **Means of Escape/Egress:** A means of escape/egress is a continuous and unobstructed way to exit from any point in a building or structure to a public way. Three separate and distinct parts of an escape/egress are (Table 44E).
- The exit access
- The exit
- The exit discharge

(iv) **Internal Staircases (Table 44F)**

(v) **Protected Staircases:** Provisions given for internal staircases should apply to protected staircases. Furthermore, additional safeguards should be provided as under (Table 44G).

(vi) **External Staircases:** External staircases serving as a required means of egress should be of permanent fixed construction (Table 44H).

(vii) **Horizontal Exits:** A horizontal exit implies that the occupants will be transferred from one side of a partition to the other. Essential fire safety provisions for horizontal exits are as follows (Table 44I):

(viii) **Exit Doors (Table 44J)**

(ix) **Corridors and Passageways (Table 44K)**

(x) **Compartmentation (Table 44L)**

(xi) **Ramps (Table 44M)**

(xii) **Service Shafts/Ducts (Table 44N)**

(xiii) **Openings in Separation Walls and Floors (Table 44O)**

(xiv) **Fire Stop or Enclosure of Openings (Table 44P)**

44.1.4 Non-Structural Elements of Fire Safety

(i) **Underground Static Water Tank for Firefighting** Provisions should be made for a dedicated firefighting tank, of suitable capacity as per NBC P-IV, that should remain full at all times. However, special attention should be given to calculating the actual capacity of the water tank to ensure its compatibility to the installed firefighting system. A four-way collecting head should be provided at an easily accessible location near the tank (Table 44Q).

(ii) **Automatic Sprinkler System (Table 44R)**

(iii) **Emergency and Escape Lighting (Table 44S)**

DOI: 10.1201/9780367460884-46

TABLE 44C: Structural Elements of Fire Safety for Open Spaces

1. In and around the hospital building to facilitate the free movement of patients and emergency/fire vehicles.
2. Kept free of obstructions and should be motorable.
3. Adequate passageway and clearance for firefighting vehicles.
4. Width of such entrances should not be less than 4.5 m with clear head room not less than 5 m.
5. Width of the access road should be a minimum of 6 m.
6. Turning radius of 9 m should be provided for fire tender movement.
7. Covering slab of storage/static water tank should be able to withstand the total vehicular load of 45 tons equally divided as a four-point load (if the slab forms a part of path/driveway).
8. Open space around the building should not be used for parking and/or any other purpose.
9. Set back area shall be a minimum 4.5 m.
10. Width of the main street on which the hospital building abuts should not be less than 12 m and when one end of this street joins another street, the street should not be less than 12 m wide.
11. Roads should not terminate in dead-ends.

TABLE 44D: Structural Elements of Fire Safety for Basements

1. Type-1 construction and material used should conform to Class A material.
2. Used only for parking vehicles and should be protected with automatic sprinkler systems.
3. Each basement should be separately ventilated, and each vent should have a cross-sectional area (aggregate) not less than 2.5% of the floor area.
4. System of air inlets and smoke outlets should be provided and clearly marked as "AIR INLET" and "SMOKE OUTLET".
5. Clear headroom of at minimum 2.4 m.
6. Minimum ceiling height of any basement should be 0.9 m and a maximum of 1.2 m above.
7. Access to the basement should be separate from the main and alternative staircases providing access and exit from higher floors. Where the staircase continues, in the case of buildings served by more than one staircase, the staircase should be of an enclosed type serving as a fire separation between the basement and higher floors.
8. Open ramps should be permitted if they are constructed within the building line and surface drainage does not enter the basement.
9. The staircase of the basement should be of enclosed type having fire resistance of not less than 2 hours and should be situated at the periphery of the basement. The staircase should communicate with the basement through a lobby provided with fire resisting, self-closing doors of 2 hours resistance.
10. For multi-story basements, one intake duct may serve all basement levels, but each level and basement compartment should have a separate smoke outlet duct or ducts. The ducts should have the same fire resistance rating as the compartment itself.
11. Mechanical extractors should be designed to permit 30 air changes per hour in case of a fire emergency.
12. Mechanical extractors should have an alternate source of electricity supply.
13. Ventilation ducts should be integrated with the structure of the building and should be made out of brick masonry or reinforced cement concrete as far as possible. Wherever this duct intersects the transformer area or an electrical switch board, fire dampers should be provided.
14. The basement should not be permitted below the ward block of a hospital.
15. No cut outs to upper floors should be permitted in the basement.
16. An openable window on the external wall should be fitted with locks that can be easily opened.
17. All floors should be compartmented by a separation wall with a 2-hour fire rating such that each compartment should have a surface area not exceeding 750 sq m. Floors that are fitted with sprinkler systems may have their surface areas increased by 50%. In a long building fire, the separation wall should be at distances not exceeding 40 m.
18. Lifts/Elevators should not normally communicate with basements; if, however, lifts are in communication, the lift lobby of the basement should be pressurized. A positive pressure between 25 and 30 Pascal (Pa) should be maintained in the lobby, and a positive pressure of 50 Pa should be maintained in the lift shaft.

TABLE 44E: Structural Elements of Fire Safety for Means of Escape/Egress

1. A means of escape/egress involves vertical and horizontal travel and should include intervening room spaces, doorways, hallways, corridors, passageways, balconies, ramps, stair enclosures, lobbies, and horizontal exits leading to an adjoining building at the same level (Figure 44M).
2. The exits in health care facilities should be limited to doors leading directly outside the building, internal staircases, smoke-proof enclosures, ramps, horizontal exits, external exits, and exit passages.
3. Exits should be so arranged that they may be reached without passing through another occupied unit.
4. Vertical evacuation of occupants within a health care facility is difficult and time consuming. Therefore, horizontal movement of patient is of primary importance.

TABLE 44F: Structural Elements of Fire Safety for Internal Staircases

1. Internal staircases should be constructed with non-combustible materials
2. Internal stairs should be constructed as self-contained units along an external wall of the building constituting at least one of its sides and should be completely closed (Figures 44N–44P).
3. A staircase should not be arranged around a lift shaft.
4. Hollow combustible construction should not be permitted.
5. The construction material should have 2 hours of fire resistance.
6. Minimum width of stairs shall be 2 m.
7. Width of the tread should not be less than 300 mm.
8. The height of the riser should not be less than 150 mm, and the number of stairs per flight should not exceed 15.
9. Handrails should be provided at a height of 1,000 mm, which is to be measured from the base of the middle of the treads to the top of the handrails.
10. Banisters or railings should be provided such that the width of staircase is not reduced.
11. Minimum head room in a passage under the landing of a staircase and under the staircase should be 2.2 m.
12. The staircase should be continuous from the ground floor to the terrace, and the exit door at ground level should open directly to the open spaces or a large lobby.
13. The number of people in between floor landings of staircases should not be less than the population on each floor for the purpose of the design of the staircase.
14. Fire/Smoke check doors should be provided for a minimum of a 2-hour fire-resistance rating.
15. Lift openings and any other openings should not be permitted.
16. No electrical shaft and panel, AC ducts, gas pipelines, etc. should pass through or open onto the staircases.
17. No combustible material should be used for decoration/wall paneling in the staircases.

TABLE 44G: Structural Elements of Fire Safety for Protected Staircases

1. The staircases should be enclosed by walls having 2 hours of fire resistance.
2. The external exit doors at ground floor should open directly onto open spaces or a lobby, and fire and smoke check doors should be provided.
3. Protected staircases should be pressurized. Under no circumstances should they be connected to a corridor, lobby, or staircase that is unpressurized.
4. Pressurization systems should be incorporated into protected staircases where the floor area is more than 500 sq m. The difference in pressurization levels between the staircase and lobby/corridor should not be greater than 5 Pa. Where a 2-stage pressurization system is in use, the pressure difference should be
   a. In normal conditions—Minimum 8 Pa to 15 Pa
   b. In emergency conditions—50 Pa
5. The pressurization system should be interconnected with the automatic/manual fire alarm system for actuation.

TABLE 44H: Structural Elements of Fire Safety for External Staircases

1. External staircases should be protected by a railing or guard. The height of such a guard/railing should not be less than 1,200 mm.
2. External staircases should extend vertically from the ground to either a point 3 meters above the top-most landing of the stairway or the roof line, whichever is lower, and at least 3 meters horizontally.
3. All openings below and outside the external staircases should be protected with a requisite fire resistance rating.
4. External staircases should be arranged to avoid any discomfort/obstruction for persons with a fear of heights that keeps them from using the staircases.
5. External staircases should be arranged to ensure a clear direction of egress to the street.
6. External staircases should be continuous from the ground floor to the terrace level.
7. The entrance to the external staircases should be separate and remote from internal staircases.
8. External staircases should have a straight flight with a width not less than 2 m, a tread not less than 300 mm, and a riser not more than 150 mm, and the number of risers should be limited to 15 per flight.
9. The handrail should have a height not less than 1,000 mm and not exceeding 1,200 mm.
10. Banisters should be provided with a maximum gap of 150 mm.
11. Stair treads should be uniformly slip-resistant and should be free of projections or lips that could trip stair users.

(Continued)

TABLE 44H: (Continued)

12. External staircases used as fire escapes should not be inclined at an angle greater than 45o from the horizontal.

13. Unprotected steel frame staircases should not be acceptable means of egress; however, steel staircases in an enclosed compartment with a fire resistance of 2 hours will be accepted as means of escape.

14. Elevators constitute a desirable supplementary facility though they are not counted as required exits. Patient's lifts should have sufficient space for a stretcher trolley.

TABLE 44I: Structural Elements of Fire Safety for Horizontal Exits

1. Width of the horizontal exits should be same as the exit doorways.

2. A horizontal exit should be equipped with at least one fire/smoke door of self-closing type with a minimum of 2 hours fire resistance. Furthermore, they should have direct access to the fire escape staircase for evacuation (Figure 44Q).

3. A refuge area of 15 sq m or an area equivalent to 0.3 sq m per person for the number of occupants on two consecutive floors, whichever is more, should be provided on the periphery of the floor or preferably on an open-air cantilever projection with at least one side protected with suitable railings/guards and a height not less than 1 m.

4. Within the aggregated area of corridors, patient rooms, treatment rooms, lounges, dining area, and other low hazard areas on each side of the horizontal exit, a single door may be used in a horizontal exit given that the exit serves one direction only.

5. Where there is a difference in the level between areas connected by a horizontal exit, ramps not more than 1 in 10 m slope should be provided. Steps should not be used.

6. Doors should be accessible at all times from both sides.

7. A horizontal exit involving a corridor of 8 ft or more in width serving as a means of egress from both sides of the doorway should have the opening protected by a pair of swinging doors arranged to swing in the opposite direction from each other.

8. An approved vision panel is required in each horizontal exit. Centre mullions are prohibited.

9. The total exit capacity of other exits (stairs, ramps, and doors leading outside the building) should not be reduced to below one-third of the amount that is required for entire area of the building.

TABLE 44J: Structural Elements of Fire Safety for Exit Doors

1. Every door and every principal entrance that also serves as an exit should be designed and constructed so that the way of exit travel is obvious and direct (Figure 44R).

2. Width of the doors should be a minimum of 2 m, and other requirements of the door should comply with the NBC.

3. Doors should not be equipped with a latch or lock that requires the use of tool and/or key from the egress side. Mental hospitals are permitted to have door locking arrangements.

4. Where door locking arrangements are provided, provision should be made for the rapid removal of patients by such reliable means such as the remote control of locks or the keys of all locks being made readily available to staff who are in constant attendance.

5. Doors in fire-resistant walls should be so installed that they may be normally kept in an open position but should close automatically. Corridor doors opening into the smoke barrier should not be less than 2,000 mm in width. Provisions should also be made for double-swing single/double-leaf type doors.

6. The fire-resistance rating of doors should meet the fire-resistance rating of construction material.

TABLE 44K: Structural Elements of Fire Safety for Corridors and Passageways

1. The minimum width and height of corridors and passageways should be 2.4 m. The exit corridor and passageways should have a width not less than the aggregate required width of exit doorways leading from them in the direction of travel to the exterior. Corridors should be adequately ventilated.

2. Corridor walls should form a barrier to limit the transfer of smoke, toxic gases, and heat.

3. Transfer grills, regardless of whether they are protected by fusible link operated dampers, should not be used in corridor walls or doors.

4. Openings, if required in corridor walls for a specific use, should be suitably protected.

5. Fixed wired glass opening vision panel should be permitted in corridor walls, provided that they do not exceed 0.84 sq m in area and are mounted in steel or other approved metal frames.

TABLE 44L: Structural Elements of Fire Safety for Compartmentation

1. In buildings or sections occupied by bedridden patients where the floor area is over 280 sq m, facilities should move patients in hospital beds to the other side of a smoke barrier from any part of such a building or section not directly served by approved horizontal exits from the floor of a building to outside.

2. Any section of the building more than 500 sq m should be suitably compartmented with fire resistance of not less than 2 hours.

3. Every building story used by inpatients for sleeping or treatment should be divided into not less than two smoke compartments

(Continued)

TABLE 44L: (Continued)

4. Every building story having an occupant load of 50 or more persons, regardless of use, should be divided into two smoke compartments.

5. The size of each smoke compartment should not exceed 500 sq m.

TABLE 44M: Structural Elements of Fire Safety for Ramps

1. All ramps should comply with the applicable requirements for stairways regarding enclosure, capacity, and limiting dimensions except in certain cases where steeper slopes may be permitted with inclination less than 1 in 8 (under no condition should slopes greater than 1 in 8 be used).

2. Ramps should be surfaced with approved non-skid and non-slippery material.

TABLE 44N: Structural Elements of Fire Safety for Service Shafts/Ducts

1. Service shafts/ducts should be enclosed by walls with 2 hour and doors with 1 hour fire resistance ratings. All such ducts/shafts should be properly shielded, and facilities should be available to control fires along these shafts/ducts at all levels (Figure 44S).

2. A vent opening at the top of a service shaft should have an area between one-fourth and one-half of the area of the shaft.

3. Refuge chutes should have openings at least 1 m above the roof level for venting purpose, and they should have an enclosure wall of noncombustible material with a fire-resistance rating of 2 hours. They should not be located within the staircase enclosure or service shaft and be as far away from the exit as possible.

4. The inspection panels and doors of air conditioning shafts should be well-fitted, with a fire resistance rating of 1 hour.

TABLE 44O: Structural Elements of Fire Safety for Openings in Separation Walls and Floors

1. At the time of designing openings in separation walls and floors, particular attention should be given to all factors that will help limit the spread of fire through these openings, and the fire ratings of these structural members should be maintained.

2. For type 1 to 3 construction, a doorway or opening in a separation wall on any floor should be limited to 5.6 sq m in area with a maximum height/width of 2.75 m. Every wall opening should be protected with fire resistant doors having the fire rating of not less than 2 hours in accordance with accepted standards.

3. Every vertical opening between the floors of a building should be suitably enclosed or protected as necessary to prevent the spread of fire, smoke, and fumes such that there is a reasonable level of safety for the occupants using the means of egress. A clear height of 2,100 mm in the passage/escape path of occupants should be ensured, thereby limiting damage to the building and its contents.

TABLE 44P: Structural Elements of Fire Safety for Fire Stop or Enclosure of Openings

1. Where openings are permitted for external walls, they should not exceed three-quarters of the area of the wall and should be protected with fire resisting assemblies or enclosures with a fire resistance equivalent to that of the wall in which these are situated.

2. All openings in the floors should be protected by vertical enclosures extending above and below such openings. The walls of such enclosures should have a fire resistance of not less than 2 hours, and all openings therein should be protected with a fire resistant assembly.

3. For type 4 constructions, openings in separation walls or floors should be fitted with 2-hour fire resistant assemblies.

4. Openings in the walls and floors that provide access to building services such as cables, electrical wiring, telephone cables, plumbing pipe, etc. should be protected by enclosures in the form of ducts/shafts with a fire resistance of not less than 2 hours.

5. The inspection doors for electrical shafts and ducts should have a fire resistance rating not be less than 2 hours, and all other service shafts and ducts should have a fire resistance rating of not less than 1 hour.

6. Medium and low voltage wiring in shafts/ducts should either be armored or run through a metal conduit.

TABLE 44Q: Non-Structural Elements of Fire Safety for Underground Static Water Tanks for Firefighting

1.	Fire Pump Room	Provisions should be made to have a centralized room to house the pumps that supply water to the various firefighting systems. The pumps should be as per NBC P-IV (Figure 44T).
		Jockey Pump: An electrically driven centrifugal single/two stage pump of 280 LPM capacity should be installed to maintain the system pressure up to 7 kg/cm². They should be activated automatically whenever the pressure falls below 5.5 kg/cm².
		Main Fire Pump: An electrically driven centrifugal multistage pump of 2850 LPM capacity should be installed to feed the fixed firefighting system. Provisions should be made for an alternate electric supply with a change over switch for this pump.
		Diesel Fire Pump: A diesel-driven prime mover multistage pump of 2850 LPM capacity should be installed to feed the fixed firefighting system in case of failure to the main fire pump.
2.	Yard Hydrant	Provision should be made to install yard hydrants throughout the premises. The distance between two successive hydrants should not exceed 45 m (Figure 44U).

(Continued)

TABLE 44Q: (Continued)

3. Wet Rising Mains   A vertical rising main of G.I. C class steel pipeline with an internal diameter of 100 mm should be provided from the ground floor to the highest floor of the hospital along with hydrant outlets fitted at the height of 0.9 m from the flooring at each floor (Figure 44V).

First aid hose reels with a diameter of 25 mm and length of 45 m should be provided at each floor fitted with a 6.5-mm diameter shut-off type nozzle.

An air release valve should be provided at the top of the rising main.

A fire service inlet should be provided at the ground floor.

4. Hose Box   A glass front cabinet containing two RRL type delivery hoses, each 15 m in length and with a diameter of 63 mm instantaneous coupling fitted with associated branch pipe, should be provided (Figure 44W).

TABLE 44R: Non-Structural Elements of Fire Safety for Automatic Sprinkler Systems

1. The entire building including the basements should be fitted with sprinklers connected to a gong bell/fire detection panel, which should be located in the central control room.

2. The entire building including the basement should be fitted with an automatic fire detection and alarm system comprising smoke detectors and manual call points, which should be connected to the fire alarm panel in the central control room.

3. The sprinkler, fire detection, and alarm systems should be provided with an alternative source of power supply.

4. Initiation of required fire alarm system should be by manual means or by means of any detection device.

5. An internal audible alarm should be incorporated.

6. Pre-signal systems are prohibited.

7. Corridors should have an approved automatic detection system.

TABLE 44S: Non-Structural Elements of Fire Safety for Emergency and Escape Lighting

1. Emergency lighting should be powered from a source independent of the normal lighting system.

2. Emergency lights should clearly and unambiguously indicate the escape routes.

3. Emergency lighting should provide adequate illumination along escape routes to allow the safe movement of persons towards and through the exits.

4. Emergency lighting should be provided in a manner to ensure that fire alarm call points and firefighting equipment provided along the escape routes are readily located.

5. The horizontal luminance at floor level on the centre line of an escape route should be not less than 10 lux. Additionally, for escape routes that are up to 2 m in width, 50% of the route width should be lit to a minimum of 5 Lux.

6. The emergency lighting should be activated within one second of the failure of the normal lighting.

7. The luminaries should be mounted as low as possible but at least 2 m above floor level.

8. Emergency lighting should be designed to ensure that a fault or failure in any open luminary does not further reduce the effectiveness of the system.

9. Emergency lighting luminaries and their fittings should be of a nonflammable type.

10. The emergency lighting system should be capable of continuous operation for a minimum of 1 and a half hours (90 minutes).

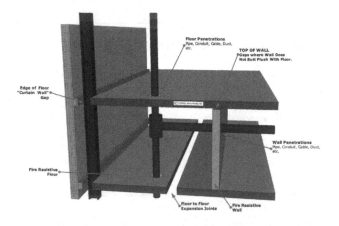

FIGURE 44A Fire-Resistant Wall Integrated into the Flooring (Courtesy: www.nachi.org/gallery/general-3/fire-resistive-walls-and-floors-1).

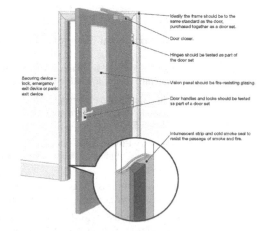

FIGURE 44B Fire-Resistant Door (Courtesy: www.ifsec-global.com/global/fire-doors-for-beginners/).

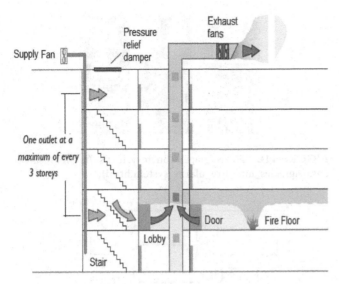

FIGURE 44C Pressurized Lobby, Corridor, and Staircase (Courtesy: www.linkedin.com/pulse/stairwell-pressurization-systems-ashique-muhammed?trk=public_profile_article_view).

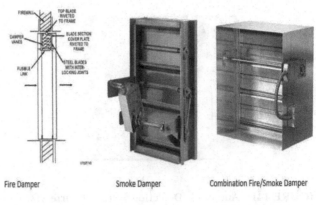

FIGURE 44F Fire and Smoke Damper (Courtesy: https://wginc.com/the-importance-of-fire-and-smoke-dampers-in-your-buildings-fire-protection-system/).

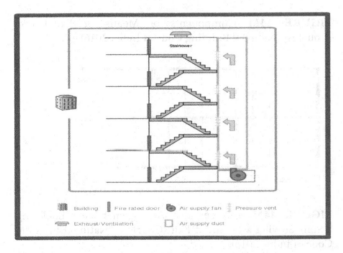

FIGURE 44D Pressurized Shaft (All Vertical Openings) (Courtesy: https://ecostruxure-building-help.se.com/topics/show.castle?id=10753&locale=ru-RU&productversion=1.6).

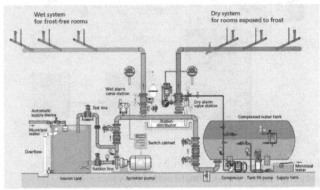

FIGURE 44G Automatic Sprinkler System (Courtesy: www.enggcyclopedia.com/2011/11/fire-sprinklers/).

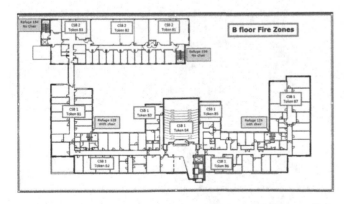

FIGURE 44E Refuge Areas (Courtesy: www.nottingham.ac.uk/nursing/sonet/rlos/healthsafety/fire-safety/resources.html).

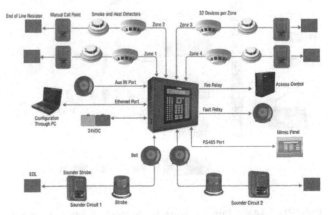

FIGURE 44H Automatic Detection System (Courtesy: https://suresafety.com/fire-alarm-and-etection-system).

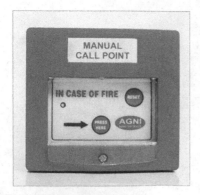

FIGURE 44I Automatic Detection System (Courtesy: www. star-tech.co/products/manual-call-point-mcp).

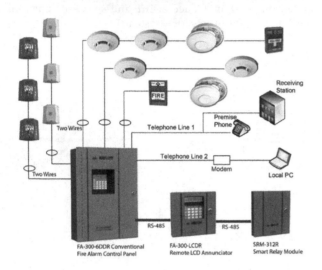

FIGURE 44J Fire Alarm System (Courtesy: https:// securityvaultsystems.com/fire-alarm-systems-fas/).

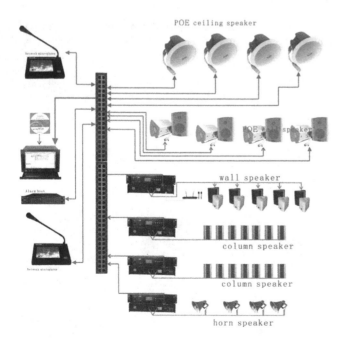

FIGURE 44K Public Address System (Courtesy: www. alibaba.com/product-detail/public-address-system-TCP-IP-SIP_60829660026.html).

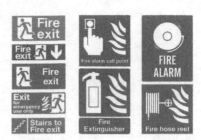

FIGURE 44L Fire Signage (Courtesy: https://noblefiresafety. com/signages_and_fire_alarm_system.html).

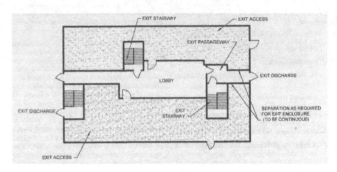

FIGURE 44M Components of Means of Exit/Egress (Courtesy: National Building Code of India, 2016).

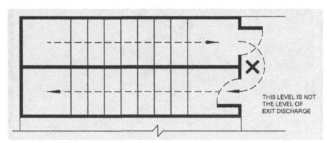

FIGURE 44N Unacceptable Arrangement for Enclosing a Stair Serving a Required Exit (Courtesy: National Building Code of India, 2016).

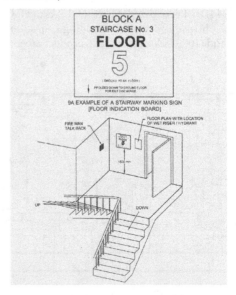

FIGURE 44O Sign Marking and Requirements in Exit (Courtesy: National Building Code of India, 2016).

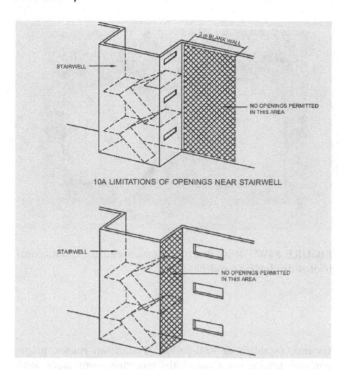

10A LIMITATIONS OF OPENINGS NEAR STAIRWELL

FIGURE 44P Opening Restrictions on Stairwell Walls (Courtesy: National Building Code of India, 2016).

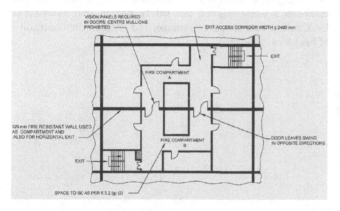

FIGURE 44Q Concept of Horizontal Exit (Courtesy: National Building Code of India, 2016).

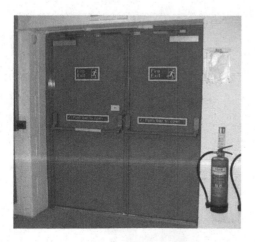

FIGURE 44R Fire Exit Door (Courtesy: www.indiamart. com/trioindia/emergency-exit-and-fire-resistant-door.html).

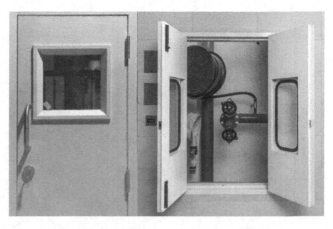

FIGURE 44S Firefighting Shaft with Door (Courtesy: https://globemetaldoor.com/shaft_door.html).

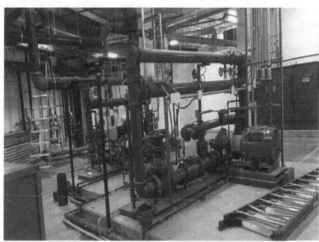

FIGURE 44T Fire Pump Room (Courtesy: www.csemag. com/articles/fire-pump-systems-design-and-coordination/).

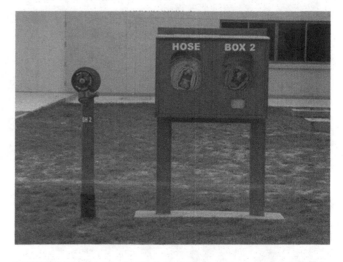

FIGURE 44U Yard Hydrant (Courtesy: www.indiamart. com/proddetail/yard-fire-hydrant-system-15792883012.html).

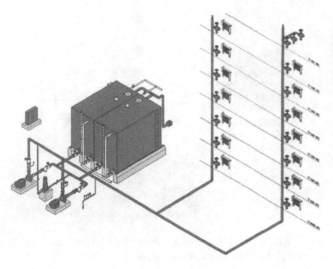

FIGURE 44V   Wet Risers (Courtesy: www.highrisefirefighting.co.uk/wr.html).

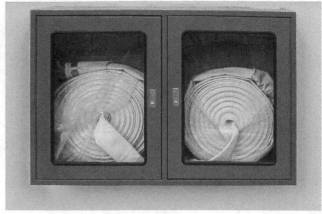

FIGURE 44W   Hose Box (Courtesy: www.istockphoto.com/photos/fire-hydrant-and-hose-box).

44.2 Summary

Planning and designing fire safety in hospitals is a critical process that ensures the protection of patients, staff, and the health care facility itself. Fire safety measures in hospitals are essential to mitigate the risks associated with fire incidents and to facilitate swift and safe evacuation in case of emergencies. Key considerations in the planning and designing process include the installation of fire detection and suppression systems, establishing well-defined evacuation routes, incorporating fire-resistant materials, ensuring compliance with fire safety codes and regulations, and providing staff training on fire prevention and response. By prioritizing these factors and engaging experts in fire safety engineering, hospitals can establish a well-designed fire safety system that safeguards lives, minimizes property damage, and ensures the continuity of health care services.

45 ECOLOGICAL ASPECTS OF PLANNING AND OPERATIONS

45.1 Introduction

The health care sector in India is growing at a rapid pace and contributing immensely to the growth of the quality of services. The sector is expected to grow several-fold in the next decade. Although this augurs well for the country, there is an imminent need to introduce green concepts and techniques in this sector, which can aid growth in a sustainable manner.

45.2 Definitions

There are many definitions of a green hospital. The Office of the Federal Environmental Executive defines a green or sustainable building as "the practice of increasing the efficiency with which buildings and their sites use energy, water, and materials, and reducing building impacts on human health and the environment, through better siting, design, construction, operation, maintenance, and removal—the complete building life cycle".

The United States Environmental Protection Agency defines green building as "the practice of creating structures and using processes that are environmentally responsible and resource-efficient throughout a building's life cycle from siting to design, construction, operation, maintenance, renovation, and deconstruction. This practice expands and complements the classical building design concerns of economy, utility, durability, and comfort. Green building is also known as a sustainable or high-performance building".

According to Health care without Harm,

A green and healthy hospital is the one that promotes public health by continuously reducing its environmental impact and ultimately eliminating its contribution to the burden of disease. A green and healthy hospital recognizes the connection between human health and the environment and demonstrates that understanding through its governance, strategy, and operations. It connects local needs with environmental action and practices primary prevention by actively engaging in efforts to foster community environmental health, health equity and a green economy.

According to the Indian Green Building Council, a green hospital building can be defined as one that enhances patient well-being and aids the curative process while utilizing natural resources in an efficient, environmentally friendly manner.

The WHO has defined green hospitals as a hospital that is responsive to local climate conditions with optimized energy use.

45.3 Focus Areas for Green Hospital Design

1. Lighting
2. Indoor Air Quality, Passive and Active Measures
3. Green Housekeeping
4. Clean and Green Interior Building Materials
5. Gardens and Landscape

In the architectural planning and design of green hospitals, an overarching consideration must be given to ensure that the floor plate facilitates efficiency. An efficient floor plate design will reduce the construction footprint of a hospital—thus benefitting both the owner (lowered construction costs) and the patient (fast, smooth, and efficient transit through the hospital).

45.3.1 Lighting

A good hospital design should maximize daylight and optimize the artificial lighting requirement. Daylighting is the controlled admission of natural light from the sky (direct and diffused) into a building to reduce the use of electrical energy for lighting (Figure 45A). Benefits of daylighting and views in hospitals are

- Daylighting has been proven to have positive effect/s on patients in hospitals.
- Enhances health and well-being of patients and reduce the stress levels of hospital employees, thus improving quality of care.
- Combats seasonal affective disorder, or winter depression, through view connectivity to natural vistas.
- Improves facility's overall operational efficiency.

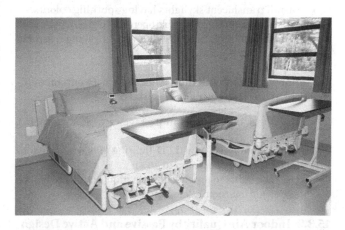

FIGURE 45A Daylight in Patient Care Area (Courtesy: www.ucl.ac.uk/bartlett/environmental-design/news/2021/mar/daylight-hospitals-health-and-wellbeing-impacts-patients).

> **Do You Know?**
> (a) Humans synthesize 90% of their body's requirements of Vitamin D naturally from the skin's exposure to sunlight.
> (b) Buildings can save up to 20% of cooling energy load by optimally substituting artificial lighting with daylighting.

Artificial lighting is required in sensitive areas of the hospital—including operating theatres, medical dispensaries, interior corridors, and passages. However, with rising energy costs and high initial investment, it is imperative to reduce operational costs of lighting in hospitals by combining natural lighting and energy-efficient artificial lighting. The recommended lighting levels for hospitals is given in Table 45A.

DOI: 10.1201/9780367460884-47

TABLE 45A: Recommended Lighting Levels for Hospitals

Type of Room	LPD (Lighting Power Density) (W/sq. ft)
Emergency	2.7
Recovery	0.8
Nurse Station	1.0
Examination/Treatment	1.5
Pharmacy	1.2
Patient Room	0.7
Operating Room	2.2
Nursery	0.6
Medical Supply	1.4
Physical Therapy	0.9
Radiology	0.4
Laundry-Washing	0.6

The following are a few of the passive design aspects to enhance natural lighting in hospitals:

- Install glazing facades to have both view and daylight minus the heat.
- Install translucent skylights having soothing colours.
- Have transparent and operable openings to green courtyards.
- Consider ledge seating at windows—engaging nature in the curative process.

The following are a few of the design aspects to enhance efficiency of artificial lighting in hospitals:

- Use occupancy sensors in passageways, storage rooms, labs, etc.
- Install energy-efficient LED lighting to save on indoor lighting energy costs (up to 40%).
- Use task lights to provide illumination in task areas such as consulting rooms, labs, and wards.

45.3.2 Indoor Air Quality by Passive and Active Design

As restoring and safeguarding health is the main purpose of health care facilities, indoor environmental quality is considered critical to green hospitals. Requirements for a good indoor environment and outdoor fresh air requirements for ventilation of health care facilities are given in Box 45A and Table 45B.

Box 45A: Must Do's for a Good Indoor Environment

- Install permanent entry-way systems, for example, slotted systems, grates, or grilles, at all primary entrances to capture dust particles.
- Use certain species of indoor plants that not only produce oxygen but also reduce indoor pollutants such as volatile organic compound (VOC) from the air.
- Improve fresh air by providing courtyard spaces with native and adaptive plant species that are free from any allergic effects.
- Use zero-VOC interior materials.

TABLE 45B: Outdoor Fresh Air Requirements for Ventilation of Health Care Facilities (In Cubic Feet per Minute—CFM)

Application	Estimated Maximum Occupancy (Person/100 m²)	Outdoor Air Requirements (Fresh Air) cfm/ person	cfm/ ft²	
Patient Rooms	10	25	—	Procedures generating contaminants may require higher rates
Medical Procedure	20	15	—	
Operating Rooms	20	30	—	
Recovery & ICU	20	15	—	
Autopsy Rooms	20	—	0.50	Air should not be recirculated into other spaces
Physical Therapy	20	15	—	—

45.4 Green Housekeeping

Accumulation of dust, soil, and microbial contaminants on surfaces is a potential source of health care–associated infections (HCAIs). Effective and efficient cleaning methods and schedules are therefore necessary to maintain a clean and healthy environment in health care buildings. Currently, housekeeping policies and procedures increasingly focus on making a positive environmental impact. Typical measures include

- Use of cleaning products/chemicals that meet environmental standards.
- Training of personnel on safe handling and disposal of hospital waste.
- Recycling waste, wherever feasible.

Do You Know?

Lack of proper insulation in the roof, walls, etc., can lead to patient discomfort in summer months through solar heat conductance. High-performance insulation, such as extruded polystyrene and poly urethane foam, in the hospital building envelope can significantly reduce energy consumption.

45.5 Clean and Green Interior Building Materials

- Hospitals may inadvertently contribute to illness by exposing patients and staff to a host of pathogenic germs and toxins that enter the hospital premises through the medium of a large number of infected patients
- Ensure that the hospital surfaces have the property of repelling or resisting the growth of pathogenic germs and bacteria. Patented interior surfaces are now available that resists bacterial and fungal growth. These include countertops, tiles, vinyl flooring, etc. Consider using

copper-based interior materials. Recent research shows that copper is a good material for common "touch" surfaces in hospitals (door handles, light switches, faucets, countertops, etc.) due to its microbial resistant properties.

- Use indoor flooring that does not emit/absorb/re-release indoor pollutants such as VOCs and dust.

Do you know?

(a) Gardens and landscapes are an aesthetic delight and promote wellness of patients in hospitals. Persons exposed to plants have higher levels of positive feelings (pleasantness, calm) as opposed to negative feelings (anger, fear).

(b) Research has shown that noise in hospitals poses problems for patients and leads to nursing errors. Some positive acoustic measures include better insulation between rooms, the use of vibrating/low volume communicating devices (intercom and pagers), use of quiet fans, design of back-to-back restrooms, and location.

45.6 Benefits of Green Health Care Facilities

Green health care facilities can have tremendous benefits, both tangible and intangible. The most tangible benefits are the reduction in water and energy consumption right from day one of occupancy. The energy savings could range from 20–30% and water savings could be around 30–50% (Figure 45B). The intangible benefits of green health care facilities include enhanced air quality, faster patient recovery, daylighting for patients, connectivity to outdoor environment, health and hygiene of occupants and patients, and safety benefits.

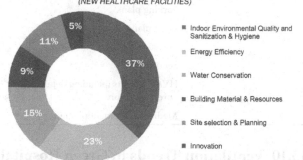

IGBC GREEN HEALTHCARE RATING SYSTEM
(NEW HEALTHCARE FACILITIES)

- Indoor Environmental Quality and Sanitization & Hygiene — 37%
- Energy Efficiency — 23%
- Water Conservation — 15%
- Building Material & Resources — 9%
- Site selection & Planning — 11%
- Innovation — 5%

FIGURE 45B Benefits of Green Health Care Facilities (Courtesy: https://igbc.in/igbc/html_pdfs/abridged/IGBC%20 Green%20Healthcare%20Facilities%20Rating%20System%20 Version%201-%20Final.pdf).

45.7 Considerations for a Green Hospital

Green hospital construction includes the implementation of specific tools and processes for the construction and operation of a hospital in an eco-friendly and sustainable manner. As a hospital is an essential part of any community, the application of green practices across all hospital operations can have a significant impact on the society. Green terminology can be implemented for hospital construction and its operations upon completion (Table 45C).

TABLE 45C: Planning and Construction Considerations for a Green Hospital

Location of the hospital	• Select a land area that is not located in the middle of the wetlands, on top of landfills, chemical dumps, or farmlands. • Select a site that is easily accessible to public transit. Access to public transportation can facilitate both the staff and patients visiting the hospital. Due to this, there is an improved community presence and reduction in carbon footprint.
Avoiding employee parking lots	• Parking spaces for hospital employees require a large area of hot black asphalt platform, which contributes to high average global temperatures. • The objective is to focus on the use of local public transport systems such as trains, buses, subways, and bike lanes.
Design interiors to receive daylight	• The interiors of the hospital rooms can be designed to receive sunshine from all directions, except from southern exposure.
Raising green roof for hospital construction	Most of the hospital facilities are large in area and can easily accommodate a green roof. A green roof facilitates the exchange of carbon dioxide and oxygen. Moreover, it has a calming effect on visitors and patients.
Automation	Sustainability and energy efficiency for a hospital facility can be best achieved with automation. It requires automation for temperature control, air-flow, electric light, and the water supply system. An automated system can sense the time of day and people's movements to control the lighting inside the building. The application of automation is not only sustainable but also saves money and reduces power consumption.
Green materials for hospital construction	• Several types of green materials can be used for different parts of hospital construction. Some of them are • **Rubber:** Rubber is a renewable material that does not require harsh chemicals for cleaning and maintenance. Hence, it is environmentally friendly and is therefore a favourable option for floors. • **Indigenous materials:** Local and regional construction materials can be preferred to avoid additional transportation. • **Recycling:** Try to set up a special unit to develop a recycling program for the chemical and toxic wastes from the laboratories.

(Continued)

TABLE 45C: (Continued)

Maintaining a clean site	• A green construction site must be clean. Proper supervision and communication with the workers can help in achieving cleanliness. • During construction, the contractor in charge should ensure that all leftover materials such as wood, rebar, drywall, flooring materials, etc. are in good shape and workable.

Use of energy-efficient systems	• Some of the core energy systems used in green buildings include:
	   • Energy-efficient lighting systems
	   • Energy-efficient medical equipment
	   • Advanced renewable energy systems
	   • Promoting daylight exposure and natural ventilation
	   • Rainwater harvesting
	   • Operation of cooling towers performed by rainwater
	   • Super-insulated roofs
	   • High-efficiency windows

45.8 National Priorities Addressed in the Rating System

The IGBC Green Health Care Rating System addresses the most important national priorities, which include water conservation, handling waste, energy efficiency, reduced use of fossil fuels, lesser dependence on usage of virgin materials, and health and well-being of patients and occupants. The rating system requires the application of national standards and codes such as the Indian Health Facility Guidelines, NBC, ECBC, MoEF guidelines, CPCB guidelines, and several others. The overarching objective is to be better than the national standards to create health care benchmarks.

(a) **Health and Well-Being of Patients & Occupants:** Health and well-being of patients and occupants are the most important aspects of the IGBC Green Health care rating system. The rating system has addressed healing architecture/evidence-based design, adequate ventilation, daylighting, infection control mechanisms, and patient well-being, which are so essential in health care facilities. The rating system also recognizes measures to minimize indoor air pollutants and infections.

(b) **Water Conservation:** Most Asian countries are water-stressed and in a country such as India, the water table has reduced drastically over the last decade. The IGBC Green Health care rating system encourages use of water in a self-sustainable manner through reduce, recycle, and reuse strategies. By adopting this rating program, green health care facilities can save potable water to an extent of 30–50%.

(c) **Handling of Consumer & Biomedical Waste:** Handling of waste in hospitals is extremely sensitive. This continues to be a challenge to the municipalities that needs to be addressed. The rating system intends to address this by encouraging buildings to have proper systems in place.

(d) **Energy Efficiency:** The health care sector is a large consumer of electrical energy. Through the IGBC Green Health care rating system, these facilities can reduce energy consumption through energy-efficient building envelopes, lighting, air conditioning systems, etc. The energy savings that can be realized by adopting this rating program can be up to 20–30%.

(e) **Reduced Use of Fossil Fuels:** Fossil fuel is a slowly depleting resource all over the world. The use of fossil fuel for transportation has been a major source of pollution. The rating system encourages the use of alternate fuel vehicles for transportation.

(f) **Reduced Dependency on Virgin Materials:** The rating system encourages projects to use recycled and reused material and discourages the use of virgin materials, thereby addressing environmental impacts associated with extraction and processing of scarce natural resources.

45.9 Certification

To achieve the IGBC Green Health care rating, the project must satisfy all the mandatory requirements and the minimum number of credit points. The project team is expected to provide supporting documents at the preliminary and final stages of submission for all the mandatory requirements and the credits attempted. The project needs to submit the details mentioned in Table 45D.

TABLE 45D: Necessary Details for Green Building Certification

General information about project, including	Project brief stating the project type, different types of spaces, occupancy, bed distribution, area provided per bed, number of floors, area statement, etc.
General drawings	Master/Site plan
	Parking plans
	Floor plans
	Elevations
	Sections
	HVAC layouts including details on pressurization
	Medical equipment planning

45.10 Ventilation Trends in Green Hospitals

Conventional systems, split air conditioners, and window air conditioners do not provide adequate fresh air ventilation. Medical procedure rooms and operating theatres require 100% exhaust, but significant energy savings can be realized even with 100% exhaust. The minimum fresh air ventilation required for all occupied spaces is mentioned in Table 45B.

45.11 Barriers to Creating "Green Hospitals"

Greg L Roberts, in his article "Shades of Green" has cited different barriers to green health facilities, which are as follows:

• **System redundancy**—Requirement of secondary and tertiary backup systems to ensure that operations do not cease during emergencies.

- **Regulatory compliance**—Health and safety regulations and building codes prevent hospitals to adopt sustainable practices.
- **Operational hours**—Health facilities function uninterruptedly throughout the year.
- **Infection control**—Hospitals require strict infection control protocols that often run counter to sustainability practices.
- **Ventilation rates**—More frequent air changes are required in a hospital than in other commercial office spaces.
- **Accreditation and licensing demands**—Compliance with central, state, and accreditation standards might prevent facilities to make environmentally sound choices.
- **Intense energy and water use**—Health care uses 2.1 times more energy per square foot than commercial buildings, and hospitals typically use 80–150 gallons of water per bed per day.
- **High-volume waste stream**—Approximately 0.5 kg of hazardous waste is generated per bed per day.
- **Chemical use**—Hazardous chemicals used to clean and disinfect, sterilize equipment, treat certain diseases, and for laboratory research and testing can be toxic and hazardous.

- **Life cycle**—The exterior of hospital buildings can last a long time, but the interior requires renovations every few years.

45.12 Summary

Planning and designing the ecological aspects of planning and operations in a hospital is an essential process that promotes sustainability, environmental responsibility, and the overall well-being of the surrounding ecosystem. Incorporating ecological considerations in hospital planning and operations involves measures such as energy-efficient building design, waste reduction and recycling programs, water conservation strategies, green landscaping practices, and sustainable procurement. By prioritizing these factors, hospitals can minimize their environmental footprint, conserve resources, reduce pollution, and create a healthier and more sustainable environment for patients, staff, and the community. The integration of ecological principles in hospital planning and operations is a testament to the commitment towards promoting environmental stewardship and supporting a greener and more resilient future.

References

Chapter	Reference
34.	TAHPI. International Health Facility Guidelines; Mechanical (HVAC) Engineering Design. www.healthfacilityguidelines.com/ViewPDF/ViewIndexPDF/Mechanical_HVAC_Engineering_Design..
	NHS. HTM 03–01: Specialized Ventilation for Health Care Premises Part A. www.england.nhs.uk/wp-content/uploads/2021/05/HTM0301-PartA-accessible-F6.pdf.
	CPWD. General Specifications for Heating, Ventilation & Air-Conditioning (HVAC) Works. 2017. https://cpwd.gov.in/publication/hvac.pdf.
	NHS. HTM 08–01: Acoustics. www.england.nhs.uk/wp-content/uploads/2021/05/HTM_08-01.pdf.
35.	TAHPI. International Health Facility Guidelines; Electrical Services. www.healthfacilityguidelines.com/ViewPDF/ViewIndexPDF/Electrical_Services.
	NHS. HTM 06–01: Electrical Services Supply and Distribution. www.england.nhs.uk/wp-content/uploads/2021/05/Health_tech_memo_0601.pdf.
	CPWD. Space for Electrical and Mechanical Services in Buildings: Companion Volume of General Specifications for Electrical Works, 2013. https://cpwd.gov.in/Publication/Space_for_Electrical_and_Machanical_Services_in_Buildings.pdf.
	CPWD. Guidelines for Substation and Power Distribution Systems of Buildings, 2019. https://cpwd.gov.in/Publication/Guidelines_for_Substation_and_power_Distribution_Systems_of_Buildings_2019.pdf.
36.	TAHPI. International Health Facility Guidelines; ELV and ICT Systems. www.healthfacilityguidelines.com/ViewPDF/ViewIndexPDF/ELV_and_ICT_systems.
	Sapling Inc. Central Clock System. https://sapling-inc.com/wireless-clocks-the-technology-within/.
	Falco G, Viswanathan A, Caldera C, Shrobe H. A master attack methodology for an AI-based automated attack planner for smart cities. IEEE Access. 2018;6:48360–48373.
	United Group. Simplified Access Control Architecture. www.unitedtecgroup.com/access-control-systems.html.
	Saitell. Semi Digital Intercom System. https://saitell.com/healthcare-intercom/semi-digital-intercom-system/.
	Advantech. Patient Infotainment System. www.advantech.com/iretail-hospitality/solutions/detail/bedside-infotainment-system-and-digital-bedside-card.
	Advantech. Queue Management System. www.advantech.com/iretail-hospitality/solutions/detail/intelligent-patient-queue-management-system.
	Scnsoft. Smart Hospital Asset Tracking. www.scnsoft.com/healthcare/iot/smart-hospital-asset-tracking.
	Honeywell. Smoke Detectors. https://buildings.honeywell.com/us/en/products/by-category/sensors/smoke-detectors.
	Security Vault Systems. Fire Alarm System. https://securityvaultsystems.com/fire-alarm-systems-fas/.
	Dsppatech. IP Network PA Solution for Hospital. www.dsppatech.com/ip-network-pa-solution-for-hospital.html.

37.   TAHPI. International Health Facility Guidelines; Public Health—Water System Design. www.healthfacilityguidelines.com/ViewPDF/ViewIndexPDF/Public_Health_Water_Systems_Design_WS.

Bureau of Indian Standards. National Building Code, 2016.

Central Public Health and Environment Engineering Organization (CPHEEO), Ministry of Housing and Urban Affairs, GoI. Manual on Water Supply and Treatment, 1999. http://cpheeo.gov.in/cms/manual-on-water-supply-and-treatment.php.

Central Public Health and Environment Engineering Organization (CPHEEO), Ministry of Housing and Urban Affairs, GoI. Manual on Operation and Maintenance of Water Supply System, 2005. http://cpheeo.gov.in/cms/manual-on-operation--and-maintenance-of-water-supply-system-2005.php.

Ministry of Water Resources, GoI. National Water Policy, 2002. http://cgwb.gov.in/documents/nwp_2002.pdf.

38.   TAHPI. International Health Facility Guidelines; Sanitary Drainage System Design. www.healthfacilityguidelines.com/ViewPDF/ViewIndexPDF/Public_Health_Sanitary_Drainage_System_Design_DS.

Bureau of Indian Standards. National Building Code, 2016.

AERB. Management of Radioactive Waste. www.aerb.gov.in/images/PDF/CodesGuides/General/RadioactiveWasteManagement/1.pdf.

39.   TAHPI. International Health Facility Guidelines; Vertical Transport System. www.healthfacilityguidelines.com/ViewPDF/ViewIndexPDF/Vertical_Transportation_System.

NHS. HBN 00–04: Circulation and Communication Spaces. www.england.nhs.uk/wp-content/uploads/2021/05/Health_Building_Note_00-04_-_Circulation_and_communication_spaces_-_updated_April_2013.pdf.

Bureau of Indian Standards. National Building Code, 2016

CPWD. Handbook on Barrier Free and Accessibility. https://cpwd.gov.in/Publication/HandbookonBarrier.pdf.

Siikonen ML, Suihkonen K. People flow and automated transportation with hospital elevators. Business Briefing: Hospital Engineering & Facilities Managements. 2005;2:41–44.

Comparison of Different Guidelines for Accessibility of Built Environment in India. https://ncpedp.org/documents/COMPARISON%20OF%20DIFFERENT%20GUIDELINES_2016.pdf.

40.   TAHPI. International Health Facility Guidelines; Pneumatic Tube System. www.healthfacilityguidelines.com/ViewPDF/ViewIndexPDF/Public_Health_Pneumatic_Tube_System_Design_PTS.

NHS. HTM 2009: Pneumatic Air Tube Transport Systems Design Considerations and Good Practice Guide. www.nwssp.wales.nhs.uk/sitesplus/documents/1178/HTM%202009%20Des.pdf.

CPWD. Pneumatic Tube Transport System. www.cpwd.gov.in/images/AzadikaAmrit/PneumaticTubesystem290921.pptx.

CPWD. General Specifications for Pneumatic Tube Transport System 2022. https://cpwd.gov.in/Publication/PTTS2022.pdf.

41.   TAHPI. International Health Facility Guidelines; Signage. https://healthfacilityguidelines.com/ViewPDF/ViewIndexPDF/iHFG_part_c_signage.

NHS. Effective Wayfinding and Signage Systems, Guidance for Healthcare Facilities, 2005. www.england.nhs.uk/wp-content/uploads/2021/05/Wayfinding.pdf.

NABH. NABH Accreditation Standards for Hospitals, April 2020. www.nabh.co/images/Standards/NABH%205%20STD%20April%202020.pdf.

Office of DGAFMS, Ministry of Defence, Government of India. Scales of Accommodation for Armed Forces Hospitals, 2003.

MoHFW, GoI. Clinical Establishment (Registration and Regulation) Act, 2010. Clinical Establishment Act Standard for Clinic/Polyclinic only Consultation. https://clinicalestablishments.gov.in/WriteReadData/9361.pdf.

Directorate General of Health Services, Ministry of Health & Family Welfare, Government of India. IPHS Guidelines for Sub District Hospital and District Hospital, 2022. https://nhsrcindia.org/sites/default/files/Volume%201_SDH-DH_0.pdf.

CPWD. Handbook on Barrier Free and Accessibility, 2014. https://cpwd.gov.in/Publication/HandbookonBarrier.pdf.

Wikipedia. Signage. https://en.wikipedia.org/wiki/Signage.

Cosign. 5 Must Have Features in Healthcare Signage. www.cosign.in/blog-post/5-must-have-features-in-healthcare-signage/.

Indiamart. Hospital Building Sign. www.indiamart.com/proddetail/hospital-building-sign-7940139033.html.

Punctual Print. Directional Sings. https://punctualprint.com/signage/exterior-signage/directional-signs/.

Gifu University Hospital. Hospital Map. www.hosp.gifu-u.ac.jp/eng/map.html.

AERB. Radiation Symbol. www.aerb.gov.in/english/radiation-symbol.

AAA Business Solutions. Hospital Wayfinding Signage. www.aaabusinesssolutions.net/hospital-wayfinding-signage-5/.

Joy Lo CW, Yien HW, Chen IP. How universal are universal symbols? An estimation of cross-cultural adoption of universal healthcare symbols. HERD: Health Environments Research & Design Journal. 2016;9(3):116–134.

Yumpu. Whipps Cross Hospital Site Map and Wayfinding System. www.yumpu.com/en/document/view/38423461/whipps-cross-hospital-site-map-and-wayfinding-system.

Firstouch Digital Solutions. Digital Signage Solutions for Hospitals. https://firstouchkiosk.com/customized-solutions/healthcare.

Beta Point. Beacon Park Hospital Signage. https://betasigns.co.uk/portfolio/beacon-park-hospital-signage/.

42.   Ministry of Environment, Forest and Climate Change, GoI. Bio Medical Waste Management Rules, 2016. https://dhr.gov.in/sites/default/files/Bio-medical_Waste_Management_Rules_2016.pdf.

Ministry of Environment, Forest and Climate Change, GoI. Bio Medical Waste Management (Amendment) Rules, 2018. https://pcb.ap.gov.in/APPCBDOCS/Tenders_Noti//WasteManagement//Bio%20medical%20waste%20management%20(amendment)%20Rules%202018.pdf.

Ministry of Environment, Forest and Climate Change, GoI. Bio Medical Waste Management (Amendment) Rules, 2019. https://cpcb.nic.in/uploads/Projects/Bio-Medical-Waste/BMW_Amended_19.02.2019.pdf.

CPCB, Ministry of Environment, Forest and Climate Change, GoI. Guidelines for Management of Healthcare Waste as per Bio Medical Waste Management Rules, 2016. https://cpcb.nic.in/uploads/Projects/Bio-Medical-Waste/Guidelines_healthcare_June_2018.pdf.

CPCB, Ministry of Environment, Forest and Climate Change, GoI. Pictorial Guide on Bio Medical Waste Management Rules, 2016 (Amended in 2018 and 2019). https://cpcb.nic.in/uploads/Projects/Bio-Medical-Waste/Pictorial_guide_covid.pdf.

VMMC and Safdarjung Hospital, Ministry of Health and Family Welfare, GoI. Bio Medical Waste Management manual. www.vmmc-sjh.nic.in/writereaddata/Biomedical%20wast%20Managment%20manual.pdf.

Sachin P, Jagadish MM, Sanjay D, Patond S. Assessment of knowledge, attitude and practice of healthcare workers towards management of biomedical waste: A cross-sectional analytical study. Annals of the Romanian Society for Cell Biology. 2021;18:6866–6873.

NABH. NABH Accreditation Standards for Hospitals, April 2020. www.nabh.co/images/Standards/NABH%205%20STD%20April%202020.pdf.

MoHFW, GoI. Clinical Establishment (Registration and Regulation) Act, 2010. Clinical Establishment Act Standard for Clinic/Polyclinic only Consultation. https://clinicalestablishments.gov.in/WriteReadData/9361.pdf.

43.   Ministry of Health and Family Welfare, GoI. Kaya Kalp: National Guidelines for Clean Hospitals, 2015. https://main.mohfw.gov.in/sites/default/files/7660257301436254417_0.pdf.

CDC. Best Practices for Environmental Cleaning in Healthcare Facilities: In Resource Limited Settings. www.cdc.gov/hai/pdfs/resource-limited/environmental-cleaning-RLS-H.pdf.

NOUS. Hospital Design for Housekeeping Service. www.nousdoc.com/Nous%20Downloads/Download%20Files/NOUS%20Covid%2019%20Housekeeping%20in%20Hospitals.pdf.

TAHPI. International Health Facility Guidelines; Housekeeping Unit. www.healthfacilityguidelines.com/ViewPDF/ViewIndexPDF/iHFG_part_b_housekeeping_unit.

44.   NDMA. NDMA Guidelines: Hospital Safety. https://nidm.gov.in/PDF/pubs/NDMA/18.pdf.

Ministry of Home Affairs, GoI, Directorate General FS, CD & HG, Fire Cell letter no. F. No. VIII-110111/02 (Adv)/2020-DGCD (F) dated 28th November, 2020. https://ndmindia.mha.gov.in/images/Hospital-Advisory-28.11.2020.pdf.

Bureau of Indian Standards. National Building Code, 2016.

Office of DGAFMS, Ministry of Defence, Government of India. Scales of Accommodation for Armed Forces Hospitals, 2003.

NABH. NABH & Fire Safety. www.nabh.co/Images/PDF/Fire_Safety_NABH.pdf.

MoHFW, GoI. Clinical Establishment (Registration and Regulation) Act, 2010. Clinical Establishment Act Standard for Clinic/Polyclinic only Consultation. https://clinicalestablishments.gov.in/WriteReadData/9361.pdf.

NHS. HTM 05–02: Fire Safety in Design of Healthcare Premises. www.england.nhs.uk/wp-content/uploads/2021/05/HTM_05-02_2015.pdf.

45.   Council IG. IGBC Green Healthcare Facilities Rating System. Version 1.0, Abridged Reference Guide. October 2020.

Roberts GL. Shades of green: The evolution of hospital sustainable design standards. Health Facilities Management. 2011;24(11):45–50.

Howard JL. The federal commitment to green building: Experiences and expectations. *Federal Executive, Office of the Federal Environmental Executive*, Washington, DC. 2003 Oct.

Bandhauer K, Gerber MA, Simon S, Smith S, Buffo C, Gitlin S. *Sustainable Design and Green Building Toolkit for Local Governments*. Environmental Protection Agency (US), 2013.

Karliner J, Guenther R. *Global Green and Healthy Hospitals*. Health Care without Harm, 2011.

Council IG. Technical Bulletin: Green Hospitals. https://igbc.in/igbc/html_pdfs/technical/Green%20Hospitals.pdf.

World Health Organization (WHO). 2010. Healthy Hospitals, Healthy Planet, Healthy people: Addressing climate change in health care settings: Discussion Draft. In *Healthy Hospitals, Healthy Planet, Healthy People: Addressing Climate Change in Health Care Settings: Discussion Draft 2010* (pp. 30–30) WHO..

Kumari S, Kumar R. Green Hospital—A necessity and not option. Journal of Management Research and Analysis. 2020;7(2):46–51.

University College London. Daylight in Hospitals: Health and Well Being Impacts on Patients. www.ucl.ac.uk/bartlett/environmental-design/news/2021/mar/daylight-hospitals-health-and-wellbeing-impacts-patients.

Unit 4
Equipment Planning and Outsourcing in Hospitals

46 MEDICAL EQUIPMENT MANAGEMENT

46.1 Introduction

As per the WHO, medical equipment is defined as medical devices requiring calibration, maintenance, repair, user training, and decommissioning—activities usually managed by clinical engineers. Medical equipment is used for the specific purposes of diagnosis and treatment of disease or rehabilitation following disease or injury; it can be used either alone or in combination with any accessory, consumable, or other piece of medical equipment. Medical equipment excludes implantable, disposable, or single-use medical devices.

Medical equipment is used in the diagnosis, treatment, and monitoring of patients. It is a major asset of the health care industry characterized by a wide range, variety, and high rate of obsolescence. Medical equipment is very expensive and represents approximately one-third to one-half of the total project cost. An overview of medical equipment management is shown in Figure 46A.

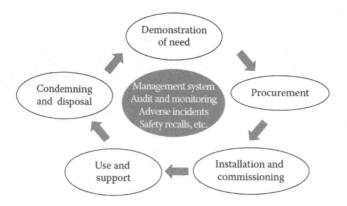

FIGURE 46A An Overview of Medical Equipment Management (Courtesy: Willson K, Ison K, Tabakov S. Medical equipment management. Taylor & Francis; 2014).

46.2 Medical Equipment Management Process

The medical equipment life cycle includes needs assessment, procurement, installation, training of staff, use of equipment, equipment maintenance and repair, and decommissioning and disposal of equipment. Figure 46B shows the activities in the life cycle of equipment under equipment management.

46.2.1 Needs Assessment

Needs assessment is a process for determining and addressing the gaps between the current situation or condition and the desired one. It is a strategic activity and a part of the planning process that aims to improve the current performance or to correct deficiencies. In case of equipment management, needs assessment is the identification and definition of prioritized requirements. It takes into account the overall objectives of the institution, existing facilities and infrastructures, long-term plan of use, and human resources (HR) development prior to purchasing a medical device.

(i) **The general approach** in performing a needs assessment is to examine what is available in the facility, region, or country and to compare it with what should be available, considering the particular demand and situation of the catchment area or target group. Part of this process includes looking at locally and globally recognized standards. The identified gap specifies the overall need. By taking into consideration possible financial and HR restrictions and prioritized epidemiological requirements, a list of the prioritized needs can be established (Table 46A and Figure 46C).

(ii) **Specific approach for needs assessment**
- **Step I: Baseline information on health service requirements (Table 46B)**
- **Step II: Baseline information on health service availability (Table 46C):** The following questions can be asked to retrieve the relevant information:
  - Where is (are) the facility(ies) located?
  - Which health services are available at the facility?
  - What range of clients does the facility cater to in terms of age, gender, geographical distribution, etc.?
  - Which specific needs do the facility (and its services) meet?
  - How does the facility receive referrals, and from whom does its referrals come?
  - How many clients does the facility see each week/month/quarter/year?
  - On average, how long do clients stay at the facility, and what are their reasons for leaving (e.g., drop-out, onward referral, etc.)?
  - How many clients each week/month, etc., are referred to other agencies?
  - What is the caseload of staff?
  - How many full-time staff does the service employ, and how much time do they have available each week for client appointments?
  - Is there any information regarding staff satisfaction or facility user satisfaction available by way of surveys?
  - How do existing clients access the facility (e.g., on foot, by public transportation, etc.)?
  - How accessible is the service by public transportation?
- **Step III: Baseline information on medical devices/equipment (Table 46D):** Key information to be collected includes the following:
  - **Infrastructure**
    - type, size, and position of premise and building(s), including the number and type of building(s)
    - availability and condition of water supply, connections, and installation (e.g., where does the water come from? what is the quality? etc.)
    - power supply, electrical connections, and installations (e.g., is an emergency generator available?)
    - waste disposal system (e.g., how is waste handled, segregated, and disposed of?)
  - **Medical equipment**
    - type and number of equipment
    - brand name
    - model

DOI: 10.1201/9780367460884-49

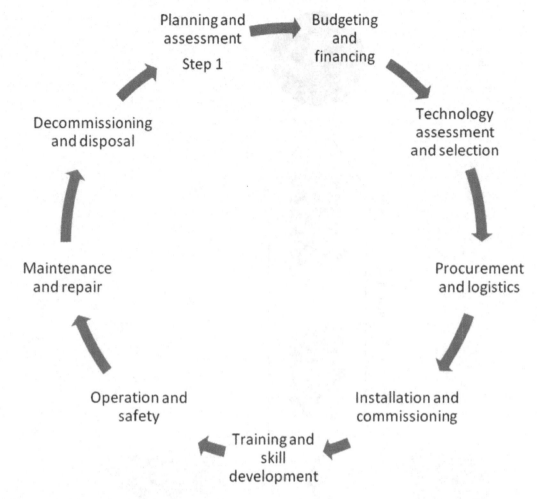

FIGURE 46B   Equipment Life Cycle (Courtesy: Kumar U, Godhia H, Srinivas N, Hoovayya P. Insights into equipment planning of a 250-bed hospital project. International Journal of Health Sciences and Research. 2014;4(10):311–21).

- year of manufacture
- date of installation
- location (medical department)
- physical condition (in operation/out of order/ repairable)
- spare parts required/available for repair
- tools available for inspection, maintenance, and repair
- medical equipment history if available (operation/ use time, maintenance/repair)
- **Health technology management**
  - type of existing management structure, including responsibilities
  - existing policy (if available)
- **Step IV: Baseline information on human resources (Table 46E):** The minimum information that should be available for collection and assessment is
  - existing posts and job descriptions
  - number of vacant posts
  - status and availability of basic, higher, or vocational education, continuous training, on-the-job training, and human resources planning
- **Step V: Baseline information on finances (Table 46F):** The minimum information that should be available for collection and assessment is
  - budget and expenses from previous periods

- current budget
- system of monitoring/controlling budget
- **Step VI: Analysis and interpretation:** Once all the information is gathered, it is possible to analyse, interpret, and draw conclusions. The analysis and interpretation should be based directly on the information gathered in the manner outlined in previous steps.
- **Step VII: Prioritization and appraisal of options:** After having analysed the information gathered in the earlier steps of the needs assessment process, and having drawn conclusions, there should now be a reasonably clear picture of the needs of the target population. Decisions regarding the actions to take will depend on several crucial and closely connected activities (Tables 46G-H). These include
  - **Prioritization**: If there are insufficient resources to meet all the identified needs, it may be necessary to rank them in order to decide which needs should be met first and which will be met later.
  - **Option appraisal**: There may be more than one way of meeting the needs identified. Various options should be considered, and the evidence in favour of each should be weighed carefully.
  - **Implementation**: When agreement has been reached about how the needs are to be met, an action plan and timetable should be drawn up, including a plan for resource allocation.

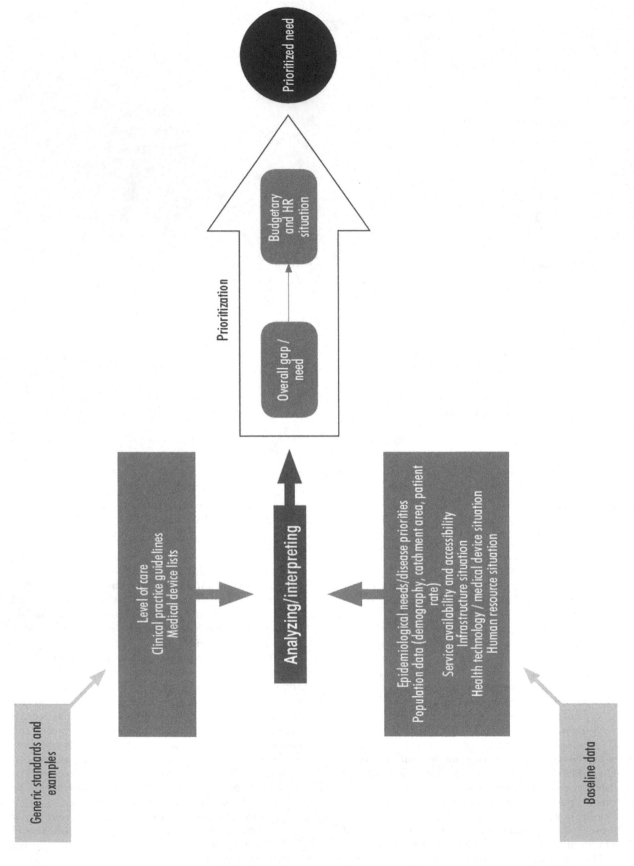

FIGURE 46C General Needs Assessment Approach (Process) (Courtesy: https://apps.who.int/iris/bitstream/handle/10665/44562/9789241501385-eng.pdf).

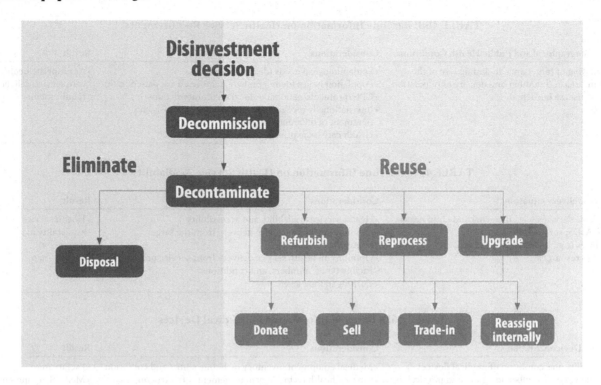

FIGURE 46D Decommissioning of Medical Equipment (Courtesy: https://apps.who.int/iris/bitstream/handle/10665/330095/9789241517041-eng.pdf).

TABLE 46A: General Needs Assessment Approach (Process)

Questions		Data Required	Tools	Result
1	What do we want/need in terms of health services?	• Population (target population, catchment area) • Health service provider availability • Epidemiological data	• "Certificate of need" process, see Appendix A • Clinical practice guidelines (CPG) • Survey questionnaires • Standards of level of care • Integrated health care technology package (iHTP)	
2	What do we have? (local conditions/limitations)	• Health service availability • Lists of available medical devices • Human resources availability	• Service availability mapping (SAM) questionnaires • Evaluation manuals/tools • Inventory management tool • Computerized maintenance management system (CMMS)	
3	Which standards/recommended best practices exist that could be applied or adapted?	• Standards/recommendations for health service delivery coverage (catchment areas) • Standards/recommendations for medical devices • Standards/recommendations for human resources required for operation/maintenance/management of medical equipment	• (essential) Medical device lists; i.e., per facility type and department or per clinical procedure	
4 = 3–2	Overall gap:			List of general needs
5	What financial/human resources do we have? (constraints)	• Budget (capital investment and operational) • Human resources		
6 = 4–5	Prioritized needs:			Prioritized list of needs

TABLE 46B: Baseline Information on Health Service Requirements

Local Geographical and Public Health Conditions	Considerations	Result
• Population of target area, including size of the region/area and number and density of population • Major disease burden	• Epidemiological needs (disease priorities) • Population issues (demography/catchment area, patient rate) • CPG/protocols/national or local recommendations • Internationally recognized standards on diagnosis and treatment of different diseases • Health care issue prioritization	• Appropriate health care service delivery requirements

TABLE 46C: Baseline Information on Health Service Availability

Service Delivery situation	Considerations	Result
• Available services (e.g., maternal and child health, HIV/AIDS, surgical, etc.) • Facilities (e.g., hospitals, clinics, etc.) • Human resources	• Health service availability and accessibility • Opinions on health service delivery from the target population • Opinions on health service delivery from service providers • Facility types, numbers, and conditions • Current staffing levels	• Health service availability map (overview) • Facility map

TABLE 46D: Baseline Information on Medical Devices

Medical Device Situation	Considerations	Result
• Availability and condition of medical devices (including type, number, location, and physical condition) • Status of electrical, water, and waste disposal systems related to medical device use	• Medical equipment inventory including status and condition • Current health technology management infrastructure (or lack thereof)	• Facility map • Medical equipment inventory (quantitative and qualitative) • Outline of health technology management infrastructure

TABLE 46E: Baseline Information on Human Resources

Human resources	Considerations	Result
Qualification and number of human resources required to cover the required health care demand (as defined by the results of Step I)	• Availability, capacity, and capability of current human resources	• Human resource data information (staffing plan) • Education and training map

TABLE 46F: Baseline Information on Finances

Financial Situation	Considerations	Result
Capacity to finance overall facility operations, including health services, health technology, and infrastructure (Steps II and III previously).	• Financial resources	• Budget

TABLE 46G: PDSA Prioritization Matrix

Finances/Resources Required to Implement Change	Likely Impact of Change	
	Low	High
Low	Soft target: Wait	Win: Go!
High	Refrain or Wait	Challenging: Wait

TABLE 46H: Key Questions for Prioritizing and Appraisal of Options

Impact
• Which changes would have the greatest positive impact in meeting needs?
• Do the identified needs relate to a local or national priority (e.g., maternal and child health, HIV/AIDS, etc.)?
• What would be the implications be of not addressing the needs?

(Continued)

Changeability
- Which things can be changed and effectively improved?
- What evidence is there of effective interventions?
- Can negative impacts be stopped or reduced?
- Are there national or local professional or organizational policies that set out guidelines on what should be done (e.g., national frameworks, national guidance, etc.)?

Acceptability
- Which of the options for change are likely to be the most acceptable to health service providers, the target population, and managers?
- What might be the "knock-on" effects, or unintended consequences, of making a change?

Resource Feasibility
- Which resources are required to implement the proposed changes?
- Can existing resources be used differently?
- Which resources will be released if ineffective actions are stopped/changed (e.g., proper management of health technology, etc.)?
- Are there other resources available that have not been given prior consideration (e.g., income generation of laboratory services, consideration of public-private partnerships, assistance from NGOs, etc.)?
- Which action will achieve the greatest impact for the resources used?

46.2.2 Budgeting and Financing

Funding for low-cost medical equipment usually comes from a departmental or service budget. Medium-cost items may require allocation of funds from the organization, and very large items often require funding to be raised externally. Funding must also be identified to cover lifetime costs, including consumables and maintenance. This requires effective liaison among equipment users, senior management, and staff in the clinical engineering, finance, and procurement services. Funding is less of a problem where depreciation and replacement of equipment form part of a long-term business plan.

46.2.3 Technical Specifications of All Medical Equipment

Once a proposal has funding, technical specification of all equipment must be prepared. The specification defines what will make a device suitable for the intended purpose. A good specification not only addresses what is needed when the item is delivered but also tries to foresee possible changes of use during its lifetime. Standardization is desirable for a number of reasons, including improvements in safety from user familiarity; simplified training; economies of scale for consumables, spares, and training; and a faster build-up of overall experience with the device.

The development of technical specifications for equipment used in more than one area, particularly where linked to standardization, therefore requires an overview greater than that of any one user. Specifications should be agreed upon among clinical, technical, and end-user groups to cover all their requirements. Apart from the need to consider the specification from different points of view such as its function, maintenance, and the costs of consumables, this also acts as a safeguard against undesirable practices that may undermine an effective, fair, and open procurement process.

46.2.4 Procurement of Equipment

(i) **Advertise/Contact all the respective vendors and call/receipt of quotations**

A list of suppliers, their address, capabilities, past experience, and reputation should be used to call and contact all the respective vendors for the quotation. Enquiries can be
- Directly to the vendors
- Quotation can be invited by letters and by advertising
- Public advertisement in reputed newspapers
- Global tenders can be invited
- The tender terms and conditions, supply period, time limit, etc. must be clearly mentioned

(ii) **Demonstration/Quotation of the equipment from the vendors**

Sealed envelopes/confidential email documents containing technical specifications, offers, price, and other financial details can be received. Vendors can also demonstrate their technology.

(iii) **Vendor analysis—Finalizing the vendor**

A comparative statement should be made mentioning the following details:
- Name of the supplier
- Details of specification
- Basic price
- Taxes, levies, and installation charges
- Freight and insurance charges
- Payment terms
- Delivery period
- Guarantee/warrantee on spares and period
- After sale service terms and conditions
- Any other conditions

All responsive offers that fulfill the needs are short-listed.

(iv) **Negotiation: Finance, maintenance services, spare parts, accessories**

Offers are discussed with the committee, and necessary negotiations are carried out by the committee with the supplier
- Asking for clarification
- Cost reduction
- Bearing the cost of site preparation
- Training of personnel, etc.

(v) **Final quote/Invoice:** After a satisfactory discussion, demonstration, and confirmation, a final invoice is sent to the vendor, and the order is placed.

(vi) **Payment policy**

If the equipment is indigenous, then payment is made on a negotiated payment policy with the respective vendor. If the equipment is to be imported, then the following documents are required:
- License: If the item is included under an open general license (OGL), then a specific import license is not required. If the item is not included in an OGL, then a specific import license in required.
- Product literature and proforma invoice: Product literature and proforma invoice mentioning price, cost-insurance-freight (CIF), free on board (FOB), and mode of transport (such as air or shipping) need to be obtained.

- Custom duty exemption: It is necessary to verify whether the item to be imported is included in the published exemption list. Exemption is usually granted to:
  - Governments, hospitals, and approved research institutes
  - Life-saving items
  - Gift on board to charitable, non-profitable organization
  - Re-import for repaired item. If the item or the hospital do not have a custom duty exemption "not manufactured in India Certificate (NMIC)", then the custom duty exemption certificate needs to be obtained
  - For minor imports, a bank draft is issued to the supplier. For major imports, a letter of credit is issued

(vii) **Delivery of the medical equipment:** The vendor should arrange for the appropriate mode of transport and confirm proper packaging. On delivery, a biomedical engineer verifies all documents as per the protocol of the hospital and verifies that the condition of the machine is free from any external damages. The company/vendor is informed regarding the procurement of the equipment who then further arranges for the installation of the equipment.

(viii) **Installation of the medical equipment:** This is performed by the biomedical engineer as per the protocol of the hospital:
  - Documents are verified
  - Machine is opened and installed
  - After satisfactory installation, it is included in the inventory and in relevant registers
  - Joint demonstration by supplier, user, and biomedical engineer is arranged
  - The item is taken to user department
  - Bill is certified and forwarded to accounting department for prompt payment

(ix) **User training:** User training is arranged for all the respective technicians and staff for all medical equipment in their respective departments by the qualified engineers from the company.

(x) **Monitoring of use and performance:** It is important that the user should make safe use of the equipment and continuously monitor the performance of the equipment. The user should also maintain a direct link with manufacture/supplier/service provider and observe any supplier's technical services. Such services should be recorded in the maintenance register. This will also provide a good learning opportunity for the in-house user. Much equipment will require daily/weekly inspections and simple maintenance. This type of maintenance is vital for the continuous, safe, effective, and reliable operation of medical equipment to obtain accurate and reliable results.

(xi) **Maintenance of equipment:** Proper maintenance of medical equipment is essential to obtain sustained benefits and to preserve capital investment. Medical equipment must be maintained in working order and periodically calibrated for effectiveness and accuracy of the results. Maintenance consists of
  - **Planned Preventive Maintenance:** Planned preventive maintenance involves maintenance performed to extend the life of the equipment and prevent its

failure. Planned preventive maintenance is usually scheduled at specific intervals and includes specific maintenance activities such as lubrication, calibration, cleaning (e.g., filters), or replacing parts that are expected to wear (e.g., bearings) or that have a finite life (e.g., tubing).
  - **Breakdown Maintenance:** Breakdown maintenance is a task performed to identify, isolate, and rectify a fault so that the out-of-order equipment, machine, or system can be restored to an operational condition. All medical equipment in use should be free from any fault or defect, and all repair work should be carried out to accepted standards by competent person(s).

46.2.5 Decommissioning and Disposal of Medical Equipment

Decommissioning is removal of medical equipment from service in a health care facility after a decision to disinvest in the medical equipment itself or in a service in which it is used. The two main pathways for decommissioning medical equipment and determining its final disposition after decontamination are permanent elimination and re-use (Figure 46D). The factors that determine which of the two pathways of the decommissioning is followed can be categorized as those intrinsic to the equipment and the infrastructure in which it operates.

Factors intrinsic to the equipment include

- unresolved performance issues,
- unresolved safety issues,
- continuous unreliability or history of serious failure,
- high cost of repairing the medical equipment (such as cost-intensive or financially unviable), and
- end of life.

Factors related to the infrastructure (decision to be made by local health care workers) are

- reorganization, closure, or relocation of the health care facility; and
- shortage of local technical support, spare parts, accessories, or consumables.

46.3 Summary

Medical equipment used for diagnostic, monitoring, and therapeutic purposes is a key component of medical treatment. Managing the equipment is one of the most important functions of a hospital for continuous, uninterrupted, and quality services. It is emphasized that state-of-the-art technology is what gives a hospital the cutting edge in maintaining the treatment standards and the advantage in meeting the exciting cutthroat competition. Proper management of equipment starting from selection, purchase, installation, use, and maintenance is important for ensuring continued readiness of the service. In addition, within the meagre medical equipment budget allotted, the proportion of funds for repair and maintenance is low, compounding the management problems. Most health managers, doctors, and nurses in developing countries are not familiar with the basic concepts of equipment management. After being procured, the equipment is installed at respective locations and appropriately documented with sufficient user training.

47 OUTSOURCING IN A HEALTH CARE ORGANIZATION

47.1 Introduction

Health care is one of the largest industries in the world, and until very recently, it lagged behind most other industries in its adoption of outsourcing. As the industry becomes more competitive, health organizations must learn to deliver excellent patient care. In most places, patients have multiple providers and health systems to choose from. It is paramount to ensure patient satisfaction, setting providers up for repeat business and referrals. However, the digital health trend is already ready to offer the consumer a very unusual project—the patient profile template. This combines the functionality, convenience, and mobility of telemedicine with the operational efficiency of an offline clinic. Unfortunately, providing excellent care requires substantial manpower and resources. Facilities must spend more, both on a recurring basis and with larger capital investments.

It is no secret that hospitals and other health care providers need to lower their expenses. The cost of health care has risen prohibitively in countries such as the United States, and somehow, this generous flow of income still is not enough. Hospitals' cost structures have become unsustainable, and as a result, nearly every provider is at least considering outsourcing; most have already taken the leap in one or more areas of their business.

The outsourcing of health care services is expanding rapidly. As opportunities expand for vendors, a better understanding of the client's decision process and the concerns involved is needed so that vendors can better take advantage of these opportunities. A framework of service outsourcing decision making is proposed, and a set of outsourcing characteristics and resulting risks that are considered by firms outsourcing are identified. A radar diagram is used to illustrate these relationships and then applied to two examples from the health care sector. This includes a discussion of how vendors might use the tool as an aid in developing sales, marketing strategies, and tactics to win outsourcing contracts in the health care sector.

IT administration is the most outsourced area, as providers continue to increase their focus on electronic health records (EHR) and data management, operations management, asset management, and billing. However, outsourcing has extended its reach well beyond IT. Commonly outsourced clinical services now include medical and technical offerings such as laboratory (pathology and microbiology), pharmacy, radiology, dialysis, magnetic resonance imaging, nuclear medicine, mental health services, physiotherapy and rehabilitation, speech and language therapy, occupational health therapy, medical tourism, and home-delivered health care. In addition to IT, non-clinical outsourced services now include facility management, sterilization, meals, patient transport, procurement, security, and more.

Outsourcing is the business practice of hiring a party outside a company to perform services or create goods that were traditionally performed in-house by the company's own employees and staff. Outsourcing is a practice usually undertaken by companies as a cost-cutting measure. As such, it can affect a wide range of jobs, ranging from customer support and manufacturing to the back office. Outsourcing means contracting out some internal activities and decision making to an external supplier. Production inputs and decision-making authority can also be outsourced. The decision to outsource an activity is one of the most complex organizational decisions. As the first part of the outsourcing process, making this decision requires identifying all the influencing factors. In addition to the risks and obstacles, the benefits of outsourcing make a thorough and accurate review of this decision inevitable. Many organizations consider only the cost criterion, ignore many quality criteria, and consider it failure for themselves in deciding to outsource activities. Although outsourcing has many benefits, it also has many risks that must be considered in the decision-making process.

Outsourcing was first recognized as a business strategy in 1989 and became an integral part of business economics throughout the 1990s. The practice of outsourcing is subject to considerable controversy in many countries. Those opposed argue that it has caused the loss of domestic jobs, particularly in the manufacturing sector. Supporters say it creates an incentive for businesses and companies to allocate resources where they are most effective and that outsourcing helps maintain the nature of free-market economies on a global scale.

Outsourcing can help businesses reduce labour costs significantly. When a company uses outsourcing, it enlists the help of outside organizations not affiliated with the company to complete certain tasks. The outside organizations typically set up different compensation structures with their employees than the outsourcing company, enabling them to complete the work for less money. This ultimately enables the company that chooses to outsource to lower its labour costs.

Outsourcing is an increasingly popular strategy that health care organizations can use to control the rising costs of providing services. With outsourcing, an external contractor assumes responsibility for managing one or more of a health care organization's business, clinical, or hospitality services. Because the contractor specializes in providing a specific service and can achieve economies of scale, they may be able to provide a service more efficiently and less expensively than the health care organization.

Outsourcing services peripheral to the organization's primary operations may also promote health care administrators and staff to concentrate more efficiently on their organization's core business.

Outsourcers must also consider the likelihood of facing quality issues. Poor quality often originates from misunderstandings around the scope of the work being provided and the full costs of these services. Health care organizations should not underestimate the amount of time and effort required to develop a successful outsourcing partnership, especially upfront. Providers and vendors must explicitly define the scope of work, the standards and objectives by which it will be measured, and the full cost of every possible agreed-upon scenario.

47.2 Outsourcing Decision-Making Factors

Cost savings and customer satisfaction were the most important factors in their decision to outsource. The decision to outsource may lead to an elimination of a number of full-related positions in the health care organization. The most significant reasons for outsourcing are to improve customer service, to reduce costs, to enable health care organizations to focus on core activities, and to increase flexibility to configure resources to meet changing market needs.

DOI: 10.1201/9780367460884-50

Apart from cost savings, outsourcing provides access to a professionally qualified and experienced workforce that can help accomplish various clinical responsibilities and other related tasks accurately and efficiently. To be ahead of competitors and meet the growing demands of the health care industry, outsourcing the previous functions to professionals trained to meet medical industry standards should be considered.

Some organizations do not achieve the expected benefits from outsourcing due to the lack of a formal outsource decision-making process including medium- and long-term cost-benefit analyses, resistance to change, and the inability to formulate and quantify requirements.

The most significant risks of outsourcing lie in the need to develop new management competencies, capabilities, and decision-making processes. These include decisions on which activities should remain within the health care organization and which should be outsourced, whether all or part of the activity should be outsourced, and how to manage relationships rather than internal functions and processes. Mistakes in identifying core and non-core activities can lead health care organizations to outsource their competitive advantages. However, what is core one day may not be core the next. Moreover, once organizational competence is lost, it is difficult to rebuild. There is a difficult decision regarding how "close to core" outsourcing should be.

Because the introduction of contract services into an organization represents an important shift in the way in which business is conducted, the provision of appropriate training for employees is an important issue. The training efforts should typically focus on employees' ability to adjust into another environment and new roles. This includes use of computerized systems, higher skills/knowledge development, and systems support. Once the decision to outsource is accepted, there is little resistance to change by the employees.

Failure to manage outsourcing relationships properly, perhaps through service level agreements, may reduce customer service, levels of control, and contact with customers. The assessment of costs to "make or outsource" should include the additional cost burden of managing the outsource relationships.

47.3 Benefits of Outsource Servicing in a Hospital

Outsourcing in health care management is a rapidly growing trend currently. This is because health care providers face tremendous pressure from competitors in the industry. Additionally, health care operations management faces many challenges for delivering high-quality health care services and maintaining service budgets. Therefore, to sustain this business, all health care organizations, including hospitals, have to gain a competitive edge and offer attractive care services to the patient community.

Patient experiences can be vastly improved across the board if outsourced staff are used, from check-in and diagnosis to recovery and discharge. Many health care providers are seeking outsourced solutions as a way to ease financial constraints and free up resources while maintaining quality service and patient care across a heavily-regulated industry. Outsourcing can help health care providers in the following ways:

- Provide access to trained professionals and industry experts at a lower cost
- Maximize staff efficiency and productivity

- Improve patient care, experiences, and outcomes
- Avoid critical and costly billing issues
- Provide employees access to better benefits at a lower cost
- Scale resources based on specific needs
- Ensure compliance with all applicable laws
- Focus on providing quality care to patients
- Manage routine and mundane administrative tasks
- Increase cost savings
- Save time/money by hiring and training support staff
- Protect patient data while complying with HIPAA regulations
- Reduce number of denied and rejected medical claims
- Drive error-free processes

For achieving maximum staff efficiency and better care outcomes, outsourcing of the non-core functions can be a blessing to hospitals. In outsourcing, some operations of an organization are assigned to another vendor or a smaller facility that has expertise and specialization in the specific area. It helps hospitals to focus on their core operations and services such as clinical diagnosis, medical care, and nursing support.

Hospital management needs to introspect the following points before outsourcing some of its operations:

- The reasons that call for outsourcing
- Challenges that the hospital is likely to face when outsourcing is implemented
- The best practices to be followed in this context
- The financial and operational implications that the hospital has to face because of outsourcing
- Determination of the correct combination of tasks or services that may be outsourced without compromising the hospital bottom-line and revenues.

The services outsourced by hospitals can be broadly classified into two areas in terms of the functions or activities that may be delegated.

- **Clinical services** that encompass both medical and technical departments. This includes
  - Laboratory and investigation services such as pathology, microbiology, magnetic resonance imaging, x-rays, nuclear medicine, and radiology
  - Treatment procedures such as dialysis and psychological counseling
  - Therapeutic interventions, for example, rehabilitation, physiotherapy, occupational therapy, speech therapy, and language therapy
  - Support services including pharmacy, medical tourism, and home-based care services enabled by health care technology
- **Non-clinical services** that need health care consulting outsourcing include
  - Integration of information technology for billing and payment systems, maintaining electronic health records, and implementing cloud computing
  - Hospital infrastructure management including equipment planning, procurement and maintenance, waste management, pest control, sterilization and cleaning services, patient transport, and security

47.4 Advantages of Outsourcing

Enhanced profitability—By outsourcing some operations, hospitals can save at least 30% of costs incurred by utilizing local resources. There can be a substantial increase in profit margins by procuring low-cost infrastructure and manpower.

Enables access to talented workforce—Apart from financial gains, outsourcing promotes access to the skilled workforce that is ready to take on various clinical responsibilities and other related tasks of varying complexity. This professionally qualified and experienced manpower is crucial in the health care sector as it is a people-driven industry. Here, patient satisfaction largely depends on the human touch and the customization provided by the hospital staff in rendering care services.

Improved sharp focus on patient care—Medical practitioners can be unburdened from the cumbersome and routine administrative tasks through outsourcing. This enables them to focus on patient needs and deliver quality care as the non-clinical tasks are largely managed by the outsourcing partner.

Decrease in staff hiring and training costs—Managing additional costs incurred by recruiting excess staff and training them decreases to a commendable extent since it is handled by the outsourcing company. In addition, hiring, training, and retention of employees are also taken care of by the outsourcing company.

Better patient experience and engagement—Since the non-core tasks are managed by the outsourcing vendor, hospitals can concentrate to a greater extent on patient care, thereby improving patient experiences, goodwill, and public image.

Reduced administration overhead—Administrative overhead constitutes a bulk portion of costs incurred and must be managed carefully. By outsourcing, excessive and unnecessary expenditure may be reduced. This amount saved may be reinvested for improving the core services and hospital facilities to improve patient experiences.

47.5 Summary

Outsourcing is an increasingly popular strategy that health care organizations can use to control the rising costs of providing services. With outsourcing, an external contractor assumes responsibility for managing one or more elements of a health care organization's business, clinical, or hospitality services. Because the contractor specializes in providing a specific service and can achieve economies of scale, they may be able to provide a service more efficiently and less expensively than the health care organization.

References

Chapter	Reference
46.	MoHFW. Biomedical Equipment Management and Maintenance Program: Technical Guidance Document for in-house Support and Monitoring of Public Private Partnership. https://nhsrcindia.org/sites/default/files/2021-05/BEMMP%20_0.pdf.
	NHSRC. Biomedical Equipment Management and Maintenance Program. https://nhsrcindia.org/sites/default/files/2021-05/Biomedical-Equipment-Revised-%2810-02-2015%29.pdf.
	ESIC. Medical Equipment Maintenance Policy. www.esic.nic.in/Publications/MEMP070812.pdf.
	WHO. Medical Equipment Maintenance Program Overview. https://apps.who.int/iris/bitstream/handle/10665/44587/9789241501538_eng.pdf?sequence=1.
	WHO. Need Assessment for Medical Devices. https://apps.who.int/iris/bitstream/handle/10665/44562/9789241501385-eng.pdf?sequence=1&isAllowed=y.
	WHO. Decommissioning Medical Devices. https://apps.who.int/iris/bitstream/handle/10665/330095/9789241517041-eng.pdf.
	Kumar U, Godhia H, Srinivas N, Hoovayya P. Insights into equipment planning of a 250-Bed hospital project. International Journal of Health Sciences and Research. 2014;4(10):311–321.
	Iadanza E, Gonnelli V, Satta F, Gherardelli M. Evidence-based medical equipment management: A convenient implementation. Medical & Biological Engineering & Computing. 2019;57(10):2215–2230.
	TAHPI. International Health Facility Guidelines; Equipment Planning. www.healthfacilityguidelines.com/ViewPDF/ViewIndexPDF/iHFG_part_q_2-equipment_planning.
	Health Facility Magazine. Medical Equipment Maintenance: Performing an Audit to Improve Efficiency and Savings. www.hfmmagazine.com/articles/1493-medical-equipment-maintenance.
	ASIAHHM. Medical Equipment Management. www.asianhhm.com/technology-equipment/medical-equipment-management.
47.	Yigit V, Tengilimoglu D, Kisa A, Younis MZ. Outsourcing and its implications for hospital organizations in Turkey. Journal of Health Care Finance. 2007;33(4):86–92.
	Young SH. Outsourcing and benchmarking in a rural public hospital: Does economic theory provide the complete answer? Rural and Remote Health. 2003;3(1):124.
	Khosravizadeh O, Maleki A, Ahadinezhad B, Shahsavari S, Amerzadeh M, Tazekand NM. Developing a decision model for the outsourcing of medical service delivery in the public hospitals. BMC Health Services Research. 2022;22(1):135. https://doi.org/10.1186/s12913–022–075091.

Power MJ, Desouza KC, Bonifazi C. *The Outsourcing Handbook—How to Implement a Successful Outsourcing Process.* London: Kogan Page; 2006.

Socrates J, Moschuris, Kondylis MN. Outsourcing in hospitals. https://bit.ly/2oukAOQ.

Power M, Bonifazi, Desouza KC. The ten outsourcing traps to avoid. Article in Journal of Business Strategy—April 2004. Quoted by Desouza KC. www.researchgate.net/publication/242345409_Ten_outsourcing_traps _to_avoid.

Dominguez LD. *Manager's Step by Step Guide to Outsourcing.* McGraw-Hill, 2006.

48 PLANNING OF HEALTH CARE FACILITIES IN INDIA

48.1 Background

The Report on the Health Survey and Development Committee, commonly referred to as the Bhore Committee Report, 1946, was a landmark report for India from which the current health policy and systems have evolved. The recommendation for a three-tiered health care system to provide preventive and curative health care in rural and urban areas by placing health workers on government payrolls and limiting the need for private practitioners became the principles on which the current public health care systems were founded. This was done to ensure that access to primary care is independent of individual socioeconomic conditions.

Although the first national population program was announced in 1951, the first National Health Policy of India (NHP) was formulated only in 1983 with its main focus on provision of primary health care to all by 2000. NHP 2002 further built on NHP 1983, with an objective of provision of health services to the general public through decentralization, use of the private sector, and increasing public expenditure on health care overall. It also emphasized increasing the use of non-allopathic forms of medicine such as ayurveda, unani, and siddha and a need for strengthening decision-making processes at the decentralized state level.

The Union Ministry of Health and Family Welfare is responsible for implementation of various programs on a national scale (for example, National AIDS Control Program, Revised National Tuberculosis Program) in the areas of health and family welfare, prevention and control of major communicable diseases, promotion of traditional and indigenous systems of medicines, and setting standards and guidelines that state governments can adapt. In addition, the Ministry assists states in preventing and controlling the spread of seasonal disease outbreaks and epidemics through technical assistance.

Public health care infrastructure in India has a mixed health care system, inclusive of public and private health care service providers. The public health care infrastructure in rural areas has been developed as a three-tier system based on the population norms. The size of a hospital depends upon the hospital bed requirement, which, in turn, is a function of the size of the population that it serves. As per the Indian Public Health Standards (IPHS), 2012, the calculation of number of beds is based on

- annual rate of admission as 1 per 50 population
- average length of stay in a hospital as 5 days.

For example, In India the population size of a district varies from 50,000 to 1,500,000. For the purpose of convenience, the average size of the district is taken as one million people. Based on the assumptions, the number of beds required for 1,000,000 people is

- No. of bed days per year: $(1,000,000 \times 1/50) \times 5 = 100,000$
- No. of beds required with 100% occupancy: $100,000/365 = 275$
- No. of beds required with 80% occupancy: $(100,000/365) \times 80\% = 220$ (Table 48A).

The Indian Public Health Standards (IPHS) classify the Public Health Care System into the following categories:

(a) **Sub-Centre**: A sub-centre (SC) is established in a plain area with a population of 5,000 people and in hilly/difficult to reach/tribal areas with a population of 3,000, and it is the most peripheral and first contact point between the primary health care system and the community. Each sub-centre is required to be staffed by at least one auxiliary nurse midwife (ANM)/female health worker and one male health worker.

(b) **Primary Health Centre**: A primary health centre (PHC) is established in a plain area with a population of 30,000 people and in hilly/difficult to reach/tribal areas with a population of 20,000 and is the first contact point between the village community and the medical officer. PHCs were envisaged to provide integrated curative and preventive health care to the rural population with emphasis on the preventive and primitive aspects of health care. The PHCs are established and maintained by the state governments under the Minimum Needs Program (MNP)/Basic Minimum Services (BMS) Program.

(c) **Community Health Centre**: Community health centres (CHCs) are established in an area with a population of 120,000 people and in hilly/difficult to reach/tribal areas with a population of 80,000. As per minimum norms, a CHC is required to be staffed by four medical specialists, that is, a surgeon, physician, gynaecologist/obstetrician, and paediatrician, supported by 21 paramedical and other staff.

(d) **Sub-District Hospital**: Sub-district/sub-divisional hospitals are in an area with a population of 100,000–500,000 people. Sub-district (sub-divisional) hospitals are below the district and above the block level (CHC) hospitals and act as First Referral Units for the Tehsil/Taluk/block population in which they are geographically located.

(e) **District Hospital**: A district hospital is a hospital at the secondary referral level responsible for a district of a defined geographical area containing a population above 5,000,000. Its objective is to provide comprehensive secondary health care services to the people in the district at an acceptable level of quality and being responsive and sensitive to the needs of people and referring centres. Every district is expected to have a district hospital. As the population of a district is variable, the bed strength also varies from 100 to 500 beds depending on the size, terrain, and population of the district. A district hospital should be in a position to provide all basic specialty services and should aim to develop super-specialty services gradually.

(f) **First Referral Units**: An existing facility (district hospital, sub-divisional hospital, and CHC) can be declared a fully operational first referral unit (FRU) only if it is equipped to provide around-the-clock services for emergency obstetric and newborn care, in addition to all emergencies that any hospital is required to provide. It should be noted that there are three critical determinants of a facility being declared an FRU: (i) emergency obstetric care including surgical interventions such as caesarean sections; (ii) care for small and sick newborns; and (iii) blood storage facility on a 24-hour basis.

A schematic diagram of the Indian Public Health Standard (IPHS) norms, which decides the distribution of health care infrastructure and the resources needed at each level of care, is shown as follows (Figure 48A).

DOI: 10.1201/9780367460884-52

TABLE 48.1: The Classification of Health Care Facilities (URDPFI Guidelines, MoUD, 2015)

Sr. No.	Category	No. of beds	Population Served per Unit	Area Requirement
1.	Dispensary	-	15,000	0.08 to 0.12 Ha
2.	Nursing home, child welfare and maternity centre	25 to 30 beds	45,000 to 1 lakh	0.20 to 0.30 Ha
3.	Polyclinic	Some observation beds	1 lakh	0.20 to 0.30 Ha
4.	Intermediate Hospital (Category B)	80 beds Initially maybe for 50 beds including 20 maternity beds	1 lakh	Total Area = 1.00 Ha (a) Area for Hospital = 0.60 Ha (b) Area for residential Accommodation = 0.40 Ha
5.	Intermediate Hospital (Category A)	200 beds Initially the provision maybe for 100 beds	1 lakh	Total Area = 3.70 Ha (a) Area for hospital = 2.70 Ha (b) Area for residential Accommodation = 1.00 Ha
6.	Multi-Specialty Hospital (NBC)	200 beds Initially the provision may be for 100 beds	1 Lakh	Total Area = 9.00 Ha (a) Area for hospital = 6.00 Ha (b) Area for residential accommodation = 3.00 Ha
7.	Specialty Hospital (NBC)	200 beds Initially the provision may be for 100 beds	1 Lakh	Total Area = 3.70 Ha (a) Area for hospital = 2.70 Ha (b) Area for residential accommodation = 1.00 Ha
8.	General Hospital (NBC)	500 Initially the provision maybe for 300 beds	2.5 lakh	Total Area = 6.00 Ha (a) Area for hospital = 4.00 Ha (b) Area for residential Accommodation = 2.00 Ha
9.	Family Welfare Centre (MPD, pg 134)	As per requirement	50,000	Total area = 500 sq m 800 sq m
10.	Diagnostic centre (MPD, pg 134)	--	50,000	Total area = 500 sq m to 800 sq m
11.	Veterinary Hospital for pets and animals (MPD, pg 134)	--	5 lakh	Total area = 2000 sq m
12.	Dispensary for pet animals and birds (MPD, pg 134)	--	1 lakh	Total area = 300 sq m
13.	Rehabilitation centres			As per requirement

Source: UDPFI Guidelines, 1996, NBC, 2005 Part 3 and MPD, 2021.

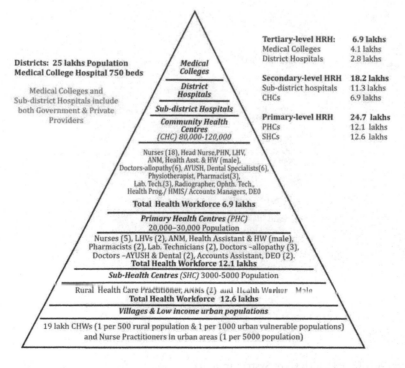

FIGURE 48.1   Health Care Facilities in India (UHC India, 2011).

48.2 Indian Public Health Standards (IPHS)

All Indian citizens can obtain free outpatient and inpatient care at government facilities. Under India's decentralized approach to health care delivery, the states are primarily responsible for organizing health services. Because of severe shortages of staff and supplies at government facilities, many households seek care from private providers and pay out-of-pocket. For low-income people, the government recently launched the tax-financed National Health Protection Scheme (Ayushman Bharat-Pradhan Mantri Jan Arogya Yojana, or PM-JAY), which allows them to also get cashless secondary and tertiary care at private facilities.

48.3 Role of Government

Responsibility for the governance, financing, and operation of the health system is divided between the central and state governments (Figure 48B). At the federal level, the Ministry of Health and Family Welfare has regulatory power over the majority of health policy decisions but is not directly involved in health care delivery.

In 2014, the government established the federal Ministry of Ayurveda, Yoga and Naturopathy, Unani, Siddha, and Homeopathy. It develops and promotes research in alternative medicine practices.

At the state level, the Directorates of Health Services and the Departments of Health and Family Welfare are responsible for

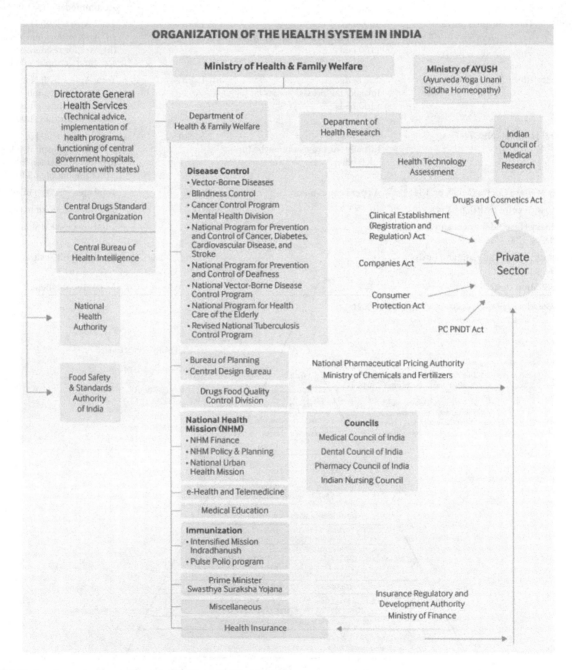

FIGURE 48.2   Organization of the Health Care System in India.

organizing and delivering health care services to their populations. These include all medical care from primary care and pharmacies to secondary and tertiary hospital care.

48.4 How Is the Delivery System Organized and How Are Providers Paid?

Regarding the physician education and workforce, medical education is provided by both state-led institutions and private colleges. In some states, private medical colleges charge approximately 16 times the fees charged by government colleges. Private fees for a five-year course typically range from INR 3 million to INR 5 million (USD 42,000–70,000) for undergraduate education.

The Medical Council of India establishes standards for undergraduate medical education, accredits undergraduate and postgraduate medical education programs, determines equivalencies for foreign medical graduates, and maintains a general directory for all certified physicians.

Primary care: Under the Health and Wellness Centres program, 150,000 sub-centres (the lowest tier of the health system) across the country are being upgraded to provide comprehensive primary health care services, free essential medicines, and free diagnostic services. Nutritional support will also be provided to all beneficiaries with tuberculosis at a rate of INR 500 (USD 7) per month during treatment. Other primary health care providers include primary health centres (PHCs) and community health centres. No patient registration is required. PHCs are the first point of contact between a village community and a medical officer. These centres provide curative and preventive services to 20,000–30,000 people and serve as a referral unit for six sub-centres with four to six beds each. Community health centres serve as a referral centre for four PHCs and provide facilities for obstetric care and specialist consultations.

Outpatient specialist care: Community health centres also provide outpatient specialist care and are required to have four medical specialists (surgeon, general practitioner, gynaecologist, and paediatrician) supported by paramedical and other staff. They must also have 30 beds, a laboratory, x-ray services, and other facilities. Each centre covers 80,000 to 120,000 people. All outpatient specialized services not provided at community centres are referred to district hospitals.

After-hours care: The India Public Health Standards determine which health care facilities are required to operate 24 hours a day, seven days a week. Depending on the facility type, specific services—such as basic obstetrics—are made available at all times, while others are daytime-only procedures. After-hours care by telephone is not well established in India. However, officials are exploring the acceptability and feasibility of mobile phone consultations as a means of improving health care access in rural India and addressing workforce shortages and resource constraints.

Hospitals: Public hospitals account for only approximately 10% of the total number of hospitals throughout the country. Patients using the public health system can be referred to a district hospital, which is the terminal

referral centre. District hospitals offer services similar to community health centres, such as emergency care, maternity services, and newborn care, but serve larger urban centres. Under the National Health Protection Scheme, some district hospitals will be upgraded to tertiary care facilities to improve access to specialized services and strengthen physician workforce capacity.

Mental health care: National health initiatives have established psychiatric centres within specialized public hospitals. With the launch of the National Health Protection Scheme, comprehensive mental health care will also be available for beneficiaries at newly established health and wellness centre programs. Despite recent policy measures to strengthen mental health care, resources are extremely limited. Across India, there is only one trained psychiatrist for every 250,000 people and fewer than one mental health worker for every 100,000 people. In addition, few hospital beds are dedicated to inpatient psychiatric care. Most private insurance plans typically do not provide comprehensive coverage for such care. In the few that cover it, covered treatment options usually focus on short-term psychotherapy rather than on long-term management.

Long-term care and social supports: The central government launched the National Programme for Health Care of the Elderly in 2011 with the aim of improving workforce capacity for long-term care and providing dedicated health care facilities and services to senior citizens (ages 65+ years) at all levels of the health care delivery system. Such services are meant to be provided for free for elderly people through state primary and secondary facilities.

Some states have launched their own activities to increase access to palliative care. In Kerala, for example, the state was the first to establish a palliative-care policy, which subsequently resulted in a network of more than 60 facilities that provide low-cost and community-based hospice and palliative care. This implementation model has resulted in similar policies and projects that have been launched in Assam, Maharashtra, Punjab, Haryana, and Karnataka by state governments and nongovernmental organizations.

48.5 Summary

The regionalization of health care in India has emerged as a pivotal strategy to address the country's vast and diverse health care needs. India's vast population and geographical expanse have necessitated the development of regional health care systems tailored to local requirements. Regionalization focuses on decentralizing health care services, optimizing resource allocation, and promoting equitable access to quality care across different regions. It involves establishing specialized medical centres, upgrading infrastructure, and training health care professionals at the regional level. By tailoring health care services to local contexts, regionalization aims to bridge the gaps in health care delivery, reduce regional disparities, and improve health outcomes. This approach empowers regions to design and implement health care policies, fostering a more comprehensive and responsive health care system for India's diverse population.

References

The guidelines can be downloaded from the following links:

Sub-Centres
https://nhm.gov.in/images/pdf/guidelines/iphs/iphs-revised-guidlines-2012/sub-centers.pdf

Primary Health Centre (PHC)
https://nhm.gov.in/images/pdf/guidelines/iphs/iphs-revised-guidlines-2012/primay-health-centres.pdf

Community Health Centre (CHC)
https://nhm.gov.in/images/pdf/guidelines/iphs/iphs-revised-guidlines-2012/community-healthcentres.pdf

Sub-District and Sub-Divisional Hospital
https://nhm.gov.in/images/pdf/guidelines/iphs/iphs-revised-guidlines-2012/sub-district-subdivisional-hospital.pdf

District Hospital
https://nhm.gov.in/images/pdf/guidelines/iphs/iphs-revised-guidlines-2012/district-hospital.pdf
www.commonwealthfund.org/international-health-policy-center/countries/india 1/23

49 PRIMARY HEALTH CENTRES

49.1 Introduction

A primary health centre is the cornerstone of rural health services. It is a first port of call to a qualified doctor of the public sector in rural areas for the sick and those who directly report to or are referred from sub-centres for curative, preventive, and promotive health care. A typical primary health centre covers a population of 20,000 in hilly, tribal, or difficult areas and a population of 30,000 in plain areas with 6 indoor/observation beds. It acts as a referral unit for 6 sub-centres and refers out cases to CHC (30-bed hospital) and higher order public hospitals located at the sub-district and district levels. However, as the population density in the country is not uniform, the number of PHCs depends upon the case load. A PHC should become a 24-hour facility with nursing facilities.

Select PHCs, especially in large blocks where the CHC/FRU is over one hour away, may be upgraded to provide 24-hour emergency hospital care for a number of conditions by increasing the number of medical officers; preferably, such PHCs should have the same IPHS norms as for a CHC.

The overall objective of IPHS for PHCs is to provide health care that is quality-oriented and sensitive to the needs of the community. These standards also help monitor and improve the functioning of PHCs.

49.2 Objectives of the Indian Public Health Standards for Primary Health Centres

The overall objective of IPHS is to provide health care that is quality-oriented and sensitive to the needs of the community. The objectives of IPHS for PHCs are

- To provide comprehensive primary health care to the community through PHCs.
- To achieve and maintain an acceptable standard of quality of care.
- To make the services more responsive and sensitive to the needs of the community.

49.3 Categorization of Primary Health Centres

From the service delivery angle, PHCs may be of two types, depending upon the delivery case load: Type A and Type B.

(a) **Type A PHC**: PHC with delivery load of less than 20 deliveries in a month
(b) **Type B PHC:** PHC with delivery load of 20 or more deliveries in a month

49.4 Physical Infrastructure

The PHC should have a building of its own. The surroundings should be clean. The details are as follows:

(a) **Location**: It should be centrally located in an easily accessible area. The area chosen should have facilities for electricity, all-weather road communication, adequate water supply, and a telephone. At a place where a PHC is already located, another health centre/sub-centre should not be established to avoid the waste of human resources. PHCs should be away from garbage collection, cattle sheds, water logging areas, etc. PHCs should have a proper boundary wall and gate.

(b) **Area**: It should be well-planned with the entire necessary infrastructure. It should be well lit and ventilated with as much use of natural light and ventilation as possible. The plinth area will vary from 375 to 450 sq m depending on whether an OT facility is opted for.

(c) **Signage:** The building should have a prominent board displaying the name of the centre in the local language at the gate and on the building. A PHC should have pictorial, bilingual, directional, and layout signage of all the departments and public utilities (toilets, drinking water). Prominent display boards in the local language providing information regarding the services available/user charges/fees and the schedule of the centre. Relevant IEC material should be displayed at strategic locations. A citizen charter including patient rights and responsibilities should be displayed at OPD and the entrance in the local language.

(d) **Entrance with barrier-free access**: A barrier-free access environment should be provided for easy access to non-ambulant (wheel-chair, stretcher), semi ambulant, visually disabled, and elderly persons as per the guidelines of GOI. Ramps as per specification, handrails, adequate lighting, etc. must be provided in all health facilities and retrofitted in older ones that lack these features. The doorway leading to the entrance should also have a ramp facilitating easy access for elderly and physically challenged patients. An adequate number of wheelchairs, stretchers, etc. should also be provided.

49.5 Space Requirements

(a) **Waiting Area**
  (i) This should have adequate space and seating arrangements for waiting clients/patients as per patient load.
  (ii) The walls should carry posters imparting health education.
  (iii) Booklets/leaflets in the local language may be provided in the waiting area for the same purpose.
  (iv) Toilets with adequate water supply separate for males and females should be available.
  (v) Waiting area should have an adequate number of fans, coolers, benches, and chairs.
  (vi) Safe drinking water should be available in the patient's waiting area.
  (vii) There should be proper notice displaying departments of the centre, available services, names of the doctors, user fee details and a list of the members of the Rogi Kalyan Samiti/Hospital Management Committee.
  (viii) A locked complaint/suggestion box should be provided, and it should be ensured that the complaints/suggestions are investigated at regular intervals and addressed.
  (ix) The surroundings should be kept clean with no waterlogging and vector breeding places in and around the centre.

DOI: 10.1201/9780367460884-53

(b) Outpatient Department
- The outpatient room should have separate areas for consultation and examination.
- The area for examination should have sufficient privacy.
- In PHCs with an AYUSH doctor, necessary infrastructure such as a consultation room for AYUSH Doctor and AYUSH drug dispensing area should be made available.
- OPD rooms should have provision for ample natural light and air. Windows should open directly to the external air or into an open verandah.
- Adequate measures should be taken for crowd management, for example, one volunteer to call patients one-by-one, token system.
- One room for immunization/family planning/counselling.

(c) Wards
- 5.5 m × 3.5 m each.
- There should be 4–6 beds in a PHC. Separate wards/areas should be earmarked for males and females with the necessary furniture.
- There should be facilities for drinking water and separate clean toilets for men and women.
- The ward should be easily accessible from the OPD to obviate the need for a separate nursing staff in the ward and OPD during OPD hours.
- Nurse station should be located in such a way that health staff can be easily accessible to the OT and labour room after regular clinic timings. Proper written handover should be given to incoming staff by the outgoing staff.
- Dirty utility room for dirty linen and used items.
- Cooking should not be allowed inside the wards for admitted patients.
- Cleaning of the wards, etc. should be carried out at regular intervals and at such times that do not interfere not only with the work during peak hours but also times of eating.
- Labour Room, OT, and toilets should be regularly monitored.

(d) Operating Theatre (Optional): To facilitate conducting selected surgical procedures (e.g. vasectomy, tubectomy, hydrocelectomy, etc.)
- It should have a changing room, sterilization area, operating area, and washing area.
- Separate facilities for storing of sterile and unsterile equipment/instruments should be available in the OT.
- The plan of an ideal OT has been annexed showing the layout.
- It would be ideal to have a patient preparation area and post-operative area. However, in view of the existing situation, the OT should be well-connected to the wards.
- The OT should be well-equipped with all the necessary accessories and equipment.
- Surgeries such as laparoscopy/cataract/tubectomy/vasectomy should be able to be carried out in these OTs.
- OT should be fumigated at regular intervals.
- One of the hospital staff should be trained in autoclaving, and the PHC should have a standard operative procedure for autoclaving.

- OT should have power back up (generator/invertor/UPS). OT should have restricted entry.
- Separate footwear should be used.

(e) Labour Room
- A room with dimensions **3.8 m × 4.2 m** is essential.
- Configuration of newborn care corner.
- Clear floor area should be provided in the room for the newborn corner. It is a space within the labour room, 20–30 sq ft in size, where a radiant warmer (functional) will be kept.
- Oxygen, suction machine, and simultaneously accessible electrical outlets should be provided for newborn infants in addition to the facilities required for the mother. Both an oxygen cylinder and suction machine should be functional with their tips cleaned and covered with sterile gauze, etc. to be in ready-to-use condition. They must be cleaned after use and kept in the same way for the next use.
- The labour room should be provided with a good source of light and preferably shadow-less.
- Resuscitation kit including Ambu Bag (paediatric size) should be placed in the radiant warmer.
- Provision of handwashing and containment of infection control if it is not a part of the delivery room.
- The area should be away from air draughts and should have a power connection for plugging in the radiant warmer. There should be separate areas for septic and aseptic deliveries.
- The labour room should be well-lit and ventilated with an attached toilet and drinking water facilities. Facilities for hot water should be available.
- Separate areas for dirty linen, baby wash, toilet, and sterilization.
- Standard treatment protocols for common problems during labour and for newborns are to be provided in the labour room.
- The labour room should have restricted entry. Separate footwear should be used.
- All the essential drugs and equipment (functional) should be available.
- Cleanliness should always be maintained in the labour room by regular washing and mopping with disinfectants.
- The labour room should be fumigated at regular interval (**desirable**).
- Delivery kits and other instruments should be autoclaved where such facility is available.
- If the labour room has more than one labour table, then the privacy of the women must be ensured by having screens between 2 labour tables.

(f) Minor OT/Dressing Room/Injection Room/Emergency
- This should be located close to the OPD to cater to patients for minor surgeries and emergencies after OPD hours.
- It should be well-equipped with all the emergency drugs and instruments.
- Privacy of the patients should be ensured.

(g) Laboratory
- (3.8 m × 2.7 m).
- Sufficient space with workbenches and a separate area for collection and screening should be available.
- Should have marble/stone table tops for platform and wash basins.

(h) **General Store**
- Separate area for storage of sterile and common linen and other materials/drugs/consumables, etc. should be provided with adequate storage space.
- The area should be well-lit, ventilated, and rodent/pest free.
- Sufficient number of racks should be provided.
- Drugs should be stored properly and systematically in a cool (away from direct sunlight), safe, and dry environment.
- Inflammable and hazardous material should be secured and stored separately.
- Near expiry drugs should be segregated and stored separately.
- Sufficient space with separate storage cabins for AYUSH drugs should be provided.
- Dispensing-cum-store area: 3 m × 3 m.

(i) **Infrastructure for AYUSH doctor**
Based on the system of medicine being practiced, appropriate arrangements should be made for the provision of a doctor's room and a dispensing room-cum-drug storage.

(j) **Waste disposal pit**: As per GOI/Central Pollution Control Board (CPCB) guidelines.

(k) Cold chain room size: 3 m × 4 m.

(l) Logistics room size: 3 m × 4 m.

(m) Generator room size: 3 m × 4 m.

(n) Office room size: 3.5 m × 3.0 m.

(o) Dirty utility room for dirty linen and used items.

(p) **Boundary wall/Fencing (Essential)**: Boundary wall/fencing with a gate should be provided for safety and security.

Layout for 24x7 PHC

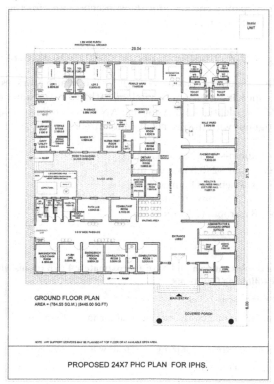

GROUND FLOOR PLAN
AREA = (784.55 SQ.M.) (8445.00 SQ.FT)

PROPOSED 24X7 PHC PLAN FOR IPHS.

(q) **Environmentally friendly features** (Desirable): The PHC should be, as far as possible, environmentally friendly and energy-efficient. Rain-water harvesting, solar energy use, and use of energy-efficient bulbs/equipment should be encouraged.

(r) **Other amenities (Essential)**
- Adequate water supply and water storage facility (overhead tank) with pipe water should be made available.
- Computer (Essential): Computer with Internet connection should be provided for the management information system (MIS).
- Lecture Hall/Auditorium (Desirable): For training purposes, a lecture hall or small auditorium for 30 persons should be available.
- Public address system and a blackboard should also be provided.

The suggested layout of a PHC is given in **Figure 49A**. The layout may vary according to the location and shape of the site, levels of the site, and climatic conditions. The prescribed layout may be implemented in PHCs yet to be built, whereas those already built may be upgraded after getting the requisite alteration/additions. The funds may be made available as per budget provision under relevant strategies mentioned in the NRHM/RCH-II program and other funding projects/programs.

49.6 Residential Accommodation (Essential)

Decent accommodation with all amenities such as 24-hour water supply, electricity, etc. should be available for the medical officer, nursing staff, pharmacist, laboratory technician, and other staff. If the accommodation cannot be provided for any reason, then the staff may be paid house rent allowance, but in this case they should be staying in the near vicinity of PHC so that they are available 24 x 7, in case of need.

49.7 Summary

The establishment of a PHC in India holds immense significance in advancing the nation's health care landscape. PHCs play a crucial role in providing primary care services, preventive measures, and health education to communities at the grassroots level. These centres act as the first point of contact for individuals seeking health care, particularly in rural and underserved areas. By offering essential medical services, immunizations, maternal and child health care, and disease management, PHCs contribute significantly to improving health outcomes and reducing the burden on secondary and tertiary health care facilities. The accessibility and affordability of primary care through PHCs empower communities, promote early intervention, and ultimately pave the way for a healthier and more resilient nation. Designing a PHC that is accessible, patient-friendly, and equipped with necessary facilities enhances health care delivery and patient experience. Moreover, incorporating sustainable and eco-friendly elements promotes a healthier environment.

50 SUB-CENTRES

50.1 Introduction

In the public sector, a health sub-centre is the most peripheral and first point of contact between the primary health care system and the community. A sub-centre interfaces with the community at the grass-root level, providing all the primary health care services. It is the lowest rung of a referral pyramid of health facilities consisting of the sub-centres, PHCs, community health centres, sub-divisional/sub-district hospitals, and district hospitals. The purpose of a health sub-centre is largely preventive and promotive, but it also provides a basic level of curative care. As per population norms, there should be one sub-centre established for every 5,000 population in plain areas and for every 3,000 population in hilly/tribal/desert areas.

50.2 Objectives of the Indian Public Health Standards for Sub-Centres

- To specify the minimum assured (essential) services that the sub-centre is expected to provide and the desirable services which the states/UTs should aspire to provide through this facility.
- To maintain an acceptable quality of care for these services.
- To facilitate monitoring and supervision of these facilities.
- To make the services provided more accountable and responsive to people's needs.

50.3 Types of Sub-Centres

Type A: Type A sub-centre will provide all recommended services except that the facilities for conducting delivery will not be available here. However, the ANMs have been trained in midwifery, and they may conduct normal delivery in case of need. If the requirement for this increases, then the sub-centre may be considered for up-gradation to type B.

Type B (MCH Sub-Centre): This would include the following types of sub-centres:

i. Centrally or better located sub-centres with good connectivity to catchment areas.
ii. They have good physical infrastructure preferably with their own buildings, adequate space, residential accommodation, and labour room facilities.
iii. They already have a good case load of deliveries from the catchment areas.
iv. There are no nearby higher level delivery facilities.

50.4 Physical Infrastructure

A sub-centre should have its own building. If this is not immediately possible, premises with adequate space should be rented in a central location with easy access to the population. The states should also explore options of getting funds for space from other health programs and other funding sources.

50.5 Location of the Centre

For all new upcoming sub-centres, the following may be ensured:

- Sub-centre is to be located within the village for providing easy access to the people and safety of the ANM.

- As far as possible, no person has to travel more than 3 km to reach the sub-centre.
- The sub-centre village has some communication network (road communication/public transport/post office/telephone).
- Sub-centre should be away from garbage collection, cattle sheds, water logging areas, etc.
- While finalizing the location of the sub-centre, the concerned Panchayat should also be consulted.

50.6 Building and Layout

- Boundary wall/fencing with a gate should be provided for safety and security.
- In the typical layout of the sub-centre, the residential facility for ANM is included; however, it may happen that some of the existing sub-centres may not have residential facilities for ANM. In this case, some housing should be available for rent in the sub-centre headquartered village for accommodating the ANM.
- Residential facility for a health worker (Male), if the need is felt, may be provided by expanding the sub-centre building to the first floor. The entrance to the sub-centre should be well-lit and easy to locate. It should have provision for easy access for disabled and elderly persons. Provision of a ramp with railings is to be made for use of wheelchairs/stretcher trollies, wherever feasible.
- The minimum covered area of a sub-centre along with a residential quarter for ANM will vary depending on land availability, type of sub-centre, and resources.
- Separate entrance for the sub-centre and for the ANM quarters may be ensured.

50.7 Residential Accommodations

This should be made available to the health workers with each one having 2 rooms, a kitchen, bathroom, and water closet (WC). Residential facility for one ANM is as follows, which is contiguous with the main sub-centre area:

- Room—1 (3.3 m × 2.7 m)
- Room—2 (3.3 m × 2.7 m)
- Kitchen—1 (1.8 m × 2.5 m)
- WC (1.2 m × 9.0 m)
- Bathroom (1.5 m × 1.2 m)

Type B sub-centre should have approximately 4 to 5 rooms with the following facilities:

- Waiting room
- One labour room with one labour table and newborn corner
- One room with two to four beds (in case the number of deliveries at the sub-centre is 20 or more, four beds will be provided)
- One room for store
- One room for clinic/office
- One toilet facility each in the labour room, ward room, and waiting area (essential)

DOI: 10.1201/9780367460884-54

Residential Facility for a minimum of 2 staff and desirably for 3 staff should be provided at Type B (MCH) sub-centres.

50.8 Summary

The establishment of a sub-centre in India plays a vital role in ensuring accessible and decentralized primary health care services to remote and underserved areas. These centres act as the backbone of rural health care and are the first point of contact for individuals seeking medical assistance. Sub-centres provide essential health care services, immunizations, antenatal care, family planning, and basic health education to communities at the grassroots level. They facilitate early intervention, disease prevention, and health promotion, contributing to improved health outcomes and reduced health care disparities. The presence of sub-centres strengthens the health care infrastructure, enhances community engagement, and fosters a healthier population, making them an indispensable component of India's primary health care system.

51 COMMUNITY HEALTH CENTRES

51.1 Introduction

Health care delivery in India has been envisaged at three levels, namely, primary, secondary, and tertiary. The secondary level of health care essentially includes community health centres (CHCs), which constitute the first referral units (FRUs) and the sub-district and district hospitals. The CHCs were designed to provide referral health care for cases from the PHC level and for cases in need of specialist care, approaching the centre directly. 4 PHCs are included under each CHC, which thus caters to approximately 80,000 people in tribal/hilly/desert areas and 120,000 people for plain areas.

A CHC is a 30-bed hospital providing specialist care in medicine, obstetrics, and gynaecology, surgery, paediatrics, dental, and AYUSH. There are 4,535 CHCs functioning in the country as of March 2010 as per the Rural Health Statistics Bulletin 2010. These centres are, however, fulfilling the tasks entrusted to them only to a limited extent. The launch of the National Rural Health Mission (NRHM) gives us the opportunity to have a fresh look at their functioning.

51.2 Objectives of the Indian Public Health Standards for Community Health Centres

- To provide optimal expert care to the community.
- To achieve and maintain an acceptable standard of quality of care.
- To ensure that services at CHCs are commensurate with universal best practices and are responsive and sensitive to the client needs/expectations.

51.3 Physical Infrastructure

The CHC should have 30 indoor beds with one operating theatre, labour room, x-ray, ECG, and laboratory facility. In order to provide these facilities, the following are the guidelines.

51.4 Location of the Centre

All the guidelines under this sub-head may be applicable only to centres that are to be newly established, and priority is to be given to operationalise the existing CHCs. To the extent possible, the centre should be located at the centre of the block headquarter in order to improve access to the patients. The area chosen should have the facility for electricity, all-weather road communication, adequate water supply, a telephone, etc. It should be well-planned with the entire necessary infrastructure. It should be well-lit and ventilated with as much use of natural light and ventilation as possible. CHCs should be away from garbage collection, cattle sheds, water logging areas, etc.

The CHC should be, as far as possible, environment friendly and energy-efficient. Rain-water harvesting, solar energy use, and use of energy-efficient CFL bulbs/equipment should be encouraged. Provision should be made for horticulture services including an herbal garden. The building should have areas/spaces marked for the following:

(a) **Entrance Zone**
  (i) Signage

- Prominent display boards in the local language providing information regarding the services available and the schedule of the institution.
- Directional and layout signage for all departments and utilities (toilets, drinking water, etc.) should be appropriately displayed for easy access.
- All signage should be bilingual and pictorial.
- A citizen charter should be displayed at the OPD and entrance in the local language including patient's rights and responsibilities.
- On-the-way signage of the CHC and location should be displayed on all approach roads.
- Safety, hazards, and caution signs should be displayed prominently at relevant places, for example, radiation hazards for pregnant woman in x-ray.
- Fluorescent fire exit signage at strategic locations.

(ii) Barrier-free access environment for easy access to non-ambulant (wheelchairs, stretchers), semi-ambulant, visually disabled, and elderly persons as per the "Guidelines and Space Standards for barrier-free built environment for Disabled and Elderly Persons" of the Government of India. A ramp as per specification, handrails, proper lighting, etc. must be provided in all health facilities and retrofitted in older ones that lack these features.

(iii) Registration-cum-enquiry counters.

(iv) Pharmacy for drug dispensing and storage.

(v) Clean public utilities separate for males and females.

(vi) Suggestion/complaint boxes for the patients/visitors and information regarding the person responsible for redressal of complaints.

51.5 Outpatient Department

(a) The facility should be planned keeping in mind the maximum peak hour load and should have a scope for future expansion. Name of the department, doctor, schedule, and user fees/charges should be displayed.

(b) Layout of the Outpatient Department should follow the functional flow of patients: **Enquiry → Registration → Waiting → Sub-Waiting → Clinic → Dressing room/Injection Room → Billing → Diagnostics (lab/X-ray) → Pharmacy → Exit**.

(c) **Clinics for Various Medical Disciplines**: These clinics include general medicine, general surgery, dental, obstetrics and gynaecology, paediatrics, and family welfare. Separate cubicles for general medicine and surgery with a separate area for internal examination (privacy) can be provided if there are no separate rooms for each.

(d) The cubicles for consultation and examination in all clinics should provide for a doctor's table, chair, patient's stool, follower's seat, wash basin with handwashing facilities, examination couch, and equipment for examination. The room should have, for the admission of light and air, one or more apertures, such as windows and fan lights, opening directly to the external air or into an open verandah. The windows should be on two opposite walls.

DOI: 10.1201/9780367460884-55

(e) **Family Welfare Clinic:** The clinic should provide educative, preventive, diagnostic and curative facilities for maternal, child health, school health, and health education. Importance of health education is being increasingly recognized as an effective tool of preventive treatment. People visiting the hospital should be informed of personal and environmental hygiene, clean habits, the need for taking preventive measures against epidemics, family planning, non-communicable diseases, etc. Treatment room in this clinic should act as an operating room for IUCD insertion and investigation, etc. It should be in close proximity to obstetrics and gynaecology. Family welfare counselling room should also be provided.

(f) **Waiting room for patients**.

(g) The **pharmacy** should be located in an area conveniently accessible from all clinics. The dispensary and compounding room should have two dispensing windows, compounding counters, and shelves. The pattern of arranging the counters and shelves should depend on the size of the room. The medicines that require cold storage and blood required for operations and emergencies may be kept in refrigerators.

Emergency Room/Casualty: At the moment, emergency cases are being attended in OPD during OPD hours and in inpatient units afterwards. It is recommended to have a separate earmarked emergency area to be located near the entrance of a hospital, preferably having 4 rooms (one for doctor, one for minor OT, one for plaster/dressing) and one for patient observation (at least 4 beds).

51.6 Treatment Rooms

- Minor OT
- Injection Room and Dressing Room
- Observation Room

51.7 Wards: Separate for Males and Females

(a) **Nurse Station:** The nurse station should be centred such that it serves all the clinics from this place. The nurse station should be spacious enough to accommodate a medicine chest/a work counter (for preparing dressings, medicines), handwashing facilities, sinks, dressing tables with a screen in between, and colour-coded bins (as per the IMEP guidelines for community health centres). It should have provision for hub cutters, needle destroyers, and examination and dressing tables.

(b) **Patient Area:** Enough space between beds. Toilets should be separate for males and females. Separate space/room for patients needing isolation should be provided.

(c) **Ancillary Rooms**
- Nurses restroom.
- There should be an area separating OPD and the indoor facility.

Operating theatre/Labour room
- Patient waiting area.
- Pre-operative and post-operative (recovery) room.
- Staff area.
- Separate changing room for males and females.

- Storage area for sterile supplies.
- Operating room/labour room.
- Scrub area.
- Instrument sterilization area.
- Disposal area.
- Newborn care corner/Newborn care stabilization unit.

Public utilities: These should be separate for males and females for both patients and paramedical and medical staff. Disabled friendly WCs with wash basins as specified under the Guidelines should be provided for a disabled friendly environment.

51.8 Physical Infrastructure for Support Services

(a) **Central Sterilization Supply Department (CSSD)**
(b) **Laundry**
- Storage should be separate for dirty and clean linen.
- Outsourcing is recommended after appropriate training of washer man regarding segregation and separate treatment for infected and non-infected linen.

(c) **Engineering Services**
- Electricity/telephones/water/civil engineering may be outsourced.
- Maintenance of proper sanitation in toilets and other public utilities should be given the utmost attention. Sufficient funding for this purpose must be kept, and the services may be outsourced.

(d) **Water Supply**
- Arrangements should be made to supply 10,000 L of potable water per day to meet all the requirements (including laundry) except for firefighting. Storage capacity for 2 days requirements should be on the basis of this consumption. Round-the-clock water supply should be made available to all wards and departments of the hospital.
- Separate reserve emergency overhead tank should be provided for an operating theatre.
- Necessary water storage overhead tanks with pumping/boosting arrangement should be provided.
- The laying and distribution of the water supply system shall be according to the provisions of IS: 2065–1983 (a BIS standard).
- Cold and hot water supply piping should be run in concealed form embedded into walls with full precautions to avoid any seepage.
- Geyser in OT/LR and one in the ward should also be provided.
- Wherever feasible, solar installations should be promoted.

(e) **Emergency Lighting:** Emergency portable/fixed light units should also be provided in the wards and departments to serve as an alternative source of light in case of power failure. Generator back-up should be available in all facilities. Generator should be of good capacity. Solar energy wherever feasible may be used. Generator 5 KVA with POL for immunization cold chain maintenance should be used.

(f) **Telephone:** Minimum two direct lines with intercom facility should be available.

51.9 Administrative Zone

Separate rooms should be available for

- Offices
- Stores

51.10 Residential Zone

- Minimum 8 quarters for doctors.
- Minimum 8 quarters for staff nurses/paramedical staff.

- Minimum 2 quarters for ward boys.
- Minimum 1 quarter for driver.

If the accommodation cannot be provided for any reason, then the staff may be paid house rent allowance, but in this case, they should be staying in the near vicinity of the CHC so that they are available 24 × 7 in case of need.

Function and Space Requirements for Community Health Centres: It is suggested that considering the land cost and availability of land, the CHC building may be constructed in two floors (Figures 51A and B).

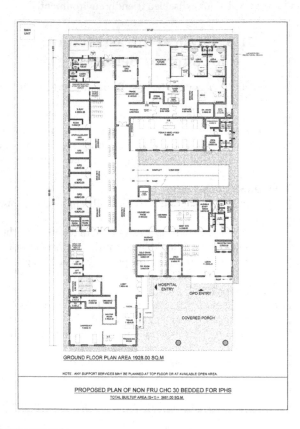

GROUND FLOOR PLAN AREA 1928.00 SQ.M

NOTE : ANY SUPPORT SERVICES MAY BE PLANNED AT TOP FLOOR OR AT AVAILABLE OPEN AREA.

PROPOSED PLAN OF NON FRU CHC 30 BEDDED FOR IPHS
TOTAL BUILTUP AREA (G+1) = 3681.00 SQ.M.

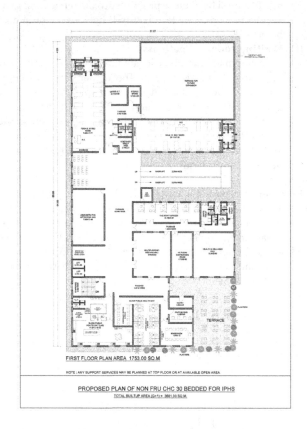

FIRST FLOOR PLAN AREA 1753.00 SQ.M

NOTE : ANY SUPPORT SERVICES MAY BE PLANNED AT TOP FLOOR OR AT AVAILABLE OPEN AREA.

PROPOSED PLAN OF NON FRU CHC 30 BEDDED FOR IPHS
TOTAL BUILTUP AREA (G+1) = 3681.00 SQ.M.

Zone	Functions	Size for Each Sub-Function in Meters	Total Areas in Sq Meters
Entrance Zone	Registration & Record storage, Pharmacy (Issue counter/Formulation/Drug storage) Public utilities & circulation space	Registration/Record Room 3.2 × 3.2 × 2	20.48 sq m
		Queue area outside registration room 3.5 × 3	10.50 sq m
		Pharmacy cum store 6.4 × 3.2	20.48 sq m
		Pharmacy cum store for AYUSH 6.4 × 3.2	20.48 sq m
Ambulatory Zone (OPD)	Examination & Workup (Examination Room, sub-waiting), Consultation (consultation room Toilets, sub-waiting) Nurse station (Nurses desk, clean utility, dirty utility, treatment rooms, injection & dressing room), Cold Chain, Vaccines and Logistics area, ECG (with sub waiting) Casualty/Emergency, public utilities, circulation space	Space for 4 General Doctor Room	40.96 sq m
		3.2 × 3.2 × 4	20.48 sq m
		Space for 2 AYUSH doctors Room	94.72 sq m
		3.2 × 3.2 × 2	11.84 sq m
		8 specialist room with attach toilets	10.24 sq m
		3.7 × 3.2 × 8	20.48 sq m
		Treatment room 3.7 × 3.2	40.96 sq m
		Refraction room 3.2 × 3.2	10.24 sq m
		Nurse Station 6.4 × 3.2	10.24 sq m
		Casualty 6.4 × 6.4	10.24 sq m
		Dress Room 3.2 × 3.2	9.50 sq m
		Injection Room 3.2 × 3.2	31.5 sq m
		Female injection room 3.2 × 3.2	10.5 sq m
		Public Utility/Common Toilets	10.5 sq m
		Waiting Area	
		Cold Chain Room 3.5 × 3	
		Vaccine and Logistics Room 3.5 × 3	

(Continued)

Zone	Functions	Size for Each Sub-Function in Meters	Total Areas in Sq Meters
Diagnostic Zone	Pathology (Optional) Laboratory, sample collection, bleeding room, washing disinfectants storage, sub-waiting, Imaging (radiology, radiography, ultrasound), Preparation, room, changing room, toilet, control, Dark room, treatment room, sub waiting, public utilities	Area specification is recommended	180 sq m
Intermediate Zone (inpatient Nursing units)	Nurse station (Nurse desk, clean utility, treatment room, pantry, store, sluice room, trolley bay)	Nurse station 6.4 × 6.4	40.96 sq m
	Patient area (bed space, toilets, Day space, Isolation Space)	4 wards each with 6 beds (2 male wards and 2 female wards) size (6.2 × 6.2) × 4 4 private room (2 each for male and females) with toilets 6.2 × 3.2 × 4 2	153.76 sq m 79.36 sq m
	Ancillary rooms (Doctor's restroom, Nurses duty room, Public utilities, circulation space.)	isolation rooms with toilet (one each for male and female) 6.2 × 3.2 × 2	39.68 sq m
Critical Zone (Operational Theatre/ Labour room	Patient area (Preparation, Paranaesthesia, post-operative resting) Staff area (Changing Resting) Supplies area (trolley bay, equipment storage, sterile storage) OT/Lr area (Operating/Labour room, scrub, instrument sterilization, Disposal) public utilities, circulation space	Area specification is recommended	240 sq m
Service Zone	Dietary (Dry Store, Day Store, Preparation, Cooking. Delivery, pot wash, Utensil wash, Utensil store, trolley park) C.S.S.D. (Receipt, wash, assembly, sterilization, sterile storage. Issue) Laundry (Receipt, weigh, sluice/wash, Hydro extraction, tumble, calendar, press) Laundry (clean storage, Issue), Civil engineering (Building maintenance, Horticulture, water supply, drainage and sanitation), Electrical engineering (substation & generation, Illumination, ventilation), Mechanical engineering, Space for other services like gas store, telephone, intercom, fire protection, waste disposal. Mortuary.	Services like Electrical engineering Mechanical engineering and Civil engineering can be privately hired to avoid permanent space in the CHC building	Area specification is recommended
Administrative Zone	General Administration, general store, public utilities circulation space	Area specification is recommended	60 sq m
Total Circulation Area/Corridors			191.15 sq m
Total Area			1503.32 sq m

51.11 Summary

The establishment of a CHC in India plays a pivotal role in providing accessible and comprehensive health care services to communities, particularly in rural and underserved areas. CHCs serve as a critical link between primary health care and specialized care by offering a wide range of medical services, preventive measures, and health education. These centres focus on community engagement, empowering individuals to make informed decisions about their health and well-being. By promoting early intervention, disease prevention, and health promotion, CHCs contribute significantly to improving health outcomes and reducing health care disparities. The presence of CHCs strengthens the health care infrastructure at the grassroots level, ensuring equitable access to quality care and fostering healthier communities across India.

52 DISTRICT HOSPITALS

52.1 Introduction

India's Public Health System has been developed over the years as a 3-tier system, namely primary, secondary, and tertiary level of health care. District Health System is the fundamental basis for implementing various health policies, delivery of health care and management of health services for defined geographic area. District hospital is an essential component of the district health system and functions as a secondary level of health care which provides curative, preventive and promotive health care services to the people in the district. Every district is expected to have a district hospital linked with the public hospitals/health centres down below the district such as sub-district/sub-divisional hospitals, community health centres, primary health centres, and sub-centres.

The Government of India is strongly committed to strengthen the health sector for improving the health status of the population. A number of steps have been taken to that effect in the post-independence era. One such step is strengthening of referral services and provision of specialty services at district and sub-district hospitals. Various specialists like surgeon, physician, obstetrician and gynaecologist, paediatrician, orthopaedic surgeon, ophthalmologist, anaesthetist, ENT specialist and dentist have been placed in the district headquarter hospital.

The district hospitals cater to the people living in urban (district headquarters town and adjoining areas) and the rural people in the district. District hospital system is required to work not only as a curative centre but at the same time should be able to build interface with the institutions external to it including those controlled by non-government and private voluntary health organizations. In the fast changing scenario, the objectives of a district hospital need to unify scientific thought with practical operations which aim to integrate management techniques, interpersonal behaviour, and decision-making models to serve the system and improve its efficiency and effectiveness. By establishing a telemedicine link with district to referral hospital (Medical College) with video-conferencing facility (desirable), the quality of secondary and limited tertiary care can be improved considerably at district hospitals.

52.2 Objectives of the Indian Public Health Standards for Sub-Centres

The overall objective of IPHS is to provide health care that is quality oriented and sensitive to the needs of the people of the district. The specific objectives of IPHS for District Hospitals are

- To provide comprehensive secondary health care (specialist and referral services) to the community through the District Hospital.
- To achieve and maintain an acceptable standard of quality of care.
- To make the services more responsive and sensitive to the needs of the people of the district and the hospitals/centres from where the cases are referred to the district hospitals.

52.3 Grading of District Hospitals

The size of a district hospital is a function of the hospital bed requirement, which in turn is a function of the size of the population it serves. In India the population size of a district varies from 35,000 to 3,000,000 (Census 2001). Based on the assumptions of the annual rate of admission as 1 per 50 populations and average length of stay in a hospital as 5 days, the number of beds required for a district having a population of 10 lakhs will be around 300 beds. However, as the population of the district varies a lot, it would be prudent to prescribe norms by grading the size of the hospitals as per the number of beds:

- Grade I: District Hospital Norms for 500 beds
- Grade II: District Hospital Norms for 400 beds
- Grade III: District Hospital Norms for 300 beds
- Grade IV: District Hospital Norms for 200 beds
- Grade V: District Hospital Norms for 100 beds.

52.4 Physical Infrastructure

(a) **Size of the hospital**: The size of a district hospital is a function of the hospital bed requirements, which, in turn, is a function of the size of the population it serves. In India the population size of a district varies from 50,000 to 1,500,000. For the purpose of convenience the average size of the district is taken in this document as one million population. Based on the assumptions of the annual rate of admission as 1 per 50 population and average length of stay in a hospital as 5 days, the number of beds required for a district having a population of 10 lakhs will be as follows:
- The total number of admissions per year = 1,000,000 × 1/50 = 20,000
- Bed days per year = 20,000 × 5 = 100,000
- Total number of beds required when occupancy is 100% = 100000/365 = 275 beds
- Total number of beds required when occupancy is 80% = 100000/365 × 80/100 = 220 beds

52.5 Area and Space Norms of Hospitals

(a) **Land Area**: Minimum land area requirements are as follows:
- Up to 100 beds = 0.25 to 0.5 hectare
- Up to 101 to 200 beds = 0.5 hectare to 1 hectare
- 500 beds and above = 6.5 hectare (4.5 hectare for hospital and 2 hectare for residential)

(b) **Size of hospital as per number of Beds**
  (i) **General Hospital**—80 to 85 sq m per bed to calculate total plinth area. The area will include the service areas such as waiting space, entrance hall, registration counter etc. In addition, hospital service buildings such as generators, manifold rooms, boilers, laundry, kitchen, and essential staff residences are required on the hospital premises. In case of specific requirements of a hospital, flexibility in altering the area may be kept.
  (ii) **Teaching Hospital**—100 to 110 sq m per bed to calculate total plinth area.

DOI: 10.1201/9780367460884-56

(c) **Facilities**
  (i) Operating Theatre
    • One OT for every 50 general inpatient beds
    • One OT for every 25 surgical beds
  (ii) ICU beds = 5 to 10% of total beds
  (iii) Floor space for each ICU bed = 25 to 30 sq m (this includes support services)
  (iv) Floor space for Paediatric ICU beds = 10 to 12 sq m per bed
  (v) Floor space for High-Dependency Unit (HDU) = 20 to 24 sq m per bed
  (vi) Floor space Hospital beds (General) = 15 to 18 sq m per bed.
  (vii) Beds space = 7 sq m per bed
  (viii) Minimum distance between centres of two beds = 2.5 m (minimum)
  (ix) Clearance at foot end of each bed = 1.2 m (minimum)
  (x) Minimum area for apertures (windows/Ventilators opening in fresh air)
    • 20% of the floor area (if on same wall)
    • 15% of the floor area (if on opposite walls)

52.6 Hospital Building: Planning and Layout

Hospital Management Policy should emphasize on hospital buildings with earthquake proof, flood proof and fire protection features. Infrastructure should be eco-friendly and disabled (physically and visually handicapped) friendly. Local agency Guidelines and Bylaws should strictly be followed. See Figures 52A to 52D.

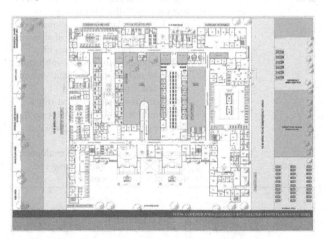

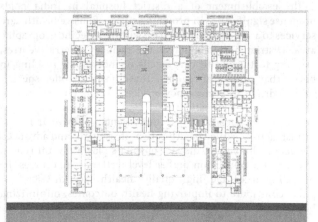

TABLE 52A: Hospital Building—Planning and Layout

Appearance and upkeep	• The hospital should have a high boundary wall with at least two exit gates. • Building shall be plastered and painted with uniform colour scheme. • There shall be no unwanted/outdated posters pasted on the walls of building and boundary of the hospital. • There shall be no outdated/unwanted hoardings in hospital premises. • There shall be provision of adequate light in the night so hospital is visible from approach road. • Proper landscaping and maintenance of trees, gardens etc. should be ensured. • There shall be no encroachment in and around the hospital.
Signage	• The building should have a prominent board displaying the name of the Centre in the local language at the gate and on the building. Signage indicating access to various facilities at strategic points in the Hospital for guidance of the public should be provided. For showing the directions, colour coding may be used. • Citizen charter shall be displayed at OPD and Entrance in local language including patient rights and responsibilities. • Hospital lay out with location and name of the facility shall be displayed at the entrance. • Directional signage for Emergency, all the Departments and utilities shall be displayed appropriately, so that they can be accessed easily. • Florescent Fire Exit plan shall be displayed at each floor. • Safety, hazard, and caution signs displayed prominently at relevant places. • Display of important contacts like higher medical centres, blood banks, fire department, police, and ambulance services available in nearby area. • Display of mandatory information (under RTI Act, PNDT Act, MTP Act, etc.).

52.7 General Maintenance

Building should be well maintained with no seepage, cracks in the walls, no broken windows and glass panes. There should be no growth of algae and mosses on walls etc. Hospital should have anti-skid and non-slippery floors.

TABLE 52B: General Maintenance

Condition of roads, pathways, and drains	• Approach road to hospital emergency shall be all weather motorable road. • Roads shall be illuminated in the nights. • There shall be dedicated parking space separately for ambulances, Hospital staff and visitors. There shall be no stagnation/over flow of drains. • There shall be no water logging/marsh in or around the hospital premises. • There shall be no open sewage/ditches in the hospital.

(Continued)

TABLE 52B: (Continued)

Environmentally friendly features	• The Hospital should be, as far as possible, environment friendly and energy efficient. • Rain-Water harvesting, solar energy use and use of energy-efficient bulbs/equipment should be • encouraged. Provision should be made for horticulture services including herbal garden. • A room to store garden implements, seeds etc. will be made available.
Barrier-free access	For easy access to non-ambulant (wheel-chair, stretcher), semi-ambulant, visually disabled, and elderly persons infrastructure as per "Guidelines and Space Standards for barrier-free built environment for Disabled and Elderly Persons" of Government of India, is to be provided. This will ensure safety and utilization of space by disabled and elderly people fully and their full integration into the society. Provisions as per "Persons with Disability Act" should be implemented.
Administrative block	Administrative block attached to main hospital along with provision of MS Office and other staff will be provided. Block should have independent access and connectivity to the main hospital building, wherever feasible.

52.8 Circulation Areas

Circulation areas comprise corridors, lifts, ramps, staircases, and other common spaces etc. The flooring should be anti-skid and non-slippery.

TABLE 52C: Circulation Areas

Corridors	• Corridors shall be at least 3M Wide to accommodate the daily traffic. • Size of the corridors, ramps, and stairs shall be conducive for manoeuvrability of wheeled equipment. • Corridors shall be wide enough to accommodate two passing trolley, one of which may have a drip attached to it. • Ramps shall have a slope of 1:15 to 1:18. It must be checked for manoeuvrability of beds and trolleys at any turning point
Roof Height	The roof height should not be less than approximately 3.6 m measured at any point from floor to roof.

52.9 Entrance Areas

Barrier free access environment for easy access to non-ambulant (wheel-chair, stretcher), semi ambulant, visually disabled, and elderly persons as per "Guidelines and Space Standards for barrier free built environment for Disabled and Elderly Persons" of CPWD/Min of Social Welfare, GOI. Ramp as per specification, Hand- railing, proper lightning etc. must be provided in all health facilities and retrofitted in older one which lacks the same. The various types of traffic shall be grouped for entry into the hospital premises according to their nature. An important consideration is that traffic moving at extremely different paces (e.g. a patient on foot and an ambulance) shall be separated. There can be four access points to the site, in order to segregate the traffic:

- **Emergency:** for patients in ambulances and other vehicles for emergency department.
- **Service:** for delivering supplies and collecting waste and for removal of dead
- **Main:** for all others

52.10 Residential Quarters

All the essential medical and para-medical staff will be provided with residential accommodation. If the accommodation cannot be provided due to any reason, then the staff may be paid house rent allowance, but in that case they should be staying in near vicinity, so that essential staff is available 24 x 7.

52.11 Disaster Prevention Measures

For all new upcoming facilities in seismic zone 5 or other disaster prone areas building structure and the internal structure of Hospital should be made disaster proof especially earthquake proof, flood proof and equipped with fire protection measures.

TABLE 52D: Disaster Prevention Measures

Earthquake-proof measures	Structural and non-structural should be built in to withstand quake as per geographical/state Govt. guidelines. Non-structural features like fastening the shelves, almirahs, equipment etc. are even more essential than structural changes in the buildings. Since it is likely to increase the cost substantially, these measures may especially be taken on priority in known earthquake prone areas.
Firefighting equipment	Fire extinguishers, sand buckets, etc. should be available and maintained to be readily available when there is a problem.
Disaster management plan	Every district hospital shall have a dedicated disaster management plan in line with state disaster management plan. Disaster plan clearly defines the authority and responsibility of all cadres of staff and mechanism of mobilization resources. All health staff should be trained and well conversant with disaster prevention and management aspects. Regular mock drill should be conducted. After each drill the efficacy of disaster plan, preparedness of hospital and competence of staff shall be evaluated followed by appropriate changes to make plan more robust.

52.12 Summary

The establishment of a district hospital in India holds immense significance in providing comprehensive health care services to a wide population base within a specific geographic area. District hospitals act as the primary referral centres, catering to the health care needs of individuals residing in both urban and rural regions. These hospitals offer specialized medical care, emergency services, surgical interventions, diagnostics, and inpatient facilities, thereby addressing a broad range of health care requirements. With their robust infrastructure, skilled health care professionals, and advanced medical technologies, district hospitals play a pivotal role in reducing the burden on higher-level tertiary care centres. By providing accessible, high-quality health care, district hospitals contribute to improving health outcomes, minimizing health care disparities, and ensuring the well-being of the communities they serve.

53 ALTERNATIVE MEDICINE

53.1 Introduction

Department of AYUSH, Ministry of Health and Family Welfare, Government of India has launched National AYUSH Mission (NAM) during 12th Plan for implementing through States/UTs. The basic objective of NAM is to promote AYUSH medical systems through cost-effective AYUSH services, strengthening of educational systems, facilitate the enforcement of quality control of Ayurveda, Siddha and Unani and Homeopathy (ASU&H) drugs and sustainable availability of ASU&H raw materials.

It envisages flexibility of implementation of the programs which will lead to substantial participation of the State Governments/UT. The NAM contemplates establishment of a National Mission as well as corresponding Missions in the State level. NAM is likely to improve significantly the Department's outreach in terms of planning, supervision, and monitoring of the schemes.

53.2 Vision

- To provide cost effective and equitable AYUSH health care throughout the country by improving access to the services.
- To revitalize and strengthen the AYUSH systems making them as prominent medical streams in addressing the health care of the society.
- To improve educational institutions capable of imparting quality AYUSH education.
- To promote the adoption of Quality standards of AYUSH drugs and making available the sustained supply of AYUSH raw materials.

53.3 Objectives

- To provide cost effective AYUSH Services, with a universal access through upgrading AYUSH Hospitals and Dispensaries, co-location of AYUSH facilities at Primary Health Centres (PHCs), Community Health Centres (CHCs) and District Hospitals (DHs).
- To strengthen institutional capacity at the state level through upgrading AYUSH educational institutions, State Govt. ASU&H Pharmacies, Drug Testing Laboratories and AYUSH enforcement mechanism.
- Support cultivation of medicinal plants by adopting Good Agricultural Practices (GAPs) to provide sustained supply of quality raw materials and support certification mechanism for quality standards, Good Agricultural/Collection/Storage Practices.
- Support setting up of clusters through convergence of cultivation, warehousing, value addition and marketing and development of infrastructure for entrepreneurs.

53.4 Minimum Space for Provision of Quality AYUSH Health Care Facilities

(a) **Primary Health Centre (PHC) level**
 - One Doctor Room- $3.2 \times 3.2 \times 2$ m
 - Pharmacy-cum-store for AYUSH- 6.4×3.2 m
(b) **Community Health Centre (CHC) level**
 - Doctor Room: $3.2 \times 3.2 \times 2$ m for 2 AYUSH Doctors
 - Pharmacy cum store for AYUSH- 6.4×3.2 m
 - In addition to the previously stated, the space required for specialized therapy follows:

Panchkarma/Thokkanam Therapy Centre	- 4 therapy rooms (each of 200 sq ft) — 800 sq ft - 10 beds in pre-existing wards—500 sq ft - Kitchen—200 sq ft - Office cum record room—200 sq ft - **Total: 1700 sq ft**
Kshar Sutra Therapy Centre	- Operating theatre—200 sq ft - Sterilization room—200 sq ft - Recovery room—200 sq ft - 10 beds in pre-existing wards—500 sq ft - Office cum record room—200 sq ft - **Total: 1300 sq ft**
Regimental Therapy of Unani (Ilaj Bil Tadbeer) Centre	- Therapy section (4 rooms each of 200 sq ft) — 800 sq ft - 10 beds in pre-existing wards—500 sq ft - Office cum record room—200 sq ft - **Total: 1500 sq ft**
Yoga & Naturopathy Therapy Centre	- Yoga hall—1,200 sq ft - Therapy section—600 sq ft - Office cum record room—200 sq ft - Kitchen—200 sq ft - **Total: 2200 sq ft**
District Hospital level	- 6 therapy rooms (each 200 sq ft)—1,000 sq ft - 2 OPD rooms—200 sq ft - 10 beds in pre-existing wards—500 sq ft - Kitchen (existing kitchen may be can be utilized)—200 sq ft - Office cum record room—200 sq ft - **Total: 2300 sq ft**

DOI: 10.1201/9780367460884-57

TABLE 53A: Specifications for 50 Bedded AYUSH Hospital (National AYUSH Mission, 2019)

SI. No.	PARTICULARS	CARPET AREA in Sq. Ft. for 50 bed
1.	ADMINISTRATIVE BLOCK	1000
2.	Hospital Superintendent	250
3.	RMO	150
4.	Administrative Officer	150
5.	Record Room & Office	600
6.	Sanitary block (M/F)	150x2
	OPD & IPD	
1.	CMO office room with attached toilet	300 (150x2)
2.	Canteen, Kitchen & store	500
3.	Statistics Dept. with computer facilities with Central Medical Record section	200
4.	Clinical laboratory for investigation	300
5.	OT Complex (1 theaters + side Theatre + wash + Changing + Autoclave + Staff + recovery room)	1000
6.	Labour room +Duty room	200+150=350
7.	Panchakarma/Thokkanam/Ilaj-bid-Tadbir Theatre (Therapy block) (Toilet, bath & circulation area)	1000 (500x2) M'F + 500=1500
8.	Central store for linen etc.	300
9.	Medicine store for AyurvedaHomoeopathy/Unam/Siddha	1000
10.	Dispensing room for Ayurveda/Homoeopathy/Unani/Siddha.	300
11.	Resident doctors Duty rooms with Toilets	600 (150X4)
12.	4 wards of 10 beds each and Private rooms (10 Nos.)	2000(500x4) + 2000(10x200)=4000
13.	Nurses duty room	100
14.	Laboratory for pathological examinations	200
15.	Storeroom for linen and equipment	200
16.	Accommodation for Rehabilitation therapies including Physiotherapy and Occupational therapy, Electrotherapy, Diathermy, Ultraviolet and Infrared treatment, Hydrotherapy	200
17.	Separate adequate area for Yoga and Naturopathy practice + Toilets	400+100
18.	Registration & Record room	200
19.	Waiting hall for patients and attendants	600
20.	Examination rooms (Cubicles) and case demonstration room for Ayurveda and Homoeopathy in the outdoors	150 each × 10 (6 Ayurveda, 4 Homoeopathy)
21.	Staff room with lockers	200
22.	Dressing room	100
23.	Audiometry room	100
24.	Optometry Room	150
25.	Central Casualty Department accommodation for Resuscitation services (2 Beds)	400

53.5 Summary

The establishment of an AYUSH (Ayurveda, Yoga, and Naturopathy, Unani, Siddha, and Homeopathy) Centre in India holds significant value in promoting holistic health care practices and integrating traditional systems of medicine into the mainstream health care system. AYUSH centres offer a wide range of natural therapies, herbal remedies, yoga, and lifestyle interventions to enhance physical, mental, and spiritual well-being. These centres play a crucial role in preserving and promoting traditional healing practices, while also complementing conventional medical treatments. By embracing AYUSH principles, these centres provide alternative treatment options, personalized care, and preventive measures to individuals seeking natural and holistic health care approaches. The presence of AYUSH centres fosters a comprehensive and integrative health care system in India, catering to the diverse needs and preferences of the population, ultimately contributing to improved health outcomes and overall wellness.

References

Chapter	Reference
49.	IPHS for Primary Health Centres. 2012, https://nhm.gov.in/images/pdf/guidelines/iphs/iphs-revised-guidlines-2012/primay-health-centres.pdf
50.	https://nhm.gov.in/images/pdf/guidelines/iphs/iphs-revised-guidlines-2012/sub-centers.pdf
51.	https://nhm.gov.in/images/pdf/guidelines/iphs/iphs-revised-guidlines-2012/community-healthcentres.pdf
52.	https://nhm.gov.in/images/pdf/guidelines/iphs/iphs-revised-guidlines-2012/district-hospital.pdf
53.	(National AYUSH Mission, 2011). http://ayush.gov.in/sites/default/files/4197396897-Charakasamhita%20ACDP%20%20english_0.pdf AYUSH stands for Ayurveda, Yoga, Unani, Siddha and Homeopathy.

Unit 6
Legal and Patient Safety Aspects

54 LAWS AND LEGISLATION IN HOSPITALS

54.1 Introduction

Health care in India features a universal health care Siddha, system run by the constituent states and territories. The constitution charges every state with raising the level of nutrition and the standard of living of its people and improvement of public health as among its primary duties. Law is an obligation on the part of society imposed by the competent authority, and noncompliance may lead to punishment in the form of monetary fine or imprisonment or both.

In a survey conducted at Mumbai, eight out of ten doctors feel that the laws that govern the practice of health care in India are outdated and even higher majority feels that there are too many laws and licenses that are required to keep their practice going. A survey among 297 doctors across specializations says that there are about 50 different laws that govern the practice of health care in India. The study conducted by Medscape India, a non-profit trust of doctors, revealed that 78% of doctors feel that many of the laws that govern medical practice are outdated. Licenses have to be procured by doctors running a hospital every year.

54.2 Medical Laws in India

The earliest civilization known to us is the Indus urban culture of 3000 to 2000 BC. "The renowned medical historian Henry Siegrist[2] believed that public health facilities of Mohenjo Daro were superior to those of any other community of the ancient orient. Since the ancient times, certain duties and responsibilities have been cast on persons who adopt this sacred profession. This is exemplified by Charak's Oath (1000 BC) and Hippocratic Oath (460 BC)".

The earliest known code of laws of health practices were the laws formulated around 2000 BC by Hammurabi, the great king of Babylon. The first ever code of medical ethics called the Hippocratic oath was established 2500 years ago, in the 5th century BC, by Hippocrates—the Greek physician. He is remembered till today as the "Father of western medicine".

The process of establishment of health care system also necessitated creation of legislative framework for practitioners of medicine. In the earlier period of the British rule in India, the physicians and surgeons brought by the East India Company and after 1857 by the British Government, needed some discipline and regulations. The Medical Council of India, now NMC, a national level statutory body for the doctors of modern medicine, was constituted after the enactment of Indian Medical Council Act 1933. The first legal recognition and registration for the Indian systems of medicine came when the Bombay Medical Practitioner Act was passed in 1938.

54.3 Prerequisites for Medical Practice in India

A duly qualified medical professional, i.e. a doctor has a right to seek to practice medicine, surgery, and dentistry by registering with the medical council of the state of which they are a resident, by following the procedure as prescribed under the medical act of the state.

The state medical council has the power to warn, refuse to register/remove from the name of a doctor who has been sentenced by any court for any nonbailable offence or found to be guilty of infamous conduct in any professional respect. The state medical council has also the power to re-enter the name of the doctor in the register.

54.4 Emergency Health Care and Laws

The supreme court has shown consideration by declaring that, the fundamental right to life covered within its scope the right to emergency health care. The landmark judgment that marked this momentous event is that of Parmanand Katara V, Union of India (Supreme Court 1989). In this case, a scooterist severely injured in a road accident was refused for admission when taken to nearest hospital on the excuse that hospital was not competent to handle medicolegal cases.

The supreme court, in its judgment, pronounced that the obligation of medical professionals to provide treatment in cases of emergencies overrode the professional freedom to refuse patients. According to the right to emergency treatment, the status of a fundamental right under Article 21 (fundamental right of life), the court categorically stated that "Article 21 of constitution casts the obligation on the state to preserve life. Interestingly, the supreme court went on to say that not only government hospitals but also "every doctor whether at a government hospital or otherwise has the professional obligation to extend his/her service with due expertise for protecting life.

54.5 Criminal Liability in Medical Profession

The criminal law for doctors is somewhat different than for ordinary persons. This is because it allows a doctor to cause injury to the patient for preventing a greater harm. The crucial area of criminal law for a doctor is offences affecting life. These offences are mainly murder, simply hurt, grievous hurt, and miscarriage or abortion. A doctor may be charged for any of these offences in general. However, the criminal law arms a doctor with three formidable defences namely: (1) informed consent, (2) necessity, and (3) good faith.

There are various criminal liabilities in medical practice related to different sections of Indian Penal Code, the code of criminal procedure and different acts like MTP, PCPNDT, Transplantation of Human Organ Act, etc.

54.6 Laws Governing the Commissioning of a Hospital

These laws ensure that the hospital facilities are created after due process of registration, the facilities created are safe for the public using them, have at least the minimum essential infrastructure for the type and volume of workload anticipated; and are subject to periodic inspections to ensure compliance (Table 54A).

DOI: 10.1201/9780367460884-59

TABLE 54A: Laws Governing the Commissioning of a Hospital

1. Atomic Energy Act 1962
2. Delhi Lift Rules 1942, Bombay Lift Act 1939
3. Draft Delhi Lifts and Escalators Bill 2007
4. Companies Act 1956
5. Indian Electricity Rules 1956
6. Delhi Electricity Regulatory Commission (Grant of consent for captive power plants) Regulations 2002
7. Delhi Fire Prevention and Fire Safety Act 1986, and Fire Safety Rule 1987
8. Delhi Nursing Home Registration Act 1953
9. Electricity Act 1998
10. Electricity Rules 1956
11. Indian Telegraph Act 1885
12. National Building Code 2005
13. Radiation Protection Certificate from BARC
14. Society Registration Act
15. Urban Land Act 1976
16. Indian Boilers Act 1923
17. The Clinical Establishment (Registration and Regulation) Act, 2010

54.7 Laws Governing the Qualification/ Practice and Conduct of Professionals

These regulations ensure that staff employed in the hospital for delivery of health care are qualified and authorized to perform certain technical jobs within specified limits of competence and in accordance with standard codes of conduct and ethics, their credentials are verifiable from the registering councils; and in case of any professional misconduct the councils can take appropriate action against them (Table 54B).

54.8 Laws Governing the Sale, Storage of Drugs, and Safe Medication

These laws control the usage of drugs, chemicals, blood, blood products, and prevent misuse of dangerous drugs, regulate the sale of drugs through licenses, prevent adulteration of drugs, and provide for punitive action against the offenders (Table 54C).

54.9 Laws Governing the Management of Patients

These are the laws setting standards and norms for conduct of medical professional practice, regulating/prohibiting performance of certain procedures, prevention of unfair practices,

TABLE 54B: Laws Governing the Qualification/Practice and Conduct of Professionals

1. The Indian Medical Council Act 1956 & the National Medical Commission Act, 2019
2. Indian Medical Council (Professional Conduct, Etiquette, and Ethics Regulations 2002)
3. Indian Medical Degree Act 1916
4. Indian Nursing Council Act 1947
5. Delhi Nursing Council Act 1997
6. The Dentist's Act 1948
7. AICTE Rules for Technicians 1987
8. The Paramedical and Physiotherapy Central Councils Bill 2007
9. The Pharmacy Act 1948
10. The Apprenticeship Act 1961

TABLE 54C: Laws Governing the Sale, Storage of Drugs, and Safe Medication

1. Blood Bank Regulation Under Drugs and Cosmetics (2nd Amendment) Rules 1999
2. Drugs and Cosmetics Act 1940 and Amendment Act 1982
3. Excise permit to store the spirit, Central Excise Act 1944
4. IPC Section 274 (Adulteration of drugs),
5. Sec 275 (Sale of Adulterated drug), Sec 276 (Sale of drug as different drug or preparation)
6. Sec 284 (negligent conduct regarding poisonous substances)
7. Narcotics and Psychotropic Substances Act
8. Pharmacy Act 1948
9. Sales of Good Act 1930
10. The Drug and Cosmetics Rule 1945
11. The Drugs Control Act 1950
12. VAT Act/Central Sales Tax Act 1956
13. GST Act

TABLE 54D: Laws Governing the Management of Patients

1. Birth and Deaths and Marriage Registration Act 1886
2. Drugs and Magic Remedies (Objectionable) Advertisement Act
3. Guardians and Wards Act 1890
4. Indian Lunacy Act 1912
5. Law of Contract Section 13 (for consent)
6. Lepers' Act
7. PNDT Act 1994 and Preconception and Prenatal Diagnostic Tech (prohibition of sex selection) Rules 1996 (Amendment Act 2002)
8. The Epidemic Disease Act 1897
9. Transplantation of Human Organ Act 1994, Rules 1995
10. The Medical Termination of Pregnancy Act 1971
11. Medical Termination of Pregnancy Rules 2003
12. The Mental Health Act 1987

and control of public health problems/epidemic disease. They deal with the management of emergencies, medicolegal cases, and all aspects related thereto including dying declarations, conducting autopsies, and types of professional negligence (Table 54D).

54.10 Laws Governing Environmental Safety

These laws are aimed at protection of the environment through prevention of air, water, surface, noise pollution; and includes punishment of offenders (Table 54E).

TABLE 54E: Laws Governing Environmental Safety

1. Air (prevention and control of pollution) Act 1981
2. Biomedical Waste Management Handling Rules 1998 (Amended on 2000)
3. Environment Protection Act and Rule1986, 1996
4. NOC from Pollution Control Board
5. Noise Pollution Control Rule 2000
6. Public Health Bylaw 1959
7. Water (prevention and control of pollution) Act 1974
8. Delhi Municipal Corporation (malaria and other mosquito borne diseases) Bylaw 1975
9. The Cigarettes and Other Tobacco Products (prohibition of advertisement and regulation of trade and commerce, production, supply, and distribution) Bill 2003
10. Prohibition of Smoking in Public Places Rules 2008
11. IPC Section 278 (making atmosphere noxious to health), Sec 269 (negligent act likely to spread infection or disease dangerous to life, unlawfully or negligently)

54.11 Laws Governing Employment and Management of Manpower

This group deals with the laws regulating the employment of manpower, their salaries and benefits, service rules and system of redressal of grievances and disputes (Table 54F).

54.12 Laws Governing Medicolegal Aspects

These are the laws governing the doctor-patient relationship, legal consequences of breach of contract and medicolegal aspects of negligence of duty (Table 54G).

54.13 Laws Governing the Safety of Patients, Public, and Staff within the Hospital Premises

These laws deal with safety of facilities and services against any accidental hazards that may endanger the lives and the liability of management for any violation (Table 54H).

TABLE 54F: Laws Governing Employment and Management of Manpower

1. Bombay Labour Welfare Fund Act 1953
2. Citizenship Act 1955
3. Delhi Shops and Establishment Act 1954
4. Employee Provident Fund and Miscellaneous Provision Act 1952
5. Employment Exchange (compulsory notification of vacancies) Act 1959
6. Equal Remuneration Act 1976
7. ESI Act 1948
8. ESI Rules 1950
9. Indian Trades Union Act 1926
10. Industrial Dispute Act 1947
11. Maternity Benefits Act 1961
12. Minimum Wages Act 1948
13. Negotiable Instrument Act 1881
14. Payment of Bonus Act 1956
15. Payment of Gratuity Act 1972
16. Payment of Wedges Act 1936
17. Persons with Disabilities Act 1995
18. PPF Act 1968
19. SC and ST ACT 1989
20. Shops and Factories Act (for national holiday)
21. TDS Act
22. The Essential Service Maintenance Act 1981
23. The Payment of Gratuity Act 1972
24. Workmen's Compensation Act 1923

TABLE 54G: Laws Governing Medicolegal Aspects

1. Consumer Protection Act 2019
2. Indian Evidence Act
3. Law of privileged communication
4. Law of torts
5. IPC Section 52 (good faith),
6. IPC Sec 80 (accident in doing lawful act)
7. IPC Sec 89 (for insane and children)
8. IPC Sec 90 (consent under fear)
9. IPC Sec 92 (good faith/consent)
10. IPC Sec 93 (communication in good faith).

54.14 Laws Governing Professional Training and Research

There are the laws meant to regulate the standards of professional education and training of doctors, nurses, technician and controlling research activities (Table 54I).

54.15 Laws Governing Business Aspects

Some rules are applicable to hospital in relation to its business aspects are listed on the screen. In our country, the Companies Act, 1956 primarily regulates the formation, financing, functioning, and winding up of companies. The Act prescribes regulatory mechanism regarding all relevant aspects including organizational, financial, and managerial aspects of companies (Table 54J).

TABLE 54H: Laws Governing the Safety of Patients, Public, and Staff within the Hospital Premises

1. The Radiation Surveillance Procedures
2. Radiation Protection Rules 1971
3. AERB Safety Code no. AERB/SC/Med-2(rev-1) 2001
4. Arms Act 1950
5. Boilers Act 1923
6. Explosive Act 1884 (for diesel storage)
7. Gas Cylinder Rules 2004
8. Insecticide Act 1968
9. IPC Section 336 (act endangering life or personal safety of others), Sec 337 (causing hurt by act endangering life or personal safety of others), Sec 338 (causing grievous hurt by act endangering the life and personal safety of others).
10. NOC from chief fire office
11. Periodic fitness certificate for operation of lifts
12. Petroleum Act and Storage Rules 2002
13. Prevention of Food Adulteration Act 1954
14. The Indian Fatal Accidents Act 1955
15. Prevention of violence and damage or loss to property) Act 2008 and violence against doctors

TABLE 54I: Laws Governing Professional Training and Research

1. MCI (NMC) rules for MBBS, PG and internship training
2. National board of examination rules for DNB training
3. ICMR rules governing medical research
4. NCI rules for nursing training
5. Ethical Guidelines for Biomedical Research on Human Subjects, 2000

TABLE 54J: Laws Governing Business Aspects

1. Contracts Act 1982
2. Copyright Act 1982
3. Custom Act 1962
4. FEMA 1999
5. Gift Tax Act 1958
6. Income Tax Act 1961
7. Insurance Act 1938
8. Sales of Good Act 1930

TABLE 54K: Licenses/Certifications Required for Hospitals

Sl. No.	Licenses/Certifications	Frequency
1.	Registration under societies registration act	Initially
2.	Inspection for electrical installation/substation	Initially
3.	NOC from local municipal office for any bylaw	Initially
4.	License for storage of petrol/diesel on form XV under the petroleum rules 2002	2 yearly
5.	Income tax exemption certificate	3 yearly
6.	NOC from Delhi fire services	Before implementation
7.	Registration for operation of X-ray installation with AERB	Every 2 years
8.	Drug License for medical store, IPD pharmacy, OPD pharmacy	Every 5 years
9.	License to operate blood bank under rule 122G of drug and cosmetic act	Every 5 years
10.	Registration under PNDT Act 1994	Every 5 years
11.	Income tax registration/PAN	Once only
12.	Registration for VAT/Sales tax	Once only
13.	Registration for EPF	Once only
14.	Registration for ESI coverage of employee	Once only
15.	Registration under rule 34, MTP Act 1971	One-time registration
16.	Registration Delhi nursing Home Act 1953	Yearly
17.	Indemnity insurance policy	Yearly
18.	Standard fire and special perils policy	Yearly
19.	Authorization for generation of BMW under BMW handling rule 1996	Yearly renewal
20.	License for operating lift under	Yearly renewal

54.16 Licenses/Certifications Required for Hospitals

There are certain licenses and permits required to open a hospital in India. A hospital administrator should be aware about the licenses that are essentially required and to renew them as and when required. However, a hospital is not a simple building with physicians, nurses, medical devices, operating theatres, and intensive care units, but it requires basic legal obligations while installing this system. Thus, doctors planning to open a hospital should follow the legal protocols and register their business via a dedicated platform (Table 54K).

54.17 Summary

Policy in health care is vitally important as it sets a general plan of action used to guide desired outcomes and is a fundamental guideline to help make decisions. The purpose of health care policy and procedures is to communicate to employees the desired outcomes of the organization.

Central and state regulations aim to address several health care system objectives, promote quality health care services, reduce health care costs/promote access to care, and protect consumers in the market for health insurance/other coverages. Health legislation is very few compared to the size of and problems in the health care sector. There is a need for having a comprehensive health care act, framed in order to gear the entire health care sector to the established objectives. Most of the common medicolegal situations arise out on noncompliance with these rules and regulations. If a hospital or doctor acquaints well with these rules and regulations and follows them sincerely, he/she would be on the right side of the law.

55 ENHANCING PATIENT SAFETY BY DESIGN

55.1 Introduction

Patient safety is a framework of organized activities that creates cultures, processes, procedures, behaviours, technologies, and environments in health care that consistently and sustainably lower risks, reduce the occurrence of avoidable harm, make error less likely and reduce its impact when it does occur

Recent attention in health care has been on the actual architectural design of a hospital facility, including its technology and equipment, and its effect on patient safety. To address the problems of errors in health care and serious safety issues, fundamental changes of health care processes, culture, and the physical environment are necessary and need to be aligned, so that the caregivers and the resources that support them are set up for enabling safe care. The facility design of the hospital, with its equipment and technology, has not historically considered the impact on the quality and safety of patients, yet billions of dollars are and will be invested annually in health care facilities.

55.2 Why Design for Patient Safety?

Since the release of the Institution of Medicine report To Err Is Human, patient safety improvements have remained elusive, despite a host of interventions. Recent studies have demonstrated no significant improvement for a number of health care-associated conditions including the failure to reduce postoperative, bloodstream, and catheter-associated urinary tract infections.

It has become increasingly clear that the problem of patient safety does not lie solely in the hands of clinicians or frontline health care staff. The health care system has many inherent latent conditions (holes and weaknesses) that interact in complex ways that result in adverse events. A growing body of research shows that features in the built environment such as light, noise, air quality, room layout, and others contribute to adverse patient

safety outcomes like health care-associated infections, medication errors, and falls in health care settings. The Conceptual Model of Physical Environment Elements as Latent Conditions in Patient Safety is shown in Figure 55A as follows. It is based on Vincent, Taylor-Adams, and Stanhope's work and Reason's work, and it shows the role of the physical environment elements as the latent conditions that contribute to patient safety.

Given the massive investment anticipated in health care facility construction in the years to come, there is an urgent need to identify and eliminate built environment latent conditions that impact patient safety during the planning, design, and construction of health care facilities. Design teams themselves are often unfamiliar with the possible built environment impact on patient safety and even less familiar with ways to incorporate these concerns into the design process. While fields such as aviation and other high-risk industries have been able to harness human factors, engineering, and cognitive science that result in the preferred human response and, consequently, improved safety, no similar method currently exists for the design of new health care facilities or major renovation projects.

55.3 The Role of Hospital Design in Patient Safety and Factors Influencing the Built Environment

Hospital design refers to the physical environment that includes the indoor environment (e.g., noise, air quality, and lighting), the interior design (e.g., furniture, fixtures, and materials) and the configuration (e.g. relative locations and adjacencies of spaces) of a hospital. According to the model of system accidents proposed by Reason, hospital design may impact patient safety, directly or indirectly, as a latent failure and a barrier. With human factors in mind, there are several aspects of the built environment that should be considered. In a review of the literature by Henriksen and colleagues, the following

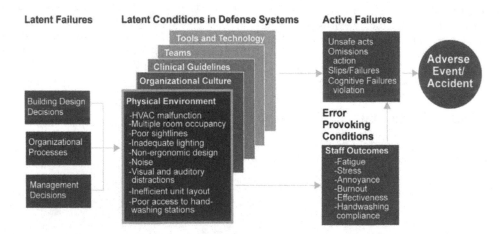

Conceptual model based on Reason's model showing the role of the environment as a latent condition or barrier to adverse events in healthcare settings. From "Designing for Patient Safety: Developing a Patient Safety Risk Assessment" by Joseph, A., & Taylor, E., 2010, Presentation at the 2010 Guidelines for Design and Construction of Health Care Facilities Workshops, Chicago.

FIGURE 55A   Conceptual Model of Physical Environment Elements as Latent Conditions in Patient Safety.

DOI: 10.1201/9780367460884-60

design elements were identified as critical in ensuring patient safety and quality care, based on the six quality aims of the Institute of Medicine's report, Crossing the Quality Chasm: A New Health System for the 21st Century:

- **Patient-centredness**, including
  - using variable-acuity rooms and single-bed bedrooms
  - ensuring sufficient space to accommodate family members
  - enabling access to health care information
  - having clearly marked signs to navigate the hospital
- **Safety**, including
  - applying the design and improving the availability of assistive devices to avert patient falls
  - using ventilation and filtration systems to control and prevent the spread of infections
  - using surfaces that can be easily decontaminated
  - facilitating handwashing with the availability of sinks and alcohol hand rubs
  - preventing patient and provider injury
  - addressing the sensitivities associated with the interdependencies of care, including work spaces and work processes
- **Effectiveness**, including
  - use of lighting to enable visual performance
  - use of natural lighting
  - controlling the effects of noise
- **Efficiency**, including
  - standardizing room layout, location of supplies and medical equipment
  - minimizing potential safety threats and improving patient satisfaction by minimizing patient transfers with variable-acuity rooms
- **Timeliness**, by
  - ensuring rapid response to patient needs
  - eliminating inefficiencies in the processes of care delivery
  - facilitating the clinical work of nurses
- **Equity**, by
  - ensuring the size, layout, and functions of the structure meet the diverse care needs of patients

Hospital design cannot, however, be considered in isolation regarding patient and staff safety. In almost all safety situations, hospital design interacts with a host of other factors, such as the culture of the organization, tasks and processes in place, and tools and technology. This paper primarily focuses on the role of hospital design while recognizing the contributing role played by other critical factors.

55.4 Direct Impacts of Hospital Design on Patient Safety

Aspects of hospital design such as air quality, lighting, patient room design and other interior design elements can directly impact safety outcomes such as health care associated infections, patient falls and medical errors.

55.4.1 Air Quality and Health Care-Associated Infections

Airborne infections are spread when dust and pathogens are released during hospital construction and are caused by contamination and malfunction of hospital ventilation systems.

Studies in hospitals show that fungal load in the air may be linked to humidity, temperature, and construction activity. High-efficiency particulate air (HEPA) filters can be highly effective in preventing airborne infections in hospitals. Air contamination is least in laminar airflow rooms with HEPA filters, and this approach is recommended for such areas as operating-room suites and ultraclean rooms for immunocompromised patients. Yavuz et al. found lower rates of sternal surgical site infections in the newer operating rooms with laminar floor ventilation systems and automatically closing doors compared with the older operating rooms with standard plenum ventilation and doors that did not close properly.

55.4.2 Single Bedrooms and Health Care-Associated Infections

In general, the reported evidence shows that single-bed patient rooms with high-quality HEPA filters and with negative or positive pressure ventilation are more effective in preventing air-borne pathogens. The evidence also shows that multi-bed bedrooms are more difficult to decontaminate and have more surfaces that act as a reservoir for pathogens. On the basis of the study findings, the 2006 American Institute of Architects Guidelines for Design and Construction of Health care Facilities has adopted the single-bed bedroom as the standard for all new construction in the United States. In addition, several other professional and scientific bodies in the United Kingdom, the United States, and Europe have published ICU design guidelines that include similar design measures to control nosocomial infections.

55.4.3 Lighting Conditions and Patient Outcomes

A large body of literature reports different psychological and physiological effects of lighting in hospitals, some of which may be directly related to patient safety. For example, "ICU psychosis" in adult patients can be partly attributed to bright or constant lighting conditions in ICUs that lack night/day cues. A similar phenomenon has been described among children in paediatric ICUs. In addition, the mortality rate may be higher in dull patient rooms, with sex having differential effects. Furthermore, poor lighting conditions may negatively impact physiological developments among infants. Those studies suggest that lighting conditions should be considered more carefully in the design of patient care areas of a hospital.

55.4.4 Lighting Conditions and Medical Errors

Performance on visual tasks gets better as light levels increase. Buchanan et al. found that errors in dispensing medications in a high volume outpatient pharmacy were significantly lower at an illumination level of 146 foot-candles (2.6%) as opposed to the baseline level of 45 foot candles (3.8%). In Alaska, Roseman and Booker found that 58% of all medication errors among hospital workers occurred during the first quarter of the year when daylight hours were less. Studies in offices have indicated the importance of appropriate lighting levels for complex tasks requiring excellent vision, but no such study has been reported in hospitals.

55.4.5 Noise in Hospitals and Patient Outcomes

Noise levels in most hospitals are higher than World Health Organization recommendations. The level of noise in the ICU ranges from 50 to 75 dB, with peaks of up to 85 dB. Parthasarathy and Tobin reported that 20% of all arousals and awakenings among ICU patients are related to noise. They argued that sleep disruption can induce sympathetic activation and elevation of blood pressure, which may contribute to patient morbidity. "ICU psychosis" in adult ICUs and in paediatric ICUs has also been partly attributed to a high level of noise in these areas. Common sources of noise in hospitals may include telephones, alarms, trolleys, ice machines, paging systems, nurse shift change, staff caring for other patients, doors closing, staff conversations, and patients crying out or coughing.

55.4.6 Hospital Design and Patient Falls

A report by the Joint Commission on Accreditation of Health care Organizations cited the physical environment as a root cause in 50% of patient falls, but studies have shown contradictory evidence on the topic. A recent review and meta-analysis of randomized controlled trials did not find any evidence for the independent effectiveness of environmental modification programs on patient falls. Some studies, however, have shown that most patient falls occurred in the patient room and that bedrails were the only design element linked strongly with falls. Other studies have shown that comprehensive multi-intervention strategies that include environmental modifications could be effective in reducing falls. Among specific interior design elements, flooring can contribute to the incidence of falls and the severity of injuries upon impact. Donald et al. reported fewer falls of geriatric patients on vinyl floors compared with carpeted floors in a rehabilitation ward. That study lacked sufficient power, however. Healey, on the other hand, reported that patients suffer more injuries when they fall on vinyl floors compared with carpeted floors. Simpson et al. reported that subfloors may impact the injury from falls, with the risk of fracture being lower for wooden subfloors compared with concrete subfloors.

55.5 Impact of the Environment on Staff Working Conditions

A poorly designed physical environment creates latent conditions such as staff stress, fatigue, annoyance, burnout, and lack of handwashing compliance that may potentially lead to adverse events in hospitals.

55.5.1 Noise in Hospitals and Staff Outcomes

Studies have shown that noise is strongly related to stress and annoyance among nurses, and that noise-induced stress is related to emotional exhaustion and burnout among critical care nurses. Health care staff have reported that the excessively high noise levels at work interfere with their work and impact patient comfort and recovery. Blomkvist and colleagues examined the effects of changing the acoustic conditions (using sound-absorbing versus sound-reflecting ceiling tiles) on the same group of nurses in a coronary ICU. During the periods of improved acoustic conditions, many positive outcomes were observed among staff, including improved speech intelligibility, reduced perceived work demands and perceived pressure and strain. There is convincing evidence that noise is a latent condition for errors in hospitals and strategies must be adopted to reduce noise.

55.5.2 Variable Acuity and Patient Room Transfers

Patients are transferred from one room to another as often as three to six times during their short stay in hospital in order to receive the care that matches their level of acuity. Delays,

communication discontinuities, loss of information and changes in computers and systems during patient transfer may contribute to increased medical errors, loss of staff time and productivity. Hendrich and colleagues developed an innovative demonstration project called the Cardiac Comprehensive Critical Care at Clarian Methodist Hospital in Indianapolis to address patient transfer and associated errors. The authors reported significant post-move improvements in many key areas: patient transfers decreased by 90%, medication errors by 70%, and there was also a drastic reduction in the number of falls. This path-breaking project demonstrated the potential impact of acuity-adaptable care in dealing with patient flow and safety issues while improving the model of care.

55.5.3 Unit Layout and Staff Effectiveness

Nurses spend a lot of time walking, which includes the time to locate and gather supplies and equipment and to find other staff members. One study found that 28.9% of nursing staff time was spent walking. This came second only to patient-care activities, which accounted for 56.9% of staff time. Unnecessary walking leads to a waste of precious staff time and adds to fatigue and stress among staff. Studies seem to suggest that bringing staff and supplies physically and visually closer to the patient may help reduce walking. To take advantage of the idea, many hospitals incorporate decentralized nurses' stations and supplies' servers next to patient rooms (as opposed to locating everything at a single central location). Hendrich and colleagues argued that such a layout may help reduce walking and supply trips. As a result, nursing time may increase significantly allowing for a reduction in budgeted staffing care hours while increasing the time spent in direct patient care activities.

55.5.4 Accessibility to Handwashing Stations and Handwashing Compliance

Surface transmission of pathogens accounts for a majority of nosocomial infections, and low handwashing frequency among health care staff (generally below 50%) is a key factor contributing to this problem. Design factors that discourage handwashing include: difficulty of access, poor visibility, poor height placement, lack of redundancy, and wide spatial separation of resources that are used sequentially while washing hands.

55.6 Design Tools to Enhance Patient Safety

Failure Modes and Effects Analysis (FMEA): FMEA is a systematic, proactive approach to evaluating a system, design, or process in order to identify potential failures; to evaluate relative effects and consequences of the failures; to identify the parts that are most in need of change; and to reduce or eliminate the failures, errors, and problems before they reach patients.

Balanced Scorecard: The balanced scorecard is a relatively new approach to strategic management that integrates an organization's key initiatives, methodologies, and critical perspectives. The scorecard measures organizational performance across four balanced perspectives: financial, customers, internal business processes, and learning and growth. The balanced scorecard "enables companies to track financial results while simultaneously monitoring progress in building the capabilities and acquiring the intangible assets they need for future growth".

Work Sampling (Time-Motion Study): Work sampling is a method of measuring time that workers spend in various activity categories. Another closely related method is time-motion study, which is a systematic study of work systems to optimize and standardize work system and methods, determine the time standard for a specific task or operation, and train the workers in the optimized method.

Link Analysis: Link analysis is an ergonomics method of identifying and representing links (or relationships) between interface components of workspace to determine the nature, frequency, and importance of the links. The term link can refer to movements of attentional gaze or position between system components (eye, body, foot movement links), communication with other components (visual, auditory, tactile communication links, e.g., nurse-to-physician communication), and control links (e.g., access and use of bedside computer).

Process Analysis (Process Chart/Flowchart): Process analysis is a systematic quality improvement method to identify the steps/tasks of a process that lead from a certain set of inputs to an output. A process analysis often involves the production of a process chart or flowchart, which is a graphical representation of the steps that occur during the performance of a task or a series of tasks.

Simulation: Gaba (2004) defines simulation as a "technique, not a technology, to replace or amplify real experiences with guided experiences, often immersive in nature, that evoke or replicate substantial aspects of the real world in a fully interactive fashion". Often a simulator as used in this context refers to a "device that presents a simulated patient (or part of a patient) and interacts appropriately with the actions taken by the simulation participant".

Root Cause Analysis: Root cause analysis (RCA) is a non-statistical method of analysis to identify conditions that can lead to harm. It is a reactive process responding to a close call or sentinel event that involves a multidisciplinary team to identify and eliminate the contributing causal factors of systems, risks, and process (not individual performance) that contribute to patient safety problems.

55.7 Safe Design Roadmap/CEO Checklist

Poorly designed and operated health care environments contribute to adverse events and subsequent patient harm, such as health care–associated infections, medication errors, and patient falls. A large and growing body of evidence indicates that the physical environment impacts patient and staff safety, as well as stress and satisfaction, staff effectiveness, and organizational resource outcomes in hospitals and other health care settings. Facility replacement and renovation projects provide an opportunity to identify and eliminate built environment latent conditions that lead to active failures impacting patient safety. The purpose of the safe design roadmap is to provide CEOs and their leadership teams with a facility project management tool that captures the opportunities to use physical environmental features to help improve patient safety outcomes.

CEOs and their teams are encouraged to read through the entire roadmap and supporting documents (Design Frameworks and Considerations) as one of the first facility strategic and business planning activities. Individual facility life-cycle phase variables can then be considered at the appropriate project phase to support timely decision making and avoid costly project changes. The tool provides a patient safety communication roadmap that drives facility project decision making to maximize facility investments and realize improved patient safety outcomes. Following the questions, additional detail is provided about the varied design phases and supporting information to answer the questions.

Prior to starting anything, it is important to evaluate whether there is a leader-led safety culture program and performance improvement initiative. Evaluate whether there is open communication within the organization about near misses, mistakes, and errors, and whether staff work within a system of accountability that supports safe behavioural choices. Establish how analyses and solutions developed around these events are shared within the organization.

55.8 15 Key Safety Questions to Ask through the Facility Project Life Cycle

- What is your current safety status for each risk category regarding patient morbidity and mortality?
- What financial impact do current patient harm, patient readmissions secondary to harm, and patient satisfaction have on your Centers for Medicare and Medicaid Services (CMS) and other reimbursement rates, as well as associated litigation and claim costs?
- Is safety a topic included in the visioning session to launch the facility project?
- What known physical environment safety features are currently missing in the present facility? Based on available research, what features need to be included?
- What cultural transformation or clinical or business reengineering efforts are needed to maximize facility safety feature investments?
- Is safety a focus of your operations plan? What culture and processes of care delivery are needed to complement safety features?
- Are specific resources needed, such as mock-up rooms or virtual tools, to integrate safety culture, process, and environmental feature changes?
- Does the functional program accommodate safety features/goals?
- Does the team that you have hired have expertise in patient safety?
- Does the design support the desired safety concepts of operation from all perspectives: patients, family and visitors, the community, staff, material movement, and equipment and technology use?
- Has a comprehensive safety-training program been developed for staff, patients, and family members? Have stakeholders (including patients and the community) been informed through marketing and press releases about the safety-focused design?
- Have the baseline, pre-occupancy safety outcome measures been captured for those variables expected to be impacted by the proposed safety features?
- Has the post-occupancy evaluation processes been defined to include evaluation of the safety features?
- Have the post-occupancy evaluations of safety features been completed at the appropriate times?
- Have the lessons learned been documented and shared broadly?

55.9 Summary

Hospital design may help improve patient safety directly by reducing nosocomial infections, patient falls, medication errors, and, sometimes, even by reducing patient morbidity and mortality. Hospital design may also help improve patient safety indirectly by reducing staff stress, staff walking and patient transfer, and by improving handwashing compliance. In contrast, very little has been reported recently on the role of hospital design as a barrier to adverse events in hospitals. Although research on the links between hospital design and safety has increased over the past few years, there is still a need for more focused studies. Some reported contradictions on these links also need to be resolved. Meanwhile, the growing body of evidence in the field may already have an impact on how hospitals should be designed in the coming years.

References

Chapter	Reference
54.	Singh MM, Garg US. Laws applicable to medical practice and hospitals in India. International Journal of Research Foundation of Hospital and Healthcare Administration 2013;1(1):19–24.
	Sinha TK. *Times of India*. Mumbai Edition. June 12, 2012, p. 5.
	Henry SE. *A History of Medicine, Vol II, Early Greek, Hindu and Persian Medicine.* (2, pp. 142–143). Oxford University Press, 1987.
	Rangarajan LN. *Kautilya's Arthashastra*, 1st Edition. Penguin Books, 27 August 1992, pp. 130–131.
	Kosambi DD. *The Culture and Civilisation of Ancient India in Historical Outline*. Vikas Publication 1970, p. 160.
	Chattopadhyay D. *Science and Society in Ancient India*. Research India Publication, 1979, p. 22.
	Ramasubban R. *Public Health and Medical Research in India: Their Origins Lender the Impact of British Colonial Policy'*. SAREC, 1982, R.4.
	Singh J, et al. *Medical Negligence and Compensation*, 3rd Edition. (pp. 2–4). Bharat Law Publication.
	Joshi SK. *Quality Management in Hospitals*, 1st Edition. (pp. 368–369). Jaypee Brothers Medical Publishers.
55.	https://cdn.who.int/media/docs/default-source/patient-safety/gpsap/global-patient-safety-action-plan-2021-2030_third-draft_january-2021_web.pdf?sfvrsn=6767dc05_15
	Gurses AP, Ozok AA, Pronovost PJ. Time to accelerate integration of human factors and ergonomics in patient safety. BMJ Quality & Safety. 2012;21:347–351.
	Burroughs TE, Waterman AD, Gallagher TH, Waterman B, Jeffe DB, Dunagan WC, Garbutt J, Cohen MM, Cira J, Fraser VJ. Patients concerns about medical errors during hospitalization. Joint Commission Journal on Quality and Safety. 2007;33(1):5–14.
	Reiling J, Hughes RG, Murphy MR. The impact of facility design on patient safety. Patient safety and quality: An evidence-based handbook for nurses. 2008 Apr.
	Donaldson MS, Corrigan JM, Kohn Lt K. *To Err is Human: Building a Safer Health System*. Institute of Medicine, Committee on Quality of Health Care in America. 2000.
	Agency for Healthcare Research and Quality. *National Scorecard on Rates of Hospital-Acquired Conditions 2010 to 2015: Interim Data from National Efforts to Make Health Care Safer*. Rockville, MD: Agency for Healthcare Research and Quality; December 2016.
	Landrigan CP, Parry GJ, Bones CB, Hackbarth AD, Goldmann DA, Sharek PJ. Temporal trends in rates of patient harm resulting from medical care. New England Journal of Medicine. 2010;363(22):2124–2134.
	Levinson DR, General I. *Adverse Events in Hospitals: National Incidence among Medicare Beneficiaries*. Department of Health and Human Services Office of the Inspector General, 2010.
	Freeman W. Designing for Patient Safety: Developing Methods to Integrate Patient Safety Concerns in the Design Process. In: *Proceedings of the AHRQ Conference on Designing for Patient Safety*; 2002 Feb 11-12; Atlanta, GA. Atlanta, GA: Centers for Disease Control and Prevention; 2002.
	Reason J. Human error: Models and management. BMJ. 2000;320(7237):768–770.
	Joseph A, Rashid M. The architecture of safety: Hospital design. Current Opinion in Critical Care. 2007;13(6):714–719.
	Ulrich RS, Zimring C, Zhu X, DuBose J, Seo HB, Choi YS, Quan X, Joseph A. A review of the research literature on evidence-based healthcare design. HERD: Health Environments Research & Design Journal. 2008;1(3):61–125.
	Vincent C, Taylor-Adams S, Stanhope N. Framework for analysing risk and safety in clinical medicine. BMJ. 1998;316(7138):1154–1157.
	Reason J. *Making the Risks of Organizational Accidents*. Ashgate Publishing, 1997.
	Leape LL. Error in medicine. JAMA. 1994;272(23):1851–1857.
	Weinger MB, Pantiskas C, Wiklund ME, Carstensen P. Incorporating human factors into the design of medical devices. JAMA. 1998;280(17):1484.
	Norman DA. *The Psychology of Everyday Things*. Basic Books, 1988.
	Henriksen K, Isaacson S, Sadler BL, Zimring CM. The role of the physical environment in crossing the quality chasm. Joint Commission Journal on Quality and Patient Safety. 2007;33(11):68–80.

Richardson WC, Berwick DM, Bisgard J, Bristow L, Buck C, Cassel CK. *Crossing the Quality Chasm: A New Health System for the 21st Century*. Washington, DC: National Academies Press; 2001.

Opal SM, Asp AA, Cannady PB, Morse PL, Burton LJ, Hammer PG. Efficacy of infection control measures during a nosocomial outbreak of disseminated aspergillosis associated with hospital construction. Journal of Infectious Diseases. 1986;153(3):634–637.

Oren I, Haddad N, Finkelstein R, Rowe JM. Invasive pulmonary aspergillosis in neutropenic patients during hospital construction: Before and after chemoprophylaxis and institution of HEPA filters. American Journal of Hematology. 2001;66(4):257–262.

Humphreys H, Johnson EM, Warnock DW, Willatts SM, Winter RJ, Speller DC. An outbreak of aspergillosis in a general ITU. Journal of Hospital Infection. 1991;18(3):167–177.

Panagopoulou P, Filioti J, Farmaki E, Maloukou A, Roilides E. Filamentous fungi in a tertiary care hospital: Environmental surveillance and susceptibility to antifungal drugs. Infection Control and Hospital Epidemiology. 2007;28(1):60–67.

Kumari DN, Haji TC, Keer V, Hawkey PM, Duncanson V, Flower E. Ventilation grilles as a potential source of methicillin-resistant *Staphylococcus aureus* causing an outbreak in an orthopaedic ward at a district general hospital. Journal of Hospital Infection. 1998;39(2):127–133.

Lutz BD, Jin J, Rinaldi MG, Wickes BL, Huycke MM. Outbreak of invasive Aspergillus infection in surgical patients, associated with a contaminated air-handling system. Clinical Infectious Diseases. 2003;37(6):786–793.

McDonald LC, Walker M, Carson L, Arduino M, Aguero SM, Gomez P, McNeil P, Jarvis WR. Outbreak of *Acinetobacter* spp. bloodstream infections in a nursery associated with contaminated aerosols and air conditioners. Pediatric Infectious Disease Journal. 1998;17(8):716–722.

Clark T, Huhn GD, Conover C, Cali S, Arduino MJ, Hajjeh R, Brandt ME, Fridkin SK. Outbreak of bloodstream infection with the mold *Phialemonium* among patients receiving dialysis at a hemodialysis unit. Infection Control & Hospital Epidemiology. 2006;27(11):1164–1170.

Hahn T, Cummings KM, Michalek AM, Lipman BJ, Segal BH, McCarthy PL. Efficacy of high-efficiency particulate air filtration in preventing aspergillosis in immunocompromised patients with hematologic malignancies. Infection Control & Hospital Epidemiology. 2002;23(9):525–531.

Friberg S, Ardnor B, Lundholm R, Friberg B. The addition of a mobile ultra-clean exponential laminar airflow screen to conventional operating room ventilation reduces bacterial contamination to operating box levels. Journal of Hospital Infection. 2003;55(2):92–97.

Yavuz SS, Bicer Y, Yapici N, Kalaca S, Aydin OO, Camur G, Kocak F, Aykac Z. Analysis of risk factors for sternal surgical site infection: Emphasizing the appropriate ventilation of the operating theaters. Infection Control and Hospital Epidemiology. 2006;27(9):958–963.

Urlich R, Zimring C, Quan X, Joseph A, Choudhary R. *The Role of the Physical Environment in the Hospital of the 21st Century*. Center for Health Design, 2004.

Vincent JL, Bihari DJ, Suter PM, Bruining HA, White J, Nicolas-Chanoin MH, Wolff M, Spencer RC, Hemmer M. The prevalence of nosocomial infection in intensive care units in Europe: Results of the European Prevalence of Infection in Intensive Care (EPIC) Study. JAMA. 1995;274(8):639–644.

Mulin B, Rouget C, Clément C, Bailly P, Julliot MC, Viel JF, Thouverez M, Vieille I, Barale F, Talon D. Association of private isolation rooms with ventilator-associated *Acinetobacter baumanii pneumonia* in a surgical intensive-care unit. Infection Control & Hospital Epidemiology. 1997;18(7):499–550.

Facilities Guidelines Institute. *Guidelines for Design and Construction of Healthcare Facilities*. The American Institute of Architects, 2006.

O'Connell NH, Humphreys H. Intensive care unit design and environmental factors in the acquisition of infection. Journal of Hospital Infection. 2000;45(4):255–262.

Gelling L. Causes of ICU psychosis: The environmental factors. Nursing in Critical Care. 1999;4(1):22–26.

Hughes J. Hallucinations following cardiac surgery in a paediatric intensive care unit. Intensive and Critical Care Nursing. 1994;10(3):209–211.

Beauchemin KM, Hays P. Sunny hospital rooms expedite recovery from severe and refractory depressions. Journal of Affective Disorders. 1996;40(1–2):49–51.

Beauchemin KM, Hays P. Dying in the dark: Sunshine, gender and outcomes in myocardial infarction. Journal of the Royal Society of Medicine. 1998;91(7):352–354.

Brandon DH, Holditch-Davis D, Belyea M. Preterm infants born at less than 31 weeks' gestation have improved growth in cycled light compared with continuous near darkness. Journal of Paediatrics. 2002;140(2):192–199.

Boyce P, Hunter C, Howlett O. *The Benefits of Daylight through Windows*. Rensselaer Polytechnic Institute, 2003.

Buchanan TL, Barker KN, Gibson JT, Jiang BC, Pearson RE. Illumination and errors in dispensing. American Journal of Hospital Pharmacy. 1991;48(10):2137–2145.

Booker JM, Roseman C. A seasonal pattern of hospital medication errors in Alaska. Psychiatry Research. 1995;57(3):251–257.

Rashid M, Zimring C. A review of the empirical literature on the relationships between indoor environment and stress in health care and office settings: Problems and prospects of sharing evidence. Environment and Behavior. 2008;40(2):151–190.

Busch-Vishniac I, West J, Barnhill C, et al. Noise levels in John Hopkins Hospital. Journal of the Acoustical Society of America. 2005;118:3629–3645.

Gabor JY, Cooper AB, Crombach SA, Lee B, Kadikar N, Bettger HE, Hanly PJ. Contribution of the intensive care unit environment to sleep disruption in mechanically ventilated patients and healthy subjects. American Journal of Respiratory and Critical Care Medicine. 2003;167(5):708–715.

Parthasarathy S, Tobin MJ. Sleep in the intensive care unit. Applied Physiology in Intensive Care Medicine. 2009:191–200.

Ulrich RS, Lawson B, Martinez M. Exploring the Patient Environment: An NHS Estates Workshop. The Stationery Office, 2003.

Cropp AJ, Woods LA, Raney D, Bredle DL. Name that tone: The proliferation of alarms in the intensive care unit. Chest. 1994;105(4):1217–1220.

Joint Commission on Accreditation of Healthcare Organizations. Root causes of patient falls. Sentinel event statistics [graph] 2006. http://www.jointcommission.org/NR/rdonlyres/FA5A080F-C259-47CC-AAC8-BAC3F5C37D84/0/se_rc_patient_falls.jpg.

Oliver D, Connelly JB, Victor CR, Shaw FE, Whitehead A, Genc Y, Vanoli A, Martin FC, Gosney MA. Strategies to prevent falls and fractures in hospitals and care homes and effect of cognitive impairment: Systematic review and meta-analyses. BMJ. 2007;334(7584):82.

Hignett S, Masud T. A review of environmental hazards associated with in-patient falls. Ergonomics. 2006;5–6:605–616.

Alcée D. The experience of a community hospital in quantifying and reducing patient falls. Journal of Nursing Care Quality. 2000;14(3):43–53.

Becker C, Kron M, Lindemann U, Sturm E, Eichner B, Walter-Jung B, Nikolaus T. Effectiveness of a multifaceted intervention on falls in nursing home residents. Journal of the American Geriatrics Society. 2003;51(3):306–313.

Brandis S. A collaborative occupational therapy and nursing approach to falls prevention in hospital inpatients. Journal of Quality in Clinical Practice. 1999;19(4):215–220.

Drahota A, Gal D, Windsor J. Flooring as an intervention to reduce injuries from falls in healthcare settings: An overview. Quality in Ageing and Older Adults. 2007;8(1):3–9.

Donald IP, Pitt K, Armstrong E, Shuttleworth H. Preventing falls on an elderly care rehabilitation ward. Clinical Rehabilitation. 2000;14(2):178–185.

Healey F. Does flooring type affect risk of injury in older in-patients? Nursing Times. 1994;90(27):40–41.

Simpson AH, Lamb S, Roberts PJ, Gardner TN, Evans JG. Does the type of flooring affect the risk of hip fracture? Age and Ageing. 2004;33(3):242–246.

Topf M, Dillon E. Noise-induced stress as a predictor of burnout in critical care nurses. Heart & Lung: The Journal of Critical Care. 1988;17(5):567–574.

Morrison WE, Haas EC, Shaffner DH, Garrett ES, Fackler JC. Noise, stress, and annoyance in a pediatric intensive care unit. Critical Care Medicine. 2003;31(1):113–119.

Bayo MV, García AM, García A. Noise levels in an urban hospital and workers' subjective responses. Archives of Environmental Health: An International Journal. 1995;50(3):247–251.

Blomkvist V, Eriksen CA, Theorell T, Ulrich R, Rasmanis G. Acoustics and psychosocial environment in intensive coronary care. Occupational and Environmental Medicine. 2005;62(3):e1.

Hendrich AL, Lee N. Intra-unit patient transports: Time, motion, and cost impact on hospital efficiency. Nursing Economics. 2005;23(4):157.

Hendrich AL, Fay J, Sorrells AK. Effects of acuity-adaptable rooms on flow of patients and delivery of care. American Journal of Critical Care. 2004;13(1):35–45.

Cook RI, Render M, Woods DD. Gaps in the continuity of care and progress on patient safety. BMJ. 2000;320(7237):791–794.

Tucker AL, Spear SJ. Operational failures and interruptions in hospital nursing. Health Services Research. 2006;41(3p1):643–662.

Burgio LD, Engel BT, Hawkins A, McCormick K, Scheve A. A descriptive analysis of nursing staff behaviors in a teaching nursing home: Differences among NAs, LPNs, and RNs. Gerontologist. 1990;30(1):107–112.

Shepley MM, Davies K. Nursing unit configuration and its relationship to noise and nurse walking behavior: An AIDS/HIV unit case study. AIA Academy Journal. 2003;6:12–14.

Shepley MM. Predesign and post occupancy analysis of staff behavior in a neonatal intensive care unit. Children's Health Care. 2002;31(3):237–253.

Rashid M. A decade of adult intensive care unit design: A study of the physical design features of the best-practice examples. Critical Care Nursing Quarterly. 2006;29(4):282–311.

Joseph A. The Impact of the Environment on Infections in Healthcare Facilities. Center for Health Design, 2006.

Larson EL, Albrecht S, O'Keefe M. Hand hygiene behavior in a pediatric emergency department and a pediatric intensive care unit: Comparison of use of 2 dispenser systems. American Journal of Critical Care. 2005;14(4):304–311.

Lankford MG, Zembower TR, Trick WE, Hacek DM, Noskin GA, Peterson LR. Influence of role models and hospital design on the hand hygiene of health-care workers. Emerging Infectious Diseases. 2003;9(2):217.

Boyce JM. Antiseptic technology: Access, affordability, and acceptance. Emerging Infectious Diseases. 2001;7(2):231.

Kaplan LM, McGuckin M. Increasing handwashing compliance with more accessible sinks. Infection Control & Hospital Epidemiology. 1986;7(8):408–410.

Vernon MO, Trick WE, Welbel SF, Peterson BJ, Weinstein RA. Adherence with hand hygiene: Does number of sinks matter? Infection Control & Hospital Epidemiology. 2003;24(3):224–225.

Vietri NJ, Dooley DP, Davis Jr CE, Longfield JN, Meier PA, Whelen AC. The effect of moving to a new hospital facility on the prevalence of methicillin-resistant *Staphylococcus aureus*. American Journal of Infection Control. 2004;32(5):262–267.

Trick WE, Vernon MO, Welbel SF, DeMarais P, Hayden MK, Weinstein RA, Chicago Antimicrobial Resistance Project. Multicenter intervention program to increase adherence to hand hygiene recommendations and glove use and to reduce the incidence of antimicrobial resistance. Infection Control & Hospital Epidemiology. 2007;28(1):42–49.

INDEX

Note: Page numbers in *italic* indicate a figure and page numbers in **bold** indicate a table on the corresponding page.

Printed in the United States
by Baker & Taylor Publisher Services

Printed in the United States
by Baker & Taylor Publisher Services